Management of
Essential

HYPERTENSION: The New Low-Dose Era

2nd Edition

by

F. Gilbert McMahon, M.S., M.D., FACP

Director of The Clinical Research Center and the Tulane Therapeutic Annex
Fellow, American College of Physicians
Fellow, Nation High Blood Pressure Council
Clinical Professor of Medicine, Tulane University School of Medicine
Adjunct Professor of Pharmacology, Tulane University School of Medicine
Adjunct Professor of Pharmacy and Therapeutics, Xavier University, New Orleans
Past President, American Society for Clinical Pharmacology and Therapeutics
President, Pan American Medical Association, Section on Drugs

FUTURA PUBLISHING COMPANY, INC.
Mount Kisco, New York
1984

Notice:

Every effort has been made to ensure that drug doses and recommendations in this book are as up to date and accurate as possible at the time of publication. However, due to the constant developments in medicine, readers are strongly advised to check the product information sheets that accompany any drugs they plan to administer to be sure that they have the latest information concerning revised recommended dosages, contraindications, and the like.

DEDICATION

- *To Dr. Harvey Sadow*, without whose encouragement this new edition would not have been written.
- *To the Tulane Medical Students* who collaborated with me:

Steve Browne	*Louis Ridgway*
Mike Dale	*Meredith Schmieg*
Jonathan Degnan	*Stefanie Schultis*
Robert Enelow	*Mark Tucker*
Ladson Hinton	*Chuck Wilder*
Don Miller	*Keith Wood*
Neil O'Conner	

- *To industry* without whose drugs we'd still be giving bromides and reassurance, weeds and seeds for this endemic disease.
- *To my wife, Mary Ann*, and *children, Sean, Tina, Anne Marie*, and *Christopher*, for their generous emotional support once again.

F. Gilbert McMahon, M.D.

ACKNOWLEDGMENTS

First, I must thank the thirteen bright young medical students without whose enthusiasm and assistance this book would not have been possible. Certainly, part of my motivation came from the immense satisfaction that comes from many academicians, physicians and lay people who told me they benefited from the first edition; the elderly gentleman who read my book in the New York Public Library Consumers' Section and phoned me to ask for a recommendation for a blood pressure doctor in his city; the two women professors from Warsaw, Poland, who turned around at a Paris International Hypertension Meeting and asked me to autograph their copies; the physician in Brussels who told me his medical student son and his friends use my text; and the 56,000 physicians who got my first edition.

I am most grateful for the advice given me by the three very knowledgeable experts in this field, who generously critiqued several chapters of this book: Dr. Ed Freis, Dr. Ray Gifford and Dr. Bob Temple.

I am particularly grateful to my publisher, Steve Korn, and his efficient staff for their most competent assistance throughout these many months.

I wish to acknowledge the many physicians and scientists who supplied me with books and publications, new materials and information about various drugs:

Rudi Hoffman, Dick Davies, McFate Smith, Leigh Thompson, Ezra Lamdin, John Fischetti, Bob Spangenberg, George Maha, John Irvin, Geraldine Mantell, Wolf Michaelis, Norman Lavy, Howard Miller, John Muldane, Sveto Vanov, Bob Fiorentini, Colin Taylor, Mike Vinocur, Barry Rofman, Mirza Beg, Martin Kaplan, Joan Leader, Steve Hulley, David Poorvin, Elmer Funk, Leonard Gonasun, Renee Isen, Stanley Fishman, Juan Guerrero, Nadim Kassem, William Cady, Jeffrey Friedman, Bob Coniff, Bob Keenan, Michael Fernandes, Keith Rottenberg, Paul Hornyak, Ted

Hughes, Eric Michelson, Lawrence Wexler, Richard Weber, Richard Friedlander, Sam Tisdale, Jim Brinckhoff, Richard Riley, Jim Page, Irv Shemano, Irwin Reich, Mike Grozier, Heinz Morr, Pat Hernandez, Zack Finkelberg, Melinko Medakovic, Dan Azarnoff, Russ Taylor, Sharon Jacobs, Ed Neiss, Al Ling, Bob Hodges, Charles Defesche.

The word processing, typing, and proofreading were accomplished by a team of people who worked patiently, generously and competently on this project: Glenda Middlebrooks, Eric Jeanise, Karen Palao. In many ways this task impacted on everyone at our Clinical Research Center, particularly on Dr. Jerome Ryan, our Medical Director, to whom I am always grateful. Finally, Drs. Adesh Jain, Ron Michael and Anand Hiremath of our group generously contributed substantial assistance with Chapter XIV on New Drugs.

TABLE OF CONTENTS

- **Dedication, Acknowledgments and Preface**
- **Chapter I: *SYNOPSIS***

What is Hypertension?	1
The Risks	3
Left Ventricular Hypertrophy	8
The Natural Course of the Disease	11
Initial Medical Evaluation of the Patient with Mild Hypertension	12
The Non-Drug Treatment of Hypertension	13
Individualized or Stepped-Care Therapy for Mild Hypertension	14
Which Second Drug Should be Added?	18
Fixed-Combination Therapy	19
Sexual Dysfunction from Antihypertensive Agents	20
The Therapeutic Goal	21
The Role of Renin	22
Who Should Have a PRA Determination?	23
Malignant Hypertension and Hypertensive Emergencies	24
Management of Azotemic Hypertension	29
Management of Refractory Hypertension	29
Drug Doses in the Presence of Liver or Renal Insufficiency	30
Therapeutic Principles	30

- **Chapter II: *THE NON-DRUG TREATMENT OF HYPERTENSION***

Introduction	37
The Role of Sodium Restriction	38
The Role of Weight Reduction	45
The Role of Physical Training and Exercise	51
Does Physical Training Help Lower Blood Pressure?	51
The Role of Potassium	54
The Role of Dietary Fat and Vegetarian Diets	58
The Role of Relaxation, Meditation, and Biofeedback	61
The Role of Calcium	63
The Effect of Alcohol	64
The Effect of Coffee	66
The Effect of Cigarettes	66

- **Chapter III: *DIURETICS—THE THIAZIDE, THIAZIDE-LIKE, AND LOOP DIURETICS***

Introduction	75
When Should the Physician Consider Thiazides for Hypertension?	80
How Effective are Thiazides in Essential Hypertension?	83
Indications for Thiazides	85
Formulations	85
Hydrochlorothiazide Dosage	85
Chlorthalidone Dosage	86
Metolazone Dosage	86
Mechanism of Action	86
Drug Interactions	88
Contraindications	89
Warnings	90
Use in Pregnancy	90
Efficacy in Blacks	91

Use in Children and Adolescents 92
Use in the Elderly 92
Precautions 94
Management of Overdose or Exaggerated Response 95
Absorption, Distribution, Metabolism and Excretion 95
Adverse Reactions 96
The Nature of Thiazide Reactions 98
    A. Pharmacological 98
    B. Unpredictable Adverse Reactions to Thiazides 110
Metolazone 112
Indapamide 114
Furosemide 115
    Formulation 121
    Oral Dose in Hypertension 121
    Mechanism of Action 121
    Drug Interactions 122
    Contraindications 125
    Warnings 125
    Use in Pregnancy 126
    Precautions 127
    Absorption, Metabolism, Excretion 129
    Adverse Reactions 129
Nature of Furosemide Reactions 133
    A. Pharmacological 133
    B. Unpredictable Adverse Reactions to Furosemide 136

● **Chapter IV:** *POTASSIUM SUPPLEMENTS*
Introduction 157
Potassium Homeostasis 160
Hypokalemia as Distinguished from Potassium Deficiency 161
Who is at Risk for Potassium Deficiency? 163
Role of Diet in Potassium Regulation 164
The Appropriate Indications for Potassium Supplements 168
What is the Proper Dose for KC1 Supplements? 168
How Safe are Potassium Supplements? What are the Side
    Effects and Toxicity? 169
Diuretic-induced Cardiac Arrhythmias 177

● **Chapter V:** *POTASSIUM-RETAINING DIURETICS*
Introduction 183
Amiloride 185
    Indications 188
    Formulation 188
    Dose in Hypertension 188
    Mechanism of Action 188
    Drug Interactions 188
    Contraindications 189
    Use in Pregnancy 189
    Precautions 190
    Management of Overdosage or Exaggerated Response 190
    Absorption, Distribution, Metabolism and Excretion 191
Triamterene 192
    Indications 193
    Formulation 194
    Dose in Hypertension 194
    Mechanism of Action 194
    Drug Interactions 194
    Contraindications 195
    Warnings 195
    Use in Pregnancy 196
    Precautions 196

Adverse Reactions 197
Absorption, Metabolism, Excretion 197
The Nature of Adverse Reactions to Triamterene 198
Spironolactone 200
Introduction 200
Indications 202
Formulation 202
Dose in Hypertension 202
Mechanism of Action 202
Drug Interactions 203
Contraindications 203
Warnings 204
Use in Pregnancy 204
Precautions 204
Management of Overdosage or Exaggerated Response 205
Absorption, Distribution, Metabolism and Excretion 205
Adverse Reactions 205
The Nature of Spironolactone Reactions 206

● **Chapter VI: _THE CENTRALLY ACTING ALPHA$_2$ AGONISTS_**

Introduction 215
Mechanism of Action 216
Absorption, Distribution, Metabolism, Excretion 218
Dose in Hypertension 219
When Should the Physician Consider Clonidine for Hypertension? 219
Use of Clonidine in Special Subgroups of Hypertensive Patients 225
Hypertensive Urgencies 228
How Effective is Clonidine? 229
Precautions 231
Drug Interactions 231
Post-Treatment Syndrome 232
Adverse Reactions 234
Methyldopa 234
Introduction 234
Indications for Use 235
Formulations 239
Dose in Hypertension 239
Low Dose Methyldopa 239
Mechanism of Action 240
Drug Interactions 242
Interference with Laboratory Tests 245
Contraindications 245
Warnings 245
Methyldopa and Pregnancy 247
Precautions 247
Absorption, Metabolism, Excretion 248
Adverse Reactions 249
Use of Methyldopa in Renal Disease 254
Guanabenz 255
Introduction 255
Indication 258
Formulation 258
Dose in Hypertension 258
Mechanism of Action 258
Drug Interactions 259
Contraindications 259
Use in Pregnancy 259
Precautions 260
Management of Overdosage or Exaggerated Response 260
Absorption, Distribution, Metabolism and Excretion 260
Adverse Reactions 261

ix

● **Chapter VII:** *BETA-ADRENERGIC BLOCKING DRUGS AND ALPHA-BETA BLOCKERS*

Introduction 277
Beta-Receptor Blockage 286
Mechanism of Action 288
Absorption, Metabolism, Excretion 291
Drug Interactions 293
Warnings 296
Adverse Reactions 298
Nature of Adverse Effects of Beta-Blockers 300
    A. Pharmacological 300
    B. Unpredictable Adverse Reactions to Beta-Blockers 306
Use in Pregnancy 308
Precautions 309
Contraindications 310
Management of Overdosage or Exaggerated Response 310
Important Differences among the Beta-Blockers 312
    Atenolol 312
    Metoprolol 312
    Nadolol 313
    Pindolol 313
    Propranolol 314
    Timolol 314
Labetalol 316
    Introduction 316
    Indications 319
    Dose in Hypertension 320
    Mechanism of Action 320
    Drug Interactions 324
    Contraindications 324
    Warnings 324
    Use in Pregnancy and Postpartum 325
    Absorption, Metabolism, Excretion 325
    Overdosage 326
    Precautions 326
    Adverse Reactions 326

● **Chapter VIII:** *ALPHA-ADRENERGIC BLOCKING AGENTS*

Prazosin 339
    Introduction 339
    Drug Interactions 345
    Warnings 345
    Use in Pregnancy 346
    Management of Overdose 346
    Side Effects 347
    Receptor Classification 348
Trimazosin 350
    Formulation 351
    Dose in Hypertension 351
Phenoxybenzamine HCL, Phentolamine HCL 352
    Introduction 352

● **Chapter IX:** *ORAL, DIRECT VASODILATORS*

Hydralazine 357
    Introduction 357
    Formulation 364
    Dose in Hypertension 364
    Mechanism of Action 365
    Drug Interactions 366
    Contraindications 367
    Warnings 367

Use in Pregnancy 368
Precautions 368
Management of Overdose or Exaggerated Response 368
Absorption, Distribution, Metabolism, Excretion 369
Adverse Reactions 370
Minoxidil 377
Introduction 377
Formulation 378
Dose in Hypertension 378
Mechanism of Action 379
Drug Interactions 380
Contraindications 380
Warnings 380
Use in Pregnancy 381
Absorption, Metabolism, Excretion 381
Adverse Reactions 381

● **Chapter X:** *CALCIUM CHANNEL BLOCKERS*
Introduction 393
Calcium Channel Blocker Monotherapy 396
Which One is Best for Hypertension? 398
Comparison with Beta-Blocker Monotherapy 398
Combination Therapy 401
Approved Indications for Calcium Channel Blockers 403
Nifedipine 403
Verapamil 403
Diltiazem 405
Dose in Hypertension 405
Mechanism of Action 405
Drug Interactions 407
Contraindications 410
Warnings 410
Use in Pregnancy 412
Precautions 413
Management of Overdose or Exaggerated Response 414
Absorption, Metabolism, Excretion 414
Adverse Reactions 416

● **Chapter XI:** *CONVERTING ENZYME INHIBITORS AND ANGIOTENSIN II BLOCKERS*
Captopril 425
Introduction 425
Formulation 433
Dose in Hypertension 433
Mechanism of Action 434
Drug Interactions 435
Interference with Laboratory Tests 436
Contraindications 436
Warnings 436
Use in Pregnancy 437
Precautions 438
Absorption, Metabolism, Excretion 438
Adverse Reactions 440
Enalapril 441
Dose in Hypertension 445
Saralasin 445
The Saralasin Test 447

● **Chapter XII:** *PERIPHERAL ADRENERGIC BLOCKING AGENTS*
Rauwolfia Alkaloids and Derivatives 457
Introduction 457

Indications for Reserpine 459
Formulation 459
Dose in Hypertension 459
Mechanism of Action 460
Drug Interactions of the Rauwolfia Compounds 460
Contraindications 461
Warnings 462
Use in Pregnancy 462
Precautions 462
Management of Overdose or Exaggerated Response 463
Absorption, Distribution, Metabolism, Excretion 463
Adverse Reactions 464
The Nature of Rauwolfia Reactions 464
Guanadrel 465
Introduction 465
Formulation 469
Dose in Hypertension 469
Mechanism of Action 469
Drug Interactions 470
Contraindications 470
Warnings 471
Use in Pregnancy 471
Precautions 472
Management of Overdose or Exaggerated Response 472
Absorption, Metabolism, Excretion 472
Adverse Reactions 473
The Nature of Guanadrel Reactions 474
Guanethidine 476
Introduction 476
Indications for Guanethidine 477
Formulation 477
Dose in Hypertension 477
Absorption, Metabolism, Excretion 477
Mechanism of Action 478
Contraindications 479
Warnings 479
Adverse Reactions 479
Drug Interactions 479
The Nature of Guanethidine Reactions 480
Bethanidine 483
Introduction 483
Indications for Bethanidine 483
Formulation 483
Dose in Hypertension 484
Mechanism of Action 484
Drug Interactions 484
Contraindications 485
Warnings 485
Use in Pregnancy 485
Precautions 485
Management of Overdose 486
Absorption, Metabolism, Excretion 486
Adverse Reactions 486
Nature of Bethanidine Reactions 486
Desbrisoquine 487

● **Chapter XIII: *POTENT PARENTERAL AGENTS***
I. Sodium Nitroprusside 495
Introduction 495
Formulation 498

Dose in Hypertension 498
Mechanism of Action 499
Drug Interactions 500
Contraindications 501
Warnings 501
Use in Pregnancy 501
Precautions 502
Management of Overdose or Exaggerated Response 502
Absorption, Metabolism, Excretion 503
Adverse Reactions 504
II. Diazoxide 506
Introduction 506
Formulation 512
Dose in Hypertension 512
Mechanism of Action 512
Drug Interactions 514
Contraindications 514
Warnings 515
Use in Pregnancy 516
Management of Overdose or Exaggerated Response 517
Absorption, Metabolism, Excretion 517
Adverse Reactions 518
The Nature of Diazoxide Reactions 519
Use of Diazoxide as an Oral Hyperglycemic 522
III. Trimethaphan Camsylate 522
Indications for Trimethaphan 522
Pharmacological Effects 523
Dosage and Administration 523
Formulation 524
Drug Interactions 524
Contraindications 524
Warnings 525
Use in Pregnancy 525
Precautions 525
Management of Overdose or Exaggerated Response 526
Labetalol 526

- **Chapter XIV: *NEW DRUGS***

Introduction 535
Alpha-Adrenergic Agonists 536
Catapres Transdermal Therapeutic System 536
Guanfacine 538
Urapidil 539
Tiamenidine 539
Alpha-Adrenergic Blockers 539
Indoramin 539
Introduction 539
Indications for Indoramin 540
Formulation 540
Dose in Hypertension 541
Mechanism of Action 541
Drug Interactions 542
Contraindications 542
Use in Pregnancy 543
Management of Overdosage 543
Absorption, Metabolism, Excretion 544
Precautions and Adverse Reactions 544
Tiodazosin 545
Beta-Adrenergic Blockers 547
Betaxolol 547
Sotalol 547

Oxprenolol 547
    Use in Pregnancy 548
Pronethalol and Alprenolol 549
Bevantolol 550
Calcium Channel Blockers 551
Nitrendipine 551
Nicardipine 551
Diuretics 552
Indacrinone 552
Piretanide 553
Muzolimine 554
Serotonin Antagonist 554
Ketanserin 554
Vasodilators 555
Guancydine 555
Pinacidil 556

● **Index** 563

PREFACE: THE NEW-LOW DOSE ERA

This book is for *physicians, medical students, nurses and pharmacists* involved in the care of hypertensive patients. It is concerned only with *treatment of essential hypertension*, not the general subject of hypertension. What began as an update has resulted in a completely new text.

Some five-year-old dogmas for treating hypertension must be modified:

> "treat all patients with mild hypertension with drugs;"
> "drug therapy is always needed for a lifetime;"
> "always start treatment with thiazides;"
> "always give full doses of thiazides;"
> "reducing blood pressure will reduce mortality to normal."

The treatment of hypertension has changed significantly. Non-drug modalities of therapy, which are inexpensive and safe, have become popular. Moderate reduction of salt intake can decrease blood pressure about 10/5 mm Hg. Weight reduction of 1 kg (2.2 lb) appears to lower blood pressure about 2.5/1.5 mm Hg. Numerous other forms of life-style modification have been studied but have not yet been clearly established as capable of long-term blood pressure reduction.

Many new drugs and new classes of drugs have been introduced, such as converting enzyme inhibitors, calcium channel blockers, and several agents which exhibit dual mechanisms of action, such as alpha-plus beta-adrenergic blockade.

Probably the single most important change in the past five years, however, has been the evolution of the "Low-Dose Era" of antihypertensive drug therapy. No class of drugs better demonstrates this than the thiazide diuretics. Five years ago most authorities recommended and used full doses to achieve optimal blood pressure reduction. The routine initial dose of hydrochlorothiazide or chlorthalidone was 100 mg, and 300 mg was not unusual. Two things have changed our thinking. Therapeutic efficacy has been clearly established for once-a-day doses of 25 and 50 mg of chlorthalidone or hydrochlorothiazide and 12.5 mg/day is effective in many elderl or black patients. Furthermore, the biochemical side effects, such as hypokalemia and the associated potentially serious cardiac arrhythmias, are minimized at these lower doses. It is now recognized that long-term use of thiazides produces subtle but important laboratory abnormalities which are risk factors for cardiovascular disease. Hypercholesterolemia (thiazides produce a 5–7% increase), hypertriglyceridemia, hyperuricemia and hyperglycemia, even when slight or perhaps still within the "normal" range, may, over a period of years, counteract the antihypertensive benefit of thiazides. A large 1983 U. S. Navy Hospital report found an 11% incidence of hypokalemia (K < 3.5 mEq/L) with 50 mg/day hydrochlorothiazide, compared with a 2.8% incidence using 25 mg/day. Others have confirmed this fact that hypokalemia and the other biochemical side effects of thiazides are indeed dose-related. The era of low-dose thiazides is here!

We should have learned from our experience with rauwolfias. We originally gave patients doses of 1.0 to 5.0 mg/day, and they suffered serious depression, sedation, rhinitis and ulcers. Today we give only 0.1 or 0.25 mg/day and side effects are quite trivial.

We might have learned from our hydralazine experience. Today we give 50 to 200 mg/day instead of 400 to 1,000 mg/day, and the result is milder, more manageable side effects with satisfactory efficacy. Methyldopa is now being given in doses of 125 to 250 mg twice daily instead of gram doses, with good blood pressure reduction in many patients. The incidence of both pharmacologic side effects (e.g., drowsiness) and immunologic side effects (positive Coombs' test) has thereby been greatly reduced.

The fixed combination of clonidine with 15 mg chlorthalidone, when given at bedtime, usually reduces blood pressure for 24 hours with minimization of bothersome side effects. Propranolol is now used in once-daily long-acting doses of 80 mg instead of the gram doses formerly used in Europe. The potassium-sparing drug, amiloride, today is used at 2.5 mg doses instead of the previous 5–10 mg/day doses. The effectiveness of captopril, at doses of 12.5 and 25 mg three times daily in mild hypertension, has been demonstrated in a recent Veterans Administration multiclinic study. The dose of atenolol has been reduced from 100 to 200 mg/day to 25 and 50 mg/day, and effectiveness is maintained.

Because the side effects of antihypertensive drugs are often dose-related and because efficacy can often be achieved by using one or two drugs each at low doses, physicians, drug companies, and the FDA need to reevaluate their traditional recommendations on appropriate doses of these agents.

The Oslo study (1980), the Australian report (1982) and the Levinson, Khatria, and Freis report (1982) have established that mild high blood pressure doesn't always have a gradually-increasing, relentless course. Some mildly hypertensive patients experience spontaneous decrements to diastolic levels of less than 90 mm Hg when followed for periods of one to three years. Also, many mild or moderately severe hypertensive patients can have their doses successfully reduced if they have been under stable control for a year or so. However, tapering or eliminating even one agent of a multiple dose regimen should be done with careful monitoring.

Additionally, even after many large, controlled, international and domestic multiclinic studies, it has still not been proven to the satisfaction of many authorities that coronary heart disease (acute myocardial infarction or sudden death) can be prevented by successfully reducing levels of 90–99 mm Hg diastolic pressure. Strokes or transient ischemic attacks, aortic aneurysms, renal disease, retinopathy, left ventricular hypertrophy, pulmonary edema and congestive heart failure (all complications of hypertension) can be prevented by drug therapy, but results have been controversial insofar as preventing coronary artery disease—an atherosclerotic complication. Many clinicians have felt that the actuarial data indicate that the benefit of lowering blood pressure is synonymous with decreasing risks. But the long-term Framingham Study data show that the risk of developing an acute myocardial infarction among patients with mild hypertension depends on the presence and severity of the *other major risk factors in addition to hypertension.* The person who smokes cigarettes, has hypercholesterolemia and a strong family history of cardiovascular disease has a far greater risk for an acute myocardial infarction than a patient with a similar degree of hypertension but without additional risk factors. The former patient needs his cholesterol reduced, his smoking stopped, *and* his blood pressure lowered. The latter patient, if his diastolic pressure is 100–114 mm Hg, should receive low doses of drugs together with moderate salt restriction and weight reduction (if obese). If his diastolic range is

90–95 mm Hg, non-drug therapy alone should be energetically pursued for perhaps three to six months before considering long-term drug therapy.

Finally, we've learned that not every patient with mild to moderate hypertension should best be started with thiazides. Besides using non-drug measures for many very mild cases, most authorities feel that many patients should be given beta-blockers as initial monotherapy, particularly the young white patient with recent onset of hypertension or patients with tachyarrhythmia or recent myocardial infarction. The elderly patient and the black patient, for instance, respond much better to thiazides. Clonidine monotherapy is often preferable to beta-blocker therapy in elderly patients because of better safety and effectiveness. Converting enzyme inhibitors and beta-blockers are less effective in black than white patients. A fixed combination drug is often the treatment of choice for patients with moderate hypertension. The single tablet combination of a thiazide with a beta-blocker is often effective. Initial therapy of hypertension should be individualized, depending upon sound clinical knowledge of the whole patient, all the clinical circumstances present, and a thorough knowledge of the drugs.

At the present time proper management of the hypertensive patient requires a multifactorial approach: reduce the blood pressure but don't allow the cholesterol, triglycerides, uric acid and glucose levels to rise significantly. The Oslo Study (1982) concluded that morbidity from cardiovascular disease was significantly lowered when lipids were reduced and smoking stopped, while antihypertensive therapy alone failed. Attention must be given to other risk factors in addition to hypertension. Cholesterol, HDL-cholesterol, cigarette smoking, obesity, inactivity, type A personality (highly competitive), left ventricular hypertrophy, the presence of diabetes mellitus—each of these contributes to the atherosclerotic process and coronary heart disease. As William Castelli (Framingham Report, 1983) has so aptly put it: "reversibility of the atherosclerotic process" should be the therapeutic goal. Achievement of this goal must involve a multifactorial approach.

CHAPTER I

SYNOPSIS

WHAT IS HYPERTENSION?

Hypertension in the adult is defined by most
authorities and by The American Heart Association as
that arterial pressure exceeding 140/90 mm Hg.

Hypertension is mankind's most common serious disease. It affects approximately 15 to 25% of all adults surveyed. The average physician in general practice, family practice, or in internal medicine can expect to see 20 to 40 patients each week with hypertension. Hypertension in the adult is defined by most authorities and by The American Heart Association as that arterial pressure exceeding 140/90 mm Hg. Not everyone accepts this definition, however, and the World Health Organization (WHO) as well as the U. S. Health Survey (the "HANES" Survey) defines normotension as blood pressure less than 140/90 mm Hg and hypertension as that pressure greater than 160/95 mm Hg WHO regards pressures in between these two levels as being borderline. Actuarial data indicate that life expectancy is reduced at all ages and in both sexes when the diastolic pressure exceeds 90 mm Hg. Of course blood pressure varies from moment to moment throughout the day; therefore, it is essential, before establishing the diagnosis, that a patient's blood pressure be determined under relaxed conditions and on multiple occasions. Generally, the patient should be resting quietly and comfortably for five to ten minutes before taking the blood pressure. Usually the patient should be examined on at least three separate occasions at perhaps weekly intervals before establishing the diagnosis in mild cases. Home blood pressures generally run lower than office or clinic pressures. Most families with a hypertensive member ought to own a reliable sphygmomanometer, preferably a good aneroid or mercurial type and have someone taught how to operate it properly.

Since hypertension increases with age and is found in 50% of people over 65 years, target organ damage increases with age. Although systolic hypertension (> 160/ < 90 mm Hg) is fairly frequent (occurring in 25–30% of patients over 75 years)[1] in the elderly, both diastolic and systolic hypertension is the usual finding in these patients. Messerli et al[2] have found the following characteristics among elderly hypertensive patients compared with a matched group of similar but young hypertensive patients: decreased cardiac output, heart rate, stroke volume, intravascular volume, renal blood flow and plasma renin activity, together with increased peripheral vascular resistance, left ventricular septal thickness and left ventricular mass. Therefore, most elderly hypertensives have left ventricular hypertrophy. Therapeutically, one must attempt not only to reduce their arterial pressure, but also to reverse this hypertrophy (as well as any other target organ damage) through appropriate antihypertensive drug administration.

The 1975 Medical Directors of Insurance Companies' Report[3] on home blood pressures taken on 158,906 people, ages 30 to 69 years, showed that 25.3% had diastolic pressures of 90 mm Hg or greater and 17.4% had diastolic pressures of 100 mm Hg or greater. The Community Hypertension Evaluation Clinic Program surveyed 1,049,225 persons' blood pressures and found 24.7% had diastolic levels greater than 90 mm Hg and 11.6% had diastolic levels greater than 95 mm Hg.[4] In addition, the "Hanes" survey report (U. S. Health Survey[5]) also concluded from its health statistics screening data that 60,000,000 U. S. adults have hypertension, and that 40,000,000 of them have mild hypertension (diastolic pressure 90–99 mm Hg).

60,000,000 U. S. adults have
hypertension, and that 40,000,000 of them have mild
hypertension (diastolic pressure 90–99 mm Hg).

It is convenient and quite conventional to classify hypertension as being "mild," "moderate" or "severe," depending on the level of diastolic pressure and the degree of target organ involvement. Recently there is much discussion about "low-mild" (diastolic pressure 90-94 mm Hg) with important therapeutic implications. Throughout this book we shall use the three classes shown in Table I. Otherwise, we shall cite specific ranges of pressure.

"Labile" hypertension is a poor word, since all blood pressure is labile, whether within normal or hypertensive ranges. "Borderline"

TABLE I
A WORKING CLASSIFICATION OF THE SEVERITY OF HYPERTENSION

Classification	Diastolic Pressure (mm Hg)
Mild	90–104
Moderate	105–119
Severe	>120

---

hypertension is a descriptive phrase used for those patients with blood pressures that don't consistently run high, i.e., $> 140/90$ mm Hg. Most U. S. authorities define adult hypertension as that pressure which exceeds 140 mm Hg systolic and/or exceeds 90 mm Hg diastolic during most of the waking day.

THE RISKS

Life expectancy decreases as blood pressure rises. Mortality increases for both men and women (Tables II and III) fairly stepwise as diastolic or systolic-diastolic pressures rise. The higher the level of either systolic or diastolic pressure, the greater the risk of developing target organ disease secondarily. Attention is called to the 30–39 year age group of men with blood pressures of 138-147/88-94 mm Hg (low—mild hypertension) because these young men have a mortality ratio of 190%, almost twice normal. Target organs include the heart, kidneys, central nervous system, and major arteries. Manifestations of cardiac involvement include the development of angina pectoris, acute myocardial infarction, left ventricular hypertrophy, acute pulmonary edema, congestive heart failure and sudden coronary death. Involvement of the kidneys secondary to hypertension produces nocturia as the initial symptom and albuminuria (more than 250 mg per 24 hours) as the first objective sign. Ultimately, renal involvement leads to azotemia and renal failure. Involvement of the central nervous system includes the development of transient ischemic attacks and cerebrovascular accidents. Involvement of the major arteries includes the development of dissecting aneurysms and atherothrombotic obstruction of the abdominal aorta and major peripheral arteries.

TABLE II
MORTALITY EXPERIENCE ACCORDING TO
VARIATIONS IN SYSTOLIC AND DIASTOLIC PRESSURES

With and Without Known Minor Impairments
All Ages Combined—By Number of Policies

Ratios (Percent) of Actual to Expected Mortality

Diastolic Blood Pressure (Fifth Phase-mm)	Men	Women		Systolic-Diastolic Combination	Men	Women
Under 68	84%	86%	A	Under 128 mm with Under 83 mm	84%	90%
68–72	85	88	B	128–137 mm with 78–87 mm	111	108
73–77	92	96	C	138–147 mm with 83–92 mm	140	125
78–82	99	103	D	148–157 mm with 88–97 mm	176	146
83–87	118	114	E	158–167 mm with 93–102 mm	226	195
88–92	136	132	F	Over 167 mm with Over 97 mm	269	216
93–97	169	167	G	148–167 mm with 78–87 mm	159	151
98–102	200	181	H	128–147 mm with 93–102 mm	154	130
103–107	258	208				
108–112	244	(195)				
Over 112	221	(220)				

From: Blood Pressure Study 1979,[6] reprinted with permission.

TABLE III
MORTALITY EXPERIENCE FOR MEN ACCORDING TO
BLOOD PRESSURE WITHOUT KNOWN MINOR IMPAIRMENTS
RATIO (PERCENT) OF ACTUAL TO EXPECTED MORTALITY

	Blood Pressure	
Age	138–147/88–94	148–157/93–97
20–29	122%	*
30–39	195	255%
40–49	160	233
50–59	141	169
60–69	133	162

* Insufficient policies to determine mortality ratio.
From: Blood Pressure Study 1979,[6] reprinted with permission.

What are the risk factors which lead to the development of cardiovascular disease? Table IV lists both the major and minor factors. The three classical major risk factors in cardiovascular disease include hypertension, hyperlipidemia and cigarette smoking. Hypertension is the most important independent risk factor for both atherothrombotic and hemorrhagic stroke.[7,8] The Framingham Study demonstrated that in the 45–74 age group, peripheral vascular disease is twice as common in hypertensives as normotensives; coronary heart disease is three times more common; congestive heart failure is four times as common; and stroke is seven times more common. Even though hypertension increases the incidence of stroke and congestive heart failure the most, the hypertensive patient is at greatest risk to develop coronary heart disease. The incidence of coronary heart disease in hypertensive patients is greater than the combination of all the other cardiovascular complications.[9]

Roberts[10] has recently reviewed the frequencies of systemic hypertension and cardiomegaly in various cardiovascular conditions and has identified a clear association between hypertension and such events as sudden coronary death and acute myocardial infarction. Systemic hypertension acts as a major risk factor in the development of cardiovascular disease by accelerating the deposit of atherosclerotic plaques in major arteries and also by weakening the media of arteries, thereby causing aneurysms which may subsequently tear or rupture.

TABLE IV
RISK FACTORS FOR CARDIOVASCULAR DISEASE

A. Major Correctable:
- Hypertension
- Cigarette smoking
- Elevated cholesterol and/or reduced HDL-cholesterol
- Target organ damage (heart, brain, kidneys, major arteries)
- Obesity

B. Major Non-Correctable
- Strong family history of hypertension, stroke, heart disease
- Diabetes mellitus
- Male
- Age

Minor:
- Black—for stroke and hypertension
  White—for coronary
- Elevated serum uric acid/gout
- Type A personality

Besides hypertension, other risk factors increase the risk of cardiovascular disease. The Framingham Studies[9] demonstrate clearly that the risk of an acute myocardial infarction among patients with mild hypertension depends on the number and extent of other major risk factors present (Figure 1). An example may be persuasive. A 40-year-old man with a systolic pressure of 165 mm Hg but with no other risk factors present has about a 2% chance of sustaining an acute myocardial infarction over a six-year interval. With his systolic pressure reduced to 135 mm Hg, the risk is reduced to about 1%. In other words, if this man had been treated successfully with thiazide diuretics, e.g., the most one could expect from treatment is a reduction in his risk of 1%. On the other hand, if this man had multiple serious risk factors present, such as cigarette smoking, left ventricular hypertrophy, elevated cholesterol, and decreased glucose tolerance, together with his systolic pressure of 165 mm Hg, his risk of developing serious cardiovascular disease increases to 28%. When this high risk individual has his blood pressure reduced to 135 mm Hg, the risk is now significantly reduced to 21%. Freis concludes from these kinds of data that "if antihypertensive treatment is beneficial in reducing the risk of myocardial infarction, it is most beneficial in patients with multiple risk factors."[11] He therefore recommends that patients with diastolic blood pressures of 90–99 mm Hg *not* be treated unless other risk factors are present. Gifford[12] and

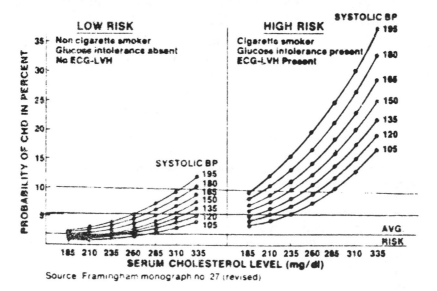

Figure 1: Probability of developing coronary heart disease in 6 years. 40-year-old men. Framingham study. 16 year follow-up.

many other authorities, impressed by the results of The Hypertension Detection and Follow-up Program (HDFP), as well as by the Australian Therapeutic Trial, disagree and would treat *all* patients with mild hypertension.

The HDFP group concluded from their study of 10,940 patients with diastolic pressure >90 mm Hg that "Stepped-Care" (SC) treatment reduced overall cardiovascular mortality by 26%, compared to a "Referred Care" (RC) group after five years.[13] The SC group all received diuretics and other Step-2 drugs as needed at special hypertension centers until their diastolic pressures were reduced below 90 mm Hg. They also received careful dietary and other formalized medical instructions to lower cholesterol and stop cigarette smoking. The RC patients were treated at their usual medical facilities with whatever routine care was available for hypertension and for reducing other risk factors. Patients were seen more frequently in the SC than in the RC group. It is beyond our scope to expound adequately on this study, but its conclusions have stirred controversy and criticism, e.g., no placebo control group was used and diagnoses were based on death-certificate diagnoses. Nevertheless, the participants concluded and many authorities concur that intensive drug treatment of mild hypertension was proven to reduce cardiovascular mortality in 20.3% of those patients with mild hypertension (diastolic: 90–104 mm Hg).

Many authorities concur that intensive drug treatment of mild hypertension was proven to reduce cardiovascular mortality in 20.3% of those patients with mild hypertension (diastolic: 90–104 mm Hg).

The Australian Therapeutic Trial reported results of placebo versus drug treatment of 3,427 patients with mild hypertension (diastolic 95–109 mm Hg) without clinical evidence of target organ disease and followed four years.[14] Results indicated that drug therapy reduced both mortality and morbidity from cardiovascular disease. There were fewer cases of ischemic heart disease, and strokes were reduced by half. The 1970 Veterans Administration Trial showed that the treatment of patients with mild hypertension clearly diminishes the incidence of congestive heart failure, renal damage, cerebral vascular accidents and accelerated hypertension (sequelae of hypertension per se); there was no prevention of coronary artery disease or myocardial infarction (sequelae of atherosclerosis per se). The same conclusions were reached in the U. S. Public Health Service Hospital Trial.[15]

McGee[16] applied multivariant analysis techniques to the 18-year Framingham Study data and prepared a series of tables giving the probabilities of developing cardiovascular disease (CVD). Madhavan and Alderman,[17] using similar techniques, published the probability of hypertensive patients' developing CVD in 15 years by sex and by level of risk (Table V). For example, a 35-year-old male with no risk factors other than a systolic pressure of 165 mm Hg has a 10% chance of developing CVD in 15 years. If his systolic pressure is reduced to 135 mm Hg, his chance declines to 6%. The question then becomes whether or not it is worthwhile giving medication with its attendant side effects and subtle biochemical effects for 15 years in order to reduce one's chances of CVD by only 4%. Gifford would treat this patient arguing that at age 50 years, his atherosclerosis will have been accelerated significantly, he is still relatively young, and manifestations of cardiovascular disease will ultimately appear. On the other hand, if this 35-year-old male is at high risk, he has a 76% chance of developing CVD within 15 years. Certainly all agree that every effort must be made to minimize risk, including giving antihypertensive drugs to reduce his systolic pressure 30 mm Hg and also his risk by 13%.

Table V further indicates that a) lowering the blood pressure of women (at low or high risk) is less beneficial than for men; b) lowering the blood pressure of young men is more beneficial than for elderly men; and c) the benefit of blood pressure reduction varies substantially depending on the constellation of other risk factors.

LEFT VENTRICULAR HYPERTROPHY

The therapeutic goal for treating hypertension is not only to normalize blood pressure, but also to prevent or reverse target organ damage. With the advent of M-mode and two-dimensional echocardiography, left ventricular hypertrophy (LVH) can be detected much earlier than by electrocardiogram, x-ray or physical examination. As many as 40 to 50% of unselected patients with mild hypertension have shown evidence of LVH by echocardiogram. Elderly hypertensives (over 65 years) usually have LVH.[2,18,19] The association is closely linked to the level of blood pressure, particularly systolic.

TABLE V
PROBABILITY (PER 100) OF CARDIOVASCULAR DISEASE (CVD) DEVELOPING IN 15 YEARS BY SEX, STARTING AGE, AND LEVELS OF RISK AND THE POTENTIAL BENEFIT FROM BLOOD PRESSURE REDUCTION**

Systolic Blood Pressure (mm Hg)	Men						Women					
	Low Risk at Age, yr			High Risk at Age, yr			Low Risk at Age, yr			High Risk at Age, yr		
	35	45	55	35	45	55	35	45	55	35	45	55
195	15	32	47	86	95	97	7	18	32	42	66	82
180	12	27	41	81	93	96	6	15	27	36	60	77
165	10	22	35	76	90	94	5	12	23	31	54	71
135	6	15	24	63	82	88	3	8	16	22	42	59

Potential Benefit*

	Men						Women					
	Low Risk at Age, yr			High Risk at Age, yr			Low Risk at Age, yr			High Risk at Age, yr		
	35	45	55	35	45	55	35	45	55	35	45	55
195→135	9(60)	17(53)	23(49)	23(27)	13(14)	9(9)	4(57)	10(56)	16(50)	20(48)	24(36)	23(28)
180→135	6(50)	12(44)	17(41)	18(22)	11(12)	8(8)	3(50)	7(47)	11(41)	14(39)	18(30)	18(23)
165→135	4(40)	7(32)	11(31)	13(17)	8(9)	6(6)	2(40)	4(33)	7(30)	9(29)	12(22)	12(17)

* Figures in parentheses are the relative benefit expressed as a percent of the original probability of having CVD; arrow indicates reduced to.

** From Madhavan, S. and Alderman, M.,[17] reprinted with permission. (*Archives of Internal Medicine*, 141:1584, 1981. Copyright 1981. American Medical Association.)

The presence of LVH is an important accompaniment of cardiovascular disease. Framingham data indicate that from electrocardiographic (ECG) evidence, the presence of LVH is a very ominous sign, resulting in increased incidences of coronary heart disease, stroke, heart failure, and peripheral vascular disease.[20]

It appears that not all antihypertensive drugs can reduce LVH, even though blood pressure may be reduced within normal limits. Hydrochlorothiazide failed to do so after 18 months' follow-up[21] in one study and after a six months' follow-up of eight patients in another study.[21] Clonidine with chlorthalidone (Combipres®) succeeded in reducing LVH among 10 of 20 patients we studied who had both ECG and echocardiographic evidence of LVH.[22] Our patients were monitored monthly for the first three months, then every third month for two years. Responders were controlled by mean doses of 0.6 mg/day of clonidine with chlorthalidone. Both the posterior wall and intraventricular septal thickness were significantly reduced after three months (many after only one month). We were not able to distinguish responders from non-responders by blood pressure level or duration, by age, sex, weight, other concurrent illnesses, response to therapy, etc. Methyldopa given with hydrochlorothiazide (Aldoril®), or given alone, has also been shown to reduce LVH.[21,23] Atenolol has also been shown to reduce left ventricular mass after eight weeks of treatment.[23,24] Others have shown propranolol and nadolol to reduce LVH in small numbers of patients treated for eight weeks.[25]

Converting enzyme inhibitors are also reported to reduce LVH. Captopril given with or without chlorthalidone to 20 patients reduced LVH significantly in 13 patients by the eighth week and even further after 16 weeks when repeat echocardiograms were done. Blood pressure was reduced in all 20 patients comparably, but seven failed to show reduction of LVH. Enalapril reduced LVH in six of seven patients treated after three months of monotherapy.[26]

M-mode echocardiogram can best detect
early LVH. When present, it must be treated
aggressively with drugs.

In summary, if mild hypertension has been present for several years, or if moderate hypertension has been present for several months, it is prudent to evaluate the patient for the presence of LVH. The ECG is readily available, but the M-mode echocardiogram can best detect early LVH. When present, it must be treated aggressively with drugs and results monitored after one or two months. It appears that alpha-agonists like clonidine and methyldopa, converting enzyme inhibitors and beta-blocking agents are the preferred drugs. Although blood pressure may be satisfactorily reduced by one of these drugs, it appears that only 50% of patients with LVH will show significant reductions of myocardial mass. Thus far, there is no clear way to distinguish responders from non-responders.

THE NATURAL COURSE OF THE DISEASE

Because hypertension is known to increase with age, it is generally felt that the untreated disease relentlessly and insidiously escalates over a period of 15–30 years in 100% of individuals. Hypertension usually becomes evident between the ages of 20 and 40 years, and over the subsequent two decades its hypertensive complications, viz., cerebrovascular accidents, renal failure, aneurysms, left ventricular hypertrophy and heart failure were believed to be ultimately inevitable. In addition, it has been generally felt that the atherosclerotic complications of hypertension, viz., coronary heart disease, acute myocardial infarction and sudden deaths occur, in time, as a result of the hypertension. About 1% or less of patients with essential hypertension develop accelerated or malignant hypertension. Most physicians are of the impression that both the hypertensive and atherosclerotic complications of hypertension can be prevented by reducing blood pressure with drug therapy.

However, it is recognized today that the natural course of hypertension is not nearly so relentless. Indeed, many patients with mild hypertension (diastolic pressures of 90–99 mm Hg), whether treated or not, may become normotensive without therapy for many months or even a few years. The Australian Therapeutic Trial Report in 1982 indicated that 48% of patients followed three years without treatment experienced drops in blood pressures from the original level of 95–109 mm Hg down to below 90 mm Hg without any treatment whatsoever. On the other hand, 12% of patients in this trial experienced increases in blood pressure to above 110 mm Hg when no antihypertensive medications were used. In a five-year study from Finland[27] of 1,080 untreated hypertensive patients (with mean pressures of 162/104 mm Hg in males, 167/104 mm Hg in females), spontaneous declines in blood pressure were noted in 50% (503/1080) of patients. Decrements were 8/10 mm Hg in males and 11/12 mm Hg in females. The Oslo Study[28] of mild hypertensives found 27% of untreated patients experienced a mean increase of 5 mm Hg diastolic pressure over a five-year interval. The U. S. Public Health Service study of 389 patients treated either with placebo or active drug indicated that 24 of 196 untreated patients developed progressive hypertension (12.2%). Other studies also support the conclusion that 2–5% per year of untreated patients with essential hypertension experience a significant rise in their blood pressure. Levinson and Freis,[29] after treating 24 mildly hypertensive patients with diuretics alone, reported that 11 (46%) were still normotensive off treatment for six months and 5 (21%) were normotensive after 12 months.

It is clearly established that hypertension increases with age and that when large populations of mild hypertensive patients are followed periodically for several years, mean blood pressures tend to drift upward. Nevertheless, when such populations are subdivided, it seems that a significant segment of untreated mildly hypertensive individuals sustain significant declines without any therapy. Such experiences demonstrate the wisdom of exercising care in establishing the initial diagnosis of mild hypertension through multiple examinations. Conservative management of mild essential hypertensive patients for three to six months before initiating therapy is prudent. Risk, however, is determined not only by the initial level of blood pressure, but also by the presence of other risk factors, including those that may be aggravated by giving drugs.

INITIAL MEDICAL EVALUATION OF THE PATIENT WITH MILD HYPERTENSION

Once the diagnosis of mild essential hypertension is established, how much of a workup should be done? Because the therapeutic goal should be reduction not only of blood pressure, but also the treatment or prevention of target organ damage, one must look carefully at these organs. Because other risk factors such as elevated cholesterol and low HDL-cholesterol, cigarette smoking, left ventricular hypertrophy each clearly increase risk of cardiovascular disease, attention to these is needed. The primary purpose of the medical history and physical examination of the patient with essential hypertension is to determine (a) whether other risk factors are present, and (b) whether target organ damage has occurred. Therefore, the physician should take a medical history for such risk factors as: cigarette smoking, family history of hypertension, stroke, or heart disease, diabetes mellitus, gout, level of physical activity, and whether or not the patient is a type A personality (domineering, impatient, competitive).

The medical history for target organ damage should include such questions as: the duration of hypertension; presence of nocturia; transient ischemic attacks; symptoms of dyspnea, orthopnea, angina pectoris, or previous myocardial infarction; and whether peripheral edema has been occurring.

The physical examination of the hypertensive should include, in addition to blood pressure: the patient's body weight; presence of a diastolic cervical bruit, abdominal, flank or paravertebral bruit; whether retinopathy is present in the refracted pupils; the presence of a visible systolic apical thrust or percussible left ventricular hypertrophy; the presence of a third heart sound (suggests congestive heart failure) or fourth heart sound (suggests left ventricular hypertrophy); the presence of pulmonary rales or edema, or abdominal or peripheral edema.

Routine laboratory tests should include: a complete blood count, urinalysis, serum cholesterol, HDL-cholesterol, fasting blood glucose, uric acid and creatinine. An ECG should be obtained for purposes of establishing baseline information, as well as the possible presence of left ventricular hypertrophy or changes due to ischemia or previous myocardial infarction. Patients over 40 years of age should get a chest x-ray. Serum potassium should be obtained if the patient has been on thiazides, or because they may be prescribed. Liver function tests are of importance when hepatic disease is suspected, and the use of drugs which are metabolized by the liver may be employed.

THE NON-DRUG TREATMENT OF HYPERTENSION

Table VI lists the various non-drug interventions that have been reported and indicates whether or not sufficient data exist to establish efficacy of each. Moderate salt restriction reduces pressure about 10/5

TABLE VI
THE THERAPEUTIC EFFICACY OF VARIOUS NON-DRUG
INTERVENTIONS (OR ADVERSE EFFECTS) AMONG
PATIENTS WITH HYPERTENSION
(See Chapter II for a full discussion of each)

Intervention	Efficacy in Reducing Blood Pressure
1. Moderate sodium restriction	Proven efficacy
2. Weight reduction in obese	Proven efficacy
3. Regular physical exercise program	Probably effective
4. Relaxation, meditation, biofeedback	Possibly effective
5. Stopping cigarettes	Possibly effective
6. Potassium therapy	Possibly effective
7. High p/s fat diet*	Possibly effective
8. Calcium supplementation	Possibly effective
9. Modest alcohol ingestion**	Possibly effective

* Polyunsaturated/saturated fat ratio.
** 2–3 alcoholic drinks/day (or < 60 oz. alcohol per month).

mm Hg. Weight reduction of 1 kg (2.2 lb) may lower pressure about 2.5/1.5 mm Hg (see Chapter II).

Moderate salt restriction reduces pressure
about 10/5 mm Hg. Weight reduction of 1 kg (2.2 lb)
may lower pressure about 2.5/1.5 mm Hg.

INDIVIDUALIZED OR STEPPED-CARE THERAPY FOR MILD HYPERTENSION

The Stepped-Care technique for the management of hypertension has performed a great service to physicians and their patients with hypertension (Figure 2). Beginning with a thiazide diuretic, approximately 50% of patients respond satisfactorily within a period of a month or two. When patients do not respond sufficiently, a so-called Step-2 drug is added to the diuretic. Figure 2 gives the various steps in the program. It has indeed served us well.

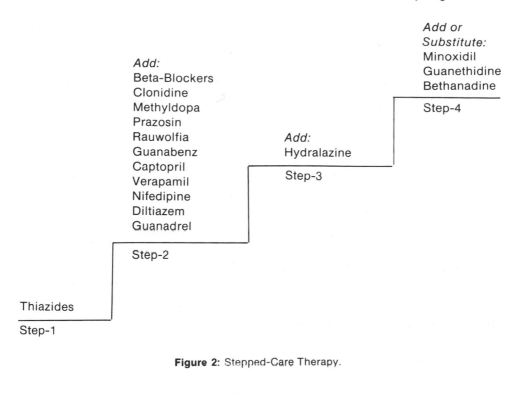

Figure 2: Stepped-Care Therapy.

Most authorities feel that therapy should be individualized
rather than regimented.

But now most authorities feel that therapy should be individualized rather than regimented. Initial therapy of mild hypertension (diastolic BP 90–99 mm Hg) should consist of a genuine effort to normalize pressure with non-drug treatment, i.e., utilizing moderate sodium restriction in all and caloric restriction in the obese.

Initial drug therapy of many patients (e.g., young whites with recent onset of mild hypertension) should begin with a beta-blocking drug. Initial therapy of most patients with moderate hypertension (diastolic 100–114 mm Hg) requires two drugs and may be initiated with a fixed combination of low doses of those drugs. Occasionally initial therapy can begin with a central agonist like clonidine or a converting enzyme inhibitor like enalapril or captopril or an alpha-blocker like trimazosin or prazosin or a calcium channel blocker like verapamil or nifedipine. Initial therapeutic choice depends upon good clinical judgment determined by careful assessment of all the clinical circumstances present, together with a thorough knowledge of the drugs.

Non-drug treatment may well include other elements involved in altering one's lifestyle (e.g., jogging or walking on a regular basis, stopping cigarette smoking, relaxation intervals, etc.) (See Chapter II, Table VII). Non-drug therapy should be the basis for treatment not only of mild hypertension but also as part of the fundamental regimen of most patients with moderate and more severe forms of hypertension.

If the diastolic blood pressure is less than 95 mm Hg and if no other risk factors are present, non-drug treatment should be continued indefinitely with the patient followed periodically. As stated above under "Risks," unless other risk factors are present in addition to mild hypertension, particularly in women, aggressive therapy has simply not been proven to reduce the chief complication of hypertension, viz., coronary heart disease. On the other hand, if the patient has left ventricular hypertrophy, smokes cigarettes, has diabetes mellitus, elevated cholesterol level, and/or a strong family history of hypertension or heart disease, he is at greater risk because of these concurrent factors and, therefore, blood pressure should be reduced by whatever means necessary, including drugs.

Today most authorities favor "individualized therapy" rather than "stepped-care" as therapy for hypertension (Table VII). Which drug should be utilized as initial monotherapy for mild hypertension? Frequently the initial drug should be a thiazide diuretic; occasionally the initial drug should be a beta-blocking agent; and occasionally the initial therapy should be a drug like clonidine, a calcium channel blocker, or a converting enzyme inhibitor. The nature of the initial monotherapy of hypertension depends on the presence or absence of other factors such as race or age, and the presence or absence of concurrent diseases such as angina pectoris or asthma. Table VII itemizes the "drugs of choice" to be utilized in instances of mild hypertension where non-drug therapy has been inadequate and lists the concurrent risk factors or other conditions which help decide the nature of the initial drug to be used. Black patients, for example, have a high incidence of low renin (expanded-plasma volume) essential hypertension. Therefore, they respond not only more briskly to thiazide diuretics but also to lower doses as well. If a patient has early hypertension, often with a fast heart rate and often noting palpitations, especially if young and if white, the

TABLE VII
INITIAL THERAPY OF CHOICE FOR MILD
HYPERTENSION DEPENDS ON THE PRESENCE OF OTHER CIRCUMSTANCES*

If Diastolic Blood Pressure Is: (mm Hg)	And Other Factors Present:	Initial Rx of Choice Is:
90–94	No Risk Factors*	Non-drug Therapy Indefinitely; some would start drugs after 3–6 months, if not controlled.
95–99	No Risk Factors*	Non-drug Therapy 3–6 months, then drugs if needed
90–94	Risk Factors Present	Non-drug Therapy 3–6 months, then drugs if needed
95–104	Risk Factors Present and Young White Recent AMI Tachyarrhythmia Hyperkinetic Heart Angina Volume-Contracted (High Renin) Gout History of Hypokalemia Migraine	Non-drug Therapy plus Beta-Blocker
95–104	Black Elderly Fluid-expanded (Low Renin) History of Hypoglycemia Asthma Congestive Heart Failure > 1° AV-Block Allergic Rhinitis	Thiazide plus Non-drug Rx

* For major and minor risk factors, see Table IV. It should be noted that patients with mild diastolic hypertension may also have left ventricular hypertrophy (best detected early via echocardiogram), in which cases drug therapy is indicated.

drug of choice initially is a beta-blocker which will specifically decrease the high cardiac output causing the hypertension. The ideal patient for initial therapy with clonidine may be a patient with a hypertensive crisis who comes to the emergency room. A patient with bouts of paroxysmal supraventricular tachycardia and mild hypertension may best respond to a cardiodepressive calcium channel blocker like verapamil. A patient with a very recent myocardial infarction and with mild hypertension may best be given a beta-blocking drug such as timolol, which has the added advantage of reducing the likelihood of having another infarction by 23%, reducing the incidence of sudden deaths by 40% and the incidence of total deaths by 39%.[30]

WHICH SECOND DRUG SHOULD BE ADDED?

Just as the selection of the initial drug depends upon such circumstances as the level of blood pressure, the presence of target organ damage, race, age, presence of other illnesses (asthma, angina, tachyarrhythmias) balanced with a substantial knowledge of the drugs, so too does the selection of the second drug depend upon similar circumstances. The most popular combination today is the use of a thiazide and a beta-blocker (a combination effective in about 85% of patients). Fortunately for sick people, however, there are numerous valuable alternatives. Clonidine, for example, is particularly valuable not only as monotherapy in hypertensive crises or as the third or fourth drug to give in refractory cases, but also as a good choice to add to the diuretic in elderly patients, in so many of whom beta-blockers are contraindicated (or simply not effective). We have found once-a-day doses of Combipres® (clonidine plus chlorthalidone) given at bedtime minimize side effects while maintaining control of blood pressure throughout the day.[22]

Beta-blockers or calcium channel blockers are the drugs of choice for many hypertensives who also have angina or certain tachyarrhythmias.

Converting enzyme inhibitors, although particularly useful in hyperreninemic types of hypertension, e.g., renovascular and other severe forms, also are effective in mild hypertension through mechanisms not yet clear. A recent V. A. Multiclinic Study[31] found 12.5 to 25 mg three times daily of captopril to be very effective in mild hypertension. When considering which of these agents to use, the new drug enalapril appears to be safer than captopril, probably because it lacks the sulfhydryl group.

Low-dose methyldopa, i.e., 125 to 250 mg twice daily, is a particularly helpful drug in older patients. Such small doses appear to minimize both the pharmacologic side effects, like drowsiness, and also the rare immunologic or "allergic" reactions as well.

FIXED-COMBINATION THERAPY

Initial therapy of moderate or severe hypertension differs from mild hypertension for which monotherapy is used initially. Frequently two and occasionally three drugs ought to be given from the outset. U. S. marketing information indicates that almost 50% of all hypertensives getting drug therapy are receiving fixed-combination drugs. These usually consist of a thiazide plus some other drug. They are clearly more convenient for the patients; frequently, compliance is better; they are often cheaper than taking two drugs separately. Often physicians initiate therapy with small doses of these combination agents, and this represents good and often necessary therapy for the long term. In view of possible adverse effects from large doses of thiazides, some fixed-combinations contain too much diuretic for patients to get their optimal dose of the second drug. It is prudent today to keep the total daily dose of diuretic to 50 mg of hydrochlorothiazide or chlorthalidone (see Chapter III).

> Theoretically, the ideal treatment of hypertension consists in producing arterial dilatation because increased peripheral vascular resistance is the chief hemodynamic abnormality found.

Theoretically, the ideal treatment of hypertension consists in producing arterial dilatation because increased peripheral vascular resistance is the chief hemodynamic abnormality found. When combination therapy is to be used, the hemodynamic and other characteristics of the various drugs should be considered (Table VIII). Perusal of this table indicates that giving two drugs, both of which reduce cardiac output (e.g., methyldopa and propranolol), or employing two drugs, both of which expand blood volume (e.g., guanethadine with hydralazine), is not rational therapy, unless additional agents are given simultaneously to counteract the added effect.

SEXUAL DYSFUNCTION FROM ANTIHYPERTENSIVE AGENTS

In general, the adrenergic blocking agents are the worst offenders; whereas the direct vasodilators, the calcium channel blockers, and the converting enzyme inhibitors are the least likely to cause difficulty.

Because libido and sexual performance appear to decrease with age and since hypertension is primarily a disease of the elderly and because psychosomatic factors play such an important role, the exact effect that drugs may have in producing sexual dysfunction is not quantifiable (in spite of the enthusiasm of many urologists conducting nocturnal penile tumescence measurements). In general, the adrenergic blocking agents (like guanethedine) are the worst offenders; whereas

TABLE VIII
HEMODYNAMIC AND OTHER CHARACTERISTICS
OF ANTIHYPERTENSIVE DRUGS

Class of antihypertensive drugs	CO	TPR	BV	PRA
1. Diuretics (chronic)	←→	↓	↓	↑
2. Adrenergic inhibitors	←→↓	−↓	↑	↓
3. Beta-blockers	↓	↑	←→	↓
4. Vasodilators	↑	↓	↑	↑
5. Converting enzyme inhibitors	←→	↓	←→	↑
6. Calcium channel blockers	↑	↓	←→	↑

Note: CO = cardiac output; TPR = total peripheral vascular resistance; BV = blood volume; PRA = plasma renin activity.

the direct vasodilators (like hydralazine), the calcium channel blockers (like nifedipine) and the converting enzyme inhibitors (like captopril) are the least likely to cause difficulty. The diuretics are intermediate. In my experience, once the possibility of impotence is discussed with an elderly (or young) male patient, a problem is likely to develop if it was not already there. Unless Congress or the Food and Drug Administration require "patient package inserts" about all possible side effects of drugs, it will continue to be my policy not to suggest such a possible side effect to male hypertensives. When, however, a patient raises the question, a candid discussion is needed and a possible change in his antihypertensive agents is indicated.

THE THERAPEUTIC GOAL

In managing the patient with hypertension, a therapeutic goal should be established from the outset. Ordinarily this means reducing arterial pressure to below 140/90 mm Hg. In Clinical practice, it is often relatively easy to reduce a patient's pressure from 180-160/110--100 to 150–140/99–94 mm Hg by using monotherapy. But we should not stop there. We should not hesitate to add a low dose of a second drug—or initiate a low dose of a fixed drug combination. Simply giving larger doses of one drug usually produces more side effects and often little added efficacy, whereas giving low doses of a second drug adds few side effects but greatly enhances efficacy.

> Simply giving larger doses of one drug usually produces
> more side effects and often little added efficacy, whereas giving
> low doses of a second drug adds few side effects
> but greatly enhances efficacy.

When the patient has hypertension together with target organ involvement, e.g., left ventricular hypertrophy or retinopathy, the therapeutic goal should be not just the normalization of pressure, but the reversal of the target organ damage. Recognizing this dual obligation and attempting to accomplish both objectives have recently become major objectives for hypertensionologists. It is still a new field, however, and precise directives are not yet available. Not all antihypertensive drugs seem to be capable of reversing left ventricular hypertrophy (see page 8) even though blood pressure is normalized. Just how much we can reverse grade I or II KW retinopathy or nephrosclerosis is not clear. How long does it take? Which drugs work? Which sub-populations of hypertensives are most likely to reverse or not reverse the target organ damage is not yet known.

Finally, the day is rapidly approaching when the means and the clinical methods for managing the hypertensive patient and his atherosclerosis will be available. Just how one can best monitor clinically the reversal of atherosclerosis is not apparent. It is difficult to quantify in the clinic such things as arterial diameter by angiography. For now, all we can do is decrease the blood pressure, stop cigarette smoking, reduce high cholesterol, reduce excess body weight, and try to reverse any target organ damage present. It may also be therapeutic to encourage physical activity and raise HDL-cholesterol. But it is already clear that the therapeutic goal for clinical pharmacologists and clinicians for the next decade will be to provide the interventions that will reverse the atherosclerotic process and the clinical methods to monitor progress.

> The therapeutic goal for clinical pharmacologists and clinicians for the next decade will be to provide the interventions that will reverse the atherosclerotic process and the clinical methods to monitor progress.

THE ROLE OF RENIN

Renin is an enzyme produced chiefly in the juxtaglomerular (JG) apparatus of the kidneys. It catalyzes the conversion of an alpha-2 globulin (renin substrate) to angiotensin I (A-I), a decapeptide. A-I is then converted to angiotensin II (A-II), an octapeptide, through the action of converting enzyme (called "ACE" or angiotensin converting enzyme) found chiefly in the lungs. A-II both raises blood pressure (since it is a most potent vasoconstrictor) and stimulates aldosterone production by the adrenal glomerulosa (Figure 3).

The renin-angiotensin-aldosterone system helps regulate blood pressure, sodium-potassium balance and blood volume. Renin production and plasma renin activity (PRA) are increased by a variety of circumstances (Table VIII). The first seven of these reduce effective blood flow to the kidneys (and JG cells).

Three subpopulations of essential hypertensives exist based on plasma renin levels:

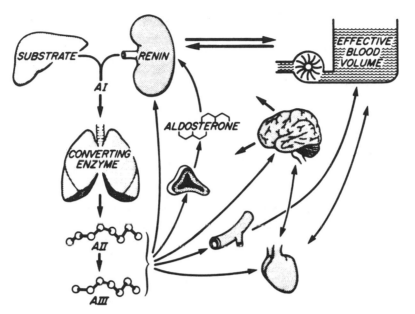

Figure 3: The Renin-Angiotension-Aldosterone System.
Reprinted by permission. (Goodfriend, T. L.: *Hypertension Essentials*. Grune and Stratton, New York, 1983, p. 19.)

Low-renin:	20–30% of total
Normal-renin:	55–70% of total
High-renin:	10–15% of total

Determination of PRA (plasma renin activity) is usually done after a renin-stimulating test such as IV furosemide. Of course patients should be off antihypertensive medications for two to three weeks and off estrogens or corticoids which can affect the results. Laragh et al[33] have constructed nomograms relating PRA to sodium excretion. A patient can therefore collect his 24-hour urine at home and have his PRA drawn in the morning. From the long list of factors (Table VIII) influencing PRA levels, a single value can be misleading unless circumstances and details of measurement are all carefully controlled.

WHO SHOULD HAVE A PRA DETERMINATION?

1. Patients who become refractory to their medications, because they may have developed renovascular disease.
2. Young patients with target organ damage and severe hypertension.

TABLE VIII
FACTORS WHICH RAISE OR LOWER RENIN PRODUCTION

High PRA*	Low PRA*
1. Erect posture for an hour or more	1. Supine position
2. Diuretic therapy	2. Low-renin essential hypertension (expanded-plasma volume)
3. Hemorrhage	3. Hyperkalemic states
4. Low sodium diet	4. After adrenergic or beta-blocking drugs
5. Dehydration	5. High salt diet or corticosteroid use
6. Vasodilator drugs	6. Increasing age
7. Congestive failure, nephrosis, cirrhosis (secondary aldosteronism)	7. Licorice digestion
8. Converting enzyme inhibitors	8. Chronic renal disease (volume-dependent)
9. Pregnancy and estrogens	9. Primary Aldosteronism
10. Renovascular or parenchymal disease	
11. Malignant hypertension	
12. Catecholamine excess (pheochromocytoma, exercise, trauma)	
13. Hypokalemia	
14. Bartter's syndrome	

---

* PRA = plasma renin activity

3. When primary aldosteronism is suspected (PRA is then low).
4. Many patients with severe hypertension.

Patients with low PRA are felt by many to have expanded plasma volume and so respond best to the antihypertensive effect of a diuretic. Black patients, for example, have a high incidence of low renin essential hypertension. They respond well not only to diuretics, but also to lower doses than white patients. On the other hand, patients with high-output hypertension, malignant hypertension, renovascular hypertension, etc. do better getting a beta- or adrenergic-blocking agent.

MALIGNANT HYPERTENSION AND HYPERTENSIVE EMERGENCIES

Malignant or accelerated hypertension is a clinical syndrome characterized by severe diastolic hypertension, usually developing insidiously over a period of a few weeks and causing retinal, cardiac and renal complications. Histopathologically, fibrinoid necrosis appears in the arterial walls. It may occur superimposed upon any other form of hypertension, but the young black male with essential hypertension is somehow predisposed. It may also appear in patients with a collagen disease, such as lupus, and also in patients with renovascular disease or with renal parenchymal disease, such as acute nephritis. Hemorrhages and exudates appear in the optic fundi reflecting fibrinoid necrosis of the retinal arterioles. Papilledema is also present. Although the incidence of malignant hypertension has usually been reported to be about 1–2% of all hypertensives, the condition is becoming less frequent. Table IX gives the major clinical characteristics of malignant hypertension and also hypertensive crises.

Treatment should begin with hospitalization, preferably in an intensive care unit where vital signs are monitored. By a brief history and physical, try to determine the cause of the emergency. Rule out convulsive disorder or acute anxiety reaction and determine the extent of target organ damage. Establish therapeutic goals, usually trying to reduce the diastolic pressure to about 100–110 mm Hg within the first two hours and normalizing it within 24 hours. Avoid medications that induce drowsiness if the patient has encephalopathy. Avoid precipitous decrements of blood pressure. Avoid vasodilators that produce reflex tachycardia in patients with angina, myocardial infarction or dissecting aortic aneurysm.

The present treatment of malignant hypertension and many hypertensive emergencies, besides utilizing rapid-acting parenteral agents (Table X) such as sodium nitroprusside and minibolus diazoxide, now includes the use of some oral drugs. When hypertension is reduced too rapidly, recent reports indicate that abnormal neurological signs may develop, renal function may deteriorate, the patient's mental status may become obtunded, focal neurological signs may develop, blindness may appear, and deaths have been reported (see Chapter XIII). Too rapid diminution of cerebral blood flow appears to be the mechanism, as reviewed by Rajagopalan and Ledingham.[34] Since malignant hypertension usually appears insidiously over several weeks, its management, though important, is not required as urgently as it is in hypertensive encephalopathy. There is time to admit the patient to the hospital, sedate him, place him on a 2 gm sodium diet, and evaluate him carefully before initiating treatment.

TABLE IX
CHARACTERISTICS OF MALIGNANT HYPERTENSION COMPARED
WITH HYPERTENSIVE ENCEPHALOPATHY

	Malignant (Accelerated)	Hypertensive Crisis (Encephalopathy)
Onset:	*Insidious—weeks	*Abrupt—hours
Blood pressure:	Diastolic: > 130 generally	Diastolic: > 140 often
Fundi:	Gr. IV KW (papilledema)	*Occasionally Gr. III or IV; always spasm and retinal sheen
Heart:	LVH; often congestive failure	LVH
Lungs:	Often pulmonary edema	Occasional pulmonary edema
Kidneys:	↑Creatinine, ↑BUN, proteinuria, hematuria, casts often present	↑Creatinine, ↑BUN may be present
CNS:	Headache, dizziness, blurred vision	*Altered consciousness, convulsions, coma, severe headache, transient ischemic attacks, blindness, neurologic deficit
GI:	Usually negative	Nausea, vomiting, abdominal pain
Treatment:	Less urgent: but admit, sedate, evaluate, then treat. Try to get diastolic < 100 mm Hg in 24–48 hours.	*Required immediately: intravenous hypotensive agent usually preferred
Prognosis:	*Untreated: 50% fatal in 6 months; 100% in 2 years	*Fatal in hours or days

* Principal distinguishing characteristics.

Oral drugs such as clonidine are being used successfully in the emergency room. Anderson et al[35] reported the results of treating 36 adult patients with hypertensive emergencies (diastolic pressure above 120 mm Hg) who were seen in his University Hospital emergency

TABLE X
**SELECTION OF PARENTERAL DRUGS TO BE GIVEN IN VARIOUS
TYPES OF HYPERTENSIVE CRISES**

Type of Hypertensive Crisis	Drug of Choice	Drugs to avoid or use cautiously
1. Acute hypertensive encephalopathy	nitroprusside diazoxide labetalol trimethaphan	rauwolfia methyldopa clonidine guanethidine propranolol
2. Intracerebral or sub-arachnoid hemorrhage	nitroprusside trimethaphan	sympatholytics labetalol
3. Acute pulmonary edema with hypertension	nitroprusside trimethaphan reserpine methyldopa furosemide	labetalol
4. Pheochromocytoma *or* 5. Monamine oxidase inhibitor with tyramines or sympathomimetics	phentolamine *or* phenoxybenzamine *or* nitroprusside, plus propranolol	sympatholytics
6. Acute glomerulo-nephritis or lupus nephritis crisis	nitroprusside diazoxide hydralazine methyldopa furosemide	trimethaphan
7. Dissecting aortic aneurysm	trimethaphan reserpine nitroprusside methyldopa furosemide	hydralazine diazoxide
8. Acute myocardial infarction or coronary insufficiency	nitroprusside	hydralazine diazoxide
9. Postoperative hypertension	nitroprusside diazoxide reserpine methyldopa	trimethaphan

room. Patients were observed for one hour to establish control pressures. Then each patient was given 0.2 mg of clonidine orally, followed by an additional 0.1 mg hourly until diastolic blood pressures were reduced below 110 or by at least 20 mm Hg. Clonidine dosage did not exceed 0.7 mg during the six hours of emergency room treatment. Patients were then hospitalized and treated with diuretics and clonidine and, when necessary, a vasodilator. Results indicated that blood pressure fell from a control value of 212 mm Hg on admission to 193 mm Hg by the first hour systolic and from 140 mm Hg initially to 105 mm Hg diastolic by the sixth hour. The average total dose used in the emergency room treatment was 0.45 mg, and only two patients of 36 treated failed to reach a 20 mm drop. Other authors have had similar good results, including Davidov,[36] who observed a 25% reduction in mean arterial pressure one hour after giving 0.3 mg clonidine, and Cohen and Katz,[37] who obtained similar reductions in 12 of 15 severely hypertensive patients.

Calcium channel blockers are also being used with success for the management of malignant hypertension and hypertensive crises in the emergency room. Dollery et al[38] recently reported successfully employing nifedipine, 30 mg orally three times a day, together with a beta-blocker and a thiazide diuretic for the management of such emergencies. The intravenous form of labetalol has also been successfully utilized in reducing severe hypertension. Some clinicians are giving oral nifedipine capsules, with the liquid squeezed out into the patient's mouth, then held sublingually, resulting in a rapid reduction in pressure.

In addition, sodium nitroprusside given by intravenous drip infusions is still popular for the emergency reduction of severe hypertension. In general, however, malignant hypertension does not require such dramatic action, although, as Table IX indicates, instances of hypertensive crises, including cases associated with convulsions or other manifestations of encephalopathy, may well require rapid reduction of blood pressure such as afforded by nitroprusside or labetalol intravenously.

The use of large bolus injections (300 mg) of diazoxide has deservedly lost popularity in the past few years in American emergency rooms. The frequent occurrence of precipitous hypotension and other serious side effects has made the use of large doses of diazoxide unpopular. On the other hand, mini-bolus injections of diazoxide (as described in Chapter XIII) are another reasonable alternative for the rapid reduction of hypertension.

MANAGEMENT OF AZOTEMIC HYPERTENSION

This is a complex therapeutic problem because most antihypertensive agents will further reduce renal plasma flow and glomerular filtration rate, and so raise the urea nitrogen and creatinine levels even higher. Exceptions are hydralazine, clonidine and methyldopa; therefore, these are suitable drugs to use in these difficult situations. Nevertheless, when one of these drugs is given together with a diuretic (high doses of furosemide are much preferred to the thiazides), the creatinine clearance is very apt to continue to deteriorate initially even as the arterial pressure gets under good control. The therapeutic goal should be to control the blood pressure (diastolic < 100 mm Hg) while maintaining urinary volume at or above 1.5 L/day (achieved with large doses of oral furosemide), during which period (1–3 months) the renal lesions may scar and significant improvement of function may return.

If hydralazine with furosemide doesn't control blood pressure, then minoxidil should be considered. Although this is a "last medical resort" drug, it is the most effective potent oral vasodilator but needs to be given with a beta-blocker and furosemide. Dialysis may otherwise be needed to reduce the increased plasma volume and lower pressure. Dialysis three times weekly controls approximately 75% of patients. If dialysis fails, drugs such as clonidine may be given in addition to dialysis. Bilateral nephrectomy is the last resort and occasionally is needed to reduce the hypertension and its complications.

MANAGEMENT OF REFRACTORY HYPERTENSION

If the usual triple-therapy (hydralazine plus hydrochlorothiazide plus a beta-blocker) fails to reduce blood pressure to $< 140/90$ mm Hg, further steps should be considered:

(1) Evaluate patient compliance to his drugs and salt restriction.
(2) Rule out secondary hypertension, e.g., renovascular disease.
(3) Substitute prazosin (or trimazosin) or a calcium channel blocker or minoxidil for hydralazine.
(4) Substitute clonidine, methyldopa, guanabenz or labetalol for the beta blocker.
(5) If creatinine is > 2.0 mg/dl, substitute furosemide for the thiazide.
(6) Consider "quadruple-therapy," by adding to the usual triple therapy either: (a) clonidine, (b) enalapril or captopril, (c) a calcium channel blocker or (d) prazosin or trimazosin or (e) guanethidine.
(7) Consider hospitalization, with the patient given a 2 gm sodium diet and bed rest together with one of the above drug regimens.

DRUG DOSES IN THE PRESENCE OF LIVER OR RENAL INSUFFICIENCY

Table XI lists how the various drug doses need to be modified in the presence of difuse-heptic disease or in patients with mild-moderate renal disease.

THERAPEUTIC PRINCIPLES

- The therapeutic objective is to prevent or reverse target organ damage by keeping blood pressure below 140/90 mm Hg for most adults.
- Teach the patient about his disease, its complications and consequences. If diastolic blood pressure is greater than 100 mm Hg, emphasize that he will likely have high blood pressure all his life.
- Teach the patient about his medications and possible side effects.
- Try to get blood pressure under stable control with tolerable side effects in 3–4 months.
- Consider home blood pressure determinations.
- Salt-restriction is important as is weight reduction in the obese.
- Geriatric patients must be treated less aggressively. Use special

TABLE XI
SHOULD THE DOSE BE CHANGED IN THE PRESENCE OF
LIVER OR KIDNEY DYSFUNCTION?

Drug	With Diffuse Liver Disease	With Mild-Moderate Renal Insufficiency
Thiazides	N.C.	↓
Furosemide	N.C.	N.C.
Spironolactone	↓?	↓
Triamterene	↓?	↓
Amiloride	N.C.	↓
Diazoxide	N.C.	↓
Nitroprusside	↓	↓
Clonidine	N.C.	N.C.
Guanethidine	↓?	↓
Hydralazine	↓?	N.C.
Methyldopa	↓	N.C.
Prazosin	↓?	N.C.
Trimazosin	?	N.C.
Rauwolfia	N.C.	↓
Guanabenz	↓	N.C.
Guanadrel	↓	↓
Propranolol	↓	N.C.
Timolol	↓	N.C.
Atenolol	N.C.	↓
Pimdolol	↓	↓?
Nadolol	N.C.	↓
Metoprolol	↓	↓
Betaxolol	N.C.	N.C.
Labetalol	↓	N.C.
Captopril	↓?	↓
Enalapril	↓	↓?
Verapamil	↓	↓?
Nifedipine	↓	?
Diltiazem	↓	↓?

↓ = Decreased
↓? = Probably decreased
N.C. = Not Changed

care to avoid orthostatic or depression-inducing drugs. Smaller doses of thiazides and other drugs are usually adequate.

• Use the lowest effective doses of antihypertensive agent needed, e.g., hydrochlorothiazide and chlorthalidone 12.5, 25 or 50 mg/day; methyldopa 125–250 mg twice daily; clonidine 0.1 mg plus chlorthalidone (15 mg) once daily at bedtime; atenolol 25–50 mg once daily, etc.

- Identify and try to minimize other risk factors, e.g., stop cigarette smoking, reduce cholesterol levels, etc.
- Drug therapy of stable mild-moderate hypertensives may be reduced, perhaps annually, for a few weeks to determine responsiveness at lower doses. An occasional patient may require no drugs for many months; however, all such patients need to be followed regularly.
- Advise the patient from the outset that initially you will likely be changing drugs and doses several times to find the best long-term therapy for him to take.
- With mild hypertensives, try to get the blood pressure to normal levels with non-drug interventions. If, however, diastolic blood pressure is greater than 95 mm Hg after three to six months, drugs should ordinarily be added, particularly if other risk factors are present.
- Identify those patient characteristics which, *for initial monotherapy*, suggest that the patient will probably do better receiving a diuretic drug, or a beta-blocker, or clonidine, or a converting enzyme inhibitor, or a calcium channel blocker.
- Be alert for drug interactions, such as:
    - (a) Methyldopa, clonidine or rauwolfia with alcohol or other CNS depressants.
    - (b) Tricyclic antidepressants with many peripheral adrenergic-blocking agents.
    - (c) Hypokalemia in patients receiving digitalis and diuretics.
- Measure blood pressure in the erect as well as reclining or seated positions, particularly when giving adrenergic-blocking agents.
- After regulation is achieved, see "mild-moderate" patients three or four times a year. See "severe" patients no less often than monthly until regulated.
- Always write out your dosage instructions for the patient. Try to use the simplest regimen possible. Clonidine, enalapril, atenolol, nadolol, propranolol-LA and metoprolol, as well as chlorthalidone and hydrochlorothiazide, can each be given once a day.

REFERENCES:

1. Kannel, W. B., Dawber, J. R., and McGee, D. L.: Perspectives on Systolic Hypertension: The Framington Study. *Circulation*, **61**:1179–1182, 1980.
2. Messerli, F. H., Ventura, H. O., et al: Essential hypertension in the elderly: Haemodynamics, intravascular volume, plasma renin activity, and circulating catecholamine levels. *Lancet*, **II**:983–985, 1983.
3. Medical Directors of Insurance Company's Report, 1975.
4. Stamler, J., Stamler, R, Riedlinger, W. F., Algera, G., and Roberts, R. H.: Hypertension screening of 1 million Americans. Community Hypertension Evaluation Clinic (CHEC) Program, 1973–1975. *JAMA*, **235**(21):2299–2306, 1976.
5. *U. S.Health Survey*, DHEW Publication No. (HRA)-77-1310, Vital Health Studies.
6. Mortality experience according to blood pressure after treatment. *Blood Pressure Study 1979*, Society of Actuaries and Association of Life Insurance Medical Directors of America, Chicago.
7. Cressman, M. D., and Gifford, R. W.: Hypertension and stroke. *J. Am. Coll. Cardiol.*, 1(2):521–527, 1983.
8. Kannel, W. B., Wolf, P. A., Verter, J., et al: Epidemiologic assessment of the role of blood pressure in stroke: The Framingham Study. *JAMA*, **214**:301–310, 1970.
9. Kannel, W. B., and Sorlie, P.: Hypertension in Framingham. In O. Paul (Ed.): *Epidemiology Control of Hypertension*, Stratton, New York, 1975, pp. 553–592.
10. Roberts, W. C.: Cardiovascular consequences of systemic hypertension: A morphologic survey. In P. Sleight and E. D. Freis (Eds.): *Hypertension*, Butterworths International Medical Reviews, Butterworth Scientific, London, 1983, pp. 78–91.
11. Freis, E. D.: Should mild hypertension be treated? *N. Engl. J. Med.*, **307**:306– 309, 1982.
12. Gifford, R. W.: Mild hypertension: Should it be treated? *Postgrad. Med.*, **7** (5): 19–24, 1982.
13. Hypertension Detection and Follow-up Program Cooperative Group: Five year findings of the Hypertension Detection and Follow-up Program. I. Reduction in mortality of persons with high blood pressure, including mild hypertension. *JAMA*, **242**:2562–2571, 1979.
14. Management Committee of the Australian Hypertension Trial: The Australian Therapeutic Trial in Mild Hypertension. *Lancet*, 1:1261–1267, 1980.
15. Smith, W. M.: Treatment of mild hypertension: Results of a ten-year intervention trial. *Clin. Res.*, 40(Suppl 1):98–105, 1977.
16. McGee, D., and Gordon, T.: Results of the Framingham Study applied to four other U. S.-based epidemiologic studies of cardiovascular diseases. *The Framingham Study: An Epidemiological Investigation of Cardiovascular Disease* (sec 31). Publication No. (NIH) 76-1083. Washington, DC, 1976, U. S. Department of Health, Education, and Welfare.
17. Madhavan, S., and Alderman, M. H.: The potential effect of blood pressure reduction on cardiovascular disease. *Arch. Int. Med.*, **141**:1583–1588, 1981.
18. Culpepper, W. S., Sodt, P. C., Messerli, F. H., Rusckhaupt, D. G., and Arcilla, R. A.: Cardiac status in juvenile borderline hypertension. *Ann. Intern. Med.*, **98**: 1–7, 1983.
19. Devereux, R. B., Savage, D. D., Droyer, J., and Laragh, J.: Left ventricular hyper-

trophy and function in high, normal and low-renin forms of essential hypertension. *Hypertension*, 4:524–531, 1982.

20. Kannel, W. B.: Prevalence and noted history of electrocardiographic left ventricular hypertrophy. Preceedings of a Symposium: Left Ventricular Hypertrophy in Essential Hypertension. *Am. J. Med.*, 75(3A):4–11, 1983.
21. Wollam, G. L., Hall, W. D., et al: Time course of regression of left ventricular hypertrophy in treated hypertensive patients. Proceedings of a Symposium: Left Ventricular Hypertrophy in Essential Hypertension. Mechanisms and Therapy. *Am. J. Med.*, pp. 100–110, September 26, 1983.
22. McMahon, F. G.: Some new aspects of modern Catapres® therapy in the United States. In Block, K. D. (Ed.): *Catapresan®*, Aulendorf: Editio Cantor, 1983.
23. Drayer, J., Weber, M. A., Gardin, J. M., and Lipson, J. L.: Effect of long-term antihypertensive therapy on cardiac anatomy in patients with essential hypertension. Proceedings of a Symposium: Left Ventricular Hypertrophy in Essential Hypertension. Mechanisms and Therapy. *Am. J. Med.*, pp. 116–120, September 26, 1983.
24. Ibrahim, M. M., Madkour, M. A., and Mossallam, R.: Factors influencing cardiac hypertrophy in hypertensive patients. *Clin. Sci.*, 61:105s–108s, 1981.
25. Hill, L. S., Monaghan, M., Richardson, R. J.: Regression of left ventricular hypertrophy during treatment with antihypertensive agents. *Br. J. Clin. Pharmacol.*, 7(Suppl 2):255–260, 1979.
26. Fouad, F. M., Tarazi, R. C., and Bravo, E. L.: Symposium on the renin-angiotensin-aldosterone system: Treatment of hypertension and heart failure; cardiac and hemodynamic effects of enalapril. *Hypertension*, 1(Suppl. 1):135–141, 1983.
27. Nissinen, A., Tuomilehto, J., et al: North Karelia (Finland) Hypertension Detection Project: Five-year follow-up of hypertensive cohort. *Hypertension*, 5(4): 564–572, 1983.
28. Helgeland, A.: Treatment of mild hypertension: A five-year controlled drug trial. The Oslo Study. *Am. J. Med.*, 69:725–732, 1980.
29. Levinson, P. D., Khatri, I. M., and Freis, E. D.: Persistence of normal BP after withdrawal of drug treatment in mild hypertension. *Arch. Intern. Med.*, 142: 2265–2268, 1982.
30. Norwegian Multicenter Study Group: Timolol induced reduction in mortality and reinfarction in patients surviving acute myocardial infarction. *N. Engl. J. Med.*, 304:801–807, 1981.
31. Veteran's Administration Multiclinic Study Group for Antihypertensive Agents. *Hypertension*, 5(5):1, 1983.
32. Goodfriend, T. L.: *Hypertension Essentials*. Grune and Stratton, New York, 1983, p. 19.
33. Laragh, J. H., Sealey, J. E., and Atlas, S. A.: The renin system for understanding human hypertension: Evidence for blood pressure control by a bipolar vasoconstriction—volume mechanism. Prorenin as a determinant of renin secretion. *Clin. Exp. Hypertens.*, 4(11-12):2303–2337, 1982.
34. Rajagopalan, B., and Ledingham, J. G. G.: Management of the hypertensive crisis. In P. Sleight and E. D. Freis (Eds.): *Hypertension*. Butterworths International Medical Reviews, Butterworth Scientific, London, 1983, pp. 271–292.

35. Anderson, R. J., Hart, G. R., Crumpler, C. P., Reed, W. G., and Mathews, C. A.: Oral clonidine loading in hypertensive urgencies. *JAMA*, **246**(8):848–850, 1981.
36. Davidov, M., Kakaviatos, H., and Finnerty, F. A.: The antihypertensive effect of an imidazoline compound. *Clin. Pharmacol. Ther.*, 8:810–816, 1967.
37. Cohen, I. M., and Katz, M. A.: Oral clonidine loading for rapid control of hypertension. *Clin. Pharmacol. Ther.*, **24**(1):11–15, 1978.
38. Murphy, M., Scriven, E., and Dollery, C.: Role of nifedipine in treatment of hypertension. *Br. Med. J.*, **287**(6387):257–259, 1983.

THE NON-DRUG TREATMENT OF HYPERTENSION

THE ROLE OF
- A. SODIUM RESTRICTION
- B. WEIGHT REDUCTION
- C. PHYSICAL TRAINING AND EXERCISE
- D. POTASSIUM SUPPLEMENTS
- E. DIETARY FAT AND VEGETARIAN DIETS
- F. RELAXATION, MEDITATION, AND BIOFEEDBACK
- G. CALCIUM SUPPLEMENTATION

THE EFFECT OF
- H. ALCOHOL
- I. COFFEE
- J. CIGARETTES

INTRODUCTION:

Can mild hypertension, i.e., diastolic 90–99 mm Hg, be adequately treated by means other than life-long drug therapy?

Concern has been expressed about the side effects, the cost, and possible subtle adverse reactions to drugs being given over several decades to patients who are otherwise in good health. For example, many beta-adrenergic blocking agents raise serum triglycerides and reduce high-density lipoproteins, both of which have been shown epidemiologically to be correlated with an increased risk of coronary heart disease. Impaired glucose tolerance, hyperuricemia, lipid disturbances, and hypokalemia have all been associated with the long-term administration of thiazide diuretics. Can mild hypertension, i.e., diastolic 90–99 mm Hg, be adequately treated by means other than life-long drug therapy? How helpful is non-drug therapy in the management of patients with diastolic pressures greater than 100 mm Hg? Which of the non-drug modalities has been demonstrated clearly to reduce blood pressure over the long haul? How does non-drug therapy compare with drug therapy insofar as efficacy and side effects are concerned? Is it even worth the effort needed to attempt to change the eating habits and the lifestyles of most patients with mild hypertension?

In Chapter I (Table VI) we summarize those non-drug modalities which we regard as "proven effective" (sodium restriction and weight reduction). We categorized physical activity as "probably effective" and all the others as "possibly effective." Our conclusions were derived from the information which follows.

THE ROLE OF SODIUM RESTRICTION

It has been well established since the 1940s that sodium restriction can lower blood pressure in most hypertensive patients.[1-3] Kempner showed that even severe hypertension could be reduced with a diet of rice and fruit.[1] This diet required extreme restriction of sodium and was very difficult to adhere to over long periods. With the advent of thiazide diuretics in the 1950s, many physicians permitted these drugs to replace sodium restriction in the treatment of patients with hypertension. Today the pendulum is swinging back with physicians and patients once again recognizing the importance of at least moderate sodium restriction for virtually all hypertensive patients.

Numerous studies have been published implicating salt as a factor in the pathogenesis of essential hypertension. Simply stated, the thesis is that the amount of sodium ingested is directly proportional to extracellular fluid volume and to systemic blood pressure in individuals with a hereditary renal inability to handle salt loads. Epidemiologic studies have shown that in unaccultured populations with low levels of salt ingestion, hypertension is rare (Table I). As urbanization and other adaptations to modern life occur, the amount of salt ingested increases

TABLE I
AS SALT INTAKE (OR EXCRETION) INCREASES,
THE PREVALENCE OF HYPERTENSION INCREASES
(ADULT SUBJECTS)

Population	Sodium Chloride Intake (mEq/day)	Sodium Chloride Excretion (mEq/day)	Hypertension Prevalence (%)
Yanomamo Indians[4]	—	1.0	None
Carajos Amazonians[5]	Very Low	—	None
Pukapukans[6]	60	—	3
New Guinea Highlands[7,8]	—	15	3
American Eskimos[9]	80	—	4
United States Whites[10]	100–300	50–200	15–20
Raratongans[6]	125	—	28
United States Blacks[10,11]	100–300	50–200	25–35
Northeast Japan[12]	435	—	30–40

and hypertension becomes more prevalent. The implication of salt in the pathogenesis of essential hypertension has led experts to urge individuals with a family history of essential hypertension to accustom themselves and their children to diets restricted in salt.

In this discussion, it is important to remember these values:

$$1 \text{ gram NaCl (salt)} = 17.1 \text{ mEq Na}^+$$
$$1 \text{ gram Na}^+ \text{ (sodium)} = 43.5 \text{ mEq Na}^+$$
$$1 \text{ level teaspoon salt} = 2{,}300 \text{ mg Na}^+ = 100 \text{ mEq Na}^+$$

The average American consumes approximately 10–20 grams of salt (NaCl) each day on a typical diet.[13] This is equal to 170–350 mEq Na$^+$ per day. One-third of this amount is added from a salt-shaker while cooking or at the table, and two-thirds comes from the natural sodium content of foods or processing.

The pendulum has swung too far in favor of drug therapy, leading many physicians to abandon sodium restriction. In general, salt restriction is beneficial to all patients with essential hypertension. Rarely, a hypertensive patient with impaired renal function, particularly medullary disease associated with papillary necrosis, pyelonephritis, or cystic disease of the medulla, will tend to lose salt and require sodium replacement. But, for the vast majority of patients with essential hypertension, salt intake needs to be reduced.

> Data suggest that a moderate dietary reduction
> from 10 to 5 grams of salt per day should drop
> blood pressure approximately 10/5 mm Hg.

TABLE II
DIETARY SODIUM RESTRICTION LOWERS BLOOD PRESSURE

| Reference | No. of Patients | Baseline | | Sodium Restriction | | Duration of Diet |
		Urinary Sodium (mEq/24 hr)	Blood Pressure (mm Hg)	Urinary Sodium (mEq/24 hr)	Blood Pressure (mm Hg)	
Parijs et al[14] 1973	17	191	147/98	93	138/92	4 wks.
Morgan et al[15] 1978	31	195	160/97	157	156/93	24 mos.
MacGregor et al[16] 1982	19	162	154/97	86	144/92	4 wks.
Watt et al[17] 1983	18	143	137/83	87	136/82	4 wks.
Morgan et al[18] 1981	24	172	?/96	68	?/88	8 wks.
	24	148	?/113	75	?/102	8 wks.
Parfrey et al[19] 1981	41	293	160/101	19	146/96	5 days
	36	244	189/120	22	165/109	5 days

Recent reports have shown that moderate dietary sodium restriction can lower blood pressure in essential hypertension (Table II). Parijs[14] did an early controlled study of moderate salt restriction. He found a significant drop in blood pressure among 17 hypertensive patients placed on a moderate salt restriction diet. The decrement was greater when these patients were given a regular diet with diuretics. This decrement, in turn, was less than the fall in blood pressure obtained when he used both a moderate salt diet and diuretics. His data suggest that a moderate dietary reduction from 10 to 5 grams of salt per day should drop blood pressure approximately 10/5 mm Hg. Morgan,[15] in 1978, reported results of treating mildly hypertensive men with a 20% sodium-restricted diet for two years. Blood pressure dropped an average of 4/4 mm Hg. MacGregor,[16] in a double-blind randomized crossover study in 1982, showed that mild hypertensives dropped their blood pressure by 10/5 mm Hg on a moderately sodium-restricted diet alone. Watt,[17] in 1983, using the same study design as MacGregor, found no significant reduction in blood pressure between his regular diet and restricted sodium intake groups. His patients, however, were normotensive on drug therapy prior to adding salt restriction.

Morgan[18] treated 24 patients whose diastolic pressures averaged 96 mm Hg with moderate sodium restriction. After two months, the diastolic pressures had fallen to 88 mm Hg. He then treated another group of 24 patients with a similar diet, and their diastolic pressure dropped from 113 to 102 mm Hg. Parfrey[19] also treated mild and severe hypertension (DBP 90–109 mm Hg and DBP 110–130 mm Hg) with sodium restriction. However, he used patients with very high sodium intake and placed them on very low sodium intakes. Blood pressures dropped significantly even though the diet lasted only five days.

Beard[20] reported results of a randomized controlled trial of 90 patients on a sodium-restricted diet who were also receiving medication for mild hypertension. He showed (Table III) that the doses used to maintain the same level of control of blood pressure could be reduced by fifty percent when sodium restriction was added. Thirty-one percent were able to stop taking medication altogether. The sodium intake used in this study was rather severe, i.e., 37 mEq Na/day and required such items as unsalted breads and baking powder (now available).

The results of these studies show that many hypertensive patients can be treated successfully with a sodium-restricted diet alone. These results suggest that, at least for mild hypertensives in whom other risk

TABLE III

LOW SODIUM DIET CAN REDUCE REQUIREMENTS FOR ANTIHYPERTENSIVE MEDICATION*

	No. of Patients	Baseline			Final			Number of Patients		
		Blood Pressure (mm Hg)	Urinary Sodium (mEq/24 hr.)	No. Of Tabs/ (day)	Blood Pressure (mm Hg)	Urinary Sodium (mEq/24 hr.)	No. Of Tabs/ (day)	Able To Stop BP Meds	Able To Reduce Dosage	On Same Dosage
Low Na+ Diet	45	142/88	150	3.6	131/82	37	1.7	14 (31%)	23 (51%)	8 (18%)
Regular Diet	45	139/86	174	3.2	133/83	161	3.1	4 (9%)	11 (24%)	30 (67%)

* From Beard et al[20] 1982; 90 hypertensives on medication with DBP 95–109 mm Hg. reprinted with permission.

factors* are not present, a moderately low salt diet should be tried before committing a patient to life-long drug therapy. It is my persuasion, however, and also the recent recommendation of the World Health Organization,[21] that if diastolic pressure isn't below 90 mm Hg after three months of such a non-drug regimen, then drug therapy ought to be initiated.

Besides helping to lower blood pressure and reduce the amount of medication needed to control blood pressure, sodium restriction also helps prevent hypokalemia and metabolic alkalosis. When large quantities of sodium are ingested, more is available in the distal renal tubule for potassium exchange under the influence of aldosterone (Figure 1). With sodium restriction, potassium supplements or potassium-retaining drugs are less likely to be needed because hypokalemia is less likely to occur.

Certainly the biggest problem with sodium restriction is patient compliance. Many physicians simply do not take the time to instruct and encourage their patients to adhere to a moderately restricted sodium diet. Kaplan recently reported[22] two techniques to help detect patient compliance. He showed that a nine-hour overnight urine collection for sodium closely correlated with a 24-hour specimen for sodium measurement. Then he showed that chloride titrator strips were quite accurate for the rapid estimation of urine sodium levels. So now it is

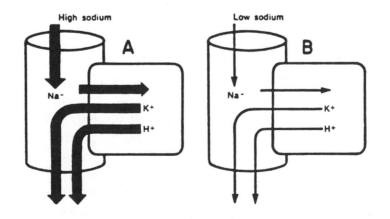

Figure 1: Individuals who ingest large amounts of salt have more sodium available for renal tubular exchange with potassium (in the presence of aldosterone), and they therefore excrete large amounts of potassium and tend to become hypokalemic.

* cigarette smoking, abnormal lipid levels, obesity, diabetes mellitus, etc.

much easier for physicians to monitor patients for compliance with dietary sodium restriction. Of course, since all patients with hypertension will not satisfactorily respond to moderate sodium restriction, it is the physician's responsibility to add a diuretic or appropriate medication if adequate pressure control is not achieved after reasonable instruction, encouragement, and checks for compliance to diet are tried.

Moderate Salt-Restricted Diet
(80–100 mEq/day sodium)

- Add no salt at table or in cooking.

- Avoid salty foods altogether (pretzels, popcorn, potato chips, peanuts, processed cheeses, and pickled foods).

- Avoid milk and milk products.

- Read labels on medications such as antacids and packaged foods such as cereals and soups so as to avoid those with high sodium contents.

- Consider using salt substitutes.

The customary approach to moderate sodium restriction begins with no salt allowed at the table or in cooking. Many patients satisfactorily use salt substitutes to flavor their food. Generally, the moderate use of salt substitutes is to be encouraged. However, since many of these products contain greater than 90% potassium chloride, their indiscriminate widespread use should be avoided. This is particularly true for hypertensives with significant renal failure and also those being treated with potassium-sparing diuretics, both of whom are at risk of hyperkalemia. The next step is to avoid all obviously salted foods— pretzels, popcorn, potato chips, peanuts and all pickled foods. These steps should be considered moderate sodium restriction (80–100 mEq Na^+/day). Specific examples of the sodium content of processed and natural foods are shown in Table IV. Several of the antacids available over the counter are particularly high in sodium content and should be avoided. To live successfully on a severely sodium-restricted diet, it is necessary for foods and drinks to be properly labeled for sodium content. The Food and Drug Administration and The American Medical Association are currently urging food and drink processors to do so.

TABLE IV
SODIUM CONTENT OF CERTAIN FOODS[23]

Food	Quantity	Sodium Content (mgs)	(mEq)
Whole milk	1 cup	120	5.3
Cheese			
— Processed	1 ounce	406	17.6
— Cottage, 2% fat	1 cup	918	40.0
Bread			
— White enriched	1 slice	117	5.3
— Buns, hot dog, enriched	1 bun	202	8.8
Corn flakes	1 cup	251	11.0
Apple pie, 9"	1/6	482	21.2
Seafood			
— Crabmeat, packed, drained	1 ounce	200	8.8
— Lobster	1 pound	1359	61.6
— Shrimp, fresh	1 pound	635	27.9
— Tuna, packed in water	1 cup	1733	76.3
Olive	1 medium	156	6.9
Meat			
— Corned beef	3 ounces	937	41.2
— Chipped beef	3 ounces	3660	161.0
— Bacon	2 ounces	386	17.0
— Bacon, Canadian	2 ounces	1072	47.2
— Ham, cured	2 ounces	427	18.8
— Bologna	2 ounces	737	32.4
Nuts, mixed, salted	1 cup	280	12.3
Butter	1 tablespoon	140	6.2
Barbecue sauce	1 tablespoon	127	5.7
Catsup, tomato	1 tablespoon	156	6.9
Mustard	1 tablespoon	195	8.8
Soup			
— Pork and beans	1 cup	1008	44.0
— Beef noodle	1 cup	1872	82.4
— Chicken noodle	1 cup	979	43.1
Dill pickle	1 large	1428	62.8

THE ROLE OF WEIGHT REDUCTION

There is still not a proven cause–effect relationship between obesity and hypertension. However, it is quite clear that being overweight is associated with a higher prevalence and a higher incidence of hypertension. The American Society of Actuaries reported that obesity was the single condition most often associated with hypertension.[24] The Evans County, Georgia study[25] showed that residents who gained 10 or more pounds over a six-year period developed hypertension (DBP > 95 mm Hg) twice as often as those who did not gain weight. If a resident were obese at the start of the study and gained no weight, he had a five times greater incidence of hypertension. If an obese resident at the start gained weight over the study period, his relative risk was eight times greater. The relative risk of developing hypertension with obesity or weight gain was much greater in whites than blacks. In the Framingham Study,[26] it was shown that men who lost 15% of their body weight dropped their systolic blood pressure by 10%. Similar men who gained 15% more weight raised their systolic pressure by 18%.

On the average, with each kilogram (2.2 lbs) weight loss, patients experienced a 2.5/1.5 mm Hg drop in blood pressure.

Ramsay et al[27] concluded from their study of obese hypertensive patients in Scotland, that, on the average, with each kilogram (2.2 lbs) weight loss, patients experienced a 2.5/1.5 mm Hg drop in blood pressure.[27]

Langford[28] reported results of withdrawing antihypertensive medications from obese (at least 20% over ideal weight) and non-obese patients. After 32 weeks, the hypertensive obese patients had both a greater incidence (i.e., relapse rate) and a more severe degree of hypertension than the non-obese patients.

It was first shown by Preble[29] in 1923 that weight reduction in obese hypertensives could lower blood pressure. It was also reported that weight reduction resulted in a greater fall in systolic pressure than diastolic and was associated with slowing of the pulse rate and increasing exercise tolerance.[30] However, Dahl[9] attributed the fall in blood pressure with weight loss to a decreased salt intake. More recent data have shown that weight reduction per se can lower blood pressure independent of salt intake in obese patients (Table V).

Reisen[31] in 1978, conducted a controlled study of weight loss in 107 obese patients with essential hypertension while salt intake remained unrestricted. His patients were at least 10% over ideal body weight and

TABLE V
WEIGHT REDUCTION IN OBESE PATIENTS LOWERS BLOOD PRESSURE

Patient Group	No. Of Patients	Weight (kg)	% Over Ideal Weight	Duration Diet (wks)	Weight Loss (kg)	Initial Blood Pressure (mm Hg)	Blood Pressure Fall (mm Hg)
Reisen[31] 1978 (obese hypertensives)							
Diet-alone group	24	86	30	8	8.8	157/106	26/20
On inadequate medication plus diet	57	85	30	8	9.8	172/113	37/23
Tuck[32] 1981 (morbid obesity)							
Moderate sodium plus low calorie diet	15	101	63	12	20.2	100*	16*
Low sodium plus low calorie diet	10	108	74	12	20.2	105*	19*
Reisen[33] 1983 (obese hypertensives)							
Obese, HBP	12	96	20	24	10	159/90	10/9

Key:
HBP = hypertensive
* = mean arterial pressure

had blood pressures > 140/90 mm Hg. He studied three groups: a non-drug-treated group on caloric restriction and a group receiving suboptimal doses of antihypertensive medications, some of whom were given a weight reduction diet, and some of whom acted as controls (the third group). After eight weeks, the "diet-only" group had a blood pressure fall of 26/20 mm Hg and had lost 8.8 kg. The drug-phase diet group had a fall of 37/23 mm Hg after losing 9.8 kg. Interestingly, only about half of each group came to within 10% of their ideal weight, while still showing remarkable falls in blood pressure. Both diet groups had unrestricted salt intakes, and their 24-hour urinary sodiums were actually higher than controls. Three-fourths of the "diet-alone" group were rendered normotensive and required no further treatment. Three-fifths of the inadequately-treated group were now normotensive (i.e., now adequately treated by medication).

Tuck[32] reported treating 25 morbidly obese patients (greater than 25% over ideal weight) with weight reduction diets for three months. He divided them into a low sodium group (40 mEq/day) and a moderate sodium group (120 mEq/day). Half the subjects had blood pressures of 140/95 mm Hg. After a weight loss of 20 kg in each group, mean blood pressure in both the low and moderate sodium intake groups fell by 19 and 16 mm Hg, respectively. Only six of the 25 patients obtained ideal weight. However, since blood pressure was significantly reduced in all subjects, a 10–30% weight reduction appears to be sufficient to lower blood pressure significantly.

Reisen[33] studied obese hypertensive patients for 24 weeks on low calorie, unrestricted salt diets. They lost an average 10 kg and had an average fall in blood pressure of 10/9 mm Hg. He theorized that the fall in blood pressure was due to a decreased total and central (cardiopulmonary) blood volume resulting in a lower venous return and cardiac output, possibly mediated by decreased catecholamine levels.

Gillum[34] studied the independent effect of both sodium-restricted and calorie-restricted diets in overweight, "borderline" hypertensives. He defined borderline hypertension as systolic blood pressure 140–159 mm Hg and diastolic blood pressure 85–94 mm Hg. Both his groups were between 10–50% overweight and all were white males. His first group dropped their blood pressures 5.4/2.4 mm Hg after losing a modest 5.2 kg (Table VI). No significant change in blood pressure occurred when the group was placed on a moderate sodium (70 mEq/day) diet afterwards. His second group was given the moderately

TABLE VI
WEIGHT REDUCTION AND SODIUM RESTRICTION INDEPENDENTLY LOWER BLOOD PRESSURE*

No. Of Patients	Baseline			Overall		Blood Pressure Fall		
	Weight (kg)	Urinary Sodium (mEq/24 hr)	Blood Pressure (mm Hg)	Weight Loss (kg)	Urinary Sodium (mEq/24 hr)	From Weight Reduction (mm Hg)	From Sodium Reduction (mm Hg)	Total (mm Hg)
10 Weeks' Weight Reduction Followed by 10 Weeks' Sodium Restriction								
28	89	167	136/83	6.2	36	5.4/2.4	0.2/0.8	5.2/1.6
10 Weeks' Sodium Restriction Followed by 10 Weeks' Weight Reduction								
59	91	175	135/84	5.8	81	5 8/4.9	3.4/1.8	9.3/6.7

* Gillum,[34] 1983 (overweight borderline hypertension), reprinted with permission. (Gillum, R. F., Prineas, R. J., et al: Nonpharmacologic therapy of hypertension: The independent effects of weight reduction and sodium restriction in overweight borderline hypertension patients. *American Heart Journal*, 105(1):130, 1983.)

sodium-restricted diet first and their blood pressures fell 5.8/4.9 mm Hg. When they then lost 4 kg weight, their blood pressure fell an additional 3.4/1.8 mm Hg, for a total drop of 9.3/6.7 mm Hg. Gillum concludes that the two approaches should be combined as the first step in the management of obese patients having, or at high risk for, essential hypertension.

A total dietary approach in treating mild hypertension can yield excellent results although long-term effects on mortality and morbidity have not yet been done. Hunt advocates a treatment plan he calls "nutritional therapy." The mainstay of his nutritional therapy is, of course, sodium restriction (20–90 mEq sodium/day). To this, he adds dietary control of total calories, cholesterol, and saturated fats, as necessary, for the basis of treatment for essential hypertension. Hunt[35] studied 3,500 patients who had had previous management of their hypertension with at least two concurrent antihypertensive medications with poor results (most still had DBP > 100 mm Hg). Their average 24-hour urine specimen, before starting his nutritional therapy, contained 234 mEq sodium. After discontinuing their medications and three months of his nutritional therapy, almost two-thirds of those patients able to restrict their sodium to less than 75 mEq/day were made normotensive (DBP 90 mm Hg) on no medication (Table VII). The long-term follow-up of those patients whose blood pressure was controlled with nutritional therapy alone is given in Table VIII.

The mainstay of non-pharmacologic treatment of hypertension and indeed the foundation of treatment for virtually all hypertensive patients are sodium restriction and weight control. Many obese patients

TABLE VII
EFFECTS OF NUTRITIONAL THERAPY ALONE FOR THREE MONTHS*

Urinary Sodium (mEq/24 hr)	Percentage of Patients Responding With DBP < 90 mm Hg, By Pretreatment DBP (mm Hg)		
	90–104	105–114	115
75	85	63	51
75–149	38	14	3
150	13	3	0

* Hunt and Margie,[35] reproduced with permission of HLS Press.

TABLE VIII
LONG-TERM EFFECTS OF NUTRITIONAL THERAPY ALONE*

Feature	Baseline	Years of Therapy			
		0.5	1	2	4
Patients (no.)	3500	1451	1310	1140	957
Diastolic BP (mm Hg)	113	96	92	94	88
Urinary Sodium (mEq/24 hr)	234	70	67	74	63
Weight Loss (Kg)	—	6.4	9.5	9.1	10.4

* Hunt and Margie,[35] reproduced with permission of HLS Press.

have difficulty in losing weight and maintaining that loss. The data from Gillum and Hunt are particularly valuable in showing that modest weight loss, together with moderate salt restriction, can substantially drop blood pressure.

THE ROLE OF PHYSICAL TRAINING AND EXERCISE

Physical exercise such as jogging, bicycling and swimming raises the heart rate, stroke volume, cardiac output, and systolic blood pressure. Diastolic pressure tends to decrease slightly in normotensives and is elevated in hypertensives. Peripheral vascular resistance, which is always elevated in patients with sustained essential hypertension, is further elevated by acute physical exercise, with stroke volume and cardiac output being little affected (as shown by Lowenthal et al[36]). However, the possible benefits of chronic physical conditioning programs have been conflicting.

DOES PHYSICAL TRAINING HELP LOWER BLOOD PRESSURE?

Vigorous physical activity has been associated with a lower incidence and prevalence of coronary artery disease[37-39] and the risk factors for this disease.[40,41] Hypertension is a major risk factor for coronary atherosclerotic disease, and physical training has been advocated as a measure to lower blood pressure. Epidemiologic studies have correlated higher levels of physical fitness with lower systolic and diastolic blood pressures.[41-43] Table IX displays the conflicting evidence about the effects of physical training on blood pressure among hypertensive patients.

Boyer[44] showed a drop in blood pressure of 13/12 mm Hg in middle-age hypertensive patients over six months with training only two days a week with minimal weight loss. Bonanno[45] found a 13/14 mm Hg fall among hypertensives on similar walk–jog type of exercise three days a week after three months. Fifteen hypertensive control patients not on exercise programs had a decline of 3/11 mm Hg in this same study. Choquette[46] studied a group of sedentary men with "borderline" hypertension (systolic 140–159 mm Hg and/or diastolic 90–95 mm Hg). Through group exercise two hours each week and 10–15 minutes of calisthenics at home each day, he found a 14/18 mm Hg fall in blood pressure. Krotkiewski[47] studied 27 obese women; six were hypertensive. Without a change in weight, six months of physical training dropped their blood pressure by 9/7 mm Hg.

Roman[48] conducted a long-term study of exercise on hypertensive females. Three months of training three days a week at a moderate intensity (70% maximum heart rate) lowered blood pressure by 21/16 mm Hg. The next three months, his patients practiced no training, and blood pressure rose to pre-study levels. Twelve months of moderate intensity training again substantially lowered blood pressure (20/18 mm Hg). An additional 12 months of more intense training (75–85% maximum heart rate) was not associated with additional blood pressure lowering. While the results of this study are impressive, the study is flawed in that changes in weight and sodium restriction were not reported. All these studies have some problems (Table IX), and all lack long-term follow-up after the experimental training period ends.

One factor limiting the usefulness of physical training in lowering blood pressure is long-term patient compliance. Ilmarinen[54] studied 166 males with multiple risk factors for coronary heart disease. On a three-year follow-up after completion of a training program, about half had decreased their exercise time and 40% had gained weight. He concludes training intervention does not alter patient lifestyle or physical activity habits over long periods. Sedgwick[55] studied 370 sedentary men for five years after a physical training course. Only one-third of the men remained on regular moderate-to-heavy exercise. Overall weight and blood pressure did not change. Pyorola[49] similarly studied 82 patients

TABLE IX

PHYSICAL TRAINING MAY LOWER RESTING BLOOD PRESSURE

Reference	No. of Patients	Duration of Training (months)	Weight Loss (kg)	Type of Training	Blood Pressure (mm Hg)			Problems
					Pre-training	Post-training	Decrease*	
Boyer,[44]	23	6	1.1	30 min. walk-jog, 2 days/week	159/105	146/93	13/12	Selected patients (referred)
Bonanno,[45]	12	3	NS**	45 min. walk-jog, 3 days/week	148/97	135/83	13/14	Exercise group had lower weight and blood pressure than controls, no definition of hypertension
Choquette,[46]	37	6	NS**	2 hr./week jog-volleyball 10-15 min./day calisthenics	136/90	122/82	14/18	All professional males, had previously joined health club (i.e., motivated)
Krotkiewski,[47]	27	6	NS**	1 hr. jog-gymnastics-bicycle/3 days/week	134/87	125/80	9/7	Recorded BP to nearest 5 mm Hg only
Romar,[48]	27 27 27 17	3 3 12 12	? ? ? ?	30 min. walk-jog, 3 days/week 70% maximum heart rate No training 70% maximum heart rate 75-85% maximum heart rate	182/113	161/97 179/113 159/95 154/97	21/16 (18/16) 20/18 5/+2	No initial weight or change of weight given; were also on low sodium diet, no urinary sodium values; antihypertensive meds stopped, but not sedatives; 60% patients had end-organ disease (WHO Stage II); large dropout rate, only 8/30 patients at 30 months.
Pyorola,[49]	82	18	0.5	3 days/week calisthenics, walking-running	135/86	123/81	12/5	84 control subjects also had 11/5 drop in blood pressure without exercise
DePlaen,[50]	6	3	2.0	3 days/week calisthenics, walking-jogging	169/108	168/111	1/+3	4 control subjects dropped 4/6 without exercise
Ressl,[51]	10	1	3.0	5 days/week with bicycle ergometry	182/98	176/98	6/0	
Rudd,[52]	19	1.5	—	3 days/week calisthenics, walking-jogging	155/95	133/85	22/10	An uncontrolled YMCA physical fitness program
Sannerstedt,[53]	5	1.5	3.2	3 days/week bicycle ergometry			−5(MAP)	Hyperkinetic hypertensives with high pulse rates and CO tended to become normalized with physical training program.

* All $p < 0.01$

** Not significant.

for 18 months after completion of a training program and found no long-term effect on blood pressure.

Stamler[56] studied the effect of diet, exercise, and weight loss on blood pressure in a large, long-term, prospective study known as the Chicago Coronary Prevention Evaluation Program. The patients were counseled on the benefits of exercise, the hazards of smoking, and were given dietary instructions to reduce total calories and total fat intake moderately, especially saturated fats and cholesterol. Patients were followed 5–10 years, and they showed sustained falls in blood pressure, serum cholesterol and weight. Among the 115 hypertensive men (baseline diastolic > 90 mm Hg), the long-term fall in blood pressure was 13/10 mm Hg. Among the group with "high normal" blood pressure (baseline diastolic 80–89 mm Hg), a fall of 7/4 mm Hg was sustained.

These studies, along with the important papers of Gillum[34] and Hunt,[35] show that the combination of dietary sodium restriction, weight reduction in the obese, and regular exercise seem to lower blood pressure, particularly in hypertensive patients. However, further controlled studies are needed in order to establish physical exercise per se as an effective hypotensive vehicle. (Table X).

THE ROLE OF POTASSIUM

The role of potassium intake in the regulation of blood pressure has attracted attention since the 1930s.[57,58] Addison[57] theorized that the high prevalence of essential hypertension in North America was due to our diet: typically high in sodium and low in potassium. In 1944, Kempner[1] reported the success of his low-sodium rice and fruit diet in treating hypertension. However, as Priddle[59] pointed out 20 years ago, as low as this rice and fruit diet was in sodium, it was also high in potassium. Meneely,[60] reviewing the high sodium/low potassium diet of civilized cultures, explains that when an entire population ingests excessive amounts of salt, but only part of that population is genetically predisposed to hypertension, epidemiologic studies might fail to find a relationship between sodium excretion and blood pressure. However, he felt a protective effect, if indeed there is any, should be demonstrable from potassium ingestion.

Sasaki[61] studied two villages in Northern Japan with similar high sodium intakes but different blood pressures. The inhabitants of the

TABLE X
LONG-TERM EFFECTS OF DIET, EXERCISE, AND WEIGHT REDUCTION*

Group	Hypertensive		"High Normal"	
	Baseline	Five-Year Follow-up	Baseline	Five-Year Follow-up
Weight (kg)	89.0	83.7	87.3	82.5
% Over Ideal Weight	30	22	28	21
Serum Cholesterol (mg/dl)	258	232	259	240
Blood Pressure (mm Hg)	146/96	133/86	130/83	123/79
BP Fall (mm Hg)	—	13/10	—	7/4

* From Stamler,[56] with permission of *The Journal of the American Medical Association,* 243 (18):1819–1823, 1980. Copyright 1980, American Medical Association.

village with lower blood pressures had a higher potassium intake. Staessen,[62] in an epidemiologic study of two Belgium towns, correlated lower systolic and diastolic pressures to high potassium excretion in men. Khaw[63] found systolic and diastolic pressures to be higher with increasing urinary sodium/potassium ratios and lower with increasing urinary potassium/creatinine ratios for adults under 45 years in the West Indies. Langford and Watson[64,65] have two studies of young girls in Mississippi showing no significant correlation between sodium excretion alone and blood pressure. However, they did correlate the ratio of urinary sodium to potassium with both systolic and diastolic pressures. Walker[66] found higher urinary potassium excretion correlated with lower diastolic blood pressure in studying 574 volunteers in Baltimore.

Bulpitt[67] has demonstrated a negative correlation between serum potassium and blood pressure in adults, and in women only, a positive correlation between serum sodium and blood pressure. Finally, Ericsson[68] recently found the mean total body potassium (K^{40}) content of his untreated hypertensives to be 13% lower than normals. Forty-two percent of his patients had total body potassium values less than 85% of the expected values.

Interventional studies have shown that supplemental potassium may lower blood pressure (Table XI). Parfrey[69,70] studied mildly hypertensive patients on a no-added-salt, potassium supplemented diet for

TABLE XI
POTASSIUM SUPPLEMENTATION MAY LOWER BLOOD PRESSURE

Reference	No. of Subjects	Weeks On Diet	Control Diet				High Potassium Diet			
			Urinary Sodium (mEq/24 hr)	Urinary Potassium (mEq/24 hr)	Urinary Na/K Ration	Blood Pressure (mm Hg)	Urinary Sodium (mEq/24 hr)	Urinary Potassium (mEq/24 hr)	Urinary Na/K Ratio	Blood Pressure Fall (mm Hg)
Parfrey[69,70] 1981	15	6	173	59	3.0	147/96	126	128	1.0	9/6**
	15	12	—	—	—	—	123	123	1.0	4/2
Mac-Gregor[71] 1982	23	4	140	62	2.2	155/99	169	118	1.4	7/4*
Khaw[72] 1982	20	4	155	78	2.1	116/72	164	130	1.3	1.1/2.4*
Iimura[73] 1981	20	3	158	41	3.9	114†	183	123	1.5	11**
Skrabal[74] 1981	20	2	210	71	3.0	125/73	28	173	0.2	2/3

† Mean Arterial Pressure
* $P < 0.05$
** $P < 0.01$

three months. He found a large fall in blood pressure at six weeks (9/6 mm Hg) that leveled out to a final 4/2 mm Hg drop in pressure. MacGregor[71] ran a double-blind, randomized, crossover study of potassium supplementation (60 mEq/day) versus placebo in mild hypertensives on an unrestricted sodium diet and found a 7/4 mm Hg fall in blood pressure. Khaw[72] did a similar study of moderate potassium supplementation (64 mEq/day), with the same study design as MacGregor, on normotensive adults, and obtained a fall of 1.1/2.4 mm Hg in blood pressure (p < 0.01). Although only a slight reduction, Khaw felt that such a reduction accomplished by dietary measures alone could have extensive epidemiologic benefit worldwide. In a small group of medically-treated hypertensives, using the same double-blind, crossover design, Mazzola[75] recently reported that small potassium supplementation (24 mEq/day) can lower blood pressure (11/2 mm Hg) over periods of only two to four weeks. Iimura[73] studied 20 hypertensives as inpatients on a rather high sodium/high potassium diet (183 and 123 mEq/day, respectively) and dropped their mean arterial pressures from 114 to 103 mm Hg.

Parfrey and Holly[70,76] studied a group of normotensive medical students who were divided into those with or without hypertensive parents. When comparing blood pressures on a low sodium diet to a low sodium/potassium supplemented diet, those students with a family history of hypertension had lower blood pressures with the added potassium while the group with no family history had higher blood pressures. This suggests a protective influence of potassium supplementations on blood pressure in those individuals familially predisposed to hypertension.

Skrabal[74] found no significant change in resting blood pressure on a diet, moderately sodium-restricted or potassium-supplemented, in normotensive subjects. He theorized there are four mechanisms by which a high potassium intake may improve blood pressure regulation and perhaps prevent essential hypertension: 1) potassium has a direct saluretic effect on the kidney,[77] leading to a decrease in the extracellular fluid space; 2) potassium increases the sensitivity of the baroreceptor response; 3) potassium prevents the increase in catecholamines (particularly norepinephrine) seen with sodium restriction; and 4) it helps improve patient compliance on a low-sodium diet, by replacing salty foods with fruits and vegetables and/or the use of salt substitutes. If results similar to these presented here are confirmed in larger groups in long-term interventional studies, the public health implications could be substantial. Clearly, longer studies of the effect of increased potassium intake among hypertensive patients are needed.

THE ROLE OF DIETARY FAT AND VEGETARIAN DIETS

Recently, the possible role of dietary fat in the management of hypertension has been studied. Several short-term interventional studies on the role of fat intake—both the quantity and quality of fat—have yielded interesting results (Table XII). Puska[78] reported the effect on blood pressure of a diet low in fat but with a high ratio of polyunsaturated fats to saturated fats (the P/S ratio). Total caloric and salt intake were kept constant. Strategic food substitutions included margarine high in polyunsaturated fatty acids, skim milk, lean meat, low-fat sausage, and low-fat cheese. After six weeks of dietary management, her patients experienced an average fall in blood pressure of 9/8 mm Hg. The fall was greater (12/11 mm Hg) among her mild hypertensives than among the normotensives (6/5 mm Hg).

Rouse[79] studied the change in blood pressure among normotensive subjects treated with a vegetarian diet supplemented with milk products and eggs, i.e., a diet free of meat, fish, and poultry. He noted that several epidemiologic studies have suggested a lowering of blood pressure by such a vegetarian diet. His diet utilized a P/S ratio of 0.8, compared to 0.4 on the customary baseline diet. He obtained a 7/3 mm Hg drop in blood pressure. Iacono[80] reported the results of feeding normotensives a high P/S ratio diet with either a normal or low overall fat content. He found significant blood pressure falls on both diets. It is believed that, since polyunsaturated fats are the precursors of vasodilatory and saluretic prostaglandins (levels of which have been shown to be low in essential hypertension[81,82]), a diet with a high P/S ratio might increase the dietary load of polyunsturated fats which should increase prostaglandin production. In fact, studies have been done giving hypertensive patients pills with either polyunsaturated fats or placebo that show a blood pressure lowering effect.[85] Of course, an easier way to achieve a diet with a high P/S ratio is to substitute vegetable oil-based margarine and cooking oil for butter and animal products. This has been shown to lower blood pressure of mildly hypertensive adults[83]

TABLE XII
DIETS THAT RESTRICT SATURATED FAT INTAKE MAY LOWER BLOOD PRESSURE

Reference	Diet	No. of Patients	Duration of Diet (wks)	BP (mm Hg)	Baseline Fat Intake (% energy intake)	P/S*	Treatment Results Fat Intake (% energy intake)	P/S*	BP Fall (mm Hg)
Puska[78]	High P/S*	35	6	138/89	39	0.27	23	0.98	9/8
Rouse[79]	Vegetarian	38	6	117/7⁻	?	0.4	?	0.8	7/3
Iacono[80]	Low fat	21	6	136/80	42	0.22	26	0.95	13/7
	Normal fat	21	6	136/80	42	0.22	37	0.97	12/4
Fleischman[83]	High P/S	28	4	148/91	?	?	?	?	8/5
Stern[84]	High P/S	30	6	144/82	?	?	?	?	11/2

* Polyunsaturated/saturated fats ratio.

and of obese hypertensive adolescents[84] (by Fleischman and Stern, respectively, Table XII). Long-term, controlled studies of a high P/S diet on blood pressure, while holding weight, sodium and potassium intake, and level of physical activity constant, are needed. Rouse's[86] recent epidemiological survey of a group of Morman omnivores vs. Seventh Day Adventist vegetarians appears in the first issue of the *Journal of Hypertension*,[86] with the results shown in Table XIII. Blood pressure was lower in the vegetarians, not because of differences in body weight or salt intake or general lifestyle. Rather the P/S ratio was significantly higher among the vegetarians. They ingested about 30% more polyunsaturated fat and about equal amounts of saturated fats, sodium, total fats and potassium.

Of course, in treating hypertensive patients, it is important to minimize all of their other risk factors for coronary heart disease (Table IV, Chapter I) as well. Several studies have shown that a high P/S diet lowers total cholesterol and low-density lipoproteins by 10–15%.[87-89]

Foods to Avoid Because of Their High Saturated Fat Content:

- Pork: sausages and hot dogs
- Milk and dairy products
- Any deep fried or French fried foods
- Eggs
- Chocolates and fudges
- Cream-based soups
- Macaroni and cheese
- Doughnuts and cookies
- Pies and pastries made with butter and milk products

Foods With High P/S Ratio:

- Vegetable oils (corn, olive, safflower, soybean)
- Nuts
- Sunflower seeds
- Margarine

TABLE XIII
EFFECT OF A VEGETARIAN DIET IN MALES WITH A HIGH
POLYUNSATURATED TO SATURATED FAT RATIO BETWEEN TWO
DIFFERENT RELIGIOUS GROUPS IN WESTERN AUSTRALIA*

	Number of Patients	Age (yrs)	Weight (kg)	P/S	Na Intake (mEq/day)	Mean Blood Pressure (mm Hg)	% With Blood Pressure >140/90 (mm Hg)
Lacto-ovo-vegetarian	47	33	69	0.83	162 ± 73	114/67	1.0
Ominorous	33	32	75	0.57	163 ± 73	121/72	8.5**

* Rouse et al[86] with permission.
** $p < 0.01$ from vegetarians.

Foods With Little Or No Fat:

- Fresh fruits and vegetables
- Fish and shellfish
- Skim milk
- Lean meat
- Low-fat sausage
- Low-fat cheese

THE ROLE OF RELAXATION, MEDITATION, AND BIOFEEDBACK

Despite intensive research, the etiology of essential hypertension remains unknown. Because stressful situations are known to elevate blood pressure, it is not surprising that relaxation is being used to treat it. Indeed, hundreds of papers have appeared during the past decade on the possible benefits of relaxation, meditation, and biofeedback techniques and their effect on reducing blood pressure. Sustained blood pressure elevations can be produced in animals by chronic exposure to various stressful stimuli. Temporary rises in blood pressure and also sustained hypertension have been found in people living in chronically stressful situations. Air traffic controllers have a 5.6 times higher incidence of hypertension than non-professional pilots.[90] Men exposed to high noise levels have also demonstrated a higher incidence of hypertension.[91] Psychogenetic stress activates the sympathetic nervous system and increases catecholamine activity. Plasma norepinephrine levels are increased in many hypertensive patients.[92] It is also common clinical experience that hospitalized hypertensive patients routinely experience a significant drop in blood pressure, often to normotensive levels, within the first two or three days of hospitalization. Their sympathetic nervous systems become less active.[93]

The two general psychological techniques utilized today may be classified as either relaxation/meditation or as biofeedback. Jacobson[94] introduced one of the most widely used progressive relaxation techniques in which the person is instructed to tense and then relax various groups of striate muscles, beginning with the hands and arms, progressing to facial muscles, and muscles in the trunk and legs. Sometimes a metronome is used to synchronize such a relaxation progression. A common feature of the "concentrative" meditation technique involves the directing of one's attention toward a "mental device"[95] or focus with which the student becomes passively absorbed. A variety of mental devices such as mantras, chants, prayers, cymbals, or indeed one's own heartbeat or breathing are used or may be used in these techniques. Their function is to reduce or eliminate conceptual thinking and to facilitate the development of an encompassing focus on the present moment and feelings of calm and relaxation. In general, there are four components of the common active ingredients of relaxation/meditation: (a) a quiet environment, (b) a decreased muscle tone, (c) a passive attitude, and (d) the restriction of one's attention to a mental device. Patients are taught to intersperse their daily activities with two daily 10–20 minute intervals of such relaxation and/or meditation.

Biofeedback, as a method of blood pressure control, involves the use of instrumentation to give moment-to-moment information to the individual patient about a specific physiologic process. The signal may be in the form of a colored light or a noise of varying intensity, etc. When individuals are given such feedback, together with appropriate incentives for controlling responses, they may be able to learn to modify such functions as heart rate, blood pressure, blood flow, skin temperature, sweating, and gastrointestinal processes.[96] Generally, a "constant cuff" method which permits continuous beat-by-beat feedback of blood pressure is utilized.

Hundreds of favorable reports have appeared in the past decade utilizing these general techniques for reducing blood pressure. Most of the studies, however, have lacked sufficient control procedures and sufficient long-term follow-ups to warrant firm conclusions about efficacy. Recently reported, Luborsky et al[97] used four groups of hypertensive treatments: medication, metronome-conditioned relaxation, metronome-conditioned mild exercise, and a fourth group utilizing biofeedback techniques. Results of this study indicate a drop in blood pressure of 22/14 mm Hg in the drug-treated group, 6.4/6.0 mm Hg in the metronome-conditioned relaxation group, 4.0/5.3 mm Hg in the metronome-conditioned mild exercise group, and a reduction of 8/+0.4 mm Hg in the biofeedback group. He suggests that methodology be developed which could predict who might benefit from these non-drug interventions.

Peter Seer[98] has published an excellent status report of psychological techniques in treating hypertension. He reviewed and critiqued results of 20 different major published studies. He concludes that without better designed clinical methodology, the unqualified acceptance of psychological techniques as an alternative to pharmacological treatment of hypertension is not yet justified. Although blood pressure reductions can be achieved with training, nevertheless, whether blood pressure reductions in real-life situations are achievable and are of sufficient clinical magnitude and are of sufficient duration have simply not been demonstrated. Seer feels that psychological approaches are a promising adjunctive but not a primary one of treating hypertension. We agree.

THE ROLE OF CALCIUM

Calcium is another dietary factor linked to hypertension. The first reports of a possible association came from studies showing an inverse relationship between hardness of water (hard water is high in calcium) and prevalence of cardiovascular disease and also diastolic blood pressure.[99,100] Then, a study showed average calcium intake in pregnancy was inversely related to the incidence of gestational hypertension among countries.[101] McCarron has published two papers where hypertensive patients, using 24-hour dietary recall surveys, reported significantly lower calcium intake than normotensive controls.[102,103] Calcium intake was 18% lower in the hypertensive group, while all other nutritional components reported were both typical and similar to controls. It has been reported that hypertensive patients have lower serum phosphorus[104,105] and lower serum ionized calcium[105] levels than matched controls. The underlying cause of these differences is unknown.

Belizan and Villar,[106] in a double-blind controlled study of calcium supplementation (1 gm/day) in healthy young adults over five months, found a fall in blood pressure of 1.2/5.6 mm Hg in females and 0.1/9.1 mm Hg in males. Baseline dietary calcium had been about 600 mg for females and 800 mg for males. The mechanism by which calcium influences blood pressure is not yet known. Studies of the effect of calcium supplementation in hypertensive patients are needed. It should be remembered that while hypertensive patients are being advised to eat dairy products only in moderation (to avoid sodium and saturated fats), these dairy products supply two-thirds of the average calcium intake.

THE EFFECT OF ALCOHOL

Numerous large epidemiologic studies have demonstrated
an association between heavy alcohol usage and
the prevalence of hypertension.

Does the moderate use of alcohol aggravate blood pressure? Studies on the immediate short-term effect of moderate alcohol ingestion indicate no effect on cardiac output or blood pressure although cutaneous blood vessels are dilated. Numerous large epidemiologic studies have demonstrated an association between heavy alcohol usage and the prevalence of hypertension. Alonzo,[107] in a study of 922 "problem drinkers," with a group of controls matched for weight and age, found the prevalence of hypertension to be 2.3 times greater among the problem drinkers. The results from the Framingham Study[108] similarly find hypertension twice as prevalent among those drinking 60 oz. alcohol per month (about four to five drinks per day) as compared to light drinkers (10–30 oz./mo. alcohol or about two or fewer drinks per day). As shown in other studies,[109,110] light drinkers have a lower prevalence of hypertension than nondrinkers (Figure 2).

Light drinkers have a lower prevalence
of hypertension than nondrinkers.

In a health survey of 84,000 people, Klatsky and Friedman[111] found higher systolic and diastolic pressures and a higher prevalence of hypertension among those men and women drinking three or more drinks per day as compared to those consuming two or fewer drinks per day. These findings were independent of age, sex, race, smoking and weight. Furthermore, their findings suggest that blood pressure increases progressively with increasing alcohol intake, once above a certain unknown "threshold level," somewhere between zero to four drinks per day. This relationship between increasing blood pressure with progressively higher alcohol intake held for whites and Orientals but not blacks; it had a greater effect on systolic than diastolic pressure; and it has been observed in several other epidemiologic studies.[108-110,112] In the only prospective study of alcohol usage on blood pressure, Dyer and Stamler[112] found the incidence of hypertension to be four times

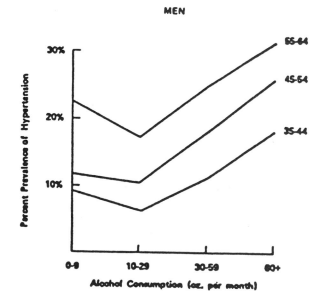

**PERCENT PREVALENCE OF HYPERTENSION
BY ALCOHOL CONSUMPTION AT EXAM. 4; FRAMINGHAM STUDY**

MEN

Figure 2: Kannel and Sorlie;[108] reproduced with permission from Stratton Intercontinental Medical Book Corporation.

greater in men who were problem drinkers or heavy drinkers (six or more drinks per day) than other drinkers and non-drinkers over a four-year period. Unfortunately, all these alcohol studies use the WHO criterion for hypertension (> 160/95 mm Hg).

THE EFFECT OF COFFEE

Does drinking coffee raise blood pressure? Is coffee safe for hypertensive patients? The usual cup of coffee contains about 100 mg of the central nervous system stimulant, caffeine. The ingestion of one to three cups of coffee has been shown to decrease drowsiness, increase concentration and the speed of performing perfunctory tasks. At higher doses, caffeine will produce a tachycardia and in sensitive individuals, a cardiac arrhythmia. Ingesting 250 mg of caffeine will produce a plasma level of about 10 μg/ml, with a resultant increase of epinephrine and norepinephrine by about 100% and 50%, respectively. A brief increase in cardiac output (and blood pressure) may occur. Vasodilatation and augmented organ volume blood flow also occur after caffeine, but the effect is short-lived. When non-coffee drinkers were given two or three cups of coffee, their blood pressure rose 14/10 mm Hg one hour after ingestion.[113] Tolerance to caffeine occurs within a few days, so abstinence for several days (up to three weeks) may be required to obtain maximal effects.

Three substantial studies all indicate that moderate coffee drinking has no adverse effect on blood pressure. Two large epidemiological studies, Framingham[114] and the IBM Corporation study,[115] plus Robertson's[116] study of the effects of chronic caffeine ingestion found no relationship between coffee drinking and blood pressure.

THE EFFECT OF CIGARETTES

Besides being a major risk factor per se for all levels of hypertension, cigarettes contain nicotine which raises blood pressure. When subjects smoked two cigarettes in one study, their blood pressure rose 10/8 mm Hg for a 15-minute duration. With a cigarette habit of 1½ or 2 packs/day, blood pressure is elevated during 7–10 hours of the day. Goodman and Gilman[117] note that "the majority of individuals (also) respond to cigarette smoking with a rise in both systolic and diastolic blood pressure." Proof is lacking, however, that abstinence from a heavy cigarette smoking habit will successfully reduce hypertension.

Nicholson et al found a strong correlation between cigarette smoking and renovascular hypertension (both arteriosclerotic and fibromuscular) when compared with a matched cohort of patients with essential hypertension.[118]

REFERENCES:

1. Kempner, W.: Treatment of hypertensive vascular disease with rice diet. *Am. J. Med.*, 4:545–577, 1948.
2. Hatch, F. T., Wertheim, A. R., et al: Effects of diet in essential hypertension III: Alterations in sodium chloride, protein, and fat intake. *Am. J. Med.*, 17:499–513, 1954.
3. Corcoran, A. C., Taylor, R. D., et al: Controlled observations on the effect of low sodium diet to therapy in essential hypertension. *Circulation*, 3:1, 1951.
4. Oliver, W. J., Cohen, E. L., et al: Blood pressure sodium intake and sodium-related hormones in the Yanomamo Indians, a "no salt" culture. *Circulation*, 52: 146, 1975.
5. Lowenstein, F. W.: Blood pressure in relation to age and sex in the tropics and subtropic. A review of the literature and an investigation in two tribes of Brazil Indians. *Lancet*, 1:389, 1961.
6. Prior, A. M., Evans, J. G., et al: Sodium intake and blood pressure in two Polynesian populations. *N. Engl. J. Med.*, 279:515, 1968.
7. Sinnet, P. F., Whyte, H. M.: Epidemiologic studies in the total highland population, Tukisenta, New Guinea. *J. Chron. Dis.*, 26:265, 1973.
8. Maddocks, I.: Blood pressure in Medlanesians. *Med. J. Aust.*, 1:1123, 1967.
9. Dahl, L. K.: Salt and hypertension. *Am. J. Clin. Nutr.*, 25:231, 1972.
10. National Center for Health Statistics, Public Health Services. *Hypertension: United States, 1974*. Advance data from Vital & Health Statistics, No. 2, 1976.
11. McMahon, F. G., Cole, P.A., et al: A study of hypertension in the inner city: A student hypertension study. *Am. Heart J.*, 85(1):65, 1973.
12. Sasuki, N.: The relationship of salt intake to hypertension in the Japanese. *Geriatrics*, 19:735, 1964.
13. Fregly, M. S., Fregly, M. J.: The estimates of sodium intake by man. In M. J. Fregly, M. R. Kare (Eds.): *The Role of Salt in Cardiovascular Hypertension*. Academic Press, New York, 1982.
14. Parijs, J., Joossens, J. V., et al: Moderate sodium restriction and diuretics in the treatment of hypertension. *Am. Heart J.*, 85:22–34, 1973.
15. Morgan, T, Gillies, A., et al: Hypertension treated by salt restriction. *Lancet*, i: 227–230, 1978.
16. MacGregor, G. A., Markandu, N. D., et al: Double-blind randomized crossover trial of moderate sodium restriction in essential hypertension. *Lancet*, i:351–354, 1982.

17. Watt, G. C. M., Edwards, C., et al: Dietary sodium restriction for mild hypertensives in general practice. *Br. Med. J.*, **286**:432–436, 1983.
18. Morgan, T. O., et al: Hypertension treated by sodium restriction. *Med. J. Aust.*, **2**: 396–397, 1981.
19. Parfrey, P. S., Markandu, N. D., et al: Relation between arterial pressure, dietary sodium intake, and renin system in essential hypertension. *Br. Med. J.*, **283**:94–97, 1981.
20. Beard, T. C., Cooke, H. M., et al: Randomized controlled trial of a no-added-sodium diet for mild hypertension. *Lancet*, **ii**:455–458, 1982.
21. Guidelines for the treatment of mild hypertension: Memorandum from a WHO/ISH meeting. *Hypertension*, **5**(3):394–397, 1983.
22. Kaplan, N. M., Simmons, M., et al: Two techniques to improve adherence to dietary sodium restriction in the treatment of hypertension. *Arch. Int. Med.*, **142**: 1638–1641, 1982.
23. Kirschmann, J. D.: *Nutritional Almanac*. McGraw-Hill Book Co., pp. 200–234, 1979.
24. Society of Actuaries, *Build and Blood Pressure Study*. Society of Actuaries, Chicago, 1959.
25. Tyroler, H. A., Heyden, S., Hames, C. G.: Weight and hypertension: Evans County study of blacks and whites. In O. Paul (Ed.): *Epidemiology and Control of Hypertension*, Stratton Intercontinental, New York, 1975.
26. Kannel, W. B., Brand, N., et al: The relationship of adiposity to blood pressure and development of hypertension. The Framingham Study. *Ann. Int. Med.*, **67**: 48–59, 1967.
27. Ramsay, L. E., Ramsay, M. H., Hettiarehehi, J., Davies, D. L., and Winchester, J.: Weight reduction in a blood pressure clinic. *Br. Med. J.*, **2**:244–245, 1978.
28. Langford, H. G.: Drug and dietary intervention in hypertension. *Hypertension*, **4** (Suppl. III):III-166–III-169, 1982.
29. Preble, W. E.: Obesity: Observation of one thousand cases. *Boston Med. Surg. J.*, **188**:617, 1973.
30. Master, A. M., Oppenheimer, A.: Study of obesity. *JAMA*, **92**:1652, 1929.
31. Reisen, E., Abel, R., et al: Effect of weight loss without salt restriction on the reduction of blood pressure in overweight hypertensive patients. *N. Engl. J. Med.*, **298**:1–6, 1978.
32. Tuck, M. L., Sowers, J., et al: The effect of weight reduction on blood pressure, plasma renin activity, and plasma aldosterone levels in obese patients. *N. Engl. J. Med.*, **304**:930–933, 1981.
33. Reisen, E., Frohlich, E. D., et al: Cardiovascular changes after weight reduction in obesity hypertension. *Ann. Int. Med.*, **98**:315–319, 1983.
34. Gillum, R. F., Prineas, R. J., et al: Nonpharmacologic therapy of hypertension: The independent effects of weight reduction and sodium restriction in overweight borderline hypertensive patients. *Am. Heart J.*, **105**:128–133, 1983.
35. Hunt, J. C., and Margie, J. D.: The influence of diet on hypertension. In J. C. Hunt, T. Cooper, E. D. Frolich, et al (Eds.): *Hypertension Update: Mechanisms, Epidemiology, Evaluation, and Management*. HLS Press, Bloomfield, New Jersey, 1980.
36. Lowenthal, D. T., Dickerman, D., Saris, S., Falkner, B., and Hare, T.: The effect

of pharmacological interaction on central and peripheral alpha-receptors and pressor response to static exercise. *Annals of Sports Medicine* (in press), 1983.

37. Morris, J. N., Chave, S. P. N., Adam, C., et al: Vigorous exercise in leisure-time and the incidence of coronary heart disease. *Lancet*, i:333–339, 1973.

38. Paffenbarger, R. S., and Hale, W. E.: Work activity and coronary heart mortality. *N. Engl. J. Med.*, 292:545–550, 1975.

39. Paffenbarger, R. S., Wing, A. L., and Hyde, R. T.: Physical activity as an index of heart attack risk in college alumni. *Am. J. Epidemiol.*, 108:161–175, 1978.

40. Hickey, N., Risteard, M., Bourke, G. J., et al: Study of coronary risk factors related to physical activity in 15,171 men. *Br. Med. J.*, iii:507–509, 1975.

41. Cooper, K. H., Pollack, M. L., Martin, R. P., et al: Physical fitness levels vs. selected coronary risk factors. *JAMA*, 236:166–169, 1976.

42. Criqui, M. H., Mebane, I., Wallace, R. B., et al. Multivariate correlates of adult blood pressures in nine North American populations: The Lipid Research Clinics Prevalence Study. *Prev. Med.*, 11:391–402, 1982.

43. Cantwell, J. D.: Running. *JAMA*, 240:1409–1410, 1978.

44. Boyer, J. L., and Kasch, F. W.: Exercise therapy in hypertensive men. *JAMA*, 211:1668–1671, 1970.

45. Bonanno, J. A., and Lies, J. E.: Effects of physical training on coronary risk factors. *Am. J. Cardiol.*, 33:760–764, 1974.

46. Choquette, G., and Ferguson, R. J.: Blood pressure reduction in "borderline" hypertensives following physical training. *Can. Med. Assoc. J.*, 108:699–703, 1973.

47. Krotkiewski, M., Mandroukas, K., Sjostrom, L., et al: Effects of long-term physical training on body fat, metabolism, and blood pressure in obesity. *Metabolism*, 28:650–658, 1979.

48. Roman, O., Camuzzi, A. L., Villalon, E., and Klenner, C.: Physical training program in arterial hypertension: A long-term prospective follow-up. *Cardiology*, 67:230–243, 1981.

49. Pyorolo, K., Karava, R, Punsar, S., et al: In O. A. Larsen, and R. O. Malmborg (Eds.): *Coronary Heart Disease and Physical Fitness.* Munksgoard, Copenhagen, 1971.

50. DePlaen, J. F., and Detry, J. M.: Hemodynamic effects of physical training in established arterial hypertension. *Acta Cardiol.*, 35:179–188, 1980.

51. Ressl, J., Chrastek, J., and Handova, R: Haemodynamic effects of physical training in essential hypertension. *Acta Cardiol.*, 32:121–133, 1977.

52. Rudd, J. L., and Day, W. C.: A physical fitness program for patients with hypertension. *J. Am. Geriatrics Soc.*, 15:373–379, 1957.

53. Sannerstedt, R., Wasir, H., Hemming, R., and Werko, L.: Systemic haemodynamics in mild arterial hypertension before and after physical training. *Clin. Sci. Mol. Med.*, 45:1455–1494s, 1973.

54. Ilmarinen, J., and Fardy, P. S.: Physical activity intervention for males with high risk of coronary heart disease. A three-year follow-up. *Prev. Med.*, 6:416–425, 1977.

55. Sedgwick, A. W., Brotherhood, J. R., et al: Long-term effects of physical training programme on risk factors for coronary heart disease in otherwise sedentary men. *Br. Med. J.*, 281:7–10, 1980.

56. Stamler, J., Farinaro, E., Mojonnier, L. M., et al: Prevention and control of hyper-

tension by nutritional-hygienic means: Long-term experience of the Chicago Coronary Prevention Evaluation Program. *JAMA*, 243:1819–1823, 1980.

57. Addison, W. L. T.: The use of sodium chloride, potassium chloride, sodium bromide, and potassium bromide in cases of arterial hypertension which are amenable to potassium chloride. *Can. Med. Assoc. J.*, 18:281–285, 1928.
58. Priddle, W. W.: Observations on the management of hypertension. *Can. Med. Assoc. J.*, 25:5–8, 1931.
59. Priddle, W. W.: Hypertension-sodium and potassium studies. *Can. Med. Assoc. J.*, 86:1–9, 1982.
60. Meneely, G. R., and Battarbee, H. D.: High sodium-low potassium environment and hypertension. *Am. J. Cardiol.*, 38:768–785, 1976.
61. Sasaki, N., Mitsuhashi, T., Fukushi, S.: Effects of ingestion of large amounts of apples on blood pressure in farmers in Akita prefecture. *Igaku Seibutsugaku*, 51:103–105, 1959.
62. Staessen, J., Bulpitt, C., Fagard, R., et al: Four urinary cations and blood pressure—a population study of two Belgian towns. International Symposium on Potassium, Blood Pressure and Cardiovascular Disease. Excerpta Medica (in press), 1983.
63. Khaw, K. T., and Rose G.: Population study of blood pressure and associated factors in St. Lucia, West Indies. *Int. J. Epidemiol.*, 11:372–377, 1982.
64. Langford, H. G., and Watson, R. L.: Electrolytes and hypertension. In O. Paul (Ed.): *Epidemiology and Control of Hypertension*. Stratton Intercontinental, New York, 1975.
65. Watson, R. L., Langford, H. G., Abernethy, J. D., et al: Urinary electrolytes, body weight, and blood pressure: Pooled cross-sectional results among four groups of adolescent females. *Hypertension*, 2(42):93–98, 1980.
66. Walker, W. G., Whelton, P. K., Saito, H., et al: Relation between blood pressure and renin, renin substrate, angiotension II, aldosterone, and urinary sodium and potassium in 574 ambulatory subjects. *Hypertension*, 1(3):287–291, 1979.
67. Bulpitt, C. J., Shipley, M. J., and Semmence, A.: Blood pressure and plasma sodium and potassium. *Clin. Sci.*, 61:85s–87s, 1981.
68. Ericsson, F., Carlmark, B., Eliasson, K., et al: Potassium in whole body and skeletal muscle in untreated primary hypertension. International Symposium on Potassium, Blood Pressure and Cardiovascular disease. Excerpta Medica (in press), 1983.
69. Parfrey, P. S., Vandenburg, M. J., Wright, P., et al: Blood pressure and hormonal changes following alteration in dietary sodium and potassium in mild essential hypertension. *Lancet*, i:59–63, 1981.
70. Holly, J. M. P., Goodwin, F. J., Evans, S. J. W., et al: Re-analysis of data in two *Lancet* papers on the effect of dietary sodium and potassium on blood pressure. *Lancet*, ii:1384–1387, 1981.
71. MacGregor, G. A., Smith, S. J., Markandu, N. D., et al: Moderate potassium supplementation in essential hypertension. *Lancet*, ii:567–570, 1982.
72. Khaw, K. T., and Thorn, S: Randomized double-blind crossover trial of potassium on blood pressure in normal subjects. *Lancet*, ii:1127–1129, 1982.
73. Iimura, O., Kyima, T., Kikuchi, K., et al: Studies on the hypotensive effect of high potassium intake in patients with essential hypertension. *Clin. Sci.*, 61:77s– 80s, 1981.
74. Skrabal, F., Auboch, J., and Hortnagl, H.: Low sodium/high potassium diet for

prevention of hypertension: Probable mechanisms of action. *Lancet,* ii:895–900, 1981.

75. Mazzola, C., and Guffanti, E.: Cardiovascular modifications after K⁺ supplementation in hypertensive patients. International Symposium on Potassium, Blood Pressure, and Cardiovascular Disease. Excerpta Medica (in press), 1983.

76. Parfrey, P. S., Condon, K., Wright, P., et al: Blood pressure and hormonal changes following alteration in dietary sodium and potassium in young men with and without a familial predisposition to hypertension. *Lancet,* i:113–117, 1981.

77. Liddle, G. W., Bennett, L. L., and Forsham, P. H.: The prevention of ACTH-induced sodium retention by the use of potassium salts: A quantitative study. *J. Clin. Invest.,* **32**:1197–1201, 1953.

78. Puska, P., Iacono, J. M. et al: Controlled, randomized trial of the effect of dietary fat on blood pressure. *Lancet,* i:1–5, 1983.

79. Rouse, I. L., Beilin, L. J., et al: Blood pressure-lowering effect of a vegetarian diet: Controlled trial in normotensive subjects. *Lancet,* i:5–10, 1983.

80. Iacono, J. M., Marshall, M. W., et al: Reduction in blood pressure associated with high polyunsaturated fat diets that reduce blood cholesterol in man. *Prev. Med.,* 4:426–443, 1975.

81. Tan, S. Y., Sweet, P., et al: Impaired renal production of prostaglandin E₂: A newly identified lesion in human essential hypertension. *Prostaglandins,* **15**:139, 1978.

82. Weber, P. C., Scherer, B., et al: Urinary prostaglandins and kallikrein in essential hypertension. *Clin. Sci.,* **57**(Suppl 5):259s, 1979.

83. Fleischman, A. I., Bierenbaum, M. L., et al: Hypotensive effect of increased dietary linoleic acid in mildly hypertensive humans. *J. Med. Soc. N. Jersey,* **76**:181–183, 1979.

84. Stern, B., Heyden, S., et al: Intervention study in high school students with elevated blood pressure. *Nutr. Metab.,* **24**:137–147, 1980.

85. Rao, R. H., Rao, U. B., and Srikantia, S. G.: Effect of polyunsaturated-rich vegetable oils on blood pressure in essential hypertension. *Clin. Exp. Hypertens.,* 3(1): 27–38, 1981.

86. Rouse, I. L., Armstrong, B. K., and Beilin, L. J.: The relationship of blood pressure to diet and lifestyle in two religious populations. *J. Hyper.,* 1:65–71, 1983.

87. Kraemer, F. B., Greefield, M., Tobery, T. A., and Reaven, G. M.: Effects of moderate increases in dietary polyunsaturated/saturated fat on plasma triglyceride and cholesterol levels in man. *Br. J. Nutr.,* 47:259–266, 1982.

88. Stein, E. A., Shapero, J., McNerney, E., et al: Changes in plasma lipid and lipoprotein fractions after alterations in dietary cholesterol, polyunsaturated, saturated, and total fat in free-living and hypercholesterolemic children. *Am. J. Clin. Nutr.,* **35**: 1375–1390, 1982.

89. Schaefer, E. J., Levy, R. I., Ernst, N. D., et al: The effects of low cholesterol, high polyunsaturated fat, and low fat diets on plasma lipid and lipoprotein cholesterol levels in normal and hypercholesterolemic subjects. *Am. J. Clin. Nutr.,* **34**:1758–1763, 1981.

90. Cobb, S., and Rose, R. M.: Hypertension, peptic ulcer and diabetes in air traffic controllers. *JAMA,* **224**:489–492, 1973.

91. Andren, L., Hansson, L., Bjorkman, M., and Jonsson, A.: Noise as a contributing factor in the development of elevated arterial pressure. *Acta Med. Scand.,* **207**: 493–498, 1980.

92. Engleman, K., Portnoy, B., and Sjoerdsma, A.: Plasma catecholamine concentrations in patients with hypertension. *Circ. Res.*, **26 & 27** (Suppl. 1)I:141–146, 1970.

93. Hossmann, V., Fitzgerald, G. A., and Dollery, C. T.: Influence of hospitalization and placebo therapy on blood pressure and sympathetic function in essential hypertension. *Hypertension*, 3:113–118, 1981.

94. Jacobson, E.: *Modern Treatment of Tense Patients.* Springfield, Ill.: Charles C. Thomas, 1970.

95. Benson, H.: *The Relaxation Response.* Morrow, New York, 1975.

96. Blanchard, E. B., Young, L. D., and Haynes, M. R.: A simple feedback system for the treatment of elevated blood pressure. *Behav. Ther.*, 6:241–245, 1975.

97. Luborsky, L., Crits-Christoph, P., Brady, J. P., et al: Behavioral versus pharmacological treatments for essential hypertension—a needed comparison. *Psychosom. Med.*, 44(2):203–213, 1982.

98. Seer, P.: Psychological control of essential hypertension: Review of literature and methodological critique. *Psychol. Bull.*, 86:(5):1015–1043, 1979.

99. Stitt, F. W., Clayton, D. G., Crawford, M. D., et al. Clinical and biochemical indicators of cardiovascular disease among men living in hard and soft water areas. *Lancet*, i:122–126, 1973.

100. Masironi, R., Kortyoham, S. R., Pierce, J. O., and Scharnschula, R. G.: Calcium content of river water, trace element concentrations in toenails and blood pressure in village population in New Guinea. *Sci. Total Environ.*, 6:41–53, 1976.

101. Belizan, J. M., and Villar, J.: The relationship between calcium intake and edema-, proteinuria-, and hypertension-gestosis: An hypothesis. *Am. J. Clin. Nutr.*, 33: 2202–2210, 1980.

102. McCarron, D. A., Morris, C. D., and Cole, C.: Dietary calcium in human hypertension. *Science*, 217:267–269, 1982.

103. McCarron, D. A.: Calcium and magnesium nutrition in human hypertension. *Ann. Int. Med.*, 98(Part 2):800–805, 1983.

104. Ljunghall, S., and Hedstrand, H.: Serum phosphate inversely related to blood pressure. *Br. Med. J.*, i:553–554, 1977.

105. McCarron, D. A.: Low serum concentrations of ionized calcium in patients with hypertension. *N. Engl. J. Med.*, 307:226–228, 1982.

106. Belizan, J. M., Villar, J., Pineda, O., et al: Reduction of blood pressure with calcium supplementation in young adults. *JAMA*, 249:1161–1165, 1983.

107. D'Alonzo, C.A., and Pell, S.: Cardiovascular disease among problem drinkers. *J. Occ. Med.*, 10:344–350, 1968.

108. Kannel, W. B., and Sorlie, P.: Hypertension in Framingham, In O. Paul (Ed.): *Epidemiology and Control of Hypertension.* Stratton Intercontinental Medical Book Corporation, New York, 1974.

109. Harburg, E., Ozgoren, F., et al: Community norms of alcohol usage and blood pressure: Tecumseh, Michigan. *Am . J. Public Health*, 70:813–820, 1980.

110. Wallace, R. B., Lynch, C. F., et al: Alcohol and hypertension: Epidemiologic and experimental consideration. *Circulation*, 64(Suppl. III):III, 41–47, 1981.

111. Klatsky, A. L., Friedman, G. D., et al: Alcohol consumption and blood pressure: Kaiser-Permanente multiphasic health examination data. *N. Engl. J. Med.*, 296: 1194–1200, 1977.

112. Dyer, A. R., Stamler, J., Paul, O., et al: Alcohol, cardiovascular risk factors and mortality: The Chicago experience. *Circulation*, 64(Suppl. III):III 20–27, 1981.

113. Robertson, D., Frolich, J. C., et al: Effects of caffeine on plasma renin activity, catecholamines and blood pressure. *N. Engl. J. Med.,***298**:181–186, 1978.
114. Dawber, T. R., Kannel, W. B., and Gordon, T.: Coffee and cardiovascular disease: Observations from the Framingham study. *N. Engl. J. Med.,* **291**:871–874, 1974.
115. Bertrand, C. A., Pomper, I., et al: No relation between coffee and blood pressure. *N. Engl. J. Med.,* **299**:315–316, 1978.
116. Robertson, D., Wade, D., et al: Tolerance to the humoral and hemodynamic effects of caffeine in man. *J. Clin. Invest.,* **67**:1111–1117, 1981.
117. *Goodman and Gilman's The Pharmacological Basis of Therapeutics.* A. G. Gilman, L. S. Goodman and A. Gilman (Eds.), Macmillan Publishing Co., New York, 1970, p. 591.
118. Nicholson, J. P., Alderman, M. H., et al: Cigarette smoking and renovascular hypertension. *Lancet,* **II**(8353):765–766, 1983.

CHAPTER III

DIURETICS
THE THIAZIDE, THIAZIDE-LIKE, AND
LOOP DIURETICS

- HYDROCHLOROTHIAZIDE
  (HYDRODIURIL,® etc.)
- CHLORTHALIDONE (HYGROTON,®)
- METOLAZONE (ZAROXOLYN,® DIULO®)
- INDAPAMIDE (LOZOL®)
- FUROSEMIDE (LASIX®)

INTRODUCTION:

The "new news" about diuretics in hypertension is:

1. Minimal effective doses have now become lower, e.g., 25 or 50 mg of chlorthalidone or hydrochlorothiazide given once daily is usually effective in satisfactorily reducing blood pressure. Indeed 12.5 mg doses are effective in many patients. Low doses produce less hypokalemia and fewer other side effects.

2. Maximal doses should be reduced to minimize occurrence of hypokalemia and the possibility of serious arrhythmias. The maximal dose of chlorthalidone or hydrochlorothiazide should ordinarily be 50 mg/day.

3. There is growing evidence that diuretics are not always the initial "drug of choice" for mild-moderate hypertension, as the stepped-care technique had led us to believe.

4. Concern is being expressed that the long-term antihypertensive benefits of diuretics may be offset by the subtle induction of biochemi-

75

cal risk factors for coronary heart disease, e.g., elevations of triglycerides, cholesterol, glucose and uric acid.

Thiazide diuretics (Table I) have been the cornerstone of modern antihypertensive therapy for the past 25 years. They owe their popularity to the fact that they work quite well, are relatively safe, are well tolerated, and are relatively inexpensive. Every physician who treats hypertension must be familiar with this class of drugs. Its unique position as the sole drug of choice in the initial treatment of hypertension is now being challenged. Some patients' treatment ought best be initiated with a beta-blocker and, occasionally, another class of antihypertensive drug, such as a calcium channel blocker, a converting enzyme inhibitor, or a centrally acting alpha-agonist. (See Chapter I for a more complete discussion.) The five classes of commonly used diuretics are:

A. The *Thiazides*, e.g., chlorothiazide, hydrochlorothiazide, polythiazide, etc.

B. The *Related-Sulfonamides* (or Thiazide-Like), e.g., chlorthalidone, metolazone, quinethazone, and indapamide.

C. The *Loop Diuretics*, e.g., furosemide, ethacrynic acid, and bumetamide.

D. The *Potassium-Sparing Diuretics*, e.g., amiloride, triamterene, and spironolactone (see Chapter V).

E. The *Isouricemic Diuretics*, e.g., indacrinone (see Chapter XIV).

INTRODUCTORY YEAR: 1958

The thiazides and thiazide-like diuretics are now being used at doses much lower than previously. Tables II and III list the efficacy of doses as low as 12.5 mg/day of hydrochlorothiazide or chlorthalidone. These are effective doses in some patients, particularly blacks and the elderly, and 25 mg is an effective dose in most patients. The decrements noted in these tables are for whites as well as blacks, and young as well as older patients. Indeed, doses as low as 6 mg/day of these diuretics are being studied (though not now recommended). The clear advantage of using these small doses of diuretics is that the laboratory abnormalities (e.g., reduction of serum potassium, elevation of uric acid, glucose, triglycerides and cholesterol) then become minimal. Recent concern about thiazide-induced hypokalemia and the development of potentially serious cardiac arrhythmias compel one to use the

TABLE I
THIAZIDE DIURETICS

Generic Name	Brand Name	Tablet Sizes (mg)	Initial Dose (mg/day)	Dose Range (mg/day)	Usual Maintenance Dose (mg/day)
Chlorothiazide	Diuril®	250, 500	250 or 500 once daily	125–1000	250–500
Hydrochlorothiazide	Hydrodiuril®, Oretic®, Esidrix®	25, 50 and 100	25 or 50 once daily	12.5–100	25–50
Chlorthalidone	Hygroton®, Thalidone®	25, 50 and 100	25 once daily	12.5–100	25
Hydroflumethiazide	Diucardin®, Saluron®	50	50 once or twice daily	25–100	50 twice daily
Bendroflumethiazide	Naturetin®	2.5, 5 and 10	5–20 once or twice daily	2.5–20	2.5–15 once or twice daily
Benzthiazide	Aquatag®, Exna®, Hydrex®	25, 50	25 to 50 twice daily	50–100	50 twice daily
Trichlormethiazide	Naqua®, Metahydrin®	2, 4	2–4 twice daily	2–4	2–4
Polythiazide	Renese®	1, 2 and 4	2–4	2–4	2–4
Cyclothiazide	Anhydron®	2	2 once daily	2–6	2
Quinethazone	Hydromox®	50	50–100 once daily	50–100	50–100
Metolazone	Zaroxolyn®	2.5, 5 and 10	2.5–5 once daily	2.5–20	2.5–5

TABLE II
ANTIHYPERTENSIVE EFFECT OF LOW DOSES OF HYDROCHLOROTHIAZIDE

Studies (Ref.)	No. Pts.	Dose (mg/day)	Pre-Treatment Blood Pressure (mm Hg)	Treatment Blood Pressure (mm Hg)	Decline in Blood Pressure (mm Hg)
Beerman et al 1978[1]	9	12.5	161/102	142/89	19/13
Berglund et al 1976[2]	40	12.5	154/108	150/105	4/3**
Beerman et al 1978[1]	9	25	161/102	138/86	23/16
Durley et al 1981[3]	7	25	163/106	139/93	24/13
Degnbol et al 1973[4]	22	25	127*	116*	11*
V. A. Cooperative Study Group 1979[5]	55	50	149/101	133/90	16/11
Alhenc-Gelas et al 1978[6]	20	50	126*	110*	16*
Beerman et al 1978[1]	9	50	161/102	138/91	23/11
McMahon 1975[7]	21	90	169/116	146/106	23/10
Multicenter Study Group 1981[8]	53	50–100	154/101	134/89	21/12
Aberg et al 1981[9]	13	50–100	166/106	148/91	18/15
Kuska et al 1981[10]	20	50–100	169/104	145/94	24/10

 * Mean blood pressure = diastolic blood pressure + 1/3 pulse pressure.
** Although only a modest reduction, these Swedish investigators obtained reductions of 4/2 mm Hg with 25 mg/day and 5/+1 mm Hg with 50 mg/day. These decrements were similar to those found when beta-blocking agents were given to the same 40 patients.

TABLE III
ANTIHYPERTENSIVE EFFECT OF LOW DOSES OF CHLORTHALIDONE

Studies (Ref.)	No. Pts.	Dose (mg/day)	Pre-Treatment Blood Pressure (mm Hg)	Treatment Blood Pressure (mm Hg)	Decline in Blood Pressure (mm Hg)
Korduner et al 1981[11]	23	12.5	183/107	156/94	27/13
Materson et al 1978[12]	20	12.5	145/101	140/97	5/4
Papadoyannis et al 1983[13]	14	12.5	160/104	145/97	15/7
Materson et al 1978[12]	20	25	148/102	133/96	15/6
Tweedale et at 1977[14]	37	25	132*	114*	18*
Carney et al 1976[15]	10	25	168/107	153/98	15/9
SHEP (NIH) Study† 1983[16]	172†	25	170/76†	—	20†
Papadoyannis et al 1983[13]	11	25	160/104	135/92	25/12
Materson et al 1978[12]	17	50	148/103	134/97	14/6
Tweedale et al 1977[14]	37	50	132	111	21*
Bengtsson et al 1975[17]	40	50	165/102	136/90	29/12
Rosenman et al 1975[18]	29	50	185/111	159/100	26/11
Sung et al 1971[19]	9	50	175/105	157/100	18/5

* Mean blood pressure = diastolic blood pressure + 1/3 pulse pressure.
† Systolic Hypertension in the Elderly Program (SHEP) preliminary report. After 3 and 6 months, about 75% of 172 elderly patients with systolic hypertension (> 160/90) achieved goal. Only 34% of patients on placebo achieved goal. See text.

smallest effective dose, because potassium loss is dose-related. There is, on the other hand, good evidence that doses above 50 mg/day of these agents produce little or no added hypotensive effect in most patients. Thus there is little reason to use doses above 50 mg in most patients.

Thiazide therapy has also been criticized recently because of the fear of subtly increasing other risk factors for coronary artery disease, viz, uric acid, triglycerides, cholesterol and glucose. The failure of epidemiologic studies in mild hypertension to demonstrate reduced incidences of coronary artery disease suggests to some authorities that the augmentation of these biochemical abnormalities may obliterate the benefit of blood pressure reduction with long-term thiazide use. Again, it is prudent to employ small doses and also to monitor changes in these laboratory values.

Preliminary results from the Heart Institute's SHEP Study (Systolic Hypertension in the Elderly Program) indicate that 25 mg/day of chlorthalidone effectively reduces systolic hypertension in 75 percent of patients compared with a 34 percent response among placebo-treated patients (see Table II).[16,20] It is noteworthy that over 40,000 age-eligible subjects had to be screened to identify 400 patients (a 1.1% yield) who were actually randomized and entered into Step-1 (diuretic vs. placebo) of the Study by May, 1982. Of 20,723 age-eligibles screened by December 25, 1981, 218 were randomized and placed in Step-I treatment. It appears that systolic hypertension ($> 160/ < 90$ mm Hg) is not a frequent finding among the elderly (> 65 yrs). When identified, however, 25 mg/day of chlorthalidone is highly effective.

When should the physician consider thiazides for hypertension?
1. As initial therapy in most hypertensive patients:[21-27]

In black patients, 70% of whom can be expected to achieve
good control on diuretics alone.

About 50 percent of hypertensive patients can be adequately controlled by a thiazide diuretic alone. This is especially true in black patients, 70% of whom can be expected to achieve good control on diuretics alone.[24-27] It is also particularly true among the elderly who often respond satisfactorily to 12.5 or 25 mg/day of chlorthalidone or hydrochlorothiazide. Most authorities still agree with the Second Joint National Committee on Detection, Evaluation, and Treatment of High Blood Pressure[28] (1975) which recommends a thiazide as the drug of choice for initial therapy for all forms of hypertension except malignant hypertension, azotemic hypertension, or hypertensive crises. Recently, the use of beta-blockers as the drug of choice for hypertension has been debated and studied extensively.[24-27, 29,30] Results of clinical trials comparing beta-blockers and thiazides do not give a clear-cut answer to which is more effective for initial use. Three large, well-controlled studies were done by the Veterans Administration Cooperative Study Group on Antihypertensive Agents addressing this question.[24,25,27] In the study reported in 1983,[27] 68 patients were given 5-10 mg/day of bendroflumethiazide and 104 patients 80-240 mg/day of nadolol. After 12 weeks of therapy, 49% of the patients on nadolol and 42% of the patients on bendroflumethiazide achieved DBP < 90 mm Hg. The DBP fell more on nadolol in whites than blacks, while it fell more on bendroflumethiazide in blacks than whites (Table IV).

The other two V.A. studies done in 1982 tested the efficacy of hydrochlorothiazide 50-100 mg/day versus propranolol 80-640 mg/day. In one study,[25] 343 patients were given hydrochlorothiazide and 340 patients propranolol. There was no significant difference between the two treatments among patients achieving goal DBP (<.90 mm Hg). Fifty-seven percent of those on propranolol and 64.1% of those on hydrochlorothiazide reached goal. Propranolol showed a larger number of white patients reaching goal (61.7% vs. 55.3%), but the difference was not significant. However, there was a significant difference found in blacks achieving goal on hydrochlorothiazide, 71.3% vs. 53.5% on propranolol.

The third V.A. study[24] found similar results, except that the percentage reaching goal on hydrochlorothiazide was significantly greater than those on propranolol (65.5% vs. 52.8%). The results showed a larger drop in systolic and diastolic blood pressure with hydrochlorothiazide; however, the systolic decrement was not statistically significant. Reductions in systolic pressure were greater for whites receiving propranolol than blacks and greater for blacks receiving hydrochlorothiazide than whites, but these racial differences were not statistically significant. Both whites and blacks had larger decreases in diastolic blood pressure with hydrochlorothiazide than with propranolol. However, in whites alone, there was no significant difference in the drop in diastolic pressure between the two drugs.

These studies suggest that the initial drug of choice in most blacks should be a diuretic, probably because of their high incidence of low-renin, expanded-volume hypertension, while the results for whites are

TABLE IV
DIURETIC VS. BETA-BLOCKER IN ANTIHYPERTENSIVE THERAPY:
A COMPARISON OF BLACK VS. WHITE RESPONSES IN MALE VETERANS

	V. A. Coop Study Group, 1983[27]		V. A. Coop Study Group, 1982[25]		V. A. Coop Study Group, 1982[24]	
	Diuretic Bendroflume-thiazide	Beta-Blocker Nadolol	Diuretic Hydrochloro-thiazide	Beta-Blocker Propranolol	Diuretic Hydrochloro-thiazide	Beta-Blocker Propranolol
No. of Patients						
Total	68	104	343	340	177	125
Black	42	61	192	197	95	57
White	36	43	151	143	82	68
Dose (mg/day)	5–10	80–240	50–200	80–640	50–200	80–640
Pre-treatment Blood Pressure						
Total group	146/101	144/101	147/101	146/102	*	*
Black	149/101	145/101	*	*	148/102	141/100
White	144/101	143/102	*	*	146/101	147/103
Post-treatment Blood pressure						
Total group	129/89	134/89	129/89	135/91	*	*
Black	130/89	139/91	*	*	128/88	136/89
White	131/91	126/86	*	*	131/89	137/91
Decline in blood pressure						
Total group	17/12	10/12	18/12	11/11	18/13	8/11
Black	19/12	6/10	20/13	8/10	20/14	5/11
White	13/10	17/16	15/11	13/13	15/12	10/12

* Information not available.

not so clear. When treating whites, age should also be considered. Young white patients with hyperkinetic hypertension should ordinarily be started on a beta-blocker, while low-dose diuretic therapy is often effective in the elderly.

2. *As part of virtually all combined antihypertensive regimens:*

A thiazide diuretic should be included in virtually all multiple drug antihypertensive regimens.

Unless specifically contraindicated, a thiazide diuretic should be included in virtually all multiple drug antihypertensive regimens because they augment the action of other antihypertensive drugs and prevent the development of tolerance to adrenergic and vasodilator drugs.[21,31,32] This frequently allows control of blood pressure with lower doses of the non-diuretic antihypertensive agents, whatever its class or mechanism of action.

Thiazides, as compared to many of the non-diuretic antihypertensives, have a relatively low incidence of subjective side effects severe enough to require discontinuation of therapy or to cause the patient to be non-compliant.

How effective are thiazides in essential hypertension?

1. A thiazide as the only drug:

Innumerable investigators have studied the antihypertensive activity of the thiazide and thiazide-like diuretics and have found them to be effective agents in the treatment of hypertension. In the studies listed in Tables II and III, a total of 525 patients were treated with low doses of a thiazide or a thiazide-like drug. The overall decrease in blood pressure caused by these agents used singly in 409 patients was 19/10 mm Hg, and the overall decrease in mean arterial pressure seen in 116 patients was 17 mm Hg. These drugs are not only more effective in blacks than in white hypertensives, but black patients also respond to lower doses.[25]

2. Thiazides as part of combination therapy:

The combination of a non-diuretic antihypertensive drug with a diuretic has been demonstrated to cause a larger decrease in blood pressure than that caused by either of the drugs alone. In several studies (Table V), 404 patients had a thiazide-type diuretic added to their previous antihypertensive therapy. An average further decrease in mean arterial blood pressure in 28 patients was 14 mm Hg, and in 376 patients

TABLE V
EFFECTS OF THIAZIDES IN COMBINATION THERAPY

Study (Ref.)	No. of Patients	First Drug	Dose (mg/day)	Blood Pressure on First Drug (mm Hg)	Thiazide†	Dose (mg/day)	Blood Pressure on Combination (mm Hg)	Amount of Decrease (mm Hg)
MacGregor et al 1982[33]	16	Captopril	450	129*	HCTZ	25	114	15
Andren et al 1982[34]	27	Captopril**	75-300	151/98	HCTZ	25-50	132/87	19/11
Pitkajarvi et al 1977[35]	12	Prazosin	3-6	151/98	HCTZ	25	145/93	6/5
Smith et al 1966[36]	60	Methyldopa	500-3000	—	CTZ	100-600	—	25/14
Mroczek et al 1972[37]	41	Methyldopa	450	163/107	CTDN	50-100	146/96	18/11
	41	Clonidine	0.45	163/107	CTDN	50-100	143/92	20/15
Igloe et al 1973[38]	40	Clonidine	0.2-0.6	171/101	CTDN	30-45	165/95	6/4
Lavenius et al 1982[39]	10	Metoprolol	100	157/100	HCTZ	12.5	150/98	7/2
	10	Metoprolol	100	157/100	HCTZ	25	143/95	14/5
	10	Metoprolol	100	157/100	HCTZ	50	143/94	14/1
Kubik et al 1978[40]	45	Metoprolol	200	173/98	CTDN	50	153/89	20/9
Weber et al 1977[41]	59	Propranolol	80-320	158/105	CTDN	50-100	140/90	18/15
Vander Elst et al 1981[42]	21	Propranolol	60-120	164/97	HCTZ	25-50	152/93	12/4
Velasco et al 1980[43]	12	Atenolol	100	119*	CTDN	50	106	13

* Mean blood pressure = diastolic + 1/3 pulse pressure.
** Six patients were on captopril alone.
† HCTZ = hydrochlorothiazide; CTDN = chlorthalidone; CTZ = chlorothiazide.

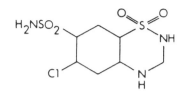

HYDROCHLOROTHIAZIDE

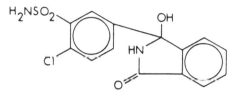

CHLORTHALIDONE

Figure 1: Thiazides and thiazide-like diuretics.

an average further decrease in blood pressure was 15/8 mm Hg. In addition to their causing additional decreases in blood pressure, the thiazides are an important part of combination therapy because they often allow dose reduction of the non-diuretic antihypertensive drugs.

Indications for Thiazides

— Hypertension
— Edema associated with congestive heart failure, hepatic cirrhosis, and corticosteroid or estrogen therapy

Formulations

Hydrochlorothiazide:	Tablets...25, 50 and 100 mg
Chlorthalidone:	Tablets...25, 50 and 100 mg
Metolazone:	Tablets...2.5, 5 and 10 mg

Hydrochlorothiazide Dosage

Frequency: once or twice daily
Initial: 12.5, 25 or 50 mg/day in a single dose
Range: 12.5–100 mg/day. To minimize biochemical abnormalities, use the smallest effective dose. Little additional effect in blood pressure reduction is found with doses larger than 50 mg/day.

Usual dose: 25–50 mg once daily or 25 mg twice daily for most adults. (Maintenance dose may be increased or decreased according to need.) Geriatric and black patients are often well maintained on 12.5 to 25 mg once daily.

Chlorthalidone Dosage

Frequency: once daily
Initial: 12.5 or 25 mg once daily
Range: 12.5–100 mg/day. To minimize biochemical abnormalities, use the smallest effective dose. Little additional effect on blood pressure is found with doses larger than 50 mg/day.
Usual dose: 25 mg once daily. (Maintenance dose may be decreased or increased according to need.)

Metolazone Dosage

Frequency: once daily
Initial: 2.5–5 mg once daily
Range: 2.5–10 mg/day. To minimize biochemical abnormalities, use the smallest effective dose. Ordinarily give no more than 10 mg/day.
Usual dose: 2.5–5 mg once daily. Dosage adjustment is usually necessary.

The recommended doses of chlorthalidone and hydrochlorothiazide are 25 mg once daily and 25–50 mg once daily, respectively. However, there is growing evidence that 12.5 mg is effective in some patients and should be tried initially in black patients and the elderly.[1,2, 11,12]

(Hydrochlorothiazide is used as a prototype below.)

Mechanism of Action

The thiazides work as diuretics and as antihypertensives. They affect the renal tubular mechanism of electrolyte reabsorption. All thiazides work in the cortical portion of the ascending tubule and at the beginning of the distal convoluted tubule, where under 10% of the filtered sodium load is reabsorbed, and so lead to the excretion of only 5–10% of this sodium load. The thiazides are equally effective in equivalent doses, but their duration of action differs. The action of most thiazides is complete within 10–12 hours.[44]

Hydrochlorothiazide increases excretion of sodium and chloride in approximately equivalent amounts. The natriuresis causes a secondary loss of potassium and bicarbonate.

Onset of the diuretic action of hydrochlorothiazide after oral use occurs in two hours and the peak action in about four hours. The diuretic activity lasts about 6–12 hours. The drug is then eliminated rapidly by the kidney unchanged.

The mechanism of the antihypertensive effect of thiazides is not clear and is a topic of great discussion. The antihypertensive effect has been attributed to:

(a) plasma volume and extracellular fluid contraction.[44-51] This is dependent upon the production of a sufficient loss of body sodium and water to deplete the extracellular fluid volume including the plasma of several liters of fluid. This reduction occurs within the first 48 hrs. of continuous effective treatment; then compensatory mechanisms are triggered to prevent any further loss of extracellular fluid.[52]

(b) sodium imbalance,[49]

(c) decreased receptor sensitivity to vasopressor substances, such as angiotensin,[53,54]

(d) direct arteriolar dilation,[49,55]

(e) decreased total peripheral resistance,[4-46,56] and

(f) possibly due to an effect on prostaglandin synthesis.[44]

Many studies have shown that the short- and long-term hemodynamic effects of thiazides are different, and there are many theories proposed to explain them.[21,45-48, 56,57] One of these theories, postulated by Tobian,[58,59] and supported by work done by Shah et al,[21] deals with what Tobian called "reverse autoregulation." Thiazides induce a reduction in extracellular fluid (ECF) which produces initially a fall in central venous pressure, venous return, and cardiac output, and there is associated with this an increase in total peripheral resistance. However, with continued treatment and maintained reduction in cardiac output and total blood flow, autoregulation occurs gradually over a period of weeks leading to a decline in total peripheral resistance. Shah et al further suggest that the resulting fall in afterload permits a rise in cardiac output toward normal. This sequence of hemodynamic events is the same as that observed by Shah et al, and it appears that they follow from a single hemodynamic effect of the thiazides, which is sustained reduction in ECF. Due to this, they feel there is no need for the theory of direct vasodilator action of the thiazides because the early fall and later return of cardiac output to normal and the early rise and later fall in total peripheral resistance can both be explained by the reduction in ECF alone.[21] Other authors feel that the direct vasodilator theory is improbable, too, mostly because the thiazides do not cause blood pressure to fall in normotensive subjects.[46,47]

Drug Interactions

1. Plus *Other Antihypertensive Drugs*

Thiazides add to or potentiate the action of all other antihypertensive drugs.

2. Plus *Lithium*[28-30,60,61]

Lithium generally should not be given with diuretics because they reduce lithium clearance and add to the risk of lithium toxicity. Lithium–thiazide treatment can be used if necessary by following the lithium levels in the plasma, alerting the patient to early indications of lithium toxicity, and making the patient aware of the importance of compliance in taking their diuretic medications. Read circulars for lithium preparations before use of such concomitant therapy.

3. Plus *Potassium Supplements*

Hypokalemia may be avoided or treated by use of potassium chloride liquid supplements or microencapsulated potassium chloride occasionally with foods having a high potassium content or by giving potassium-retaining drugs.

4. Plus *Insulin*

Insulin requirements in diabetic patients may be increased by thiazide use. Diabetes mellitus which has been latent may become manifest during thiazide administration.

5. Plus *Surgical Skeletal Muscle Relaxants*[62]

Thiazides potentiate the response of skeletal muscle relaxants used in surgery: tubocurarine, gallamine, and succinylcholine.

6. Plus *Digitalis*[63,64]

Hypokalemia induced by thiazide therapy predisposes to digitalis toxicity. Magnesium depletion may also have some effect in predisposing to digitalis toxicity and cardiac arrhythmias.

7. Plus *Oral Anticoagulants (Warfarin)*[65-70]

Thiazides decrease the hypoprothrombinemic response to oral

anticoagulants and may precipitate a bleeding diathesis when withdrawn.

8. Plus *Diazoxide*[71-73]

The hyperglycemic activity of the thiazides is potentiated by the concomitant administration of diazoxide.

9. Plus *Catecholamines*[74,75]

The vascular response to norepinephrine is decreased by thiazides and may cause resistance to catecholamine pressor agents used to treat hypotension. This does not preclude the effectiveness of the pressor agents but does require that larger doses be used. Arrhythmias may result from catecholamine administration as cardiac sensitivity to catecholamines is increased by thiazide-induced hypokalemia.

10. Plus *Corticosteroids*[76]

The potassium losing qualities of steroids may potentiate the potassium wasting qualities of the thiazides resulting in severe potassium depletion.

11. Plus *Cation-Exchange Resins*[77,78]

Colestipol may decrease absorption of thiazides if administered within one hour after the thiazide. Cholestyramine seems to have less effect on thiazide absorption.

12. Plus *Fenfluramine*

In a study done by Lake et al[79] in 1980, nine obese patients whose hypertension was not controlled by hydrochlorothiazide alone were given fenfluramine, an anorectic, in addition to the thiazide. In two weeks their blood pressures were seen to decrease by an average of 16/12 mm Hg. The mode of action was not determined.

13. Plus *Anti-inflammatory Drugs*

Steiress et al,[80] in 1982, reported thiazide treatment of ten hypertensives being attenuated by indomethacin and enhanced by sulindac. They suggest the difference was related to the different effects each drug has on renal prostoglandins.

Contraindications

— Anuria
— Hypersensitivity

Warnings

● *In Patients with Severe Renal Disease:*

Hydrochlorothiazides should be used with caution in severe renal disease. In patients with renal disease, thiazides may precipitate azotemia. Cumulative effects of the drug may develop in patients with impaired renal function. In severe renal failure, the thiazides may become ineffective because their diuretic activity begins to decline with reduced glomerular filtration rates and essentially stops when the GFR reaches approximately 20 ml/ min.[52]

● *In Patients with Impaired Hepatic Function or Progressive Liver Disease:*

Thiazides should be used with caution in patients with impaired hepatic function or progressive liver disease since minor alterations of fluid and electrolyte balance may precipitate hepatic coma.

● *In Patients with Allergies or Bronchial Asthma:*

Sensitivity reactions may occur in patients with or without a history of allergy or bronchial asthma.

● *In Patients on Other Antihypertensive Therapy:*

Thiazides may add to or potentiate the action of other antihypertensive drugs. Potentiation occurs with ganglionic or peripheral adrenergic blocking drugs.

● *In Patients with Systemic Lupus Erythematosus:*

The possibility of exacerbation or activation of systemic lupus erythematosus has been reported.

● *In Patients on Lithium Preparations:*

Lithium generally should not be given with diuretics because they reduce its renal clearance and add a high risk of lithium toxicity. Read circulars for lithium preparations before use of such concomitant therapy.

Use in Pregnancy

Routine use of diuretics during normal pregnancy is inappropriate and exposes mother and fetus to unnecessary hazard. Diuretics do not prevent development of toxemia of pregnancy, and there is no satisfactory evidence that they are useful in the treatment of toxemia.[58]

Edema during pregnancy may arise from pathologic causes or from the physiologic and mechanical consequences of pregnancy. Thiazides are indicated in pregnancy only when edema or other conditions requiring their use is due to pathologic causes, just as they are in the absence of pregnancy.

Dependent edema in pregnancy, resulting from restriction of venous return by the gravid uterus, is properly treated through elevation of the lower extremities and use of support stockings. Use of diuretics to lower intravascular volume in this instance is inappropriate. During normal pregnancy there is hypervolemia which is not harmful to the fetus or the mother in the absence of cardiovascular disease. However, it may be associated with edema and, rarely, generalized edema. If such edema causes discomfort, increased recumbency will often provide relief. Rarely this edema may cause extreme discomfort which is not relieved by rest. In these instances, a short course of diuretics may provide relief and may be appropriate. Thiazides cross the placental barrier and appear in cord blood. The use of thiazides in pregnancy requires that the anticipated benefit be weighed against the possible hazards to the fetus. These hazards include fetal or neonatal jaundice, thrombocytopenia, and possibly other adverse reactions which have occurred in the adult.

Kraus et al,[81] in a double-blind randomized trial with 1,030 pregnant women, found no adverse effects on the fetuses or infants due to the administration of 50 mg/day of hydrochlorothiazide. This view is supported by some researchers[82] while others feel that: (a) the administration of thiazides during pregnancy decreases the vascular volume and placental perfusion,[83] (b) is associated with an increased incidence of thiazide-induced pancreatitis,[84-86] (c) is deleterious to the fetus, and (d) diuretic therapy should be reserved for treatment of left ventricular heart failure associated with preeclampsia.[87]

Thiazides appear in breast milk. If use of the drug is deemed essential, the patient should stop nursing.

Efficacy in Blacks

It has been established that there are different responses to diuretics noted when black hypertensives are compared with white. Due to this, racial differences should be considered when determining therapy.[88] Many studies have been done to determine the drug of first choice in black hypertensives.[23-25,89] Moser et al (1981),[23] Seedat (1980),[90] and two studies done by the Veterans Administration Cooperative Study Group on Antihypertensive Agents[24,25] done in 1982 conclude that although effective in both races, the thiazide diuretics are more effective than beta-blockers. Not only do more black patients achieve good control than white patients, but they also respond to lower doses. A dose of 12.5 mg/day of either hydrochlorothiazide or chlorthalidone should be the initial dose in blacks, and the majority will respond to this dose. In the studies cited in Table VI, a total of 352 black hypertensives were treated with thiazides and an average decrease of 23/12 mm Hg was found.

Use in Children and Adolescents

The Task Force on Blood Pressure Control in Children appointed by the National Heart, Lung and Blood Institute reported in 1977 that "only children who manifest persistent hypertension, documented by multiple observations, should be considered for initiation of treatment."[91] They stated that drugs are not always called for, but when used, thiazide diuretics are usually the initial drug used. They suggest a "stepped-care" titration approach, beginning with low doses and working slowly to therapeutic level. Sometimes other drugs are needed, but the Task Force emphasized that when adrenergic drugs or direct vasodilators (those drugs which produce fluid accumulation) are used, it is advisable to use a diuretic concurrently.

However, Falkner et al[92] treated 15 adolescents who had sustained hypertension and had not responded to non-drug treatment with 50–100 mg/day of hydrochlorothiazide and reported only a 40% satisfactory response to the diuretic therapy.

Use in the Elderly

Whether or not to treat hypertension in the elderly is a topic still debated,[93] but most authorities prefer to treat most elderly hypertensives. Thiazides are presently the preferable drug, but calcium channel blockers like nifedipine are becoming popular with many clinicians. In 1981 Forrest[94] gave ciclopenthiazide, 0.25–0.50 mg daily, to a total of 206 patients with a mean age of 65 and found an average decrease in the blood pressure of 15/10 mm Hg. In another study of 389 patients over age 65, Goodfellow et al[95] found that the fixed combination of hydrochlorothiazide (12.5 mg) and metaprolol (100 mg) once daily gave an average decrease in blood pressure of 28/17 mm Hg.

Twenty-five mg/day of hydrochlorothiazide effectively reduces systolic hypertension in 75% of elderly patients.[16,20] Initial doses of only 12.5 mg/day should be given to elderly patients because they are indeed

TABLE VI
THE ANTIHYPERTENSIVE EFFECTS OF THIAZIDES IN BLACK HYPERTENSIVES

Studies (Ref.)	No. Patients	Drug	Dose (mg/day)	Pre-treatment Blood Pressure (mm Hg)	Post-treatment Blood Pressure (mm Hg)	Amount of Decrease (mm Hg)
Moser et al 1981[23]	17	Hydrochlorothiazide	50–150	157/106	128/91	29/15
Moser et al 1982[89]	8	Hydrochlorothiazide	50–100	166/111	134/92	32/19
V. A. Cooperative Study 1982[25]	192	Hydrochlorothiazide	50–200*			20/13
V. A. Cooperative Study 1982[24]	95	Hydrochlorothiazide	50–200	148/1C2	128/88	20/14
Holland et al 1979[86]	16	Hydrochlorothiazide	100	170/112	140/95	30/17
Seedat et al 1980[90]	24	Chlorthalidone	25	159/103	153/96	6/7

* 65% given 50 mg/day.

more sensitive to the effects of most drugs and because it will be an effective dose in many such patients.

Precautions

Periodic determination of serum potassium to detect possible deficiency should be performed at appropriate intervals.

All patients receiving thiazide therapy should be observed for clinical signs of fluid or electrolyte imbalance, namely hyponatremia, hypochloremic alkalosis, and hypokalemia. Serum and urine electrolyte determinations are particularly important when the patient is vomiting excessively or receiving parenteral fluids. Medications such as digitalis may also influence serum electrolytes. Warning signs, irrespective of cause, are: dryness of mouth, thirst, weakness, lethargy, drowsiness, restlessness, muscle pains or cramps, muscular fatigue, hypotension, oliguria, tachycardia, and gastrointestinal disturbances such as nausea and vomiting.

Hypokalemia may develop, especially with diuresis, when severe cirrhosis is present, during concomitant use of corticosteroids or ACTH, or after prolonged therapy with the thiazides.

Interference with adequate oral electrolyte intake will also contribute to hypokalemia. Hypokalemia can sensitize or exaggerate the response of the heart to the toxic effects of digitalis (e.g., increased ventricular irritability and arrhythmias).

Hypokalemia may be avoided or treated by the use of potassium supplements such as food with a high potassium content, liquid KCl, or micronized KCl.

Any chloride deficit is generally mild and usually does not require specific treatment except under extraordinary circumstances (as in liver disease or renal disease). Dilutional hyponatremia may occur in edematous patients in hot weather; appropriate therapy is water restriction rather than administration of salt, except in rare instances when the hyponatremia is life-threatening. In actual salt depletion, appropriate replacement is the therapy of choice.

Hyperuricemia may occur or frank gout may be precipitated in certain patients receiving thiazide therapy.

Insulin requirements in diabetic patients may be increased. Diabetes mellitus, which has been latent, may become manifest during thiazide administration.

Thiazide drugs may increase the responsiveness to tubocurarine.

The antihypertensive effects of the drug may be enhanced in he post-sympathectomy patient. Thiazides may decrease arterial responsiveness to norepinephrine. This diminution is not sufficient to preclude effectiveness of the pressor agent for therapeutic use.

If progressive renal impairment becomes evident, consider withholding or discontinuing thiazide therapy.

Thiazides may decrease serum PBI levels without signs of thyroid disturbance.

Calcium excretion is decreased by thiazides. Pathologic changes in the parathyroid glands with hypercalcemia and hypophosphatemia have been observed in a few patients on prolonged thiazide therapy. The common complications of hyperparathyroidism such as renal lithiasis, bone resorption, and peptic ulceration have not been seen. Thiazides should be discontinued before carrying out tests for parathyroid function.

Management of Overdose or Exaggerated Response

No specific antidotes exist. Gastric lavage, parenteral electrolytes and fluids, and general supportive measures are indicated.

Absorption, Distribution, Metabolism and Excretion[1, 96-100]

In general, thiazides are well absorbed from the gastrointestinal tract and so can be administered orally. However, the various thiazides are absorbed to different extents; hydrochlorothiazide is well absorbed while chlorothiazide is poorly absorbed. Beermann et al,[96] in 1978, gave 75 mg of hydrochlorothiazide to eight healthy volunteers without or together with a standardized meal. They found that there was a significantly greater absorption with meals (75%) vs. empty stomach (63%).

All of the thiazide diuretics are excreted by the kidneys and appear in the urine unmetabolized. Only minute quantities are excreted in the bile. The excretion rates vary also, with the excretion of hydrochlorothiazide being 33–58% complete in 24 hours and chlorthalidone 50% complete in 54 hours. The slow excretion of chlorthalidone is due to its being 90% bound to or in red blood cells while the other drugs seem to be evenly distributed throughout the body. All thiazides are concentrated in the kidneys as they are excreted.

Beermann et al[97] administered hydrochlorothiazide at four different doses (12.5, 25, 50 and 75 mg) to eight healthy volunteers to study the pharmacokinetics. They found that the peak plasma levels were highly correlated (p <0.001) with the dose of hydrochlorothiazide given, but that the mean renal plasma clearance did not vary with the dose. The diuresis after 12.5 mg exceeded that after placebo by a mean of 800 ml and the diuresis was not seen to increase further with the higher doses. The maximal natriuretic effect was also found after the 12.5 mg dose. The excretion of potassium, however, rose with increasing doses, with the maximal increment seen at the largest dose given, 75 mg. The excretion of calcium ions was significantly increased after 50 mg, while the maximal effect on magnesium excretion occurred after 25 mg. There was found to be no correlation between the peak plasma level of hydrochlorothiazide and the renal excretion of water and electrolytes. In a later study, by Beermann et al,[1] no relation was found between plasma concentration and reduction in blood pressure and/or decreasing plasma volume.

In renal disease, thiazides should be given with caution, if at all, and generally at reduced doses, since blood drug levels can be expected to be elevated and, therefore, the biological effects of the drug will be potentiated. In addition, they elevate creatinine per se by decreasing renal function.

In hepatic disease, the half-life of these drugs is essentially unaltered. However, caution must be exerted because of the possibility of precipitating hepatic coma with even minor electrolyte changes.

Adverse Reactions

Thiazide diuretics are used often in the treatment of essential hypertension either singly or in combination. They are useful because they are efficacious, relatively safe, and well-tolerated. The more common side effects of the thiazides (Table VII) are either extensions of their pharmacological properties or mild, often subjective, symptomatology. Those side effects due to the pharmacologic properties of the thiazides can be prevented by appropriate monitoring and prophylaxis; the other common reactions are usually transient or can be controlled by titrating the dosage and by more careful attention to concomitant medications and/or conditions. Adverse reactions severe enough to require the discontinuation of therapy do occur but are relatively rare. If an allergic rash develops to thiazide use, a different class of diuretic should be attempted (e.g., metolazone, furosemide, etc.).

In a cooperative study by Boston area hospitals, Miller[101] found, in 7,017 hospital admissions, there were 260 due to drug reactions (3.7% of

TABLE VII
THE INCIDENCE OF SUBJECTIVE SIDE EFFECTS FROM
LOW DOSE DIURETICS*
(AMONG 346 PATIENTS)

Side Effect†	Total No. of Patients Exhibiting Side Effect	Percent Incidence
Dizziness	25	7.2
Tiredness	21	6.1
Dryness of mouth	17	4.9
Cramps	13	3.7
I leadache	12	3.5
Nausea	12	3.5
Indigestion	9	2.6
Increased dreaming	9	2.6
Constipation	9	2.6
Sleep disturbance	8	2.3
Increased frequency of urination	7	2.0
Nervousness	7	2.0
Abdominal gas	7	2.0
Perspiration	5	1.4
Shortness of breath	5	1.4
Impotence	4	1.2
Decreased appetite	4	1.2
Weakness	4	1.2
Numbness of extremities	4	1.2
Sedation	3	0.9
Palpitations	2	0.6
Rash	2	0.6
Orthostatic hypotension	2	0.6
Change in defecation	2	0.6

* See references 5, 12, 14, 28, 102–106. Some references on the Tables on Antihypertensive Effects on Low Dose Diuretics were not used because: 1) they had no subjective side effects reported, 2) they did not ask about subjective side effects, or 3) exact numbers were not given. 75 mg was highest dosage used of hydrochlorothiazide and/or chlorthalidone. Drugs used to calculate table: hydrochlorothiazide, chlorthalidone, cyclothiazide, chlorothiazide, bendroflumethiazide, metolazone.

† Endogenous depression, lightheadness, joint stiffness, nocturia, vomiting, bronchitis, eye infection, back pain, tinnitus, pain in legs, diarrhea, chest pain, cold extremities, abdominal cramps were all seen once each (0.28%).

the total number of admissions) of which only six were due to thiazide reactions (2% of drug reactions, 0.09% of all admissions). In light of the large number of patients receiving thiazides, this clearly demonstrated the usual safety of the thiazides.

The Nature of Thiazide Reactions
A. Pharmacological (Figure 2)

1. Hypokalemia

Hypokalemia is the most common side effect of treatment with thiazides.[44,107] The volume depletion induced by thiazides leads to the production of renin and aldosterone which causes sodium to be selectively reabsorbed and potassium excreted. The hypokalemia is a direct result of this potassium excretion.[52] Some decrease in serum potassium levels is detected in almost all patients,[44] unless dietary or drug means

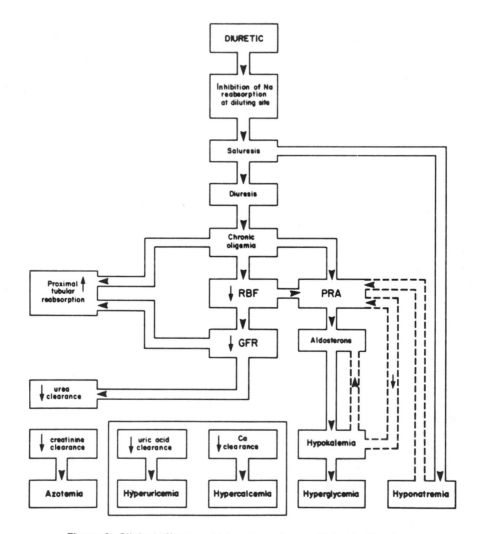

Figure 2: Clinical effects and laboratory effects of thiazide diuretics.

are used to prevent it. In a collection of studies where 215 patients were treated with 50 mg/day doses of chlorthalidone (taken from Table VIII), an average decrease of 0.4 mEq/L was noted. Only one of these 13 studies showed an average decrease below 3.5 mEq/L.

Most researchers have felt that the hypokalemia is asymptomatic unless it falls below 3.5 mEq/L, and that it is not considered severe unless it is below 3.0 mEq/L.[44,108] But today we are concerned that arrhythmias might occur with serum levels below 3.5 mEq/L. Recent studies by the British Medical Research Council, Hollifield, Caralais, Holland and others indicate that ectopic ventricular activity occurs in relation to the decline in serum potassium (see p. 109). Because of this potential risk, serum potassium levels should be monitored regularly and, when below 3.5 mEq/L, should be treated. Symptoms that may develop with continued hypokalemia are listed in Table IX.

Hypokalemia causes increased myocardial irritability to catecholamines[44,74,75] and sensitivity to digitalis[63,64,114] which may result in serious or even fatal arrhythmias. Severe potassium depletion has also been associated with causing interference with renal tubular function and impairment of glucose tolerance. When most severe, it deters the contraction of skeletal muscle.[114] Potassium deficiency has also been linked to deterioration in consciousness in patients with severe liver disease.[114] Therefore, the serum potassium of all patients on thiazides, especially those receiving digitalis or corticosteroids, must be carefully monitored and appropriate dietary changes or supplementary potassium chloride instituted for the early detection and/or prevention of the development of hypokalemia. (See Chapter IV on potassium supplements and Chapter V on potassium-sparing agents.)

Effects of Diuretics on Total Body Potassium (TBK)

Thiazide diuretics are commonly used as the sole agent or in combination with other antihypertensive agents in the long-term management of hypertension. A statistically significant mean reduction in the level of serum potassium is the usual laboratory finding after thiazides (Table VIII). The question clinicians have debated for over two decades is whether or not this reduction is clinically significant and needs replacement. One must be particularly alert to the possibility of ventricular extrasystoles or more severe arrhythmias resulting from hypokalemia which are more often associated with the higher doses of thiazides.

The usual clinical method for diagnosing potassium deficiency is

TABLE VIII

SERUM POTASSIUM AND TOTAL BODY POTASSIUM CHANGES AFTER LOW DOSE DIURETIC THERAPY

Ref.	Drug	Dose (mg/day)	No. of Patients	Duration of Therapy (wks)	Serum Potassium (mEq/L) Before	After	Decline	P Value	Total Body K40 (MEq/L) Before	After	Decline	P Value
Materson et al 1978[12]	Chlorthalidone	12.5	20	12	4.2	3.9	0.3	NS				
Carney et al 1976[15]	Chlorthalidone	25	10	4	4.1	3.9	0.2	< 0.001	†	†	†	NS
Materson et al 1978[12]	Chlorthalidone	25	20	12	4.4	4.0	0.4	< 0.05				
Tweedale et al 1977[14]	Chlorthalidone	25	37	8	†	†	0.4	< 0.05				
Durley et al 1981[3]	Hydrochlorothiazide	25	6	12	4.0	3.6	0.4	< 0.05				
Degnbol et al 1973[4]	Hydrochlorothiazide	25	22	6	4.2	3.7	0.5	< 0.001				
Materson et al 1978[12]	Chlorthalidone	50	18	12	4.4	3.7	0.7	< 0.05				
Degnbol et al 1973[4]	Hydrochlorothiazide	50	22	6	4.2	3.6	0.6	< 0.01				
Hollifield et al 1981[111]	Hydrochlorothiazide	50	38	4	4.5	3.9	0.6	< 0.001	4107	3722	385	††
Winchester et al 1980[102]	Metolazone	5	6	6	3.9	3.5	0.4	< 0.05	109**	107**	2	NS
	Metolazone	5	5	6	4.0	3.3	0.7	< 0.05	122**	111**	11	NS
	Bendroflumethiazide	5	6	6	3.9	3.5	0.4	< 0.05	109**	105**	4	NS
		5	5	6	4.0	3.8	0.2	< 0.05	122**	129**	7	NS
Healy et al 1970[112]	Furosemide	80	9	14	†	†	0.6	< 0.001				
Oh et al 1980[113]	Chlorothiazide	1000	7	12–16	4.0	3.6	0.4	†	2315	2296	19	††

* Those studies with furosemide and chlorothiazide are not low dose.
** Grams.
† Information not given.
†† Mathematically significant but not clinically (P value not given).

TABLE IX
SYMPTOMS OF CLINICALLY IMPORTANT HYPOKALEMIA*

- muscle weakness, lethargy and easy muscle fatigue
- nocturia
- muscle cramps
- bilateral calf pain
- paresthesias in the extremities
- palpitations
- loss of libido
- mental depression

---

* References: Ram, 1962,[109] Cannon et al, 1978,[110] and Sherrill et al, 1981[107]

by measuring serum potassium concentration, a very convenient but rather poor reflection of actual potassium balance.[115-117] The healthy adult body contains about 55 mEq/Kg of body weight (3,500–4,000 mEq) with the vast majority (95–98%) of it being intracellular.[114] About 2–5% is the extracellular component of which only 0.4% is in the plasma.[118] Important therapeutic (and diagnostic) decisions are based on serum levels which represent less than one-half of one percent of the total potassium pool. Total exchangeable potassium (K^{42}) involves radiation exposure, is time consuming, and is not as accurate as whole body potassium measurements which involve counting the naturally endogenous isotope, K^{40}.[116-119] Studies using K^{42} give values about 15% lower than K^{40}.[114] New methods of measuring potassium levels are being investigated, including determining red cell and muscle cell potassium content.[114]

When 50–100 mg/day doses of hydrochlorothiazide or chlorthalidone therapy are given, hypertensive patients' potassium levels fall promptly within a week. They often reach a nadir after 2–4 weeks. Thereafter, they generally remain quite stable for many months or years, at least in patients whose disease, diet and treatment regimens are relatively stable.[115-117] The majority of hypertensive patients in this situation maintain potassium levels > 3.5 mEq/L. They usually do not require either potassium-sparing drugs or potassium supplements since they are obtaining sufficient potassium from their diet, and they are retaining enough via their renal tubular sodium-potassium exchange mechanisms mediated by endogenous aldosterone. The controversy and clinical dilemma arise with those patients who do not eat an adequate diet (see Chapter II), who use excessive amounts of table salt and who may have additional risk factors (from being on digitalis preparations or corticosteroids, etc.) regarding need for potassium supplements. Cardiac toxicity of digitalis is potentiated by low intracellular potassium, whereas corticoids, being catabolic, enhance potassium loss per se. Treatment should start when a patient has values of 3.5 mEq/L, or less. In the past we felt that the majority of these patients did not require treatment.[52,108,109,120] But because an increased frequency of ectopic ventricular beats is now recognized to occur in those patients with potassium levels less than 3.5 mEq/L (see page 109), it is prudent to treat with potassium supplementation (or potassium-sparing drugs) those patients whose levels fall below 3.5 mEq/L.

Seven studies with WBK[40] counting (see Table VIII) indicate that body stores and, therefore, intracellular potassium are not sufficiently reduced to produce toxicity or warrant replacement. Nevertheless, the risk of cardiac arrhythmias appears to supercede the intracellular levels. Some steps that can be taken before using potassium supplements or potassium-sparing diuretics are:

1. use lowest dosage possible to get the desired response;[109,121]

2. change in diuretic therapy. If the patient is on long-acting diuretics (e.g., chlorthalidone), change them to an intermediate-acting diuretic because the longer-acting drugs increase the potassium loss;[44,107-109,114]

3. restrict sodium intake;[109] and,

4. increase dietary potassium intake[122] (bananas, orange juice, proteins, etc.).

When should the physician consider adding either potassium-sparing agents or potassium salts to the regimen of a hypertensive patient who is receiving diuretics?

1. *Prophylactically*, in patients who might be susceptible to potassium depletion for one or more of these reasons:

   — Secondary to co-administration of digitalis or corticosteroids with diuretics

   — Secondary to poor potassium dietary intake and/or excessive salt ingestion

   — Historically, by previous episodes of documented levels under 3.5 mEq/L (rule out primary aldosteronism)

   — Diuretic-treated patients who may become refractory because of secondary hyperaldosteronism

2. *Therapeutically*, when serum potassium is < 3.5 mEq/L, potassium chloride may be administered as either liquid or microencapsulated KCl.

The wax–matrix preparations cause an unacceptable increased risk of upper gastrointestinal lesions[123-125] (see Chapter IV). The fixed dose combinations that contain a thiazide and a potassium-sparing diuretic have become popular because they increase compliance, are effective and convenient.[52,109] The risks of hyperkalemia, e.g., cardiac arrest, should always be considered before administering potassium supplements or potassium-sparing diuretics.[110,114] Additionally, diabetics, the elderly and patients with poor renal function are at risk when KCl supplements or potassium-sparing agents are given.

Table VIII summarizes seven controlled whole-body potassium (WBK) studies found in the medical literature, ranging from 1976–1981. The technique is not generally available since it involves an expensive, highly sensitive, whole-body counter.[114] Uniquely safe, it measures a naturally occurring isotope in man, K^{40}. The counting error is less than 2.5%.[126] A 5.8% variation is reported in the WBK counts of healthy untreated individuals. The technique may involve 800 seconds' counting, comparing each subject with a reference standard of K^{40} with background activity deducted.[117]

Several generalizations are apparent from the review of these seven studies:

- Thiazides *generally* do produce statistically significant decreases in serum potassium values but not clinically significant decreases.
- Of the seven studies in which WBK was measured before and after diuretics, five showed no mathematically significant fall of WBK. The other two studies showed decreases of 0.8% and 9% which are mathematically, but not clinically, significant.
- While some believe a decrease of 1.0 mEq/L in serum potassium level is approximately equivalent to a decrease of WBK of 10%, others have found no correlation between the plasma potassium levels and the WBK.[44,113] Indeed, the recent evidence that serious arrhythmias do occur in some patients with low-normal serum potassium levels supports this lack of correlation.[111,127-129]
- Differences in dosage, how long therapy is administered, intake of sodium chloride, intake of potassium and problems with the

methods used to measure WBK make interpretation of the data difficult.[114]

2. Hyperuricemia

The uric acid retaining properties of thiazide diuretics are being investigated more thoroughly with the advent of the new uricosuric diuretics (see Indacrinone, Chapter XIV). Hyperuricemia is defined as serum uric acid levels greater than 7.0 mg/dl in males and postmenopausal females and greater than 6.0 mg/dl in premenopausal females. It has been reported that 25–35% of all untreated essential hypertensives have hyperuricemia.[109,110] Furthermore, 50% of patients treated with benzothiadiazine diuretics have elevated serum uric acid levels (above 7.0 mg/dl) due to competitive inhibition of tubular secretion of uric acid.[130] In hypertensive patients with cardiovascular disease and on chronic thiazide treatment, the incidence is still higher.[52,110,131] Some researchers feel that dosage is not related to the thiazide-induced hyperuricemia,[110] while most agree it is dose-dependent.[106,132] Bengtsson[17] found that treatment with doses of 50 mg/day or greater of hydrochlorothiazide or chlorthalidone gives an average increase of 1.53 mg/dl and with low doses (25 mg/day or less), about one-half this increase may be expected. In several studies, totaling 309 patients on low dose diuretic therapy, an average increase of only 0.8 mg/dl was observed (Table X).

The hyperuricemia that develops with thiazide diuretics is usually asymptomatic.[44,109,110] In the predisposed individual, acute gouty attacks may occur. Since only a small number of asymtomatic patients with hyperuricemia develop gout or renal uric acid stones, it is not required that all patients be treated for this condition. It is important to monitor serum uric acid levels during thiazide therapy in order to avoid an acute gouty episode or other complications of hyperuricemia. Colchine is used to treat these acute gouty attacks. Probenecid[133] or allopurinol[134] has been shown to be effective in hyperuricemia secondary to thiazides and should be considered whenever serum uric acid levels rise to 9.0 or 10.0 mg/dl.[52,107,109] The thiazide therapy should not necessarily be discontinued.[52]

Although the clinical significance is not known, it is agreed that hyperuricemia, per se, is a risk factor, though a minor one, in coronary artery disease. The significance, if any, of persistent, asymptomatic

TABLE X

EFFECTS OF LOW DOSE DIURETIC THERAPY ON SERUM URIC ACID LEVELS

Study (Ref.)	No. of Patients	Drug	Dose (mg/day)	Duration of Therapy (wks)	Pre-treatment Uric Acid (mg/dl)	Treatment Uric Acid (mg/dl)	Increase in Uric Acid (mg/dl)
Korduner et al 1981[11]	22	Chlor.	12.5	12	5.8	5.8	0
Materson et al 1977[12]	20	Chlor.	12.5	12	6.2	7.0	0.8
Eerglund et al 1976[2]	40 40	HCTZ HCTZ	12.5 25	6 6	4.7 4.7	5.3 5.5	0.6 0.8
Carney et al 1976[15]	10	Chlor.	25	4	6.6	7.0	0.4
Berglund et al 1976[2]	40	HCTZ	25	6	4.7	5.5	0.8
Materson et al 1977[12]	20	Chlor.	25	12	6.1	7.1	1.0
Bengtsson et al 1975[17]	39	Chlor.	25	12	3.8	5.3	1.5
Materson et al 1977[12]	18	Chlor.	50	12	6.1	7.6	1.5
Berglund et al 1976[2]	40	HCTZ	50	6	4.7	5.6	0.9
Alhenc-Gelas et al 1978[6]	20	HCTZ	50	3	6.1	6.9	0.8

Chlor. = chlorthalidone; HCTZ = hydrochlorothiazide

hyperuricemia among thiazide-treated hypertensives is not known but is something that deserves attention.

The new Merck drug. MK-286, appears to prevent the usual hyperuricemia. When given together with small doses of amiloride, the resultant combination diuretic approaches being an actual isokalemic, isouricemic agent which may become the agent of choice for avoiding most of these two metabolic problems.

3. Azotemia

Thiazides are usually ineffective with a serum creatinine above 2.0 mg/dl (or GFR < 25 ml/min) and their use will only exacerbate the azotemia. Metolazone (and furosemide) usually *do* work with the creatinine up to 10 mg/dl and these agents are the preferred diuretics in azotemic hypertension.

The reduction in effective plasma volume secondary to thiazide-induced diuresis tends to elevate serum creatinine and to decrease creatinine clearance, the mechanism of which is felt to be reduced renal blood flow and glomerular filtration. Sherlock and Walker[135] found that 22% of cirrhotics (persons whose homeostatic mechanism is precariously balanced) developed azotemia when thiazide therapy was instituted.

4. Elevation of Blood Glucose

Thiazide therapy has been associated with increases in serum glucose, decreases in oral glucose tolerance tests, and with the development of overt diabetes mellitus.[95,131, 132, 136] The development of nonketotic, hyperglycemic, hyperosmolar coma has also been associated with thiazide diuretics.[29,137,138] This diminished glucose tolerance is thought to be due to interference with the release of insulin from the pancreas[52] and also the hypokalemia. As the serum potassium levels rise to normal, the glucose tolerance improves. This is thought to be a dose-dependent phenomenon.[109,132] Usually, the hyperglycemia only develops when the patient's original glucose levels are high.[132] Many researchers agree that an impaired glucose tolerance may be worsened, but an unimpaired glucose tolerance may not be affected by diuretic therapy. Marks et al, in a study with 40 patients who had been on hydrochlorothiazide therapy for hypertension for no less than ten years, found that only four patients had abnormal blood glucose levels and those with a diabetic glucose tolerance test had a family history of diabetes.[139] Long-term use of thiazides usually produces a slight rise in fasting glucose levels of non-diabetics. Amery et al[140] found fasting blood sugar levels increased by an average of 9.6 mg/dl after two years of therapy. A two-year follow-up of thiazide- vs. placebo-treated veterans in a large multi-clinic study indicated that FBS exceeded 110 mg/dl in 12% more of the thiazide-treated patients than those who had been on placebo. In addition, there was no correlation between hypokalemia and hyperglycemia.[141]

Blood glucose levels should be followed in patients on chronic diuretic therapy, particularly if they have diabetes mellitus, borderline oral glucose tolerance tests, elevated fasting blood sugars, or a family history of diabetes mellitus. If hyperglycemia should develop, it is usually mild and does not call for treatment.[52] In the rare event of the development of frank diabetes, the dose of the diuretic can be lowered or the diuretic being used may be substituted with another chemically unrelated one (e.g., hydrochlorothiazide for chlorthalidane or vice versa).[52,109] Rarely will it be necessary to discontinue diuretic therapy or administer insulin to the patient.[52]

5. Hyponatremia

One of the rare complications of thiazide administration is hyponatremia,[108] but it may occur especially in edematous and/or elderly patients. The thiazides inhibit the reabsorption of sodium causing loss of both sodium and water. The normal, intact homeostatic mechanisms for sodium regulation are usually sufficient to prevent diuretic-induced hyponatremia caused by pushed doses, excessive water ingestion, greatly restricted sodium intake or other complicating factors. Thiazides can impair the diluting segment of the cortical thick ascending limb of Henle; this inhibits the ability of the patient to excrete a maximally dilute urine in response to a high intake of water and, therefore, dilutional hyponatremia may develop.[108] Although rare, hyponatremia is a real possibility.[142,143] Acute hyponatremia resulting in encephalopathy[144] and in diffuse cerebral edema[145] has been reported secondary to thiazide administration.

6. Effects on Calcium

Thiazides are sometimes used in the prophylaxis of kidney stones because they decrease the renal clearance of calcium. However, hypercalcemia, unassociated with any demonstrable pathology[109,132,146] and relieved by withdrawal of the drug,[147] has been reported. There is little clinical significance of this usually mild hypercalcemia. The doctor should, however, rule out other etiologies to be safe.[132] Some investigators have, however, associated prolonged administration of thiazides with the development of hypercalcemia, secondary hyperparathyroidism and parathyroid adenomas,[148] although this needs much more study.

7. Hypomagnesemia

Diuretics are known to cause magnesium loss, but the incidence of hypomagnesemia is not known.[149] The clinical manifestations need more study, but they include the development of cardiac arrhythmias.[150,151] Sheehan et al[149] reported five patients with hypomagnesemia on thiazide therapy. Patients deficient in potassium may be refractory to treatment if magnesium depletion is also present.[152] Magnesium deficiency is more common in alcoholic, malnourished or edematous patients.

8. Effects on Zinc

Thiazide therapy has been shown to cause an increase in urinary zinc excretion in several studies.[153-155] However, the serum zinc concentrations remain normal or even slightly increased.[153] Due to the fact that "zinc has been recognized as an essential element for human health, the diuretic-zinc problem calls for further attention."[153]

9. Effects on Lipids

It has been established that after hypertension and smoking, abnormalities in plasma lipids are major coronary risk factors. Recently, many researchers have investigated the effects of thiazide diuretics on the levels of plasma lipids.[156-166] In a joint Veterans Administration–National Heart, Lung and Blood Institute Study,[162] 1,012 patients were placed into one of two double-blind treatment groups. The active group was treated with chlorthalidone alone (or sometimes with reserpine) and the other group received matching placebo. After one year of treatment, the diuretic group showed significant increases in cholesterol levels, triglyceride, and low-density lipoprotein-cholesterol compared with placebo. HDL-cholesterol was unchanged. The Multiple Risk Factor Intervention Trial found similar rises in cholesterol but a *decrease* in HDL-cholesterol, thus modestly increasing both risk factors.[167] Most studies have obtained similar results,[159,160,162, 164,166] viz., slight decreases in HDL-cholesterol, the so-called "protective" cholesterol factor. Many authorities are concerned that the long-term benefit of thiazide in reducing one risk factor for cardiovascular disease may be at least partially offset by the 5–7% rise of cholesterol and the slight reduction of HDL-cholesterol. With the present state of information, the prudent physician should use low doses of diuretics and also periodically monitor these lipid levels.

> Many authorities are concerned that the long-term benefit of thiazides in reducing one risk factor for cardiovascular disease may be at least partially offset by the 5–7% rise of cholesterol and the slight reduction of HDL-cholesterol.

---

10. Cardiovascular Effects

Thiazides have been reported to cause orthostatic hypotension,[12,136,168] chest pain,[105,169] palpitations,[7,105, 169-171] shortness of breath,[12,105,169] flushing,[172] shock,[173] and increased heart rate[6,174]—each of these rarely, however.

Cardiac arrhythmias have also been detected in patients on diuretic therapy, attributed usually to low potassium and/or magnesium levels.[111,127,128,175] In a trial of 287 patients randomly assigned to twice daily placebo or 5 mg bendrofluazide, the British Medical Research Council (MRC),[175] found that 33% of the patients on thiazide therapy had more than five ventricular ectopic beats during the day and 23% at night, while only 20% of the placebo-treated patients had more than five ventricular ectopic beats during the day and only 9% at night. The thiazide-treated group had multifocal beats, couplets and bigeminy observed in 33% of the patients, while only 15% of the placebo patients experienced these. In a special group of 20 patients with serum potassium levels of less than 2.7 mEq/L or less after diuretic therapy, nearly 50% were found to have more than five premature beats an hour. Twelve of these patients received potassium supplementation, but only five had fewer premature beats after the potassium treatment. From these findings, the MRC concluded that thiazide therapy is associated with an increased ventricular ectopic activity. Hollifield et al,[111] Caralis et al,[127] and Holland et al[128] concluded from their investigations that there is a link between thiazide-induced hypokalemia and an increase in cardiac arrhythmias observed in patients on diuretic therapy. In Holland's fine study, ventricular ectopy even occurred in one patient with serum potassium levels of 3.7 mEq/L. He noted that 33% of his patients treated with hydrochlorothiazide (50 mg twice daily) were hypokalemic and developed ventricular ectopic activity. Hollifield et al[111] found a significant correlation between the fall in serum potassium observed and the occurrence of PVCs in 13 patients treated with hydrochlorothiazide. Cooper et al[129] studied the relationship of serum potassium levels to the incidence of arrhythmias in diuretic-treated vs. non-diuretic-treated patients with acute myocardial infarction. Significant arrhythmias occurred in those patients with potassium levels in the range of 3.5–3.9 mEq/L. They found 51.9% of the diuretic group vs. 38.8% of the non-diuretic group had arrhythmias. In view of these reports of potentially serious arrhythmias being associated with thiazide treatment, acute myocardial infarction patients who have been receiving these diuretics should receive KCl if their potassium levels are less than 4.0 mEq/L. It also appears prudent to give either potassium supplements or potassium-sparing agents to hypertensive patients with potassium levels of 3.5 mEq/L or less.

A new report with contrary findings should be mentioned. Freis' group found that cardiac arrhythmias were not reversed in hypokalemic patients after restoration of potassium levels to normal.[176] Since spontaneous, consecutive, day-to-day variations occur with ectopic atrial or ventricular arrhythmias,[177] longer monitoring intervals than 24 hours are required before valid conclusions are reached.

11. Renal Colic

Dilevette and Recalde[178] reported a case of renal colic caused by hydrochlorothiazide plus triamterene.

B. Unpredictable Adverse Reactions to Thiazides

1. Deaths

The thiazides, like all systemic medications, are capable of producing very rare fatal adverse reactions. Thiazide-related fatalities have been reported due to bone marrow aplasia[179] and cerebral edema with pulmonary congestion.[145] Other potentially fatal reactions have occurred and include the possibility of fatal anaphylactoid reactions.

2. Coma

Thiazide diuretics have been reported to cause encephalopathy[180] and coma. Acute hyponatremia, cerebrovascular insufficiency due to plasma volume contraction,[144,173] hepatic insufficiency,[135] and hyperosmolar hyperglycemia[137,138] are all reported cases of encephalopathy and coma induced by thiazides. Cirrhotics are particularly at risk of developing thiazide-induced encephalopathy. Sherlock and Walker[135] report a 22% incidence in this population and postulate as the causes a contraction of plasma volume with subsequent reduction in hepatic blood flow and further decrease in liver function.

3. Pancreatitis

The development of acute pancreatitis has been associated with the use of thiazide diuretics in both pregnant[84-86] and non-pregnant persons.[52,135,181-183] Hyperglycemic coma has also been reported due to thiazide-induced pancreatitis.[137]

4. Hepatic Injury

Thiazide-induced jaundice has been reported.[184,185] Hokkanen and Kaipainen,[186] in a study of 1,500 admissions to selected medical wards, found 55 drug-related cases of hepatic damage. Only four of the 55 cases were associated with thiazide administration.

5. Hematologic Effects of Thiazides

These are rare following thiazide administration,[52] but cases of thrombocytopenic purpura,[187-189] non-thrombocytopenic purpura and petechiae[186] have been reported. A case of hemolytic anemia,[187] thought to be due to a thiazide following hydrochlorothiazide and methyldopa, has been reported. A case of fatal bone marrow aplasia[144] has been reported following the use of polythiazide. Eosinophilia with lympadenopathy and splenomegaly has also been reported.[173]

6. Pulmonary Edema

Steinberg[190] reported two different cases of pulmonary edema which developed 45 minutes after ingestion of 50 mg hydrochlorothiazide. Beaudry and Laplante[191] reported a case of pulmonary edema due to hydrochlorothiazide that was confirmed by rechallenge with the drug.

7. Withdrawal Hypertension

Dinon et al[173] reported a case in which a patient's blood pressure was controlled (from 280/160 to 110/80) by combined therapy including a thiazide; withdrawal of only thiazide from the therapeutic regimen resulted in a hypertensive crisis, i.e., blood pressure of 300+/180 mm Hg.

8. Spastic Craniofacial Syndrome

Perchuk[192] reported eight cases of "Spastic Craniofacial Syndrome" consisting of craniofacial pain, facial muscle spasm, facial distortion, and aphasia secondary to the administration of the thiazide, bendroflumethiazide.

9. Neurological Effects

Insomnia,[193] depression,[7,170] vertigo,[7,169] lightheadedness,[7,12,171] tinnitus,[171] paresthesias,[172] dry mouth,[12,136] and tiredness[7,105, 169-171] have all been associated with the administration of thiazide diuretics, though very rarely.

10. Allergic-type Reactions

Thiazides have been reported to cause vasculitis,[194,195] photosensitivity,[196] exfoliative dermatitis,[173] interstitial nephritis, allergic purpura and glomerulonephritis,[197] fever, [173,198] and arthralgia.[198] The possibility of other very rare allergic phenomena must be remembered,[52,199] especially those of laryngeal edema and anaphylaxis. When rash, for example, occurs from a thiazide, other classes of diuretics may be tried, e.g., chlorthalidone, metolazone, amiloride, etc.

11. Blindness

Srivastave el al[200] reported a case of cortical blindness associated with prolonged coma and hyperpyrexia following ingestion of chlorothiazide. Other investigators have reported transient blurring of vision[169,171] and burning eyes.[169]

12. Non-occlusive Mesenteric Infarction

Shaufkin and Silen[201] reported two cases of thiazide-related non-occlusive mesenteric infarction.

METOLAZONE (Zaroxolyn,® Diulo®)

Metolazone is a sulfonamide derivative with diuretic, saluretic and antihypertensive activity. A single daily dose of 2.5–5.0 mg of metolazone is an effective dose in the management of hypertension. Ten mg tablets are also available but are primarily used for the treatment of edema. The antihypertensive effect of metolazone is usually apparent within three or four days after initiating therapy and the optimal effect is usually evident after three or four weeks of treatment.

The side effects of metolazone are similar to those of the thiazide diuretics. They consist primarily of biochemical effects including hy-

TABLE XI
FREQUENCY OF ADVERSE REACTIONS DUE TO
LOW-DOSE THIAZIDE THERAPY*

FREQUENT (> 5.0%)

        Hypokalemia
        Hyperuricemia
        Dizziness
        Tiredness

OCCASIONAL (0.1–5.0%)

        GI: nausea, flatulence, pancreatitis, dry mouth, indigestion, constipation, abdominal gas and cramps, change in defecation, diarrhea, vomiting
        CV: palpitations, orthostatic hypotension, chest pain, shortness of breath
        CNS: headache, tiredness, dizziness, lightheadness, depression, tinnitus, sedation
        METABOLIC: hyponatremia, dehydration, hyperglycemia
        ALLERGIC: rash, petechia, fever, arthralgia
        MISC: weakness, impotence, loss of libido, visual disturbance, cramps, burning eyes

RARE (< 0.1%)

        Erythema multiform, thrombocytopenic purpura, pancreatitis
        All others listed under Unpredictable Adverse Reactions not on table under frequent or occasional

* The data used to compute this table were gathered from the articles cited in the sections on efficacy and adverse reactions.

pokalemia, hyperglycemia, hyperuricemia, hypertriglyceridemia, and hypercholesterolemia. Azotemia and oliguria occasionally occur as with other diuretics. These changes are usually mild and have been discussed earlier in this chapter.

Metolazone and furosemide given concurrently have been reported to produce marked diuresis in some patients with edema previously refractory to other diuretics. The mechanism of action of metolazone on the renal tubule is similar to that of the thiazide diuretics. Its antihypertensive mechanism is not fully understood.

Metolazone is a relatively potent thiazide-like diuretic with a prolonged activity from 12 to 24 hours' duration or even longer. Once-a-day dosage has been shown to be effective in the management of mild hypertension. As with other diuretics, metolazone will augment the antihypertensive efficacy of other antihypertensive agents.

TABLE XII
NATURE OF REACTIONS TO THIAZIDES

Gastrointestinal
Nausea, vomiting, dry mouth, abdominal cramps, anorexia, jaundice, pancreatitis, sialadenitis, constipation, diarrhea, gastric irritation, hepatic damage, flatulence

Central Nervous System
Dizziness, vertigo, paresthesias, headache, xanthopsia, coma, insomnia, depression, tiredness, blindness, tinnitus

Cardiovascular — Pulmonary
Orthostatic hypotension, shock, chest pain, shortness of breath, palpitations, acute pulmonary edema, non-occlusive mesenteric infarction

Metabolic
Hyperglycemia, hypertriglyceridemia, hyperosmolarity, hyponatremia, hypokalemia, hypercalcemia, hyperuricemia, dehydration, glycosuria, ↑BUN, ↑Cr

Hematologic, Lymphatic
Leukopenia, bone marrow aplasia, agranulocytosis, thrombocytopenia, eosinophilia, hemolytic anemia, spenomegaly, lymphadenopathy

Hypersensitivity
Purpura, photosensitivity, rash, urticaria, necrotizing angiitis (vasculitis), fever, glomerulonephritis, anaphylactic reactions, Stevens–Johnson syndrome

Other
Male impotence, loss of libido, muscle cramps, weakness, renal colic, withdrawal hypertension, spastic craniofacial syndrome, parathyroid edema

---

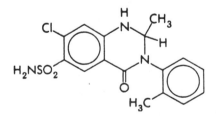

Figure 3: Structure of metolazone.

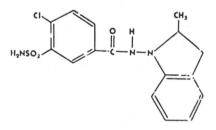

Figure 4: Structure of indapamide.

INDAPAMIDE (Lozol®)
Introductory year: 1983

Indapamide is a newly introduced sulfonamide derivative possessing both diuretic and antihypertensive activity. It is available in 2.5 mg tablets to be given once daily. It is 5 to 80 times more lipid soluble than thiazide diuretics[1] and has little or no direct effect on cardiac or kidney function. It is metabolized by the liver and, therefore, should be used very cautiously in patients with liver disease. As with the thiazide diuretics, serum uric acid increases in proportion to indapamide dosage.[2-4] However, it does appear not to alter fasting blood sugar or glucose tolerance in either diabetics or non-diabetics.[5-10] It does produce a natriuresis and kaliuresis as well as hypokalemia. Thus far no effects on lipoproteins have been noted.[9,11,12] Direct comparisons are needed.

The most frequent reactions to indapamide are similar to those with the thiazide diuretics and include the following which occur with a frequency greater than 5%: headache, dizziness, fatigue, weakness, malaise, lethargy, tiredness, muscle cramps, numbness of extremities, nervousness, tension, anxiety, irritability, agitation. Other side effects such as impotence, drowsiness, vertigo, nausea, palpitation, skin rash, etc., appear to be less frequent.

The efficacy of indapamide from published literature is contained in Table XIII. It is apparent that doses of 2.5 mg a day reduce blood pressure satisfactorily.

FUROSEMIDE
Introductory year: 1966

INTRODUCTION:

Furosemide is a potent diuretic[1-10] which can be administered either orally[10,11] or parenterally[10,12,13] (Figure 5). It is the most popular

TABLE XIII
EFFICACY OF INDAPAMIDE ALONE IN HYPERTENSION

Study (Ref.)*	No. of Patients	Dose (mg/day)	Duration of Treatment (wks)	Pre-treatment Blood Pressure† (mm Hg)	Post-treatment Blood Pressure† (mm Hg)	Decline in Blood Pressure† (mm Hg)
Hatt et al[13]	38	5.0	6½	185/97	153/81	32/16
Milliez et al[6]	22	5.0	4	166/103	155/97	11/6
Wheeley†† et al[14]	2497	2.5	12	177/104	153/90	24/14
Mimran†† et al[5]	2184	2.5	12	186/105	155/87	31/18
Passerson et al[15]	644	2.5	12	186/110	154/87	32/13
Roux†† et al[16]	11	2.5	16	162/95	146/86	16/9
Burgess et al[17]	25	2.5	24	189/116	141/85	48/31
Dunn et al[18]	14	2.5	8	175/114	142/93	33/21
Chalmers†† et al[19]	7	2.5	6	149/102	131/90	18/12
Chalmers et al[4]	16	2.5	8	162/101	150/95	12/6
Kubik et al[20]	27	2.5	8	170/109	151/99	19/10
Van Hee et al[21]	23	2.5	8	197/112	157/92	40/30
Bowker et al[22]	75	2.5	16	177/106	151/88	27/18

* See reference section to this chapter for complete information regarding sources.
† Erect blood pressure.
†† No placebo given.

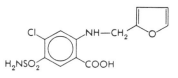

Figure 5: Structure of furosemide.

"loop" diuretic in the world and plays an important role in managing not only edematous states but also some types of hypertension.

In a patient who requires a potent diuretic but is allergic to furosemide or if furosemide is contraindicated, ethacrynic acid and bumetanide have very similar activity and may be considered.

When should the physician consider furosemide for hypertension?

1. As an adjunct in the parentheral therapy of hypertensive crisis:[13-16]

Hypertensive crisis is a life-threatening medical emergency which requires rapid, aggressive therapy. Intravenous furosemide produces rapid diuresis with sodium loss and plasma-volume contraction which helps lower blood pressure and potentiates the action of the primary antihypertensive drug such as nitroprusside, diazoxide, or hydralazine. The patient's pressure is then more easily and more rapidly controlled with lower doses of these drugs.

2. In the management of azotemic hypertension:[4,9, 17-22]

Furosemide is the diuretic of choice in patients with impaired renal function, as it produces profound diuresis without significantly decreasing renal blood flow or glomerular filtration (as do thiazides). If urine output can be maintained above one liter a day and diastolic blood pressure kept below 100 mg Hg, renal function in nephrosclerotic patients often improves significantly over a period of two or three months. Usually, the patient can then be maintained on combination therapy. Several hundred milligram oral daily doses of furosemide may be required.

3. As an alternative to thiazides in resistant hypertension:[23-25]

In some patients, thiazides do not completely stop the retention of sodium caused by other drugs in an antihypertensive regimen. This accumulation of sodium causes resistance or a pseudotolerance. The permanent or intermittent substitution of furosemide, with its more potent natriuretic action, reverses the sodium retention and restores the responsiveness to antihypertensive therapy in many of these patients.

How effective is furosemide in essential hypertension?

● *Furosemide as initial monotherapy:*

The antihypertensive effect of furosemide alone has been the topic of several studies. In eight studies[26-33] where furosemide was given alone to 147 patients, 69 patients had an average decrease in mean arterial blood pressure of 10 mm Hg and 79 other patients had an average decrease of 16/7 mm Hg (Table XIV). This is slightly higher than the 10/5 mm Hg drop when furosemide has been directly compared to thiazides in controlled studies. (See below.) However, Licht et al[34] recently found 40 mg/day doses of furosemide produced significantly less hypokalemia than 50 mg/day hydrochlorothiazide, while lowering blood pressure almost as well as the thiazide. Prevention of hypokalemia must be an important consideration in diuretic-treated hypertensives.

● *Furosemide as part of combination therapy:*

Furosemide's potent natriuretic effect results in a negative sodium balance which potentiates the antihypertensive activity of the non-diuretic agents. The antihypertensive action of furosemide-induced natriuresis is especially pronounced and therapeutically important in those patients whose hypertension has become resistant to multiple drug therapy. In 73 resistant patients where furosemide replaced a thiazide, an average decrease of 24/15 mm Hg was observed. In two studies where furosemide was added to multiple drug therapy of 31 patients, an average decrease of 21/11 mm Hg was observed (Table XIV).[7,35-38]

How effective is oral furosemide compared with thiazides in mild hypertension:

Seven controlled studies[29,31-33,39-43] are tabulated in Table XV. These are the only published reports of well-controlled studies we could find comparing these two diuretics. Based on these studies, one can conclude that thiazides are more effective in reducing blood pressure than 50 mg of furosemide in the treatment of mild hypertension. VanderElst,[39] selecting patients on fixed doses of propranolol, added either furosemide or thiazide. He found the two diuretics equipotent using this combined drug model. In six of the seven studies, the difference was statistically significant. In none of the studies was furosemide superior to thiazides.

TABLE XIV
EFFICACY OF FUROSEMIDE IN ESSENTIAL HYPERTENSION

Study (Ref.)	No. of Patients	Dose (mg/day)	Decline in Blood Pressure (mm Hg)
Olshan et al 1981[26]	12	40	8*
Mroczek et al 1978[27]	23	40–80	14/9
Tasker et al 1976[28]	16	80	16*
Anderson et al 1971[29]	16	80	9/6
Johnston et al 1970[30]	20	80	12/4
Bracharz et al 1969[31]	11	75	28/10
Bariso et al 1970[32]	9	80–160	18/7
Valmin et al 1975[33]	40	80	5*
Nielson et al 1981[13]	23	80†	60/30
Kristensen et al 1980[24]	12	40–120***	28/13
VanderElst et al 1981[39]	19	46**	13/8
Ramsay et al 1980[23]‡	16	40–80	18/7
Araoye et al 1978[40]‡	30	80	18/10
Wilson et al 1977[25]‡	5	80	34/22
Mroczek et al 1974[38]‡	22	80–640	30/20

   * Mean arterial blood pressure = diastolic + 1/3 pulse pressure.
   † 80 mg total injected to treat emergency hypertensive cases (240/140 mm Hg went to 180/110 mm Hg).
   ‡ Blood pressure after furosemide substituted for thiazides.
  ** Added to a stable dose of propranolol.
*** Added to drug therapy given for resistant hypertension.

TABLE XV
RESULTS OF SEVEN CONTROLLED COMPARISONS OF FUROSEMIDE AND THIAZIDES

Study (Ref.)	No. of Patients	Design	Thiazide Dose	Furosemide	RESULTS Thiazide (↓mm Hg)	RESULTS Furosemide (↓mm Hg)	RESULTS Statistical Significance
Arayoe & Freis et al 1978[40]	30	Crossover double-blind	HCTZ 50 mg bid × 3 months	40 mg bid × 3 months	18/10	9/8	HCTZ > F (p. < .05) NS
Holland et al 1979[41]	30	Open label, crossover study	HCTZ 50 mg bid × 4 weeks	40 mg bid × 4 weeks	25*	16*	HCTZ > F (p. < .01)
Araoye et al 1977[43]	33	Single-blind crossover	HCTZ 50 mg bid × 3 months	40 mg bid	13.1	8.8	HCTZ > F (p. < 0.05)
Finnerty et al 1977[42]	52	Parallel, double-blind, 3 clinics	HCTZ 50 mg bid × 2 years	40 mg bid × 2 years	30/16	18/13	HCTZ > F (p. < 0.05)
Valmin et al 1975[33]	34	Double-blind vs. placebo, crossover, 5 different treatments	HCTZ 12.5 mg bid × 4 weeks	12.5, 25 and 40 mg bid × 4 weeks	8/3	(12.5):4/0 (25) :7/3 (40) :6/3 vs. placebo: 4/1	(F) 12.5 = placebo (F) 25 and 40 mg = HCTZ and all three > placebo X (p. < 0.05)
Anderson et al 1971[29]	16	Crossover double-blind	HCTZ 50 mg bid × 8 weeks	40 mg bid × 8 weeks	19/12	9/6	HCTZ > F (p. < 0.01)
Bariso et al 1970[32]	10	Hospitalized, crossover, double-blind vs. placebo	CTZ 1-2 gm/day	80-160 mg/day	18.3/5.6	12.6/3.6	NS

HCTZ = Hydrochlorothiazide; CTZ = chlorothiazide; F = furosemide.
* Mean arterial blood pressure = diastolic + 1/3 pulse pressure.
** HCTZ + furosemide was added to a stable dose of propranolol.

In no way does this detract from the excellent benefit of furosemide in treating azotemic hypertension (see Chapter I) and hypertensive crises.

Formulations

Tablets .... 20, 40 and 80

mg Oral Solution 10

mg/ml Injectable .... 20 mg in 2 ml ampule

40 mg in 2 ml ampule

100 mg in 10 ml ampule

Oral Dose in Hypertension

Frequency: twice daily

Initial: 40 mg once or twice daily

Range: 20–80 mg/day. Reduce dose when adding other antihypertensive agents. In mildly azotemic patients several hundred milligrams/day may be needed.

Usual Dose: 40 mg twice daily

Mechanism of Action

Investigations into the mode of action of furosemide have utilized micropuncture studies in rats, stop–flow experiments in dogs, and various clearance studies in both humans and experimental animals. Furosemide's major diuretic activity results from the inhibition of active chloride transport in the medullary and cortical thick ascending limb of Henle.[7-10,37,44,45] (see Figure 6, p. 130.) It also has weak effects in the proximal tubule due to its mild carbonic anhydrase inhibitory activities which lead to interference with sodium transport. Furosemide is a very potent diuretic with an infinite dose response curve that can lead to an excretion of up to 30% of the filtered sodium load.[8,10] This high degree of efficacy is due to the uniqueness of its major site of action which is independent of any inhibitory effect of carbonic anhydrase or aldosterone. Thiazides produce a limited volume depletion independent of the dose; however, furosemide does not have this protective factor and can, therefore, cause dangerous volume depletion.[18]

Following oral administration, an effective diuresis will occur within 30 minutes.[10] The peak effect is produced within the first or second hour and the duration of action is between four to six hours.[8,10] This relatively short half-life makes the administration of the drug frequent. The diuresis resulting from intravenous injection commences within five minutes (somewhat later after intramuscular injection) peaks within 30 minutes and lasts for two hours.[10]

Although thiazides lose their effectiveness when the GFR decreases, furosemide remains effective because it inhibits the reabsorption of such a high percentage of sodium. If large doses are used in renal failure, a diuresis may be obtained.[18] It has been demonstrated that acute administration of large doses may lead to renal vasodilation, which increases renal blood flow.[19]

Most evidence indicates that the hypotensive effect of furosemide is a direct result of the decrease in plasma and extracellular fluid volume which leads to a decrease in cardiac output.[46] The reflex increase in peripheral resistance is not enough to compensate completely and the blood pressure declines.[46]

Drug Interactions

1. Plus *Potassium-Retaining Diuretics*

Furosemide is used with potassium-retaining diuretics such as amiloride, triamterene or spironolactone to reduce potassium loss.

2. Plus *Other Antihypertensive Agents*

Furosemide may add to or potentiate the action of the nondiuretic antihypertensive drugs. Care should be taken to reduce the dose of these drugs when furosemide is added.

3. Plus *Salicylates*

Patients receiving high doses of salicylates, as in rheumatic diseases, in conjunction with furosemide may experience salicylate toxicity at lower doses because of competitive renal excretory sites.

4. Plus *Cephalosporins*

There have been several case reports that furosemide increased the nephrotoxicity of cephaloridine or cephalothin.[47-50] Concomitant administration of furosemide to patients on cephaloridine has been shown to prolong the serum half-life of the latter.[51] Animal studies have also shown furosemide to enhance the nephrotoxicity of cephaloridine.[52,53]

5. Plus *Antidiabetic Drugs*

Furosemide has been reported to cause hyperglycemia,[54] abnormal glucose tolerance, and glucosuria.[55] Patients who are diabetic or prediabetic should have their blood glucose monitored while on furosemide and appropriate dosage changes in their antidiabetic drugs instituted if necessary.

6. Plus *Skeletal Muscle Relaxants*

Furosemide has been reported to enhance the effects of skeletal muscle relaxants, especially tubocurarine.[56] It is advisable that oral furosemide be discontinued for one week prior to any elective surgery and parenteral furosemide for two days prior to elective surgery.

7. Plus *Metolazone*

An apparent synergistic effect has been observed between furosemide and metolazone. Three patients, who failed to respond to 320 mg/day of furosemide, had a profound diuresis when 5–20 mg/day of metolazone was added to the furosemide therapy.[57,58] Black et al[58] found a synergistic hypotensive effect when metolazone and furosemide were given in two resistant hypertensive patients. However, when given to five patients with refractory heart failure, serum electrolyte levels were severely disturbed, but when the metolazone–furosemide combination was terminated, the electrolytes stabilized.

8. Plus *Corticosteroids*

Severe hypokalemia may result from the concomitant administration of furosemide and steroids due to mutual enhancement of their respective potassium-losing actions.[59]

9. Plus *Digitalis*

Furosemide-induced hypokalemia and hypomagnesemia increase myocardial sensitivity to digitalis and can precipitate digitalis toxicity[60-63] and serious cardiac arrhythmias.

Digoxin has been shown to decrease greatly the observed increase in PRA induced by furosemide.[64]

Intravenous furosemide has been shown to increase the renal excretion of digoxin.[65] No short-term effect on the serum concentration of digoxin was observed, possibly due to a large total body pool of digoxin. However, it is advisable to monitor patients for signs of digitalis toxicity if furosemide is suddenly withdrawn from concomitant therapy.

10. Plus *Lithium Salts*

Lithium generally should not be given with diuretics, as it causes sodium depletion, thereby reducing the renal clearance of lithium and increasing the risk of lithium toxicity. Lithium toxicity associated with furosemide administration[66] and with treatment with bumetamide,[67] another loop diuretic, has been reported. However, in a two-week trial, furosemide did not cause an increase in lithium concentration when given to subjects taking lithium.[68] The proposed reason for avoidance of toxicity is thought to be because lithium is reabsorbed in the proximal tubule, and there is evidence for reabsorption in Henle's loop. Therefore, the blocked reabsorption in the loop ensures a balance by decreasing the lithium reabsorption in the loop to make up for the increased reabsorption in the proximal tubule caused by sodium loss.[68] Read circulars for lithium preparations before use of such concomitant therapy.

11. Plus *Chloral Hydrate*

Uneasiness, hot flashes, diaphoresis, and variable blood pressure occurred in six patients in a coronary care unit who received chloral hydrate within the 24 hours preceding the administration of furosemide. These patients did not react to furosemide alone, furosemide with flurazepam, or chloral hydrate until the furosemide was administered.[69]

12. Plus *Clofibrate*

Excessive diuresis, muscular pain, and stiffness have been reported to occur in hyperlipoproteinemic patients with the nephrotic syndromes, secondary to the concomitant administration of furosemide and clofibrate.[70]

13. Plus *Indomethacin*

Yasujima et al[71] noted the inhibition of furosemide's antihypertensive benefit when given together with indomethacin.

14. Plus *Warfarin*

Nilsson et al,[72] in a study of 11 normal subjects given warfarin and furosemide or bumetanide, determined that they caused no significant effects on the hypoprothrombinemic response to warfarin.

15. Plus *Non-Steroidal Anti-inflammatory Drugs*

Rawles et al[73] found complete antagonism of the effect of furosemide when given to five normal subjects with flurbiprofen. One patient was given furosemide and ibuprofen. Laiwah et al[74] found the same type of antagonism when furosemide was concomitantly given with ibuprofen.

Contraindications

Furosemide is contraindicated in anuria. If increasing azotemia and oliguria occur during treatment of severe progressive renal disease, the drug should be discontinued. In hepatic coma and in states of electrolyte depletion, therapy should not be instituted until the basic condition is improved or corrected. Furosemide is contraindicated in patients with a history of hypersensitivity to this compound.

Because animal reproductive studies have shown that furosemide may cause fetal abnormalities, the drug is contraindicated in women of childbearing potential. An exception exists in life-threatening situations where the use of a diuretic is considered of paramount importance over the use of alternative drugs and where the physician has balanced this efficacy potential against the teratogenic and embryotoxic potential demonstrated to occur in animal studies.

Warnings

Excessive diuresis may result in dehydration and reduction in blood volume with circulatory collapse and with the possibility of vascular thrombosis and embolism, particularly in elderly patients. Excessive loss of potassium in patients receiving digitalis glycosides may precipitate digitalis toxicity. Care should also be exercised in patients receiving potassium-depleting steroids.

Frequent serum electrolyte, CO_2, and BUN determinations should be performed during the first few months of therapy and periodically thereafter. Correct abnormalities or withdraw the drug temporarily.

In patients with hepatic cirrhosis and ascites, initiation of therapy with furosemide is best carried out in the hospital. Sudden alterations of fluid and electrolyte balance in patients with cirrhosis may precipitate hepatic coma; therefore, strict observation is necessary during the period of diuresis. Supplemental potassium chloride or, if required, a potassium-sparing agent is helpful in preventing hypokalemia and metabolic alkalosis.

As with many other drugs, patients should be observed regularly for the possible occurrence of blood dyscrasias, liver damage, or other idiosyncratic reactions.

In those instances where potassium supplementation is required, an oral liquid preparation or a microencapsulated preparation should be used rather than enteric-coated or wax-coated potassium salts because of the reports of intestinal and upper gastrointestinal lesions, respectively, following these formulations.[75,76] The wax-matrix potassium chloride preparations have recently been shown to cause gastric lesions in two separate studies.[75,76] (See Chapter IV, Tables IV and V.)

There have been several reports, published and unpublished, concerning nonspecific small-bowel lesions consisting of stenosis, with or without ulceration, associated with the administration of enteric-coated thiazides with potassium salts. These lesions may occur with enteric-coated potassium tablets alone or when they are used with nonenteric-coated thiazides or certain other oral diuretics. These small-bowel lesions have caused obstruction, hemorrhage, and perforation. Surgery was frequently required, and deaths have occurred.

Available information tends to implicate enteric-coated potassium salts, although lesions of this type also occur spontaneously. Therefore, coated potassium-containing formulations should be administered only when indicated and should be discontinued immediately if abdominal pain, distention, nausea, vomiting, or gastrointestinal bleeding occurs.

The possibility exists of exacerbation or activation of systemic lupus erythematosus in patients taking furosemide.

Patients with known sulfonamide sensitivity may show allergic reactions to furosemide. The oral solution contains tartrazine which may cause allergic-type reactions in certain susceptible individuals. The incidence of these reactions is low, but it is frequently seen in patients who are sensitive to aspirin.

Use in Pregnancy

Because animal reproductive studies have shown that furosemide may cause fetal abnormalities, the drug is contraindicated in women of childbearing potential.

The effects of furosemide on embryonic and fetal development and on pregnant dams were studied in mice, rats, and rabbits.

Furosemide caused unexplained maternal deaths and abortions in the rabbit when 50 mg/kg (four times the maximal recommended human dose of 600 mg/day) was administered between days 12 to 17 of gestation. In a previous study, the lowest dose of only 25 mg/kg (two times the maximal recommended human dose of 600 mg/day) caused maternal deaths and abortions. In a third study, none of the pregnant rabbits survived a dose of 100 mg/kg. Data from the above studies indicate fetal lethality which can precede maternal deaths.

The results of the mouse study and one of the three rabbit studies also showed an increased incidence of hydronephrosis (distention of the renal pelvis and, in some cases, of the ureters) in fetuses derived from treated dams as compared to the incidence of fetuses from the control group.

Because of these reproductive findings and the lower LD_{50} of furosemide in newborn than in adult rats, the drug is contraindicated in women of childbearing potential. An exception exists where the use of a diuretic such as furosemide injection is considered of paramount importance over the use of alternative drugs and where the physician has balanced this efficacy potential against the teratogenic and embryotoxic potential demonstrated to occur in animal studies.

Prema et al[77] treated 21 cases of either pregnancy-induced hypertension or pregnancy edema with 40 mg/day of furosemide and compared the blood pressure drop and edema reduction observed with 42 cases of untreated pregnancy edema and pregnancy-induced hypertension. All patients were in the hospital and were advised to rest in the lateral recumbent position. There was a significant reduction in edema and fall in blood pressure noted in all women irrespective of whether or not they received diuretic therapy. The plasma electrolyte profile, urinary output, and body weight remained unaltered after the furosemide therapy. This study suggested that diuretics may not cause diuresis in women with pregnancy edema or pregnancy-induced hypertension.

Precautions

As with any potent diuretic, electrolyte depletion may occur during therapy with furosemide, especially in patients receiving higher doses and a restricted salt intake. Electrolyte depletion may manifest itself by weakness, dizziness, lethargy, leg cramps, anorexia, vomiting, and/or mental confusion.

In edematous hypertensive patients being treated with antihypertensive agents, care should be taken to reduce the dose of these drugs when furosemide is administered, since furosemide potentiates the hypotensive effect of antihypertensive medications.

Hypokalemia may develop with furosemide, especially with risk diuresis, when cirrhosis is present, or during concomitant use of corticosteroids or ACTH. Digitalis therapy may exaggerate the metabolic effects of hypokalemia, especially with reference to myocardial activity.

Asymptomatic hyperuricemia can occur, and gout may rarely be precipitated. Reversible elevations of BUN may be seen. These have been observed in association with dehydration which should be avoided, particularly in patients with renal insufficiency.

Where parenteral use of furosemide precedes its oral use, it should be kept in mind that cases of tinnitus and reversible hearing impairment have been reported. There have been some reports of cases in which irreversible hearing impairment occurred. Usually, ototoxicity has been reported when Lasix® (furosemide) was injected rapidly in patients with severe impairment of renal function at doses exceeding several times the usual recommended dose and in whom other drugs known to be ototoxic were often given. If the physician elects to use high-dose parenteral therapy in patients with severely impaired renal function, controlled intravenous infusion is advisable. (For adults, it has been reported that an infusion rate not exceeding 4 mg furosemide per minute has been used.)

Periodic checks on urine and blood glucose should be made in diabetics and even in those suspected of latent diabetes when receiving furosemide. Increases in blood glucose and alterations in glucose tolerance tests with abnormalities of the fasting and two-hour post-prandial sugar have been observed, and rare cases of precipitation of diabetes mellitus have been reported.

Furosemide may lower serum calcium levels, and rare cases of tetany have been reported. Accordingly, periodic serum calcium levels should be obtained.

Patients receiving high doses of salicylates, as in rheumatic diseases, in conjunction with furosemide may experience salicylate toxicity at lower doses because of competitive renal excretory sites.

It has been reported in the literature that diuretics such as furosemide may enhance the nephrotoxicity of cephaloridine. Therefore, furosemide and cephaloridine should not be administered simultaneously.

Sulfonamide diuretics have been reported to decrease arterial responsiveness to pressor amines and to enhance the effect of tubocurarine. Great caution should be exercised in administering curare or its derivatives to patients undergoing therapy with furosemide, and it is advisable to discontinue oral furosemide for one week and parenteral furosemide two days prior to any elective surgery.

Absorption, Metabolism, Excretion

Furosemide is quickly, well-absorbed in the gastrointestinal tract.[10] The peak plasma concentrations are achieved at approximately 1.5 hours after oral administration.[10] Huang et al[78] report that 50–100% of an oral dose is absorbed. In both fasting and post-prandial states, Kelley et al[79] report 50–60% absorption after ingestion. They reported that the peak serum concentration of furosemide after a single 80 mg tablet in the fasting state is 2.3 mg/ml and occurs 60–70 minutes post-ingestion. In the post-prandial state, the peak serum concentration is 1 mg/ml and occurs two hours after taking the tablet. Furosemide is excreted mainly unaltered by the renal tubules except in patients with very low glomerular filtration rates who then must rely on gut excretion.[10] Rupp[12] administered 40 mg of S^{35}-labeled furosemide intravenously to patients with normal renal function with 100% recovery after five days. Eighty-eight percent was excreted in the urine and 12% in the feces. In severe renal insufficiency, biliary excretion accounted for up to 86–98% of the total dose with 82–96% being excreted in the first 24 hours. Other investigators have found only 60% biliary excretion in severe renal impairment.[12] In hepatic and renal disease, the excretion of furosemide is greatly decreased.

Adverse Reactions

Furosemide is an extremely potent diuretic. The common unwanted reactions to this drug are acid-base disturbances, electrolyte disturbances, and volume depletion[18] which are extensions of its pharmacologic action of inhibiting sodium and H_2O reabsorption in the ascending loop of Henle[7,10,37,80] (Figure 6). When severe, these abnormalities are life-threatening,[81] and fatalities have been associated with the administration of furosemide.[54] Various unpredictable reactions, including sudden death, have been reported.[82,83]

In reviewing the literature, two large studies concerned with adverse reactions to furosemide administration were found. In the most recent study, Lowe et al[81] monitored 2,580 medical inpatients, 585 of which were on furosemide therapy. Of these 585, 123 patients (21.0%) had 177 adverse reactions. The most common adverse reactions were volume depletion (14.5%), hyperuricemia (9.2%), and hypokalemia (3.6%). The other adverse effects observed were rare and included hyponatremia, gastrointestinal upsets and glycosuria. Most of the adverse reactions were mild, with only three potentially life-threatening reactions, but no

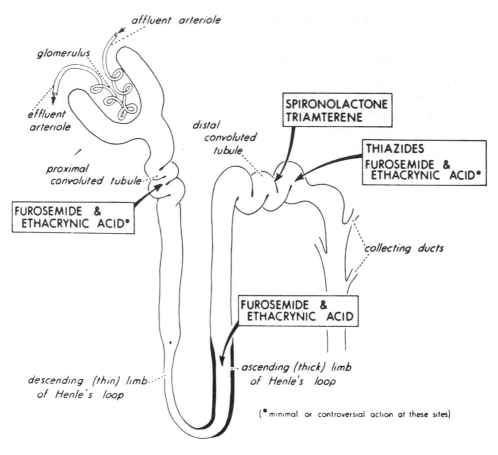

Figure 6: Diuretics — sites of action.

deaths were reported. The incidence of the adverse reactions seemed to be dose-dependent. Furosemide given up to 40 mg/day caused 13.5% of the adverse reactions, given up to 80 mg caused 26.3%, and 43.6% were observed with furosemide administered in doses over 80 mg/day.

Greenblatt et al[54] monitored 2,367 hospitalized patients from the initiation of furosemide therapy until either discharge or death. They reported 239 (10% of patients administered furosemide) adverse reactions of which 218 (91.2%) were extensions of furosemide's pharmacologic properties, and 21 (8.8%) were unpredictable reactions. Fourteen life-threatening reactions occurred, and they had five deaths (some not drug-induced) (Tables XVI, XVII and XVIII). Arndt and Hershel[84] found nine out of 3,497 (2.6%) receiving furosemide to have allergic skin reactions, but they did not look for other adverse effects.

TABLE XVI
USAGE OF FUROSEMIDE IN HOSPITALIZED PATIENTS*

Characteristic	% of patients
Indication for therapy:	
Congestive heart failure	77.7
Fluid retention due to cirrhosis	7.7
Fluid retention due to neoplastic disease	1.9
Hypertension	1.4
Anuria	0.1
Other and unspecified	11.2
Total	100.0
Total dose of furosemide:	
Less than 100 mg	34.4
100 to 450 mg	30.3
451 mg or more	29.1
Could not be calculated	6.2
Total	100.0
Daily doses of furosemide:†	
Less than 35 mg	36.8
35 to 55 mg	33.6
56 mg or more	21.4
Could not be calculated	8.2
Total	100.0
Route of furosemide administration:	
Intravenous	35.5
Intramuscular	6.9
Oral only	56.7
Not specified	0.9
Total	100.0
Drug therapy concurrent with furosemide:††	
Other "potassium-wasting" diuretics (thiazides, mercurials, ethacrynic acid, etc.)	23.4
Potassium supplements or "potassium-sparing" diuretics (i.e., potassium chloride, spironolactone, triamterene)	64.8
Digitalis glycosides	69.2
Corticosteroids or antineoplastic agents	15.7
Antihypertensive drugs (methyldopa, hydralazine, guanethidine, clonidine, diazoxide, etc.)	7.3

* From Greenblatt, D. J., Duhme, D. W., et al,[54] Clinical toxicity of furosemide in hospitalized patients. *American Heart Journal,* 94(1).8, 1977, reprinted with permission.
† Calculated as the total dose divided by the number of days of therapy.
†† Many patients received more than one class of drug concurrently.

TABLE XVII
ADVERSE REACTIONS TO FUROSEMIDE††

Adverse Reactions	No. of Patients	% of Patients
Volume depletion:		4.6
Elevation in BUN or serum creatinine only	68	
Elevation in BUN with other adverse reactions*	27	
• Hyponatremia or hypochloremia	(12)	
• Hyperuricemia	(6)	
• Hypotension	(4)	
• Hyperglycemia	(2)	
• Gastrointestinal disturbance	(2)	
• Alkalosis	(1)	
Other manifestations of volume depletion	14	
• Hypotension†	(10)	
• Excess diuresis or loss of body weight	(4)	
Total		
Hypokalemia:		3.6
As the only manifestation of toxicity	59	
With other adverse reactions	26	
• Hyponatremia or hypochloremia	(16)	
• Volume depletion	(4)	
• Cardiac arrhythmias	(3)	
• Gastrointestinal disturbance	(3)	
Total		
Electrolyte or metabolic disturbances:		1.5
• Hyponatremia	11	
• Hypochloremia	1	
• Hyponatremia and hypochloremia	12	
• Hyperuricemia	8	
• Metabolic alkalosis	3	
• Hyperglycemia	1	
Total	36	
Other adverse reactions:		0.4
• Rash	4	
• Central nervous system disturbances	3	
• Flushing	1	
• Dry mouth	1	
Total		
Total with adverse reaction:	239	10.1

†† Based on a Boston Collaborative Survey by Greenblatt, D. J., Duhme, D. W., et al,[54] Clinical toxicity of furosemide in hospitalized patients. *American Heart Journal,* 94(1):8, 1977, reprinted with permission.

  * Does not include four patients with volume depletion and hypokalemia (see Hypokalemia).
 ** Does not include patients with electrolyte or metabolic disturbances together with hypokalemia or volume depletion.
  † Does not include four patients with elevation in BUN and hypotension.

TABLE XVIII
NATURE OF REACTIONS TO FUROSEMIDE

Gastrointestinal	nausea, vomiting, diarrhea, G. I. upset, non-occlusive mesenteric infarction, pancreatitis, jaundice, gastric burning
Cardiovascular-Pulmonary	volume depletion, hypotension, chest pain, arrhythmias, edema, thrombophlebitis, emboli
Central Nervous System	CNS disturbances, visual hallucinations, generalized paresthesias, headache, somnolence, vertigo, dry mouth, flushing, blurring of vision, sweet taste, weakness, fatigue, diaphoresis, thirst, light headedness, tinnitus
Allergic	rash, interstitial nephritis, cutaneous necrotizing vasculitis, bullous hemorrhagic lesions, erythema multiform, exfoliative dermatitis, phototoxic blisters, pruritus, urticaria
Metabolic	hypokalemia, hyponatremia, hypochloremia, alkalosis, hyperuricemia, hyperglycemia, diabetic coma, acute gout
Hematological	leukopenia, eosinophilia, thrombocytopenia, aplastic anemia, anemia agranulocytosis
Miscellaneous	sudden death, ototoxicity, rapid excessive diuresis, acute bladder spasm and urinary retention

Nature of Furosemide Reactions
A. Pharmacological

1. Hyponatremia

Furosemide induces a substantial sodium loss by blocking its reabsorption mainly in the ascending loop of Henle[7,10,37, 43,78] and can easily overwhelm the normal homeostatic mechanisms for sodium. Hyponatremia should always be considered a possibility when furosemide is administered.[10] If large amounts of water are given, a salt-restricted diet is employed, and if the patient is on furosemide therapy, hyponatremia may be likely.[37] Lowe et al[81] observed in 585 medical inpatients on furosemide treatment that only six patients (1%) had developed hyponatremia. They also found, as with all other adverse side effects studied, that the incidence was dose-related. Four out of the six patients with hyponatremia were taking the largest doses administered (> 80 mg/day). "Inappropriate" antidiuretic hormone secretion has been associated with furosemide-induced hyponatremia.[85] Severe hyponatremia is life-threatening and fatalities have been reported.[54]

2. Hypokalemia

Hypokalemia is a potentially lethal condition because it increases myocardial sensitivity to catecholamines[86] and to digitalis,[61] thereby increasing the risk of arrhythmias. Both Lowe et al[81] and Greenblatt et al[54] observed the incidence of hypokalemia to be 3.6%. Many authorities agree the hypokalemia caused by furosemide is less severe and occurs less often than that associated with thiazide therapy,[5,10,27,40-42,87] although the nature of the illness and the doses are important. However, furosemide-induced hypokalemia has precipitated hospital admissions and both non-fatal and fatal arrhythmias.[54,88] Sherlock and Walder[89] reported that the incidence of hypokalemia and other electrolyte disturbances due to furosemide is significantly increased in cirrhotic patients.

3. Hypochloremia

Hypochloremia is another life-threatening electrolyte disturbance precipitated by furosemide therapy. Even though it is occasionally seen alone, hypochloremia is usually associated with metabolic alkalosis and often with other disturbances of fluid and electrolyte homeostasis. The hypochloremic metabolic acidosis does not interfere with the effectiveness of furosemide[7] (Table XVII).

4. Hyperuricemia

Furosemide, like the thiazides, has been associated with the development of hyperuricemia.[8,10,20, 90-92] It has been reported that 25–35% of all untreated essential hypertensives have hyperuricemia.[8,20,40]

Lowe et al[81] found a 9.2% incidence of hyperuricemia, but only two patients developed symptoms of gout. Wertheimer et al[93] reported that 31 out of 44 patients (71%) treated for eight weeks with 40 mg of furosemide twice daily had a statistically significant rise in uric acid. It is important to monitor serum uric acid during furosemide therapy because hyperuricemia, per se, is considered a minor risk factor in coronary artery disease, and acute gouty attacks precipitated by furosemide have been reported.[94,95]

5. Excessive Diuresis

Exaggerated diuretic responses after 40 mg furosemide (usually intravenous) have been reported. Greenblatt et al[54] report two life-threatening cases—1,500 ml in five hours and 2,000 ml in seven hours. Both were associated with severe plasma volume contraction and hypotension. Furosemide also produces a slowly progressing volume depletion[18] which can cause hypotension; anginal chest pains, probably due to decreased coronary flow; and progressive azotemia, probably due to decreased renal blood flow. Both Greenblatt et al[54] and Lowe et al[81] found volume depletion to be the most common adverse effect they observed, 4.6% and 14.5% respectively.

6. Hyperglycemia

Hyperglycemia[10,54] associated with furosemide has been reported, but the incidence has not been determined.[87] Deterioration of the glucose tolerance test and glucosuria[55] has also been noted to occur with furosemide therapy. Lowe et al[81] reported one case of glycosuria attributed to furosemide. Robinson et al,[87] in a study of six normal patients and two non-insulin dependent diabetic subjects—all of whom were given 80 mg furosemide a day—found that furosemide had minimal effects on the glucose utilization of all the patients. Kalder et al[96] reported no significant change in the oral glucose tolerance tests of ten asymptomatic diabetics placed on 40 mg/day of furosemide.

Non-ketotic diabetic coma[97] and precoma[28] have been associated with furosemide, and a direct pancreatotoxic effect of the drug is suggested by furosemide-induced acute pancreatitis.[98,99]

7. Effect of Calcium

Furosemide induces a calciuric effect.[10,100,101] It is sometimes used to treat hypercalcemia,[100,101] as opposed to thiazides which can cause hypercalcemia.[8,10]

8. Effects on Magnesium

Furosemide has been reported to cause hypomagnesemia, but the incidence is unknown.[10,102,103] The clinical manifestations do not seem to be clinically frequent except for the development of cardiac arrhythmias[103,104] which is rare. Sheehan et al[102] reported 14 cases of furosemide-induced hypomagnesemia.

9. Effects on Lipids

It has been established that after hypertension and smoking, abnormalities of plasma lipids are major coronary risk factors. Joos et al[105] gave 12 healthy male subjects 80 mg/day of furosemide for three weeks. They found total plasma triglycerides and total plasma cholesterol levels to have increased significantly. The VLDL fraction was elevated by furosemide, but the LDL was not. The effects of furosemide on plasma lipids, especially HDL-cholesterol, need further study.

10. Decreased Absorption of Water and Electrolytes

MacKenzie et al[106] report decreased absorption of sodium, potassium, chloride, bicarbonate, and water following the administration of furosemide. The clinical significance of this finding (if confirmed) is yet to be determined.

B. Unpredictable Adverse Reactions to Furosemide

1. Sudden Death

Sudden death within one minute after injection of furosemide due to cardiac or respiratory arrest has been reported after both intravenous[79] and intramuscular[83] administration. Physicians should be prepared to deal with anaphylactoid-type reactions before parenteral administration of furosemide, as with any medication.

2. Ototoxicity

Ototoxicity varying from transient, mild hearing loss to permanent deafness has been reported.[8-10,107-113] Some authors feel that ototoxicity is dose-related; however, Heiland et al[111] demonstrated that the rate of intravenous administration is an important determinant. At doses of 600 mg or greater, they demonstrated transient ototoxicity in 60% of patients when administering 25 mg/min, in 40% of patients when administering 15 mg/min, and in none of the patients when administering 5–6 mg/min.

3. Allergic Reaction

In a study specifically looking for cutaneous, allergic reactions to drugs, 3,497 patients on furosemide were monitored with only nine (0.26%) developing skin reactions.[84] Greenblatt et al[54] in 2,367 patients on furosemide found four (0.17%). One or more cases of the following allergic-type reactions has been reported in the literature: interstitial nephritis,[114,115] cutaneous necrotizing vasculitis,[116] hemorrhagic bullous lesions,[117,118] erythema multiform,[119] phototoxic blisters,[120] and a patchy erythmatous rash associated with a mild bullous eruption.[81] The possibility of other allergic reactions,[9,10,107] especially anaphylaxis, must be remembered.

4. Hematologic Reactions

Eosinophilia,[54,115] leukopenia,[121] progressive thrombocytopenia,[81] and fatal thrombocytopenia[54] have all been associated with the use of furosemide.

5. Nervous System Disturbances

Greenblatt et al[54] reported three cases of central nervous system

---

TABLE XIX
LIFE-THREATENING REACTIONS TO FUROSEMIDE

— Sudden death
— Electrolyte disturbances*
— Volume depletion (acute and chronic)
— Diabetic coma
— Hematologic reactions**
— Non-occlusive mesenteric infarction

---

* Especially hypokalemia with associated arrhythmias.
** Especially thrombocytopenia; no cases of aplastic anemia secondary to furosemide were found in the literature.

TABLE XX
FREQUENCY OF ADVERSE REACTIONS DUE TO FUROSEMIDE*

Frequent (> 5.0%)
  • None

Occasional (0.5–5.0%)

• Volume depletion	• Hypokalemia	• Azotemia
• Hyponatremia	• Hypochloremia	• Hyperuricemia
• Metabolic alkalosis	• Hypotension	• GI upset
• Rash	• Arrhythmias	• Hyperglycemia
• CNS disturbance		

Rare (< 0.5%)
  • All others (Table VI)

---

* This table calculated from the 2,367 patients in the Boston Collaborative Study, by Greenblatt, D. J., Duhme, D. W., et al,[54] with permission.

disturbance. Various investigators have reported visual hallucinations,[122] generalized paresthesias,[123] headache,[36] somnolence,[36] vertigo,[124] dry mouth,[54] and flushing.[54]

6. Gastric Disturbances

Several researchers have reported cases of gastric disturbances associated with furosemide therapy.[10,39,81,125]

7. Musculoskeletal Disturbances

There have been reports of muscle pain,[39] weakness,[107] cramps,[107] and arthritic pain[97] in patients taking furosemide.

8. Mesenteric Infarction

The potentially fatal condition, non-occlusive mesenteric infarction, has been associated with furosemide administration.[126]

9. Edema

Edema due to water retention from furosemide-induced activation of homeostatic mechanisms for water conservation has been reported.[127-129]

10. Acute Bladder Obstruction

Stretching of the bladder beyond a point at which the patient may void with resulting acute urinary retention has been associated with the diuresis produced by furosemide.[124]

REFERENCES:
Thiazide Diuretics

1. Beermann, B., and Groschinsky-Grind, M.: Antihypertensive effect of various doses of hydrochlorothiazide and its relation to the plasma level of the drug. *Eur. J. Clin. Pharmacol.*, **13**:195–201, 1978.
2. Berglund, G., and Andersson, O.: Low doses of hydrochlorothiazide in hypertension: Antihypertensive and metabolic effects. *Eur. J. Clin. Pharmacol.*, **10**:177–182, 1976.
3. Durley, Y., Cubberley, R., and Thomas, S.: Antihypertensive effect of oral timolol maleate and hydrochlorothiazide once daily compared with hydrochlorothiazide once daily. *Am. J. Hosp. Pharm.*, **38**:1161–1164, 1981.
4. Degnbol, B., Dorph, S., and Marner, T.: The effect of different diuretics on elevated blood pressure and serum potassium. *Acta Med. Scand.*, **193**:407–410, 1973.
5. Veterans Administration Cooperative Study Group on Antihypertensive Agents: Comparative effects of ticrynafen and hydrochlorothiazide in the treatment of hypertension. *N. Engl. J. Med.*, **301**(6):293–297, 1979.

6. Alhenc-Gelas, F., Plouin, P., Ducrocq, M., Corvol, P., and Menard, J.: Comparison of the antihypertensive and hormonal effects of a cardioselective beta-blocker, acebutolol, and diuretics in essential hypertension. *Am. J. Med.*, **64**(6): 1005–1012, 1978.

7. McMahon, F. G.: Efficacy of antihypertensive agent comparison of alpha-methyldopa plus hydrochlorothiazide in combination and singly. *JAMA*, **231**:155, 1975.

8. Multicenter Diuretic Cooperative Study Group: Multiclinic comparison of amiloride, hydrochlorothiazide, and hydrochlorothiazide plus amiloride in essential hypertension. *Arch. Intern. Med.*, **141**(3):482–486, 1981.

9. Aberg, H., Frithz, G., and Morlin, C.: Comparison of captopril (SQ 14225) with hydrochlorothiazide in the treatment of essential hypertension. *Int. J. Clin. Pharmacol. Ther. Tox.*, **19**(8):368–371, 1981.

10. Kuska, J., Kokot, F., Pachelski, J., Krok, J., and Seredynski, M.: The secretion of insulin in patients with arterial hypertension, treated with hydrochlorothiazide. *Mater. Med. Pol.*, **2**(46):124–129, 1981.

11. Korduner, I., Kabin, I., and Hagbarth, G.: Low-dose chlorthalidone treatment in previously untreated hypertension. *Curr. Ther. Res.*, **29**(1):208–215, 1981.

12. Materson, B., Oster, J., et al: Dose response to chlorthalidone in patients with mild hypertension: Efficacy of a lower dose. *Clin. Pharmacol. Ther.*, **24**(2):192–198, 1978.

13. Papadoyannis, D. E., Papzachos, G. A., Karatzas, N. D., Palminteri, R., and Kilborn, J. R.: *Betaxolol in Hypertension: Comparison with Chlorthalidone*. P. L. Morselli, et al (Eds.), Raven Press, New York, 1983, pp. 339–345.

14. Tweedale, M., Ogilvie, R., and Ruedy, J.: Antihypertensive and biochemical effects of chlorthalidone. *Clin. Pharmacol. Ther.*, **22**(5 Part 1):519–527, 1977.

15. Carney, S., Gillies, A., and Morgan, T.: Optimal dose of a thiazide diuretic. *Med. J. Aust.*, **2**:692–693, 1976.

16. Systolic Hypertension in the Elderly Program (SHEP): *Heart Institute's SHEP trial has revealed no serious problems*. F-D-C Reports, June 6, 1983, p. 6.

17. Bengtsson, C., Johnsson, G., Sannerstedt, R., and Werko, L.: Effect of different doses of chlorthalidone on blood pressure, serum potassium, and serum urate. *Br. Med. J.*, **1**(5951):197, 1975.

18. Rosenman, R. H.: Combined clonidine-chlorthalidone therapy in hypertension. *Arch. Intern. Med.*, **135**:1236, 1975.

19. Sung, P., Somet, P., et al: Effects of clonidine and chlorthalidone on blood pressure and glucose tolerance in hypertensive patients. *Curr. Ther. Res.*, **13**(5): 280, 1971.

20. Smith, W. M.: Isolated systolic hypertension in the elderly. *Curr. Med. Res. Opin.*, **8**(Suppl 1), 1982.

21. Shah, S., Khatri, I., and Freis, E.: Mechanism of antihypertensive effect of thiazide diuretics. *Am. Heart J.*, **95**(5):611–617, 1978.

22. Moser, M., et al: Report of the Joint National Committee on detection, evaluation, and treatment of high blood pressure. *JAMA*, **237**(3):255, 1977.

23. Moser, M., and Lunn, J.: Comparative effects of pindolol and hydrochlorothiazide in black hypertensive patients. *Angiology*, **32**:561–566, 1981.

24. Veterans Administration Cooperative Study Group on Antihypertensive Agents: Comparison of propranolol and hydrochlorothiazide for the initial treatment of hypertension II: Results of long-term therapy. *JAMA*, **248**(16):2004–2011, 1982.

25. Veterans Administration Cooperative Study Group on Antihypertensive Agents:

Comparison of propranolol and hydrochlorothiazide for the initial treatment of hypertension I: Results of short-term titration with emphasis on racial differences in response. *JAMA*, **248**(16):1996–2003, 1982.

26. Finnerty, F., Jr.: Initial therapy of essential hypertension: Diuretic or beta-blocker? *J. Fam. Pract.*, **11**(2):199–205, 1980.

27. Veterans Administration Cooperative Study Group on Antihypertensive Agents: Efficacy of nadolol alone and combined with bendroflumethiazide and hydralazine. *Am. J. Cardiol.*, **52**(10):1230–1237, 1983.

28. The 1980 Report of the Joint National Committee on detection, evaluation, and treatment of high blood pressure. *Arch. Intern. Med.*, **140**:1280–1285, 1980.

29. Whitworth, J., and Kincaid-Smith, P.: Diuretics or beta-blockers first for hypertension? *Drugs*, **23**:394–402, 1982.

30. Diuretic or beta-blocker as first-line treatment for mild hypertension? (Editorial), *Lancet*, **ii**:1316–1317, 1982.

31. Freis, E. D., and Wilson, I. M.: Potentiating effect of chlorothiazide in combination with antihypertension agents, preliminary report. *Med. Ann. DC*, **26**:468, 1957.

32. Walter, N., Suthers, M., Friedman, A., and Johnston, C.: A comparison between spironolactone and hydrochlorothiazide with and without alpha-methyldopa in the treatment of hypertension. *Med. J. Aust.*, **1**:509–512, 1978.

33. MacGregor, G., Markandu, N., et al: Captopril in essential hypertension; contrasting effects of adding hydrochlorothiazide or propranolol. *Br. Med. J.*, **284**:693–696, 1982.

34. Andren, L., Karlberg, B., et al: Captopril and atenolol combined with hydrochlorothiazide in essential hypertension. *Br. J. Clin. Pharmacol.*, **14**:107S–111S, 1982.

35. Pitkajarvi, T., Kyostila, S., Kontro, J., and Mattila, M.: Antihypertensive drug combinations: Prazosin, hydrochlorothiazide and clonidine. *Ann. Clin. Res.*, **9**:296–300, 1977.

36. Smith, W. M., Bachman, B., et al: Cooperative clinical trial of alpha-methyldopa. *Ann. Intern. Med.*, **65**(4):657, 1966.

37. Mroczek, W. J., and Leibel, B. A.: Comparison of clonidine and methyldopa in hypertensive patients receiving a diuretic. *Am. J. Cardiol.*, **29**:712, 1972.

38. Igloe, M. C.: Antihypertensive efficacy and safety of a clonidine–chlorthalidone combination. *Curr. Ther. Res.*, **15**(8):559, 1973.

39. Lavenius, B., and Hansson, L.: A double-blind comparison of spironolactone and hydrochlorothiazide in hypertensive patients treated with metoprolol. *J. Clin. Pharmacol. Ther. Tox.*, **20**(6):291–295, 1982.

40. Kubik, M., Kendall, M., Ebbutt, A., and John, V.: Metoprolol with chlorthalidone in hypertension. *Clin. Pharmacol. Ther.*, **25**(1):25–32, 1979.

41. Weber, M., Lopez-Ovejero, J., Drayer, J., Case, D., and Laragh, J.: Renin reactivity as a determinant of responsiveness to antihypertensive treatment. *Arch. Intern. Med.*, **137**:284–289, 1977.

42. Vander Elst, E., Dombey, S., Lawrence, J., and Vlassak, W.: Controlled comparison of the effects of furosemide and hydrochlorothiazide added to propranolol in the treatment of hypertension. *Am. Heart J.*, **102**(4):734–740, 1981.

43. Velasco, M., Guevara, J., et al: Antihypertensive effect of atenolol alone or combined with chlorthalidone in patients with essential hypertension. *Br. J. Clin. Pharmacol.*, **9**:499–504, 1980.

44. Maclean, D., and Tudhope, G.: Modern diuretic treatment. *Br. Med. J.*, **286**:1419–1422, 1983.

45. de Carvalho, J., Dunn, F., Lohmoller, G., and Frolich, E.: Hemodynamic correlates of prolonged thiazide therapy: Comparison of responders and nonresponders. *Clin. Pharmacol. Ther.*, **22**(6):875–880, 1977.

46. Conway, J.: Antihypertensive effect of diuretics. *Handbook of Exp. Pharmacol.*, **39**:477–494, 1977.

47. Tarazi, R.: Diuretic drugs: Mechanisms of antihypertensive action. In G. Onesti, K. Kim, and J. Moyer (Eds.): *Hypertension: Mechanisms and Management.* Grune and Stratton, Inc., New York, 1973, p. 251.

48. Bennett, W., McDonald, W., Kuehnel, E., Hartnett, M., and Porter, G.: Commentary: Do diuretics have antihypertensive properties independent of natriuresis? *Clin. Pharmacol. Ther.*, **22**(5 Part 1):499–504, 1977.

49. Tobian, L.: Why do thiazides lower blood pressure in essential hypertension? *Annu. Rev. Pharmacol.*, **7**:399, 1967.

50. Wilson, I. M., and Freis, E.: Relationship between plasma and extracellular fluid volume depletion and the antihypertensive effect of chlorothiazide. *Circulation*, **20**:1028, 1959.

51. Leth, A.: Changes in plasma volume in patients during long-term treatment with hydrochlorothiazide. *Circulation*, **42**:479, 1970.

52. Freis, E.: Treatment of mild hypertension. *Resident and Staff Physician*, 55–69, September, 1975.

53. Freis, E., Wanko, A., et al: Mechanism of the altered blood pressure responsiveness produced by chlorothiazide. *J. Clin. Invest.*, **39**:1277, 1960.

54. Weinberger, M. H., Ramsdell, J. W., et al: Effect of chlorothiazide and sodium on vascular responsiveness to angiotensin II. *Am. J. Physiol.*, **223**:1049, 1972.

55. Tarazi, R., Duston, A., and Frohlich, E.: Long-term thiazide treatment in essential hypertension. *Circulation*, **42**:709, 1970.

56. Van Brummelen, P., Veld, A., and Schalekamp, A.: Haemodynamics during long-term thiazide treatment in essential hypertension: Differences between responders and non-responders. *Clin. Sci.*, **57**:359s–362s, 1979.

57. Van Brummelen, P., Woerlee, M., and Schlekamp, M.: Long-term versus short-term effects of hydrochlorothiazide on renal haemodynamics in essential hypertension. *Clin. Sci.*, **56**:463–469, 1979.

58. Tobian, L.: Hypertension and the kidney. *Arch. Intern. Med.*, **133**(6):959–967, 1974.

59. Tobian, L.: How sodium and the kidney relate to the hypertensive arteriole. *Fed. Proc.*, **33**(2):138–142, 1974.

60. Schwarcz, G.: The problem of antihypertensive treatment in lithium patients. *Compr. Psychiatry*, **23**(1):50–54, 1982.

61. Kerry, R., Ludlow, J., and Owen, G.: Diuretics are dangerous with lithium. *Br. Med. J.*, **281**:371, 1980.

62. Goddard, J. E., and Phillips, O. C.: The influence of nonanesthetic drugs on the course of anesthesia. *Pa. Med.*, **68**:48, 1965.

63. Jelliffe, R. W.: Effect of serum potassium level upon risk of digitalis toxicity. *Ann. Intern. Med.*, **78**:821, 1973.

64. Seller, R. H., et al: Digitalis toxicity and hypomagnesemia. *Am. Heart J.*, **79**:57, 1970.

65. O'Reilly, R. A., and Aggeler, P. M.: Impact of aspirin and chlorthalidone on the

pharmacodynamics of oral anticoagulant drugs in man. *Ann. N. Y. Acad. Sci.*, **179**: 173, 1971.

66. O'Reilly, R. A., and Aggeler, P. M.: Determinants of the response to oral anticoagulant drugs in man. *Pharmacol. Rev.*, **22**:35, 1970.

67. Buee-Hoi, N. P., Hein, D. P., et al: Effects of deux diuretiques, l'hydrochlorothiazide et l'acide ethacrynique, sur la coagulation sanguine chez le rat normal et chez le tat recevant de antivitamines K. *Acad. Sci. Paris*, **265**:2165, 1967.

68. Field, J. B., and Larsen, E. G.: Hypercoagulability and liver dysfunction induced by compounds of some heavy metals. *Acta Haematol.*, **12**:253, 1954.

69. Egeberg, O.: Effect of edema drainage on the blood clotting system. *Scand. J. Clin. Lab. Invest.*, **15**:14, 1963.

70. Vinazzer, H., and Wien, Z.: Die buinflussung du antikoaggulantientherapu durch ein diuretikum. *Inn. Med. Ihre Grenzgeb.*, **44**:323, 1963.

71. Sellers, E. M., and Koch-Weser, J.: Protein binding and vascular activity of diazoxide. *N. Engl. J. Med.*, **281**:1141, 1969.

72. Seltzer, H. S., and Allen, E. W.: Hyperglycemia and inhibition of insulin secretion during administration of diazoxide and trichlormethiazide in man. *Diabetes*, **18**: 19, 1969.

73. Wolff, F.: Diazoxide misunderstood. *N. Engl. J. Med.*, **286**:612, 1972.

74. Aleksandrow, D., Wysznackaw, W., et al: Influence of chlorothiazide upon actual responsiveness to nor-epinephrine in hypertensive subjects. *N. Engl. J. Med.*, **261**: 1052, 1959.

75. Abrams, W. B.: The mechanisms of drug induced arrhythmias. *J. Newark City Hosp.*, **2**:3, 1965.

76. Thorn, G. W.: Clinical considerations in use of corticosteroids. *N. Engl. J. Med.*, **274**:775, 1966.

77. Kauffman, R. E., and Azarnoff, D. L.: Effect of colestipol on gastrointestinal absorption in chlorothiazide in man. *Clin. Pharmacol. Ther.*, **14**:886, 1973.

78. Gallo, D. G., et al: The interaction between cholestyramine and drugs. *Proc. Soc. Exp. Biol. Med.*, **120**:60, 1965.

79. Lake, C., Ziegler, M., Coleman, M., and Kopin, I.: Fenfluramine potentiation of antihypertensive effects of thiazides. *Clin. Pharmacol. Ther.*, **28**(1):22–27, 1980.

80. Steiness, E., and Waldorff, S.: Different interactions of indemethacin and sulindac with thiazides in hypertension. *Br. Med. J.*, **285**:1702–1703, 1982.

81. Kraus, G. W., Marchese, J. R., et al: Prophylactic use of hydrochlorothiazide in pregnancy. *JAMA*, **198**(11):128, 1966.

82. Falls, N. E., Plauche, W. C., et al: Thiazide versus placebo in prophylaxis of toxemia of pregnancy in primigravid patients. *Am. J. Obstet. Gynecol.*, **88**:502, 1964.

83. Gant, N. F., Madden, J. D., et al: The metabolic clearance rate of dehydroisoandiosterone sulfate. *Am. J. Obstet. Gynecol.*, **123**(2):159, 1975.

84. Menzies, D., and Prystowsky, H.: Acute hemorrhagic pancreatitis during pregnancy and the puerperium associated with thiazide therapy. *J. Fla. Med. Assoc.*, **54**(6):564, 1967.

85. Livingston, S. H., and Gold, E. M.: Acute hemorrhagic pancreatitis in pregnancy, report of fatal cases. *Am. J. Obstet. Gynecol.*, **26**:237, 1965.

86. Minkowitz, S., Solowey, H. G., et al: Fatal hemorrhagic pancreatitis following chlorothiazide administration in pregnancy. *Am. J. Obstet. Gynecol.*, **24**:337, 1964.

87. Redman, C.: Treatment of hypertension in pregnancy. *Kidney Int.*, **18**:267–278, 1980.
88. Holland, O., Gomez-Sanchez, E., Kuhnert, L., Poindexter, C., and Pak, C.: Antihypertensive comparison of furosemide with hydrochlorothiazide for black patients. *Arch. Intern. Med.*, **139**:1015–1021, 1979.
89. Moser, M., and Lunn, J.: Responses to captopril and hydrochlorothiazide in black patients with hypertension. *Clin. Pharmacol. Ther.*, **32**(3):307–312, 1982.
90. Seedat, Y.: Trial of atenolol and chlorthalidone for hypertension in black South Africans. *Br. Med. J.*, **281**:1241–1243, 1980.
91. Task Force on Blood Pressure Control in Children: Report of the Task Force. *Pediatrics*, **59**(5 Suppl):797–820, 1977.
92. Falkner, B., Onesti, G., Lowenthal, D., and Affrime, M.: Effectiveness of centrally acting drugs and diuretics in adolescent hypertension. *Clin. Pharmacol. Ther.*, **32**(5):577–582, 1982.
93. Forrest, W.: The treatment of hypertension in older patients: A comparative study between a diuretic, a beta-receptor antagonist, and their fixed combination. *Practitioner*, **226**(4):777–778, 1982.
94. Forrest, W.: The treatment of hypertension in older patients: A double-blind, between-patient study in previously treated patients comparing a diuretic, a beta-receptor antagonist and their fixed combination. *J. Int. Med. Res.*, **9**:490–494, 1981.
95. Goodfellow, R., and Wesberg, B.: The treatment of high blood pressure in the elderly: A multi-centre evaluation of a fixed combination of metoprolol and hydrochlorothiazide ('Co-Betaloc') in general practice. *Curr. Med. Res. Opin.*, **57**: 536–542, 1981.
96. Beermann, B., and Groschinsky-Grind, M.: Gastrointestinal absorption of hydrochlorothiazide enhanced by concomitant intake of food. *Eur. J. Clin. Pharmacol.*, **13**:125–128, 1978.
97. Beermann, B., and Groschinsky-Grind, M.: Pharmacokinetics of hydrochlorothiazide in man. *Eur. J. Clin. Pharmacol.*, **12**:297–303, 1977.
98. Goodman, L. S., and Gilman, A.: *The Pharmacologic Basis of Therapeutics.* MacMillan Publishing Co., Inc., New York, 1975, p. 817.
99. Beermann, B., Groschinsky-Grind, M., et al: Absorption, metabolism, and excretion of hydrochlorothiazide. *Clin. Pharmacol. Ther.*, **19**(5):531, 1976.
100. Anderson, K. V., Bretell, H. R., et al: C^{14}-labeled hydrochlorothiazide in human beings. *Arch. Intern. Med.*, **107**:736, 1961.
101. Miller, R. R.: Hospital admissions due to adverse reactions: A report from the Boston Surveillance Program. *Arch. Intern. Med.*, **134**:219, 1974.
102. Winchester, J., Kellett, R., et al: Metolazone and bendroflumethiazide in hypertension: Physiologic and metabolic observations. *Clin. Pharmacol. Ther.*, **28**(5): 611–618, 1980.
103. Weinberger, M.: Comparison of captopril and hydrochlorothiazide alone and in combination in mild to moderate essential hypertension. *Br. J. Clin. Pharmacol.*, **14**:127S–131S, 1982.
104. Pitkajarvi, T., Ala-Laurila, P., Ruosteenoja, R., Torsti, P., and Masar, S.: Treatment of hypertension successively with a diuretic, clonidine or a beta-blocking agent and hydralazine. *Eur. J. Clin. Pharmacol.*, **12**:161–165, 1977.
105. Pitkajarvi, T.: Cyclothiazide and atenolol once daily in essential hypertension. *Ann. Clin. Res.*, **11**:1–8, 1979.

106. Fernandez, P., Zachariah, P., Bryant, D., and Missan, S.: Antihypertensive efficacy of alpha-methyldopa, chlorothiazide and supres-150 (alpha-methyldopa-chlorothiazide). *CMA J.*, **123**:284–287, 1980.

107. Sherrill, E., and Carr, A.: Chemotherapy for hypertension. *Journal of MAG*, **70**: 341–344, 1981.

108. Langlois, S: Les Diuretiques dans le traitement de l'hypertension arterielle. *Union Med. Canada*, (7):649–652, 1982.

109. Ram, C.: Diuretics in the management of hypertension. *Postgrad. Med.*, **71**(2):155–168, 1982.

110. Cannon, M., Tannenbaum, R., and LaFranco, M.: Diuretics in the treatment of hypertension. *Am. Pharm.*, **NS18**(5):34–39, 1978.

111. Hollifield, J., and Slaton, P.: Thiazide diuretics, hypokalemia, and cardiac arrhythmias. *Acta Med. Scand.*, **S647**:67–73, 1981.

112. Healy, J., McKenna, T., et al: Body composition changes in hypertensive subjects on long-term oral diuretic therapy. *Br. Med. J.*, **1**:716–719, 1970.

113. Oh, M., and Carroll, H.: The renin-aldosterone system and thiazide-induced depletion of total body potassium in essential hypertension. *Nephron*, **21**:269-276, 1978.

114. Kassirer, J., and Harrington, J.: Diuretics and potassium metabolism. A reassessment of the need, effectiveness, and safety of potassium therapy. *Kidney, Int.*, **11**: 505–515, 1977.

115. Dargie, H. J., Boddy, K., et al: Total body potassium in long-term furosemide therapy: Is potassium supplementation necessary? *Br. Med. J.*, **4**:316, 1974.

116. Wilkinson, P. R., Issler, H., et al: Total body and serum potassium during prolonged thiazide therapy for essential hypertension. *Lancet*, **1**(7910):759, 1975.

117. Edmonds, C. J., and Jasani, B.: Total body potassium in hypertension patients during prolonged diuretic therapy. *Lancet*, **2**:8, 1972.

118. Edelman, I. S., and Liebman, J.: Anatomy of body water and electrolytes. *Am. J. Med.*, **27**:256, 1959.

119. Boddy, K., King, P. C., et al: The relationship between total body potassium and exchangeable body potassium measured at 24 hours and 44 hours after administration of K^{43}. *Eur. J. Clin. Invest.*, **3**:188, 1973.

120. Lemieux, G., Beauchemin, M., Vinay, P., and Gougoux, A.: Hypokalemia during the treatment of arterial hypertension with diuretics. *CMA J.*, **122**:905–907, 1980.

121. Francisco, T., and Ferris, T.: The use and abuse of diuretics. *Arch. Int. Med.*, **142**: 28–32, 1982.

122. Kilcoyne, M.: Hypertension in adolescents: Diagnosis and treatment. *Clin. Med.*, **82**:16–23, 1975.

123. McMahon, F. G., Ryan, J. R., Akdamar, K., and Ertan, A.: The effect of potassium chloride supplements on upper gastrointestinal mucosa: Nine controlled clinical studies. (In press)

124. Barkin, J. S., Harary, A. M., Shamblen, C. E., and Lasseter, K. C.: Potassium chloride and gastrointestinal injury (letter). *Ann. Intern. Med.*, **98**:261-262, 1983.

125. Costa, F. V., Caldari, R., Ambrosioni, E., and Magnani, B.: Efficacy and tolerability of a new microencapsulated potassium chloride in hypertensive patients. *Curr. Ther. Res.*, **33**(6):1112, 1983.

126. Graybiel, A. L., and Sode, J.: Diuretics, potassium depletion, and carbohydrate intolerance. *Lancet*, **2**:265, 1971.

127. Caralis, P., Perez-Stable, E., Materson, B., and Rozanski, J.: Ventricular ectopy

and diuretic-induced hypokalemia in hypertensive patients. *Clin. Res.*, **29**(5): 832A, 1981.

128. Holland, O., Nixon, J., and Kuhnert, L.: Diuretic-induced ventricular ectopic activity. *Am. J. Med.*, **70**:762–768, 1981.

129. Cooper, W. D., Reuben, S., VandenBurg, M. J., Kaun, P., and Currie, W. J. C.: *Cardiac Arrhythmias following Acute Myocardial Infarction: Association with the Serum Potassium Level and Prior Diuretic Therapy*. International Symposium on Potassium, Blood Pressure and Cardiovascular Disease, April 2–23, 1983. Capri, Italy.

130. Freis, E. D., and Sappington, R. F.: Long-term effect of probenecid on diuretic-induced hyperuricemia. *JAMA*, **198**(2):147–149, 1966.

131. Breckenridge, A.: Hypertension and hyperuricemia. *Lancet*, **6**(15):15, 1966.

132. Hollifield, J.: Biochemical consequences of diuretic therapy in hypertension. *J. Tenn. Med. Assoc.*, **71**(10):757–758, 1978.

133. Hutchinson, J., Wilkinson, W. H., et al: Drug-induced hyperuricemia prevented by probenicid. *J. Med.*, **2**(1):45, 1971.

134. Nicotero, J. A., Scheib, B. A., et al: Prevention of hyperuricemia by allopurinol in hypertensive patients treated with chlorothiazide. *N. Engl. J. Med.*, **282**(3):133, 1970.

135. Sherlock, S., and Walker, J. G.: The complications of diuretic therapy in patients with cirrhosis. *Ann. N. Y. Acad. Sci.*, **139**:497, 1958.

136. Hutchinson, J.: The hypotensive action of ethacrynic acid. *Vas. Dis.*, **5**(2):104, 1968.

137. Diamond, M. T.: Hyperglycemic hyperosmolar coma associated with hydrochlorothiazide and pancreatitis. *N. Y. State J. Med.*, **72**(2):1741, 1972.

138. Curtis, J., and Horrigan, F.: Chlorthalidone-induced hyperosmolar hyperglycemic nonketotic coma. *JAMA*, **220**(12):1592, 1972.

139. Marks, P., Nimalasuriya, A., and Anderson, J.: The glucose tolerance test in hypertensive patients treated long term with thiazide diuretics. *Practitioner*, **225**: 392–393, 1981.

140. Amery, A., Bulpitt, C., et al: Glucose intolerance during diuretic therapy. *Lancet*, **1**:681–683, 1978.

141. Veterans Administration Cooperative Study Group on Antihypertensive Agents: Effects of treatment on morbidity in hypertension. III. Influence of age, diastolic pressure and prior cardiovascular disease. Further analysis of side effects. *Circulation*, **45**:991–1004, 1972.

142. Kochar, M. S., and Itskov, H. D.: Effects of hydrochlorothiazide in hypertensive patients and the need for potassium supplementation. *Curr. Ther. Res.*, **15**:298, 1973.

143. Fishman, M. P., and Vorheir, H.: Diuretic induced hyponatremia. *Ann. Intern. Med.*, **75**(6):853, 1971.

144. Buesford, H. R.: Polydipsia, hydrochlorothiazide and water intoxication. *JAMA*, **214**(5):879, 1977.

145. Schifrin, B. S., Spellacy, W. N., et al: Maternal death associated with excessive ingestion of a chlorothiazide diuretic. *Am. J. Obstet. Gynecol.*, **34**(2):215, 1969.

146. Duarte, C. G., Winmacker, J. L., et al: Thiazide induced hypercalcemia. *N. Engl. J. Med.*, **284**(15):828, 1971.

147. Hilker, R. R. J.: Reversible hypercalcemia associated with prolonged thiazide administration to control hypertension. *J. Occup. Med.*, **12**(11):444, 1970.

148. Balizit, L.: Recurrent parathyroid adenoma associated with prolonged thiazide administration. *JAMA*, **225**(10):1238, 1973.

149. Sheehan, J., and White, A.: Diuretic—associated hypomagnesaemia. *Br. Med. J.*, **285**:1157–1159, 1982.

150. Loeb, H., Pietras, R., Gunnar, R., and Tobin, J.: Paroxysmal ventricular fibrillation in two patients with hypomagnesemia. *Circulation*, 37:210–215, 1968.

151. Iseri, L., Freed, J., and Bures, A.: Magnesium deficiency and cardiac disorders. *Am. J. Med.*, **58**:837–846, 1975.

152. Whang, R., and Aikawa, J. K.: Magnesium deficiency and refractoriness to potassium repletion. *J. Chron. Dis.*, 30:65–68, 1977.

153. Wester, P.: Urinary zinc excretion during treatment with different diuretics. *Acta Med. Scand.*, 208:209–212, 1980.

154. Pak, C., Ruskin, B., and Diller, E.: Enhancement of renal excretion of zinc by hydrochlorothiazide. *Clin. Chim. Acta*, 39:511–517, 1972.

155. Wester, P.: Trace elements in serum and urine from hypertensive patients before and during treatment with chlorthalidone. *Acta Med. Scand.*, **194**:505–512, 1973.

156. Johnson, B.: The emerging problem of plasma lipid changes during antihypertensive therapy. *J. Cardiovasc. Pharmacol.*, 4(Suppl 2):S213–S221, 1982.

157. Fagerberg, S.: Serum lipids and some metabolic parameters after treatment with spironolactone and thiazides in hypertensive patients. *Curr. Ther. Res.*, **32**(6):872–878, 1982.

158. Leren, P., Eide, I., et al: Antihypertensive drugs and blood lipids: The Oslo study. *J. Cardiovasc. Pharmacol.*, 4(Suppl 2):S222–S224, 1982.

159. Gluck, Z., Weidmann, P., et al: Increased serum low-density lipoprotein cholesterol in men treated short-term with the diuretic chlorothalidone. *Metabolism*, **29**(3):240–245, 1980.

160. Grimm, R., Leon, A., et al: Effects of thiazide diuretics on plasma lipids and lipoproteins in mildly hypertensive patients. *Ann. Intern. Med.*, **94**:7–11, 1981.

161. Meier, A., Weidmann, P., Mordasini, R., Riesen, W., and Bachmann, C.: Reversal or prevention of diuretic-induced alterations in serum lipoprotein with beta-blockers. *Atherosclerosis*, **41**:415–419, 1982.

162. Goldman, A., and Steele, B., et al: Serum lipoprotein levels during chlorthalidone therapy: Veterans Administration–National Heart, Lung, and Blood Institute Cooperative Study on Antihypertensive Therapy: Mild Hypertension. *JAMA*, **244** (15):1691–1695, 1980.

163. Ames, R., and Hill, P.: Raised serum lipid concentrations during diuretic treatment of hypertension: A study of predictive indexes. *Clin. Sci. Mol. Med.*, **55**:311s–314s, 1978.

164. Ames, R., and Hill, P.: Antihypertensive therapy and the risk of coronary heart disease. *J. Cardiovasc. Pharmacol.*, 4(2):S206–S212, 1982.

165. Joos, C., Kewitz, H., and Reinhold-Kourniati, D.: Effects of diuretics on plasma lipoproteins in healthy men. *Eur. J. Clin. Pharmacol.*, 17:251–257, 1980.

166. Gluck, Z., Baumgartner, G., et al: Increased ratio between serum beta and alpha lipoproteins during diuretic therapy: An adverse effect? *Clin. Sci. Mol. Med.*, **55**:325s–328s, 1978.

167. Stamler, J.: Lifestyles, major risk factors, proof and public policy. *Circulation*, **58** (1):3–19, 1978.

168. Bariso, C. R., Hanenson, I. B., et al: Comparison of antihypertensive effects of furosemide and chlorothiazide. *Curr. Ther. Res.*, **12**:333, 1970.

169. Stokkeland, O. M., Sangvils, K., et al: Comparative study of metoprolol and trichlormethiazides. *Curr. Ther. Res.*, **18**(6):755, 1975.
170. Pederson, O. L.: Comparison of metoprolol and hydrochlorothiazides as antihypertensive agents. *Eur. J. Clin. Pharmacol.*, **10**(6):381, 1976.
171. Speikerman, R. E., Achor, R. W. P., et al: Antihypertensive properties of polythiazide and chlorothiazide. *JAMA*, **184**:191, 1963.
172. Hollander, W., and Wilkins, R. W.: Chlorothiazide: A new type of drug for the therapy of arterial hypertension. *Boston Med. Q.*, **8**(3):69, 1957.
173. Dinon, L. R., Kim, Y. S., et al: Clinical experience with chlorothiazide (diuril) with particular emphasis on untoward responses: A report of 121 cases studied over 15 month period. *Am. J. Med. Sci.*, **236**:533, 1958.
174. Salonen, J., and Ylitalo, P.: Antihypertensive, saluretic and hypokalaemic effects of cyclothiazide in comparison with hydrochlorothiazide with amiloride supplement. *Eur. J. Clin. Pharmacol.*, **22**:495–499, 1982.
175. New trial tightens link between thiazides and cardiac arrhythmia. *Medical World News*, **24**(2):32, 1983.
176. Papademetriou, V., Fletcher, R., Khatri, I., and Freis, E. D.: Diuretic-induced hypokalemia in uncomplicated systemic hypertension: Effect of plasma potassium correction on cardiac arrhythmias. *Am. J. Cardiol.*, **52**:1017–1022, 1983.
177. Michelson. E. L., and Morganroth, J.: Spontaneous variability of complex ventricular arrhythmias detected by long-term electrocardiographic recording. *Circulation*, **61**:690–695, 1980.
178. Delevette, A. F., and Recalde, M.: Diuretic induced renal colic. *JAMA*, **225**(8):992, 1973.
179. Srivastava, G., and Agarival, K. N.: Thiazide-induced bone marrow aplasia—report of a case. *Indian J. Pediatr.*, **34**:407, 1967.
180. Harden, R., and Russell, R.: Iatrogenically induced hypertensive encephalopathy. *Johns Hopkins Med. J.*, **145**(2):44–48, 1979.
181. Jones, M. F., and Caldwell, J. R.: Acute hemorrhagic pancreatitis associated with administration of chlorthalidone, report of a case. *N. Engl. J. Med.*, **267**:1029, 1962.
182. Shanklin, D. R.: Pancreatic atrophy apparently secondary to hydrochlorothiazide. *N. Engl. J. Med.*, **266**:1097, 1962.
183. Johnston, D. H., and Cornish, A. L.: Acute pancreatitis in patients receiving chlorthalidone. *JAMA*, **170**:2054, 1959.
184. Huesbye, K. O.: Jaundice with persisting pericholangiolitic inflammation occurring in a patient treated with chlorothiazide. *Am. J. Dig. Dis.*, **9**:439, 1964.
185. Drerup, A. L., and Alexander, W. A.: Jaundice occurring in patient treated with chlorothiazide. *N. Engl. J. Med.*, **259**:534, 1958.
186. Hokkanen, E. S., and Kaipainen, W. J.: Hepatic injury and multiple drug treatment. *Ann. Clin. Res.*, **3**:220, 1971.
187. Eisner, E. V., and Crowell. E. B.: Hydrochlorothiazide—dependent thrombocytopenia due to IgM antibody. *JAMA*, **215**(3):3, 1971.
188. Gesink, M. H., and Bradford, H. A.: Thrombocytopenic purpura associated with hydrochlorothiazide therapy. *JAMA*, **172**:556, 1960.
189. Ball, P.: Thrombocytopenia and purpura in patients receiving chlorothiazide and hydrochlorothiazide. *JAMA*, **173**:663, 1960.
190. Steinberg, A. D.: Pulmonary edema following ingestion of hydrochlorothiazide. *JAMA*, **204**(9):825, 1968.

191. Beaudry, C., and Laplante, L.: Severe allergic pneumonitis from hydrochlorothiazide. *Ann. Intern. Med.*, **78**(2):251, 1973.
192. Perchuk, E.: Spastic craniofacial syndrome precipitated by diuretics. *N. Y. State J. Med.*, **75**:91, 1975.
193. Morgan, T., Adam, W., Gillies, A., and Carney, S.: Treatment of mild hypertension. *Clin. Sci. Mol. Med.*, **55**:305S–306S, 1978.
194. Bjornberg, A., and Hakan, G.: Thiazides: A cause of necrotizing vasculitis. *Lancet*, **2**:982, 1965.
195. Kjellto, H., Stakeberg, H., et al: Possibility of thiazide induced renal necrotizing vasculitis. *Lancet*, **1**:1034, 1965.
196. Knox, J. M.: Photosensitivity—a common physical allergy. *S. Med. J.*, **57**:904, 1964.
197. Fitzgerald, E. W.: Fatal glomerulonephritis complicating allergic purpura due to chlorothiazides. *Arch. Intern. Med.*, **105**:303, 1960.
198. Smith, J. W., Seidl, L. G., et al: Studies on the epidemiology of adverse drug reactions. *Ann. Intern. Med.*, **65**(4):629, 1966.
199. Guin, J.: Photosensitive reactions to thiazide-related diuretic agents. *J. Indiana State Med. Assoc.*, **75**:720–721, 1982.
200. Srivastave, R. N., Travis, L. B., et al: Prolonged coma and visual loss: Unusual reactions to chlorothiazide. *J. Pediatr.*, **74**(1):126, 1969.
201. Shaufkin, J. B., and Silen, W.: Diuretic agents: Inciting factors in non-occlusive mesenteric infarction. *JAMA*, **229**(11):1451, 1974.

Indapamide

1. Campbell, D. P., Taylor, A. R., et al: Pharmocokinetics and metabolism of indapamide: A review. *Curr. Med. Res. Opin.*, **5**(Suppl 1):13, 1977.
2. Coutinho, C. B., Bekele, T., et al: Comparison of the safetey and efficacy of indapamide (a new antihypertensive agent) with hydrochlorothiazide. *Clin. Pharmacol. Ther.*, **28**:296, 1980.
3. Kynel, J., Oheim, K., et al: Antihypertensive action of indapamide. Comparative studies in several experimental models. *Arzneim-Forsch. (Drug Res.)*, **25**(10):1491, 1975.
4. Chalmers, J. P., Wing, L. M. H., et al: Effects of once daily indapamide and pindolol on blood pressure, plasma aldosterone concentration, and plasma renin activity in a general practice setting. *Eur. J. Clin. Pharmacol.*, **22**:191, 1982.
5. Mimran, A., Zambrowski, J. J., and Coppolani, T.: The antihypertensive action of indapamide: Results of a French multicentre study of 2184 ambulant patients. *Postgrad. Med. J.*, **57**(Suppl 2):60, 1981.
6. Milliez, P., and Tcherdakoff, P.: Antihypertensive activity of a new agent, indapamide: A double-blind study. *Curr. Med. Res. Opin.*, **3**(1):9, 1975.
7. Campbell, D. B., and Phillips, E. M.: Short term effects and urinary excretion of the new diuretic, indapamide, in normal subjects. *Eur. J. Clin. Pharmacol.*, **7**:407, 1974.
8. Lewis, P. S., Petrie, A., et al: Deterioration of glucose tolerance in hypertensive patients on prolonged diuretic therapy. *Lancet*, **i**:564, 1976.
9. Royer, R. J.: Progress in the treatment of hypertension: A multicenter study of indapamide in 442 patients. *Curr. Med. Res. Opin.*, **5**(Suppl 1):151, 1977.
10. Anavekar, S. N., Ludbrook, A., et al: A clinical trial of indapamide in the treatment of hypertension. In M. Valasco (Ed.): *Proceedings of the Second Interna-*

tional Symposium on Arterial Hypertension. Caracas, 1979, International Congress Series, 496, 206, Excerpta Medica, 1980.

11. Astacio, N., Cruz, A., and Molana, E.: Clinical study of indapamide in arterial hypertension. In M. Velasco (Ed.): *Proceedings of the Second International Symposium on Arterial Hypertension.* Caracas, 1979, International Congress Series, 496, 206, Excerpta Medica, 1980.

12. Weidmann, P., Grimon, M., et al: Studies of the antihypertensive mechanism of indapamide in man (Abstract). *Postgrad. Med. J.*, **57**(Suppl 2):18, 1981.

13. Hatt, P. Y., and Leblond, J. B.: A comparative study of the activity of a new agent, indapamide, in essential arterial hypertension. *Curr. Med. Res. Opin.*, **3**: 138, 1975.

14. Wheeley, M. St. G., Bolton, J. C., and Campbell, D. B.: Indapamide in hypertension: A study in general practice of new or previously poorly controlled patients. *Pharmacotherapeutica*, **3**(2):143, 1982.

15. Passerson, J., Pauly, N., and Desprat, J.: International multicentre study of indapamide in the treatment of essential arterial hypertension. *Postgrad. Med. J.*, **57** (Suppl 2):57, 1981.

16. Roux, P., and Courtois, H.: Blood sugar regulation during treatment with indapamide in hypertensive diabetics. *Postgrad. Med. J.*, **57**(Suppl 2):70, 1981.

17. Burgess, C. D., McKee, C. E., et al: The effect of indapamide on muscle blood flow in hypertensive patients. *Postgrad. Med. J.*, **57**(Suppl 2):23, 1981.

18. Dunn, F. C., Hillis, W. S., et al: Non-invasive cardiovascular assessment of indapamide in patients with essential hypertension. *Postgrad. Med. J.*, **57**(Suppl 2):19, 1981.

19. Chalmers, J. P., Bune, A. J., et al: Comparison of indapamide with thiazide diuretics in patients with essential hypertension. *Med. J. Aust.*, **2**:100, 1981.

20. Kubik, M. M., and Coote, J. H.: Comparison of the antihypertensive effects of indapamide and metoprolol. *Postgrad. Med. J.*, **57**(Suppl 2):44, 1981.

21. Van Hee, W., Thomas, J., and Brens, H.: Indapamide in the treatment of essential arterial hypertension in the elderly. *Postgrad. Med. J.*, **57**(Suppl 2):29, 1981.

22. Bowker, C. H., and Murphy, M. A.: A multicentre open trial of indapamide in general practice. *Postgrad. Med. J.*, **57**(Suppl 2):53, 1981.

Furosemide

1. Robson, A. O., et al: The diuretic response to furosemide. *Lancet*, **2**:1085, 1964.

2. Stokes, W., and Nunn, L.: A new diuretic: Lasix.® *Br. Med. J.*, **2**:910, 1964.

3. Verel, D., Rahmann, R., et al: A clinical trial of furosemide. *Lancet*, **2**:1088, 1964.

4. Muth, R. G.: Diuretic properties of furosemide in renal disease. *Ann. Intern. Med.*, **69**: 249, 1968.

5. vanZwieten, P.: Modern concepts in the drug treatment of arterial hypertension. *Int. J. Clin. Pharmacol. Ther. Tox.*, **18**(9):412–419, 1980.

6. Gifford, R. W., and Tarazi, R. C.: Resistant hypertension: Diagnosis and management. *Ann. Intern. Med.*, **88**:661–665, 1978.

7. Francisco, L., and Ferris, T.: The use and abuse of diuretics. *Arch. Intern. Med.*, **142**: 28–32, 1982.

8. Ram, C.: Diuretics in the management of hypertension. *Postgrad. Med.*, **71**(2):155–168, 1982.

9. Dodelson, R., Sherman, R., Gary, N., and Eisinger, R.: Diuretic therapy. *J. Med. Soc. N. J.*, **78**(11):748–750, 1981.

10. Maclean, D., and Tudhope, G.: Modern diuretic treatment. *Br. Med. J.*, **286**:1419–1422, 1983.

11. Calesnick, B., Christensen, J. A., et al: Absorption and excretion of furosemide S[35] in human subjects. *Proc. Soc. Exp. Biol. Med.,* **123**:17, 1966.

12. Rupp, W.: Pharmacokinetics and pharmacodynamics of Lasix.® *Scott. Med. J.*, **19**: 5, 1974.

13. Nielsen, P. E., Krogsgaard, A., McNair, A., and Hilden, T.: Emergency treatment of severe hypertension evaluated in a randomized study. *Acta Med. Scand.*, **208**: 473–480, 1980.

14. Freis, E. D.: Hypertensive crisis. *JAMA*, **208**(2):338, 1969.

15. Gifford, R. W., and Westbrook, E.: Hypertensive encephalopathy: Mechanisms, clinical features, and treatment. *Prog. Cardiovasc. Dis.*, **17**(2):115, 1974.

16. Finnerty, F. A.: Hypertensive encephalopathy. *Am. J. Med.*, **52**:672, 1972.

17. Mroczek, W. J.: Malignant hypertension: Kidneys too good to be extirpated. *Ann. Intern. Med.*, **80**:754, 1974.

18. Freis, E. D.: Treatment of mild hypertension. *Resident and Staff Physician*, **21**:55–69, 1975.

19. Swartz, C., and Kim, K.: Treatment of complicated hypertension. *N. Y. State J. Med.*, **5**:956–960, 1977.

20. Cannon, M., Tannenbaum, R., and La Franco, M.: Diuretics in the treatment of hypertension. *Am. Pharm.*, **NS18**(5):34–39, 1978.

21. The Joint National Committee on Detection, Evaluation, and Treatment of High Blood Pressure: The 1980 Report of the Joint National Committee on Detection, Evaluation, and Treatment of High Blood Pressure. *Arch. Intern. Med.*, **140**:1280–1285, 1980.

22. Sherrill, E., and Carr, A.: Chemotherapy for hypertension. *J. Mag.*, **70**:341–344, 1981.

23. Ramsay, L., Silas, J., and Freestone, S.: Diuretic treatment of resistant hypertension. *Br. Med. J.*, **281**:1101–1103, 1980.

24. Kristensen, B., and Skov, J.: Captopril or furosemide in drug-resistant hypertension. *Lancet*, **2**:699–700, 1980.

25. Wilson, M., Morgan, T., et al: A role of furosemide in resistant hypertension. *Med. J. Aust.*, **1**:213, 1977.

26. Olshan, A., O'Conner, D., Preston, R., Frigon, R., and Stone, R.: Involvement of kallikrein in the antihypertensive response to furosemide in essential hypertension. *J. Cardiovasc. Pharmacol.*, **3**:161–167, 1981.

27. Mroczek, W., Martin, C., Hattwick, M., and Kennedy, M.: Once-daily furosemide therapy in diuretic-treated hypertensive patients. *Curr. Ther. Res.*, **24**(7):824–830, 1978.

28. Tasker, P. R. W., and Mitchel-Heggs, P. F.: Non-ketotic diabetic pre-coma associated with high dose furosemide therapy. *Br. Med. J.*, **1**(6010):626, 1976.

29. Anderson, J., Godfrey, B. E., et al: A comparison of the effects of hydrochlorothiazide and of furosemide in treatment of hypertensive patients. *Q. J. Med.*, **40**(160):541, 1971.

30. Johnston, L. C., Santos, D. E., et al: The antihypertensive properties of furosemide on chronic oral administration. *J. Clin. Pharmacol.*, **10**:121, 1970.

31. Bracharz, H., et al: Comparative studies on the hypotensive effect of furosemide and hydrochlorothiazide. *Geriatrics Dig.*, **6**:33, 1969.
32. Bariso, C. R., Hanenson, I. B., et al: A comparison of the antihypertensive effects of furosemide and chlorothiazide. *Curr. Ther. Res.*, **12**(6):333, 1970.
33. Valmin, K., and Hansen, T.: Treatment of benign essential hypertension: Comparison of furosemide. *Eur.J. Clin. Pharmacol.*, **8**:393, 1975.
34. Licht, J. H., Haley, R. J., Pugh, B., and Lewis, S. B.: Diuretic regimens in essential hypertension: A comparison of hypokalemia effects, BP control and cost. *Arch. Intern. Med.*, **143**:1694–1699, 1983.
35. Saito, M., et al: Effects of furosemide and chlorothiazide on blood pressure and plasma renin activity. *Cardiovasc. Res.*, **10**:149, 1976.
36. Velasco, M., Arbona, J., et al: A randomized double-blind study of furosemide-reserpine in essential hypertension. *Curr. Ther. Res.*, **18**(3):395, 1975.
37. Steiner, R., and Blantz, R.: The use of diuretics in nonedematous conditions. *Med. Times*, **12/79** (Special Section):5s–13s, 1979.
38. Mroczek, W. J., Davidov, M., et al: Large-dose furosemide therapy for hypertension. *Am. J. Cardiol.*, **33**:5406, 1974.
39. VanderElst, E., Dombey, S., Lawrence, J., and Vlassak, W.: Controlled comparison of the effects of furosemide and hydrochlorothiazide added to propranolol in the treatment of hypertension. *Am. Heart J.*, **102**(4):734–740, 1981.
40. Araoye, M., Chang, M., Khatri, I., and Freis, E.: Furosemide compared with hydrochlorothiazide. *JAMA*, **240**(17):1863–1866, 1978.
41. Holland, O. B., Gomez-Sanchez, C. E., Kuhnert, L., Poindexter, C., and Pak, C.: Antihypertensive comparison of furosemide with hydrochlorothiazide for black patients. *Arch. Intern. Med.*, **139**:1015–1021, 1979.
42. Finnerty, F., et al: Long-term effects of furosemide and hydrochlorothiazide in patients with essential hypertension: A two-year comparison of efficacy and safety. *Angiology*, **28**(2):125, 1977.
43. Araoye, M., Freis, E., et al: Furosemide compared to hydrochlorothiazide in hypertension. *Circulation*, (Suppl III):55–56:30, 1977.
44. Gold, C., and Viljoen, M.: Site of renal action of xipamide. *Clin. Pharmacol. Ther.*, **25**(5) (Part 1):522–527, 1979.
45. Leary, W., and Reyes, A.: Mathematical evaluation of the effects of tizolemide, furosemide and placebo in healthy adults. *S. Afr. Med. J.*, **61**:398–401, 1982.
46. Conway, J.: Antihypertensive effect of diuretics. In F. Gross (Ed.): *Handbook of Exp. Pharmacol.*, Vol. 39, Springer-Verlag, Berlin, Heidelberg, New York, 1977, pp. 477–494.
47. Busuttil, A. A., et al: Possible cephaloridine nephrotoxicity in a neonate. *Lancet*, **1**:264, 1973.
48. Kleinknecht, D., et al: Nephrotoxicity of cephaloridine. *Ann. Intern. Med.*, **80**:421, 1974.
49. Simpson, I. J.: Nephrotoxicity and acute renal failure associated with cephalothin and cephaloridine. *N. Z. Med. J.*, **74**:312, 1971.
50. Gabriel, R., et al: Reversible encephalopathy and acute renal failure after cephaloridine. *Br. Med. J.*, **4**:283, 1970.
51. Norrby, R., Stenqvist, K., et al: Interaction between cephaloridine and furosemide in man. *Scand. J. Infect. Dis.*, **8**:209, 1976.
52. Dodds, M. G., and Foord, R. D.: Enhancement by potent diuretics of renal tubular necrosis induced by cephaloridine. *Br. J. Pharmacol.*, **40**:227, 1970.

53. Lawson, D. H., MacAdam, R. F., et al: Effect of furosemide on antibiotic-induced renal damages in rats. *J. Infect. Dis.*, **126**:593, 1972.

54. Greenblatt, D. J., Duhme, D. W., et al: Clinical toxicity of furosemide in hospitalized patients. *Am. Heart J.*, **94**(1):6, 1977.

55. Toivonen, S., and Mustala, O.: Diabetogenic action of furosemide. *Br. Med. J.*, **1**:920, 1966.

56. Medical Letter: Lasix.® *Med. Lett. Drugs. Ther.*, **9**(2):6, 1967.

57. Epstein, M., Lepp, B. A., et al: Potentiation of furosemide by metolazone in refractory edema. *Curr. Ther. Res.*, **21**(5):656, 1977.

58. Black, W. D., Shiner, P. T., and Roman, J.: Severe electrolyte disturbances associated with metolazone and furosemide. *South. Med., J.*, **71**(4):380–381, 1978.

59. Thorn, G. W.: Clinical considerations in the use of corticosteroids. *N. Engl. J. Med.*, **274**:775, 1966.

60. Beller, G. A., et al: Correlation of serum magnesium levels and cardiac digitalis intoxication. *Am. J. Cardiol.*, **33**:225, 1973.

61. Jelliffe, R. W.: Effect of serum potassium level upon risk of digitalis toxicity. *Ann. Intern. Med.*, **78**:821, 1973.

62. Schick, D., and Scheur, J.: Current concepts of therapy with digitalis glycosides, part II. *Am. Heart J.*, **87**:391, 1974.

63. Seller, R. H., et al: Digitalis toxicity and hypomagnesemia. *Am. Heart J.*, **79**:57, 1970.

64. Ferrari, M.: Effects of digoxin and digoxin plus furosemide on plasma renin activity of hypertensive patients. *Circ. Res.*, **44**(2):295, 1979.

65. McAllister, R. G., Howell, S. H., et al: Effects of intravenous furosemide on renal excretion of digoxin. *J. Clin. Pharmacol.*, **16**:110,1976.

66. Hurtig, H. I., and Dyson, W. L.: Lithium toxicity enhanced by diuresis. *N. Engl. J. Med.*, **290**:748, 1974.

67. Kerry, R., Ludlow, J., and Owen, G.: Diuretics are dangerous with lithium. *Br. Med. J.*, **281**:371, 1980.

68. Jefferson, J., and Kalin, N.: Serum lithium levels and long-term diuretic use. *JAMA*, **241**(11):1134–1136, 1979.

69. Malach, M., and Berman, N.: Furosemide and chloral hydrate—adverse drug interaction. *JAMA*, **232**(6):638, 1975.

70. Bridgman, J. F., et al: Complications during clofibrate treatment of nephrotic syndrome hyperlipoproteinemia. *Lancet*, **2**:506, 1972.

71. Yasujima, M., Abe, K., et al: Effects of indomethacin on plasma renin activity, plasma aldosterone concentration, urinary prostaglandin E excretion and blood pressure in patients with essential hypertension. *Tohoku J. Exp. Med.*, **128**:31–37, 1979.

72. Nilsson, C., Horton, E., and Robinson, D.: The effect of furosemide and bumetamide on warfarin metabolism and anticoagulant response. *J. Clin. Pharmacol.*, Feb/March:91–94, 1978.

73. Rawles, J.: Antagonism between non-steroid anti-inflammatory drugs and diuretics. *Scott. Med. J.*, **27**:037–040, 1982.

74. Laiwah, A., and Mactier, R.: Antagonistic effect of non-steroidal anti-inflammatory drugs on furosemide-induced diuresis in cardiac failure. *Br. Med. J.*, **283**:714, 1981.

75. McMahon, F. G., Ryan, J. R., Akdamar, K., and Ertan, A.: Upper gastrointestinal

lesions after potassium chloride supplements: A controlled clinical trial. *Lancet*, **2**: 1059–1060, 1982.

76. Barkin, J. S., Harary, A. M., Shamblen, C. E., and Lasseter, K. C.: Potassium chloride and gastrointestinal injury (letter). *Ann. Intern. Med.*, **98**:261–262, 1983.

77. Prema, K., Ramalakshmi, B., and Babu, S.: Diuretic therapy in pregnancy induced hypertension and pregnancy edema. *Indian J. Med. Res.*, **75**:545–553, 1982.

78. Huang, C, M., Atkinson, A. J., et al: Pharmacokinetics of furosemide in advanced renal failure. *Clin. Pharmacol. Ther.*, **16**(4):659, 1974.

79. Kelley, M. R., Cutler, R. E., et al: Pharmacokinetics of orally administered furosemide. *Clin. Pharmacol. Ther.*, **15**(2):178, 1974.

80. Mudge, G. H.: Drugs affecting renal function and electrolyte metabolism. In L. S. Goodman and A. Gilman (Eds.): *The Pharmacological Basis of Therapeutics*, 5th edition. Macmillan, New York, 1975, p. 743.

81. Lowe, J., Gray, J., Henry, D., and Lawson, D.: Adverse reactions to furosemide in hospital inpatients. *Br. Med. J.*, **2**:360–362, 1979.

82. Rance, C. P.: Cardiac arrest after intravenous furosemide. *Lancet*, **1**:1265, 1969.

83. Macherty, I.: Sudden death after intramuscular furosemide. *Lancet*, **2**:1301, 1968.

84. Arndt, K. A., and Hershel, J.: Rates of cutaneous reactions to drugs: A report from Boston Collaborative Drug Surveillance Program. *JAMA*, **235**(9):918, 1976.

85. DeRubertis, F. R., Michelis, F. M., et al: Complications of diuretic therapy: Severe alkalosis and syndrome resembling inappropriate secretion of antidiuretic hormone. *Metabolism*, **19**(9):709, 1970.

86. Abrams, W. B.: The mechanism of drug induced arrhythmias. *J. Newark City Hosp.*, **2**:3, 1965.

87. Robinson, D., Nilsson, C., Leonard, R., and Horton, E.: Effects of loop diuretics on carbohydrate metabolism and electrolyte excretion. *J. Clin. Pharmacol.*, **21**: 637–646, 1981.

88. David, D. S., and Hitzig, P.: Diuretics and ototoxicity. *N. Engl. J. Med.*, **284**(23): 1328, 1971.

89. Sherlock, S., and Walder, J. G.: The complications of diuretic therapy in patients with cirrhosis. *Ann. N. Y. Acad. Sci.*, **139**:497, 1958.

90. Hettiarachchi, J., McInnes, G., Ramsay, L., Scott, P., and Shelton, J.: Bumetamide and furosemide: Qualitative differences. *Br. J. Clin. Pharmacol.*, **4**:42–43, 1977.

91. Bogie, W., Homeida, M., Roberts, C., and Roberts, F.: Relationship between urate retention and electrolyte excretion during treatment with loop diuretics. *Br. J. Clin. Pharmacol.*, **4**:25, 1977.

92. Roberts, C., Homeida, M., and Roberts, F.: Effects of piretamide, bumetamide and furosemide on electrolyte and urate excretion in normal subjects. *Br. J. Clin. Pharmacol.*, **6**:129–133, 1978.

93 Wertheimer, L., Finnerty, F., et al: Furosemide in essential hypertension. *Arch. Intern. Med.*, **127**:934, 1971.

94. Humphreys, D. M.: Acute gout apparently precipitated by furosemide. *Br. Med. J.*, **1**:1024, 1966.

95. McSherry, J.: Acute gout complicating furosemide therapy. *Practitioner*, **201**:809, 1968.

96. Kaldor, A., Gachalyi, B., et al: Diabetogenic effect of oral diuretics in asymptomatic diabetics. *Int. J. Clin. Pharmacol. Biopharm.*, **11**(3):232, 1975.

97. Burke, G. J.: Non-ketotic, hyponatremic, normosmolar, diabetic coma and moderate furosemide therapy. *S. Afr. Med. J.*, **50**(54):2118, 1976.

98. Jones, P. E., and Oelbaum, M. H.: Furosemide induced pancreatitis. *Br. Med. J.*, 1:133, 1975.
99. Wilson, A. E., Mehra, S. K., et al: Acute pancreatitis associated with furosemide therapy. *Lancet*, 1:105, 1967.
100. Martinez-Maldonado, M., Eknoyan, G., and Suki, W. N.: Diuretics in non-edematous states. *Arch. Intern. Med.*, 131:797–800, 1973.
101. Norenberg, D.: Furosemide, hypertension and osteoporosis. (Letter) *JAMA*, **241** (3):237–238, 1979.
102. Sheehan, J., and White, A.: Diuretic-associated hypomagnesaemia. *Br. Med. J.*, **285**:1157–1159, 1982.
103. Iseri, L., Freed, J., and Bures, A.: Magnesium deficiency and cardiac disorders. *Am. J. Med.*, **58**(6):837–846, 1975.
104. Loeb, H., Pietras, R., Gunnar, R., and Tobin, J.: Paroxysmal ventricular fibrillation in two patients with hypomagnesemia. *Circulation*, **37**(2):210–215, 1968.
105. Joos, C., Kewitz, H., and Reinhold-Kourniati, D.: Effects of diuretics on plasma lipoproteins in healthy men. *Eur. J. Clin. Pharmacol.*, **17**:251–257, 1980.
106. MacKenzie, J. F., Cochran, K. M., et al: The effect of furosemide on small intestinal absorption of water and electrolytes. *Gut*, **15**:831, 1974.
107. Tuzel, I.: Comparison of adverse reactions to bumetamide and furosemide. *J. Clin. Pharmacol.*, **21**:615–619, 1981.
108. Schwartz, G. H., David, D. S., et al: Ototoxity induced by furosemide. *N. Engl. J. Med.*, **282**(25):1413, 1970.
109. Wigand, M. E., and Heidland, A.: Ototoxic side effects of high dose furosemide in patients with uremia. *Postgrad. Med. J.*, April (Suppl):54, 1971.
110. Venkateswaran, P. S.: Transient deafness from high dose furosemide. *Br. Med. J.*, 4:113, 1971.
111. Heidland, A., and Wigand, M. E.: Einflub hoher furosemiddosen auf die gehorfunktoin bei vramie. *Klin. Wochenschr.*, **48**(17):1052, 1970.
112. Rifkin, S. I., De Quesada, A. M., Pickering, M. J., and Shires, D. L.: Deafness associated with oral furosemide. *South. Med. J.*, **71**(1):86–88, 1978.
113. Peterson, V., et al: Effect of prolonged thiazide treatment on renal clearance. *Br. Med. J.*, 2:143, 1974.
114. Lyons, H., Pinn, V. W., et al: Allergic interstitial nephritis causing reversible renal failure in four patients with idiopathic nephrotic syndrome. *N. Engl. J. Med.*, **288** (3):124, 1973.
115. Fuller, T. J., Barcenas, C. G., et al: Diuretic induced interstitial nephritis. *JAMA*, **235**(18):1998, 1976.
116. Hendricks, W. M., and Ader, R. S.: Furosemide induced cutaneous necrotizing vasculitis. *Arch. Dermatol.*, **113**:375, 1977.
117. Kennedy, A. C., and Lyell, A.: Acquired epidermolysis bullosa due to high dose furosemide. *Br. Med. J.*, 1(6024):1509, 1976.
118. Ebringer, A., Adam, W. R., et al: Bullous hemorrhagic eruption associated with furosemide. *Med. J. Aust.*, 1:768, 1969.
119. Gibson, T. P., and Blue, P.: Erythema multiforme and furosemide therapy. *JAMA*, **212**:1709, 1970.
120. Furey, J. N., and Lawrence, J. R.: Phototoxic blisters from high furosemide dose. *Br. J. Dermatol.*, **94**:495, 1976.
121. Wauters, J. P.: Unusual complication of high-dose furosemide. *Br. Med. J.*, **4** (5997):624, 1975.

122. Willets, G. S.: Ocular side effects of drugs. *Br. J. Ophthalmol.*, **53**:252, 1969.
123. Matherson, B. J.: Generalized burning paresthesias due to intravenous furosemide. *J. Fla. Med. Assoc.*, **58**(6):34, 1971.
124. Syme, R. R. A.: Iatrogenic retention of urine. *Med. J. Aust.*, **1**(3):150, 1971.
125. Morgan, T., Adam, W., Hodgson, N., and Myers, J.: Duration of effect of different diuretics. *Med. J. Aust.*, **2**:315–316, 1979.
126. Sharefkin, J. B., and Silen, W.: Diuretic agents: Inciting factors in non-occlusive mesenteric infarction. *JAMA*, **229**(11):1451, 1974.
127. Churcher, A.: Diuretic induced edema. *Lancet*, **1**(7950):90, 1976.
128. Norbiato, G., Sommariva, D., et al: Diuretic induced edema. *Lancet*, **2**:1304, 1975.
129. MacGregor, G. A., Tasker, P. R., et al: Diuretic induced edema. *Lancet*, **1**:489, 1975.

CHAPTER IV

POTASSIUM SUPPLEMENTS

INTRODUCTION:

One might summarize the subject of potassium supplementation as follows:

1. Use low-dose thiazides in the management of hypertension and there will be less, if any, need for potassium supplements.
2. Identify from the outset those patients who might be at risk of potassium deficiency.
3. Try to minimize risks of potassium deficiency by dietary and other means available.
4. Treat all patients with serum potassium less than 3.5 mEq/L with the safest and best tolerated KCl supplement available, liquid KCl, microencapsulated KCl (Micro-K®), or one of the potassium-sparing agents such as amiloride or triamterene.

The appropriate use of potassium supplements includes both the therapeutic correction of hypokalemia and also its prevention. Potassium supplements are effective in restoring or maintaining serum or plasma potassium levels within the normal range. However, new and potentially serious side effects have been recently reported with the popular wax-matrix KCl formulations showing a high incidence of upper gastrointestinal pathology.

Hypokalemia, i.e., a serum level less than 3.5 mEq/L, does not, per se, indicate a deficiency in the body's potassium balance. Potassium deficiency means that state in which there is clinical evidence that potassium deficits exist in the body, appreciating the fact that 98% of potassium is intracellular. Generally when this exists, serum potassium levels are less than 3.5 mEq/L and, because we cannot ordinarily measure whole body potassium (WBK), we must depend on the clinical signs and symptoms of potassium deficiency, including electrocardiography (Table I).

TABLE I
THE SIGNS AND SYMPTOMS OF POTASSIUM DEFICIENCY

Skeletal muscle
- Weakness & hypotonia (chiefly in the legs), areflexia, flaccid paralysis, paresthesias, tetany, episodic paralysis

Smooth muscle
- Intestinal atony, ileus, constipation, abdominal cramps

Cardiac muscle
- Arrhythmias, chiefly atrial, nodal or ventricular premature contractions, atrial tachycardia, atrial flutter, idioventricular rhythms, postural hypotension

Electrocardiographic (see Figure 1)
- Flat or inverted T-waves
- Prominent U-waves
- Widened QT-interval
- Depressed ST-segment

Laboratory
- Urine: Low fixed specific gravity, resistance to anti-diuretic hormone (vasopressin), polyuria (and polydipsia)
- Blood: Hypokalemia, hypochloremia, alkalosis, azotemia

Central Nervous System
- Depression, coma, confusion, disorientation, polydipsia

Within a few days of initiating treatment with 50 to 100 mg of hydrochlorothiazide, serum potassium values begin to decline and usually reach their nadir in two to four weeks. Levels generally stabilize then in the range of 3.5–4.0 mEq/L.[1-13] How frequent is hypokalemia? A multi-clinic Veterans Administration study reported an incidence of 10% of thiazide-treated patients.[14] A recent study involving over 5,000 patients with essential hypertension from the Naval Regional Medical Center, Oakland, California,[15] indicates that 50 mg/day of hydrochlorothiazide produced 11.0% of patients with potassium values less than 3.5 mEq/L, whereas 25 mg doses produced an incidence of only 2.2%. It is clear from such studies that hypokalemia is dose-related and that it is significantly minimized by giving small doses of diuretics. Incidentally, the 25 mg doses also lowered blood pressure virtually the same as the 50 mg doses.

Total body potassium (TBK) has not been shown to fall significantly in otherwise healthy individuals taking diuretics. TBK decreases by no more than a mean of 5.5%.[17]

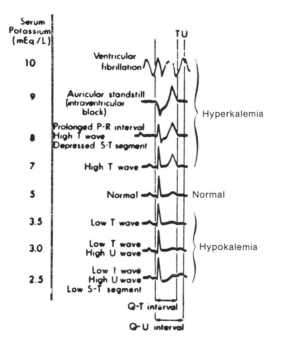

Figure 1: Effect of varying serum potassium levels on electrocardiogram (reprinted with permission[16]).

About 10 to 35% of thiazide-treated patients (receiving usually 50–100 mg/day doses of hydrochlorothiazide) develop serum levels less than 3.5 mEq/L, and some 30 to 50% of thiazide-treated hypertensive patients in the U. S. are given potassium supplements. A Boston Collaborative Drug Surveillance report among 16,000 hypertensive patients monitored indicated that 31% were receiving potassium chloride. In that report adverse reactions occurred in 5.7% of patients and consisted chiefly of hyperkalemia. Seven deaths were directly attributed to the potassium supplements. Indeed, an increasing number of medical authorities have urged that the time has come for a reassessment of the need for potassium supplements or potassium-sparing agents.[2,18-27]

On the other hand, a new concern exists today, particularly as a result of the MRFIT and OSLO studies[28,29] in which somewhat more myocardial infarctions and coronary deaths occurred in those mildly hypertensive patients who were treated with thiazides (see below). The possibility that thiazide-induced hypokalemia may result in potentially serious cardiac arrhythmias is supported further by the studies of Holland,[30] Hollifield,[31] Cooper[32] and others. (See Chapter III, Thiazides, for a further discussion.) The most prudent position for clinicians to assume today is to use minimally effective doses of thiazides in the management of hypertensive patients. Chapter III on diuretics will emphasize the efficacy of 25 and 50 mg/day doses of hydrochlorothiazide or chlorthalidone. Since hypokalemia is clearly dose-related, the maximal doses of these diuretics should no longer be 200 or 300 mg/day of hydrochlorothiazide, but generally no more than 50 mg/day.

Potassium Homeostasis

The usual American diet contains from 50–150 mEq/day of potassium. Under ordinary circumstances little is lost in the feces (5–10 mEq) or sweat (5.9 mEq/L), but the kidneys excrete from 40–140 mEq/day. Homeostasis depends upon a variety of factors, including intake, intestinal losses, sweat losses, urinary losses, and acid base balance.

Total potassium content of the body is regulated by renal excretion adjustments rather than by dietary intake. The kidney cannot conserve potassium as efficiently as it does sodium, there being an obligatory excretion from 3–15 mEq/day even in depleted patients.[33] On a zero-potassium diet a man would reduce his serum potassium to 3.0 mEq/L only after two or three weeks. Virtually all of the serum potassium is filtered at the glomerulus and most of this is then reabsorbed in the proximal tubule or loop of Henle, regardless of the state of potassium stores. Thus the amount of potassium finally appearing in the urine is determined in the distal renal tubule and collecting ducts.[34] Sodium loading is known to augment potassium excretion. When the tubule contains little sodium, little potassium is exchanged for sodium and therefore little potassium is excreted. However, when the proximal tubule is rich in sodium as with a high salt dietary intake, then large amounts of potassium are excreted in the presence of aldosterone.

Potassium is driven intracellularly by such factors as the infusion of glucose or insulin or bicarbonate. Alkalosis tends to increase intracellular potassium while acidosis lowers it. In the case of diabetic ketoacidosis, serum potassium is generally within normal limits when the patient is initially seen, although in fact there often exists a severe total body potassium deficiency. Cellular excitability is largely dependent on the ratio of intracellular to extracellular potassium. Extrarenal mechanisms, viz, insulin levels and the adrenergic nervous system, play an important role in regulating this ratio. Hypokalemia occurs with epinephrine administration or from albuterol (salbutamol) treatment of asthma or from terbutaline treatment of premature labor (both are beta-2-agonists). The hyperkalemia of exercise is aggravated by propranolol and attenuated by the alpha-antagonist, phentolamine.

Excessive gastrointestinal potassium losses occur with such clinical conditions as vomiting, diarrhea, laxative abuse and various malabsorption syndromes.

The normal urinary potassium excretion exceeds 40 mEq/day. Values of less than 40 are regarded as low. However, when the 24-hour excretion exceeds 20 mEq in the presence of hypokalemia, the diagnosis of "potassium wasting" is likely. One then should consider such conditions as primary aldosteronism, secondary aldosteronism, Cushing's syndrome, renal tubular acidosis, Fanconi's syndrome, renin-secreting kidney tumor and salt-losing nephritis.

In summary, potassium homeostasis is regulated primarily by the kidneys, principally at the level of the distal tubules under the influence of aldosterone. However, the efficiency of this process is not as effective as it is for sodium, and an obligatory excretion occurs in spite of depletion. Thiazides and other diuretics disturb potassium homeostasis by increasing urinary excretion. A patient with normal TBK will tend to be hyperkalemic if he is acidotic or hypokalemic if he is alkalotic. Since 98% of the body's potassium is intracellular, serum potassium values may not reflect accurately TBK deficiencies. Clinicians, however, can reliably use serum potassium values when taken together with the total clinical picture. The 2% of TBK found in the extracellular fluid greatly influences neuromuscular function. The most frequent clinical cause (non-drug related) of potassium depletion is gastrointestinal loss through vomiting or diarrhea. In contrast to sodium, potassium depletion may result from poor intake alone. The most frequent overall cause of potassium depletion is the effect of chronic diuretic use without adequate dietary or other potassium supplementation. Renal potassium deficiency occurs particularly in edematous patients with secondary aldosteronism. Chronic use of licorice or chronic administration of corticosteroids may also induce hypokalemia and alkalosis.

Hypokalemia as Distinguished from Potassium Deficiency

Hypokalemia and potassium deficiency are not equivalent terms. Hypokalemia, whether referring to a reduced serum or plasma potassium level (and the latter is a more meaningful measurement[14]), indicates a value below established normal ranges for healthy populations, generally less than 3.5 mEq/L. By itself such a level does not indicate that the body's potassium balance is negative or that intracellular concentrations are reduced or that total body potassium (TBK) is low.[1-3,18,35] TBK is determined usually by placing the patient inside a whole body counter and measuring endogenous isotopic K^{40}. This equipment is not generally available, but when TBK has been measured before and after long-term thiazide administration, potassium losses have amounted only to less than 6%.[17] More studies, however, need to be done to correlate signs and symptoms of potassium deficiency with diuretic usage in patients at risk. Meanwhile, it is felt that a deficit in TBK greater than 20% is needed to produce clinical evidence of potassium deficiency.[2,22] A value of 3.0 to 3.5 mEq/L is often obtained in the treatment of hypertensive patients with thiazide diuretics, particularly with doses of 50–100 mg/day of hydrochlorothiazide or similar doses of chlorthalidone. Most of the patients with this range of potassium values have no clinical signs or symptoms of TBK deficiency, but because of the recent evidence that arrhythmias can occur when levels are 3.0 to 3.5 mEq/L, these patients should receive potassium supplements or potassium-sparing agents as described in Chapter III. By potassium deficiency we mean that state in which there is clinical evidence of a potassium deficit existing in the body. Most potassium-deficient patients have serum potassium levels less than 3.5 mEq/L. It should be emphasized that all hypokalemic hypertensive patients should have primary aldosteronism ruled out before thiazides are started. Often thiazides quickly precipitate hypokalemia in such individuals.

The signs and symptoms of potassium deficiency are outlined in Table I. When potassium is reduced, skeletal, smooth and cardiac muscle function is impaired and neuromuscular conduction abnormalities are conspicuous. The patient is weak, particularly in his legs, has reduced deep tendon reflexes, complains of constipation, abdominal cramps, may experience paresthesias or even paralysis periodically and may have electrocardiographic abnormalities with or without cardiac arrhythmias. During potassium depletion, serum or plasma potassium initially decreases about 1 mEq/L for each 100–200 mEq lost, but potassium levels fall much more slowly after it reaches 2.0 mEq/L. Therefore, a serum potassium of 2–3.5 mEq/L is a reasonably accurate guide to the degree of potassium depletion, but lower levels reflect a wide range of deficits from moderate to very severe. The largest proportion of administered potassium rapidly enters cells, although renal excretion also increases promptly.

Who Is at Risk for Potassium Deficiency?

Table II lists factors which, if present in diuretic-treated patients, place them at added risk of developing potassium deficiency. Hypokalemia occurs in as many as 40% of patients given thiazide diuretics continuously. The toxicity of digitalis preparations is greatly enhanced when patients are also hypokalemic. Therefore, it is good medical practice to use potassium supplements concurrently in patients receiving both diuretics and digitalis. Edematous patients with secondary aldosteronism, e.g., cirrhosis or nephrosis, also tend to lose a great deal of potassium and tend to become hypokalemic. Many other "risk factors" are listed in Table II.

Only recently have physicians begun to appreciate the efficacy of

---

TABLE II
RISK FACTORS FOR POTASSIUM DEFICIENCY
AMONG DIURETIC-TREATED HYPERTENSIVE PATIENTS

— Patients receiving digitalis glycosides
— Patients getting beta-2-agonists, like epinephrine, albuterol (salbutamol) or terbutaline
— Patients with secondary aldosteronism, e.g., cirrhosis, nephrosis
— Patients on high sodium diets
— Patients on high doses of thiazide diuretics (100 mg or more HCTZ or chlorthalidone)
— Patients with a history of previous bouts of documented hypokalemia
— Patients ingesting "fad" diets or other diets which may be potassium-deficient
— Patients with unstable diabetes mellitus
— Patients with gastrointestinal problems as diarrhea, malabsorption syndromes, persistent vomiting, chronic laxative use, chronic enemas, intestinal or biliary drainage, fistulas and ostomies
— Patients receiving corticosteroids, or with spontaneous Cushing's syndrome, or on carbenoxolone or licorice
— Patients with protein malnutrition
— Patients with renal tubular diseases in which urine cannot be acidified
— Patients with metabolic alkalosis
— Patients who sweat excessively at work

Any of the above conditions, called "risk factors," may either *cause* potassium deficiency of itself, or its presence *adds to the risk* of potassium deficiency in hypertensive patients receiving thiazide diuretics.

---

low doses of thiazides or thiazide diuretics in treating hypertensive patients.[36-44] Doses of 25 or 50 mg/day of hydrochlorothiazide or chlorthalidone have been demonstrated to be effective in thiazide-responsive hypertensive patients. Additionally, it is now quite clear that the frequency of hypokalemia is related to the dose of thiazide administered. A study involving over 5,000 hypertensive patients reported from the Oakland, California Naval Regional Medical Center,[15] indicates that 50 mg/day of hydrochlorothiazide produced 11.0% of patients with potassium values less than 3.5 mEq/L, whereas 25 mg/day produced an incidence of only 2.2% of hypokalemia. Hollifield et al[31] also demonstrated clearly that hypokalemia is dose-related, as have many others. It is clear from such studies that hypokalemia is indeed dose-related and is dramatically minimized by giving smaller doses of diuretics.

Hypertensive patients, even on low-dose thiazides, even when restricting their dietary sodium, may still be at risk of potassium deficiency because of other coexisting factors such as edema, digitalis, protein-poor or fruit/vegetable-poor diet, unstable diabetes, chronic diarrhea, etc. It is therefore prudent to supplement KCl in these groups of hypertensives. Another strong reason for this recommendation is the concern about hypokalemia-included cardiac arrhythmias as a possible explanation for the higher incidence of coronary deaths reported in the MRFIT and the Oslo epidemiological studies.

Role of Diet in Potassium Regulation

Most patients who are on the new "low-dose" diuretic regimens and who do not have added risks for becoming potassium deficient will not require potassium supplements. It is prudent, however, to urge them to eat a good balanced diet which would likely contain 80–150 mEq of potassium. Table III gives the potassium content of various foods. Foods that are rich sources of potassium include fruits (e.g., bananas, oranges, apricots, plums, peaches, melons, and berries), milk and ice cream, meat, fowl, fish and shellfish, and vegetables (e.g., spinach, tomatoes, beets, brussel sprouts, carrots, squash, beans, celery, and mushrooms).

It is important to obtain a dietary history on all new hypertensive patients, not only with regard to total calories, but also salt (sodium) and potassium intakes. Emphasis on a high-potassium diet (and low sodium) is well worth the initial investment in time, as these patients

TABLE III
POTASSIUM CONTENT OF FOODS

Food	Approximate Amount	Potassium (mEq)
Meat (cooked)		
— Beef	1 ounce	2.8
— Ham	1 ounce	2.6
— Lamb	1 ounce	2.2
— Pork	1 ounce	3.0
— Veal	1 ounce	3.8
— Liver	1 ounce	3.2
— Sausage, pork	2 links	2.8
— Cold cuts	1 slice	2.7
— Frankfurters	1	3.0
Fowl		
— Chicken	1 ounce	3.0
— Turkey	1 ounce	2.8
Egg	1	1.8
Fish	1 ounce	2.5
Shellfish		
— Scallops	1 large	6.0
— Shrimp	5 small	1.7
Cheese		
— (American or Cheddar type)	1 slice	0.6
Peanut butter	2 tablespoon	5.0
Peanuts (unsalted)	25	4.5
Avocado	1/8	4.6
Butter or margarine	1 teaspoon	-0-
Cream		
— Half and Half	2 tablespoons	1.0
Cream Cheese	1 tablespoon	-0-
Nuts		
— Almonds, slivered	5 (2 teaspoons)	0.8
Bread	1 slice	0.7
Biscuit	1 (2" diameter)	0.7
Cornbread	1 (1½" cube)	1.7
Pancake	1 (4" diameter)	1.1
Cereals		
— Cooked	2/3 cup	2.0
— Dry, flake	2/3 cup	0.6
— Dry, puffed	1½ cups	1.5
— Shredded wheat	1 biscuit	2.2
Crackers		
— Graham	3	2.0

TABLE III (Continued)
POTASSIUM CONTENT OF FOODS

Food	Approximate Amount	Potassium (mEq)
— Soda	3	0.6
Ice Cream	1/2 cup	3.0
Flour products		
— Macaroni	1/4 cup	0.8
— Noodles	1/4 cup	0.6
— Rice	1/4 cup	0.9
Beans		
— Dried (cooked)	1/2 cup	10.0
— Lima	1/2 cup	9.5
— Green or wax (fresh or frozen)	1/2 cup	4.0
Corn		
— Canned	1/3 cup	2.0
— Frozen	1/3 cup	3.7
Parsnips	2/3 cup	9.7
Peas		
— Canned	1/2 cup	1.2
— Fresh	1/2 cup	2.5
Potato		
— Potato chips	1 ounce	3.7
— White, baked	1/2 cup	13.0
— White, boiled	1/2 cup	7.3
— Sweet, baked	1/4 cup	4.0
Whole milk	1 cup	8.8
Powdered whole milk	1/4 cup	10.0
Powdered skim milk	1/4 cup	13.5
Asparagus		
— Cooked	1/2 cup	4.7
Beet greens	1/2 cup	8.5
Broccoli	1/2 cup	7.0
Cabbage (cooked)	1/2 cup	4.2
Cauliflower (cooked)	1 cup	5.2
Celery (raw)	1 cup	9.0
Cucumber	1 medium	4.0
Mushrooms (raw)	4 large	10.6
Pepper, green or red (cooked)	1/2 cup	5.5
Radishes	10	8.0
Sauerkraut	2/3 cup	3.5
Spinach	1/2 cup	8.5
Tomatoes	1/2 cup	6.5
Tomato juice	1/2 cup	5.8
Beets	1/2 cup	5.0

Brussel sprouts	2/3 cup	7.6
Carrots (cooked)	1/2 cup	5.7
Pumpkin	1/2 cup	6.3
Squash, winter		
— Baked	1/2 cup	12.0
Apple		
— Fresh	1 small	2.3
— Juice	1/2 cup	3.1
Apricots		
— Canned	1/2 cup	6.0
— Fresh	3 small	8.0
Banana	1/2 small	4.8
Berries (fresh)		
— Blackberries	3/4 cup	3.0
— Blueberries	1/2 cup	1.5
— Strawberries	1 cup	6.3
Cherries		
— Fresh	15 small	2.7
Figs		
— Dried	1 small	2.5
— Fresh	1 large	3.0
Fruit cocktail	1/2 cup	5.0
Grapes		
— Fresh	15	3.2
Grapefruit		
— Juice	1/2 cup	4.1
Melon		
— Cantaloupe	1/2 small	13.0
— Honeydew	1/4 medium	13.0
— Watermelon	1/2 slice	5.0
Orange		
— Fresh	1 medium	5.1
— Juice	1/2 cup	5.7
— Sections	1/2 cup	5.1
Papaya	1/2 cup	7.0
Peach		
— Fresh	1 medium	6.2
Pear		
— Fresh	1 small	2.6
Pineapple		
— Juice	1/3 cup	3.0
Plums		
— Fresh	2 medium	4.1
Prunes		
— Juice	1/4 cup	3.6
Raisins	1 tablespoon	2.9
Rhubard	1/2 cup	6.5
Tangerines		
— Fresh	2 small	3.2

generally have better control of their blood pressure and fewer problems with potassium deficiency.

The Appropriate Indications for Potassium Supplements

The appropriate use of potassium supplements includes two: the therapeutic correction of hypokalemia and also its prevention. Potassium supplements are generally effective in restoring or maintaining serum potassium levels and whole body potassium levels within normal accepted ranges. Potassium chloride is clearly the potassium salt of choice in the treatment of potassium deficiencies related to long-term diuretic use. Other potassium salts such as the lactate, citrate, or acetate fail to restore the chloride deficiency or to correct the metabolic alkalosis which is associated with the hypokalemia. In severely depleted individuals, hospitalization with intravenous therapy is preferred. Intravenous rates exceeding 20 mEq/hour or concentrations exceeding 40 mEq/L are generally excessive. Careful laboratory and clinical monitoring including frequent electrocardiograms is important. When renal function is impaired, the hazard of potassium therapy is greatly increased.

The potassium chloride preparations which are best absorbed, produce the most rapid clinical effect, and possess the least potential for serious toxicity are the liquid KCl solutions. Unfortunately, these are poorly tolerated and produce a great deal of nausea, anorexia, and vomiting. Patient compliance is often poor with KCl solutions. Dietary supplements (Table III) might also be considered in the management of potassium deficiency, but ordinarily when signs or symptoms of deficiency are present, the treatment choice is the administration of potassium chloride per se. Potassium-sparing diuretics may also be indicated but should never be given together with KCl supplements. Potassium chloride supplementation is generally required for deficiency states, occasionally with intravenous therapy in hospitalized patients for severe deficiencies, but more often satisfactory treatment can be given with oral drugs on an out-patient basis. The particular potassium chloride therapy of choice is discussed below, and, as with all therapeutic decisions, benefit-to-risk ratios should determine which drug to use.

What Is the Proper Dose for KCl Supplements?

The most popularly used dose of KCl is one tablet (8mEq) taken three times a day. *Therapeutic replacement doses* and the *prophylactic doses* of KCl are much different. The former are large and the latter are relatively small. Arieff[45] recommends 100–200 mEq supplementation if the serum potassium is 3.0–3.5 mEq/L. Schwartz[46] was able to raise serum potassium levels in only 80% of thiazide-treated hypertensive patients by giving 40–60 mEq/day of liquid KCl. The other 20% failed to respond to doses as high as 100 mEq/day. Freis' group found Slow-K at doses of 96 mEq/day effectively corrected diuretic-induced hypokalemia in only 8 of 16 (50%) of their patients.[47] Potassium-sparing drugs were needed in the other eight. If a patient is ingesting the normal amount of daily potassium (50–150 mEq) but also has some added risk for developing potassium deficiency, 40 to 60 mEq/day should usually be given. The most commonly used prophylactic dose of KCl is one tablet (8 mEq) taken three times a day. Obviously, too, patients need to be encouraged to increase their intake of potassium-rich foods and to decrease their intake of sodium. Early on in treatment, potassium levels ought to be monitored, perhaps monthly, for those patients at risk to ascertain whether or not enough potassium is being provided.

How Safe are Potassium Supplements?
What are the Side Effects and Toxicity?

The usual side effects of potassium salts, occurring in about 6% of patients,[33] consist of mild gastrointestinal upset, nausea, vomiting, bad taste, salty taste, anorexia and diarrhea. Rarely, hyperkalemia may occur, usually because the salt was incorrectly given to a patient with azotemia or a patient also receiving one of the potassium-retaining drugs—situations where they are contraindicated.

Safety, of course, is a major consideration in selecting which of the myriad preparations one should utilize in the prophylaxis of potassium deficiency among thiazide-treated hypertensive patients. It is well to recall that among the most widely employed drugs in the United States in late 1964 were several enteric-coated potassium chloride preparations. Millions of patients were being treated with these enteric formulations and no one had noted any serious toxicity. At that time, there was a rather abrupt discovery of cases of severe, sometimes fatal, ulcerative or stenotic lesions of the intestinal tract associated *with enteric-coated potassium salts*. Most importantly, this association was only identified after more than six years of use of these enteric salts and only after more than seven million treatment courses had been employed.

Today we have a similar situation. Important new toxicity has appeared with the popular wax-core, slow-release KCl formulations which had previously not been recognized. In November, 1982 *Lancet* published results of our studies demonstrating new toxicity with wax-matrix KCl preparations.[48] Our studies indicate that a frequently-prescribed slow-release wax-matrix oral potassium chloride supplement (Slow-K®) produces a high incidence of upper gastrointestinal erosions and/or ulcers when compared to a new microencapsulated formulation (Micro-K®).

Our total experience now includes 225 subjects, each of whom received at least seven days of treatment with a KCl formulation or placebo. Our experience includes eight separate studies, each involving healthy normal volunteers treated for seven days, and a ninth study involving 18 hypertensive patients treated for almost two years.[49]

Our basic methodology involves, with written informed consent and after institutional peer review, admitting healthy male subjects for 11–18 days to our Clinical Research Center. Here their total dietary intake and medications were completely controlled. A normal upper gastrointestinal endoscopic examination was a prerequisite for admission to the first eight studies. Endoscopy was performed before and again after each seven-days' administration of study drugs. All subjects were placed on a red meat-free diet throughout the study and were permitted a moderate intake of caffeine-containing beverages, such as coffee or cola drinks. Every stool was examined for occult blood with Hemoccult® testing.

Table IV lists the number of subjects, duration of treatment, preparations and doses of drugs used in the eight short-term studies. Drugs were given one hour before meals with a full glass of water, except for Kaon Cl tablets which were given with the meals. Studies three, four and seven were two-week trials with endoscopy performed at weeks zero, one and two. In five of the eight studies, the anticholinergic drug, glycopyrrolate, was administered 2 mg t.i.d. to the subjects in order to produce delayed gastric emptying time,[50] a frequent clinical condition in the elderly.

The ninth study involved nine hypertensive patients who had received a slow-release, wax-matrix KCl preparation at doses of 40–80 mEq/day for a period of 19–23 months (mean of 21 months). They were admitted and endoscoped on the day of admission, as well as seven days later with their drugs having been given at the same doses they had received as out-patients. Their mean age was 65 years; two

TABLE IV
SHORT—TERM CONTROLLED STUDIES WITH ORAL KCl FORMULATIONS[49]

Study	Total No. Of Subjects	Weeks Of Treatment	KCl Formations*	KCl Dose (mEq/day)	Other Drugs*	With (+) Without (−) Glycopyrrolate
1	12	1	SK, MK	96	—	+
2	24	1	SK, MK	96	—	−
3	12	1	SK, MK	24	—	+
	8	2	SK, MK	24	—	+
4	36	1	SK, MK	24	—	−
	23	2	SK, MK	24	—	−
5	60	1	SK, MK, KL	24	pl	+
6	30	1	SK	72	Mod†	+
7	21	1	KA, MK	40**	pl	−
	14	2	KA, MK	40**	pl	−
8	30	1	K-3, SK	80	—	−

* Drug Key
1—SK   Slow-K® (wax-matrix)
2—KA   Kaon-Cl® tablets (wax-matrix)
3—K-3   A wax-matrix product
4—MK   Micro-K® (microencapsulated crystals)
5—KL   Kaon-Cl® liquid (20%)
6—Mod   Moduretic® tablets (5 mg amiloride HCl—50 mg hydrochlorothiazide)
7—pl   placebo tablets
** Given *after* meals.
† Dose of Moduretic®, one tablet twice a day.

were females and seven were males; their duration of hypertension averaged 23 years. In addition, nine control hypertensive patients, matched for sex, weight, age, concurrent diagnoses and treatment, were similarly admitted for endoscopic evaluation before and after seven days of placebo. These nine control patients, however, had never received KCl therapy.

Multiple photographs were obtained before and after seven days' therapy. All the endoscopies were performed with the gastroenterologist being blinded as to the patient's treatment. Table IV lists the chief elements in each of the eight short-term studies.

Results are shown in Tables V and VI. It is apparent that the three marketed wax-matrix KCl products (SK, KA, and K-3) produce a significantly higher incidence of erosions and/or ulcerations than do the other treatments (K-liquid, MK, and Moduretic®). It is also noteworthy

TABLE V

INCIDENCE OF EROSIONS AND ULCERS IN EIGHT STUDIES*

Study No.	No. of Subjects With Erosions/Total No. Treated							No. of Subjects With Ulcers/Total No. Treated						
	SK	KA	K-3	MK	KL	Mod	Pl	SK	KA	K-3	MK	KL	Mod	Pl
1	5/6	—	—	0/6	—	—	—	2/6	—	—	0/6	—	—	—
2	5/12	—	—	1/12	—	—	—	0/12	—	—	0/12	—	—	—
3	4/6	—	—	0/6	—	—	—	2/6	—	—	0/6	—	—	—
4	2/3	—	—	0/5	—	—	—	0/3	—	—	0/5	—	—	—
	6/17	—	—	5/19	—	—	—	0/17	—	—	0/19	—	—	—
	6/13	—	—	2/10	—	—	—	2/13	—	—	0/10	—	—	—
5	5/15	—	—	0/15	0/15	—	—	0/15	—	—	1/15	0/15	—	—
6	7/15	—	—	—	—	0/15	2/15	1/15	—	—	—	—	0/15	1/15
7	—	3/8	—	0/7	—	—	1/6	—	0/8	—	0/7	—	—	0/6
	—	1/3	—	1/6	—	—	1/5	—	0/3	—	0/6	—	—	0/5
8	2/15	—	9/15	—	—	—	—	1/15	—	6/15	—	—	—	—
Totals	42/102	4/11	9/15	9/86	0/15	0/15	4/26	8/102	0/11	6/15	1/86	0/15	0/15	1/26
Percent:	41.2	36.4	60.0	10.5	0	0	15.3	7.8	0	40.0	1.2	0	0	3.8

* From: F. G. McMahon with permission[49]

Drug Key
1—SK Slow-K® (wax-matrix)
2—KA Kaon-Cl® tablets (wax-matrix)
3—K-3 A wax-matrix product
4—MK Micro-K® (microencapsulated crystals)
5—KL Kaon-Cl® liquid (20%)
6—Mod Moduretic® tablets (5 mg amiloride HCl—50 mg hydrochlorothiazide)
7—pl placebo tablets

TABLE VI
ENDOSCOPIC FINDINGS AMONG HYPERTENSIVE PATIENTS TREATED
19–23 MONTHS WITH A WAX-MATRIX KCI SUPPLEMENT[49]

	Admission (Day 0)		Day 7 (in-patient)*	
	Erosions	Ulcers	Erosions	Ulcers
Wax-matrix, Slow-Release KCl Tablet	6/9	0/9	5/9	1/9
Matched Control Patients on Placebo	1/9	0/9	3/9	0/9

* After confinement for 7 days with continued wax-matrix KCl or placebo therapy.

that among patients who received SK with glycopyrrolate, 23 among 45 subjects developed erosions (51%) and five of 45 (11%) developed ulcers. Among SK-treated patients who did not receive glycopyrrolate, 19 of 57 (33%) developed erosions and three of 57 (5%) developed ulcers.

Table V also indicates that among the 225 subjects treated for seven days and the 45 subjects treated for an additional seven days, there was a 41.2% incidence of erosions and a 7.8% incidence of ulcers following Slow-K®. Only 10.5% of the subjects receiving Micro-K developed erosions, and only one subject developed an ulcer. Neither the liquid Kaon-Cl® nor Moduretic® produced erosions or ulcers. Among the placebo-treated subjects, erosions occurred in 15.3% and ulcers occurred in one of 26 subjects (3.8%).

The results of our long-term study (Table VI) indicate that on the day of admission, six of nine hypertensive patients who had been receiving a marketed, slow-release wax-matrix product for an average of 21 months had developed erosions. One of the nine matched-control hypertensive patients had an erosion on admission. After receiving the slow-release KCl for seven days in the research unit, one of the six patients who had had erosions now developed a gastric ulcer while the other five still had their erosions. Among the placebo-treated control patients, two more developed erosions, while none had ulcerations.

The essential elements in the design and conduct of these carefully controlled comparative studies which we consider to be critical are:

1) The utilization of sufficiently large numbers of subjects for each treatment group before valid conclusions can be drawn (15 per group is insufficient);

2) The selection of subjects with normal endoscopic examinations prior to enrollment;

3) The "total control" of the subjects, environment throughout the study, including all foods and medications;

4) The total compliance of patients, including a tongue blade/flashlight mouth inspection with each dosing and the administration of a full glass of water with study medications;

5) Endoscopists were blinded as to the nature of the drug treatment and in almost all of the 225 subjects, the "before" and "after" endoscopy was done by the same gastroenterologist;

6) The replication of results outside of our clinical unit by independent investigators; and

7) The utilization of a positive and/or negative control group in each of the studies.

The addition of the anticholinergic drug, glycopyrrolate, to produce delayed gastric emptying time is important. It had also been previously noted in laboratory animal studies that partial ligation of the esophagus or duodenum, simulating physiologic or pharmocological delay in transit of some solid KCl formulations, enhances the irritating effects of potassium on the upper gastrointestinal mucosa.

Reduced gastric motility has been directly associated with sleep,[51] pregnancy,[52] anxiety,[53] gastric surgery,[54] immobility and advancing age.[55] It has also been noted in a number of disease states, including diabetes mellitus,[54] hypothyroidism, and gastroenteritis.[56] Finally, various medications with known anticholinergic activity also delay gastric emptying, such as opiates, phenothiazines, tricyclic antidepressants, antihistamines, monoamine oxidase inhibitors and various antiarrhythmic agents. Indeed, hypokalemia itself may cause ileus and delayed gastric emptying. Our results indicate that there is a much higher incidence of serious mucosal injury when gastric emptying is delayed. Consideration of a patient's upper gastrointestinal motility is therefore warranted when prescribing a KCl supplement.

A consistently higher incidence of lesions was observed with the wax-matrix preparations regardless of whether or not glycopyrrolate was used.

A consistently higher incidence of lesions was observed with the wax-matrix preparations regardless of whether or not glycopyrrolate was used.

Wax-matrix preparations are the most frequently prescribed form of potassium supplements used in the world. They have generally been considered to be safe. The long-term effects of these drugs are not really known because, until our reports, patients were seldom endoscoped, particularly if they were asymptomatic. Our studies clearly show that symptoms, which were mild and appeared very rarely in our studies, were not related to endoscopic pathology. Certainly too, millions of people apparently consume over-the-counter antacids with great frequency. The results of our studies indicate that there exists an approximately four-fold difference in the incidence of erosive and an even greater difference in the incidence of ulcerative changes when wax-matrix formulations are compared to liquid or micronized KCl formulations. Micro-K® is clearly safer than Slow-K®. Even though information about long-term effects of these drugs is relatively sparse, there is no evidence from our studies that cyto-adaptation occurs. Certainly too, many patients who are on wax-matrix formulations or KCl formulations may coincidentally drink alcohol and ingest salicylates or other gastric-irritating substances. We feel that it is this population which is at particular risk. In our opinion, patients and doctors need to know these findings and to make the judgment when initiating long-term therapy with these drugs, whether to risk inducing upper gastrointestinal lesions with a wax-matrix formulation or to minimize this risk by taking a liquid or a microencapsulated KCl formulation, such as Micro-K®. Our conclusions from these studies are as follows:

1) Wax-matrix KCl preparations produce more upper gastrointestinal mucosal damage than microencapsulated KCl, liquid KCl, a potassium-sparing agent, or placebo.

2) Gylcopyrrolate and probably any anticholinergic agent or any illness associated with diminished gastric emptying is likely to increase the frequency and severity of KCl-induced mucosal damage.

3) The appearance of upper GI symptoms or positive Hemoccult® testing correlates very poorly with the severity of actual mucosal lesions, as demonstrated by endoscopy.

4) Long-term treatment with wax-matrix KCl is associated with more mucosal injury than is found in matched-control patients.

5) Cyto-adaptation of KCl-induced mucosal injury does not occur after 21 months of treatment in hypertensive patients.

Our studies complied with the criteria listed above. University of Miami investigators, following these same rigid criteria, confirmed our findings and their results appeared in the *Annals of Internal Medicine*.[57]

Unpublished, but widely advertised, reports attempt to refute our data and to equate the quality of our studies with theirs. Commercial advertisements of clinical studies about any drug should not be regarded with the same credulity as published material in peer-reviewed medical journals. Unfortunately, some physicians don't have time to read medical journals and see only drug advertisements. Three studies have been performed (unfortunately not published) and these are widely circulated and contained in advertisements of many medical journals.

The Utah School of Medicine study involved two doses (30 and 60 mEq/day) of a wax-polymer slow-release formulation (K-Tab). These investigators found one lesion among 15 subjects at the end of two-weeks' treatment with the low dose and found eight lesions among 15 subjects who received the high dose (60 mEq/day). The investigators concluded that lesions from the wax formulation slow-release KC1 were dose-related. Our data concur. However, we don't agree with the investigators' other conclusion, viz., that continued administration of the KC1 drugs results in spontaneous healing, via "cytoprotection" mechanism. Of their two patients with lesions after eight weeks of treatment, one persisted and the other disappeared. Our own experience among 18 hypertensive patients treated for a mean of 21 months indicates that lesions, including erosions and ulcers, do not disappear with continued administration of these KC1 formulations.

The Hershey Medical Center study (Patterson and Jeffery) and the Tucson, Arizona study (Earnest), though not published,* are nevertheless widely circulated in journal advertisments. Both studies were conducted using out-patients; both were conducted without placebo controls; and both studies utilized only six subjects per drug treatment group. Because out-patients were utilized, subjects could, if they desired, take aspirin for an occasional headache, drink alcohol (the subjects were apparently largely medical students and nurses), eat spicy snacks or extra meals, etc. They could also, if they wished, take antacids or cimetidine or whatever. Although the protocols required that pa-

---

* As of November 1, 1983.

tients *not* do these things, we simply maintained that out-patients *could* do any of these things, whereas, our own in-patients could not.

Second, we feel we have demonstrated that large numbers of subjects are essential to draw any valid conclusions. Obviously, people do develop upper gastrointestinal lesions spontaneously. Our in-patient study included 225 individual subjects. In addition, we obtained one ulcer among 26 subjects who received placebo (3.8%) and four cases of erosions among 26 patients treated with placebo (15.3%), so we are impressed that the use of placebo, as a negative control, and the utilization of the large number of patients for each treatment group are essential before valid conclusions can be rendered.

Third, our study has been duplicated, using the identical protocol, and also published by investigators at the University of Miami.[57]

Finally, a comment is needed with regard to the data from the Jick study contained in a letter to the editor of *Lancet*.[58] Among 15,791 inpatients, Jick studied those 10,710 *who had no predisposing conditions to upper GI bleeding*. In other words, he eliminated studying the very group about whom we are most concerned. We don't feel that wax-matrix KCl preparations cause serious danger in every patient, but only those particular patients who might be somehow predisposed to erosions or ulcers. This is the very population Jick eliminated and whom he ought to study. We believe it is the patient who may also drink some alcohol, injest aspirin or other ulcerogenic drugs together with wax-matrix KCl who may get into serious trouble. He should not have eliminated the cirrhotics, the patients on anticoagulants, the patients who had histories of peptic ulcer disease or gastritis. We therefore feel that Jick studied the wrong population. His conclusions about safety of these formulations are valid only for that population he surveyed—the non-risk patient.

Diuretic-induced Cardiac Arrhythmias

It has been recognized for decades that hypokalemia can cause arrhythmias, chiefly atrial, nodal or ventricular premature contractions, but also atrial tachycardia, atrial flutter and idioventricular arrhythmias. Retrospective studies indicate that from 8–28% of nondigitalized patients with hypokalemia have ventricular ectopic acitivty.[30] Holland et al, in an important prospective study of 21 thiazide-treated patients (50 mg twice daily hydrochlorothiazide for four weeks) with mild hypertension, found the following results with 24-hour Holter monitoring:

1) 7/21 developed an average increase in unifocal ventricular premature beats (VPCs) from 0.02/hr to 71.2/hr on diuretic, while their mean plasma potassium values dropped from 4.0 to 3.0 mEq/L.

2) Four of these seven patients developed multifocal VPCs and three of the four also developed couplets, one had ventricular tachycardia and two had bigeminy. Their plasma potassium levels were all 3.0 mEq/L.

3) The addition of a potassium-sparing agent abolished the four more serious arrhythmias and reduced the PVCs to 5.4/hr.

Holland concluded that some patients are sensitive even to minor potassium depletion.

Hollifield and Slaton[31] studied 38 hypertensive patients on increasing doses of hydrochlorothiazide, monitoring serum K and WBK, as well as blood pressure response and also exercise testing under EKG monitoring. Mean serum potassium values decreased with rising doses of hydrochlorothiazide as follows: 4.5–3.9–3.4–2.9 and 2.4 mEq/L after baseline, then doses of 50, 100, 150 and 200 mg/day doses, respectively. Static and dynamic exercise increased VPCs and this correlated with the reduction in serum potassium values.

Freis' group found contradictory results.[47] Correction of diuretic-induced hypokalemia did not significantly reduce the occurrence of spontaneous atrial or ventricular ectopic activity when single 24-hour Holter monitoring was done during hypokalemia and normokalemia. However, Michelson and Morganroth have reported significant day-to-day variations in such arrhythmias, so that multiple 24-hour Holter monitoring is needed.[59]

Others have also recognized an association between hypokalemia and arrhythmias. Dukes[60] reported an association between thiazide-induced hypokalemia and ventricular fibrillation noted in patients following acute myocardial infarction. Nordrehaug[61] reported an increasing incidence of ventricular fibrillation, as the serum potassium values fell in patients with acute myocardial infarction. The MRFIT study (Multiple Risk Factor Intervention Trial Research Group[28]) found that among the 1,987 patients with mild hypertension (diastolic: 90–99 mm Hg) who received "special intervention" beginning with thiazide diuretics, there was a significantly higher mortality rate from coronary heart disease than among the 2,027 other mildly hypertensive patients who received only "usual care." Patients who began with diastolic pressures > 100 mm Hg were protected by the more intensive therapy. The slightly increased cholesterol levels and diminished glucose tolerance may also have been etiologic factors. Hypokalemia, however, may have been a factor and further data analyses from this study are not yet available. Another conclusion from MRFIT derives from patients with initial presence of a variety of relatively minor ECG abnormalities. There were significantly more coronary deaths among 1,233 intensively-treated hypertensives with prior existing abnormalities of their ECG than among the 2,785 patients whose ECGs were completely normal initially. Such results suggest that hypertensive patients who have an abnormal ECG might be even more susceptible to thiazide-related hypokalemia and coronary deaths. This same type of outcome was noted in the Australian trial.[62]

One must conclude from these reports that:

1) In a dose-related manner, thiazides and thiazide-like diuretics cause hypokalemia; therefore small doses are much safer.

2) Hypokalemia appears to be associated with cardiac arrhythmias even among patients without infarction or other serious heart diseases.

3) Preexisting ECG abnormalities may predispose thiazide-treated patients to increased risk of coronary death.

4) Treat all patients whose serum potassium values drop below 3.5 mEq/L.

5) Hypokalemic patients with acute myocardial infarctions are at risk of ventricular fibrillation.

It is therefore prudent to use smaller doses of thiazides (12.5 or 25 or 50 mg/day) which, incidentally, are approximately equally effective to 100 and 200 mg doses, but produce less hypokalemia (and less disturbance in glucose, uric acid and lipids).

It is also important to identify, before initiating thiazide treatment, whether or not the patient might be at risk (and therefore needs potassium supplementation from the outset) because of a habit of eating high salt diets or because of an outdoor job that causes much sweating or because the patient is also taking digoxin or corticosteroids or because any of the risk factors listed in Table I are present.

REFERENCES

1. Wilkinson, P. R., Issler, H., et al: Total body and serum potassium during prolonged thiazide therapy for essential hypertension. *Lancet*, 1(7910):759, 1976.

2. Dargie, H. J., Boddy, K., et al: Total body potassium in long-term furosemide therapy: Is potassium supplementation necessary? *Br. Med. J.*, **4**(5940):316, 1974.
3. Lawson, D. H., Boddy, K., et al: Potassium supplements in patients receiving long-term diuretics. *Q. J. Med.*, **XLV**(179):469, 1976.
4. Jick, H., Miettinen, O. S., et al: Comprehensive drug surveillance. *JAMA*, **213**:1455, 1970.
5. Maronde, R., Milgrom, M., et al: Potassium loss with thiazide therapy. *Am. Heart J.*, **78**:16, 1969.
6. Davidson, D. G., Levinsky, N. G., et al: Maintenance of potassium excretion despite reduction of glomerular filtrate during sodium diuresis. *J. Clin. Invest.*, **37**:545, 1958.
7. Berlin, R. W., and Kennedy, T. J.: Renal tubular secretion of potassium in the dog. *Proc. Soc. Exp. Biol. Med.*, **67**:542, 1948.
8. Kosman, M. E.: Management of potassium problems during long-term diuretic therapy. *JAMA*, **230**(5):743, 1974.
9. Edmonds, C. J., and Jasani, B.: Total body potassium in hypertensive patients during prolonged diuretic therapy. *Lancet*, **2**:8, 1972.
10. Jaattela, A.: Clinical efficacy of fixed combinations of saluretic agents and potassium in sustained release from the treatment of arterial hypertension. *Eur. J. Clin. Pharmacol.*, **4**(146):146, 1972.
11. Anderson, J., Godfrey, B., et al: A comparison of the effects of hydrochlorothiazide and furosemide in the treatment of hypertensive patients. *Q. J. Med.*, **XL**(160):541, 1971.
12. Podolsky, S., and Burrows, B. S.: Scientific exhibit. American College of Physicians, Boston University, Department of Medicine, 1977.
13. Graybiel, A. L., and Sode, J.: Diuretics, potassium depletion and carbohydrate intolerance. *Lancet*, **2**:265, 1971.
14. Brown, J. J., Chinn, R. H., et al: Falsely high plasma potassium values in patients with hyperaldosteronism. *Br. Med. J.*, **1**:18, 1970.
15. Licht, J. H., Haley, R. J., Pugh, B., and Lewis, S. B.: Diuretic regimens in essential hypertension: A comparison of hypokalemic effects, BP control, and cost. *Arch. Intern. Med.*, **143**:1694–1699, 1983.
16. Burch, G. E., and Winsor, T.: *A Primer of Electrocardiography*. Lea and Febiger, Philadelphia, 1960.
17. McMahon, F. G.: *Management of Essential Hypertension*, Futura Publishing Co., Mount Kisco, N. Y. 1978, pp. 90–91.
18. McKenna, T. J., Donohoe, J. F., et al: Potassium-sparing agent during diuretic therapy in hypertension. *Br. Med. J.*, **1**:739, 1971.
19. Seldin, D. W., and Welt, L. G.: The effect of pituitary and adrenal hormones on the metabolism and excretion of potassium. *J. Clin. Invest.*, **30**:673, 1951.
20. Maronde, R., Milgrom, M., et al: Potassium loss with thiazide therapy. *Am. Heart J.*, **78**:16, 1969.
21. Welt, L. G., Hollander, W. B., et al: The consequences of potassium depletion. *J. Chronic Dis.*, **11**:213, 1960.
22. Levene, D. L.: The absorption of potassium chloride—liquid vs. tablet. *Can. Med. Assoc. J.*, **108**:1480, 1973.
23. Davidson, C., McLacklan, M. S. F., et al: Effect of long-term diuretic treatment on body potassium in heart disease. *Lancet*, **2**:1044, 1976.
24. Baron, J. H.: Potassium and diuretic therapy. *Lancet*, **2**:136, 1972.

25. *Medical Letter:* Who needs slow-release potassium tablets? New Rochelle, N. Y. **17** (18):73, 1975.

26. Maffly, R. H.: How to avoid complications of potent diuretics. *JAMA,* **235**(23): 2526, 1976.

27. MacLeod, S. M.: The rational use of potassium supplements. *Postgrad Med.,* **57** (2):123, 1975.

28. MRFIT (Multiple Risk Factor Intervention Trial), *JAMA,* **248**:1465–1477, 1982.

29. Helgeland, A.: Treatment of mild hypertension: A 5-year controlled drug trial. *Am. J. Med.,* **69**:725–732, 1980.

30. Holland, O. B., Nixon, J. V., and Kuhnert, L.: Diuretic-induced ventricular ectopic activity. *Am. J. Med.,* **70**:762, 1981.

31. Hollifield, J. W., and Slaton, P. E.: Thiazide diuretics, hypokalemia and cardiac arrhythmias. *Acta Med. Scand.,* **S647**:67–73, 1981.

32. Cooper, W. D., Reuben, S., VandenBurg, M. J., Kuan, P., and Currie, W. J. C.: *Cardiac Arrhythmias following Acute Myocardial Infarction: Association with the Serum Potassium Level and Prior Diuretic Therapy.* International Symposium on Potassium, Blood Pressure and Cardiovascular Disease, April 2–23, 1982, Capri, Italy.

33. Fourman, P.: The ability of the normal kidney to conserve potassium. *Lancet,* **1**: 1042, 1952.

34. Suki, W. N.: Disposition and regulation of body potassium: An overview. *Am. J. Med. Sci.,* **272**(1):31, 1975.

35. Burchell, H. B.: Dilemmas in potassium therapy. *Circulation,* **XLVII**:1144, 1973.

36. Beermann, B., and Groschinsky-Crind, M.: Antihypertensive effect of various doses of hydrochlorothiazide and its relation to the plasma level of the drug. *Eur. J. Clin. Pharmacol.,* **13**:195–201, 1978.

37. Berglund, G., and Andersson, O.: Low doses of hydrochlorothiazide in hypertension: Antihypertensive and metabolic effects. *Eur. J. Clin. Pharmacol.,* **10**:177–182, 1976.

38. Durley, Y., Cubberley, R., and Thomas, S.: Antihypertensive effect of oral timolol maleate and hydrochlorothiazide once daily compared with hydrochlorothiazide once daily. *Am. J. Hosp. Pharm.,* **38**:1161–1164, 1981.

39. Degnbol, B., Dorph, S., and Marner, T.: The effect of different diuretics on elevated blood pressure and serum potassium. *Acta Med. Scand.,* **193**:407–410, 1973.

40. Korduner, I., Kabin, I., and Hagbarth, G.: Low-dose chlorthalidone treatment in previously untreated hypertension. *Curr. Ther. Res.,* **29**(1):208–215, 1981.

41. Materson, B., Oster, J., et al: Dose response to chlorthalidone in patients with mild hypertension: Efficacy of a lower dose. *Clin. Pharmacol. Ther.,* **24**(2):192–198, 1978.

42. Tweeddale, M., Ogilvie, R., and Ruedy, J.: Antihypertensive and biochemical effects of chlorthalidone. *Clin. Pharmacol. Ther.,* **22**(5 Part 1):519–527, 1977.

43. Carney, S., Gillies, A., and Morgan, T.: Optimal dose of a thiazide diuretic. *Med. J. Aust.,* **2**:692–693, 1976.

44. Systolic Hypertension in the Elderly Program (SHEP): *Heart Institute's SHEP trial has revealed no serious problems.* F-D-D Reports, June 6, 1983, p. 6.

45. Arieff, A. I.: Principles of parenteral therapy. M. H. Maxwell and C. R. Kleeman (Eds.): *Clinical Disorders of Fluid and Electrolyte Metabolism,* second edition, McGraw-Hill, New York, 1972, p. 567.

46. Schwartz, A. G., and Schwartz, C. D.: Dosage of potassium elixir to correct thiazide-induced hypokalemia. *Lancet*, 11(1):702, 1974.
47. Papademetriou, V., Fletcher, R., Khatri, I. M., and Freis, E. D.: Diuretic-induced hypokalemia in uncomplicated systemic hypertension: Effect of plasma potassium correction on cardiac arrhythmias. *Am. J. Cardiol.*, 52:1017–1022, 1983.
48. McMahon, F. G., Ryan, J. R., Akdamar, K., and Ertan, A: Upper gastrointestinal lesions after potassium chloride supplements: A controlled clinical trial. *Lancet*, 2:1059–1060, 1982.
49. McMahon, F. G., Ryan, J. R., Akdamar, K., and Ertan, A.: The effect of potassium chloride supplements on upper gastrointestinal mucosa: Nine controlled clinical studies. *Clin. Pharmacol. Ther.*, 1984. (In press)
50. Hurwitz, A., Robinson, R. G., Herrin, W. F., Christie, J.: Oral anticholinergics and gastric emptying. *J. Clin. Pharmacol. Ther.*, 31:163–174, 1982.
51. Orr, W. C., Robinson, M. G.: The sleeping gut. *Med. Clin. N. Am.*, 65(6):1359–1376, 1981.
52. Wald, A., Van Thiel, D. H., et al: Effect of pregnancy on gastrointestinal transit. *Digestive Diseases and Sciences*, 27(11):1015–1018, 1982.
53. Latimer, P. R., Malmud, L. S., and Fisher, R. S.: Gastric stasis and vomiting: Behavioral treatment. *Gastroenterology*, 83:684–688, 1982.
54. Pellegrini, C. A., Broderick, W. C., Van Dyke, D., and Way, L. W.: Diagnosis and treatment of gastric emptying disorders. *Am. J. Surg.*, 145:143–151, 1983.
55. Evans, M. A., Triggs, E. J., Cheung, M., Broe, G. A., and Creasey. H.: Gastric emptying rate in the elderly: Implications for drug therapy. *J. Am. Geriatr. Soc.*, 29 (5):201–205, 1981.
56. Meeroff, J. C., Schreiber, D. S., Trier, J. S., and Blacklow, N. R.: Abnormal gastric motor function in viral gastroenteritis. *Ann. Intern. Med.*, 92:370–373, 1980.
57. Barkin, J. S., Harary, A. M., Shamblen, C. E., and Lasseter, K. C.: Potassium chloride and gastrointestinal injury (letter). *Ann. Intern. Med.*, 98:261–262, 1983.
58. Aselton, P. J., and Jick, H: Short-term follow-up study of wax matrix potassium chloride in relation to gastrointestinal bleeding (letter). *Lancet*, i:5, 1983.
59. Michelson, E. L., and Morganroth, J.: Spontaneous variability of complex ventricular arrhythmias detected by long-term electrocardiographic recording. *Circulation*, 61:690–695, 1980.
60. Dukes, M.: Thiazide-induced hypokalemia. Association with acute infarction and ventricular fibrillation. *JAMA*, 239:43, 1978.
61. Nordrehaug, J. D.: Malignant arrhythmias in relation to serum potassium values in patients with an acute myocardial infarction. *Acta Med. Scand.*, S647:101–107, 1980.
62. Management Committee, The Australian Trial in Mild Hypertension. *Lancet*, i: 1261–1267, 1980.

CHAPTER V

POTASSIUM-RETAINING DIURETICS

- AMILORIDE (MIDAMOR®)
- TRIAMTERENE (DYRENIUM®)
- SPIRONOLACTONE (ALDACTONE®)

INTRODUCTION

Amiloride, triamterene and spironolactone are mild diuretic agents
whose pharmacologic action is unique, since
they cause potassium retention.

Amiloride, triamterene and spironolactone are mild diuretic agents whose pharmacologic action is unique, since they cause potassium retention. Spironolactone is a steroid derivative and exerts its effect by competitively antagonizing aldosterone. Amiloride and triamterene share certain structural features but are chemically and mechanistically distinct from spironolactone. They do not competitively antagonize aldosterone; rather, they directly inhibit the exchange of sodium ions for potassium and hydrogen ions in those cells of the distal tubule where aldosterone exerts its action. In clinical practice, these three drugs are primarily used in combination with the more powerful diuretics, such as thiazides or furosemide, for the purpose of preventing or correcting hypokalemia which the latter agents may produce when used to treat hypertension or edema-forming states. The potassium-sparing compounds are especially useful in edematous conditions, with their associated secondary hyperaldosteronism, which often makes patients refractory to usual diuretic therapy. While these three drugs are weak diuretics by themselves, they also augment the action of the thiazide or loop diuretics. Amiloride and spironolactone exert a moderate hypotensive effect alone while triamterene has a milder effect. Spironolactone alone may be effective in treating hypertensive patients with diabetes

183

mellitus or gout when these diseases have been aggravated by the hyperglycemic or hyperuricemic effect of the thiazide or loop diuretics. The side effects and risk of potential toxicity appear to be more severe with spironolactone while they are fairly mild with either triamterene or amiloride. The potentially most serious complication from the use of these drugs is hypekalemia. The guidelines in Table I should be followed to minimize this risk.

Finally, spironolactone has a role in treating primary hyperaldosteronism, a relatively rare condition characterized by hypertension and hypokalemic alkalosis. The usual etiology is an isolated adrenal adenoma, but some cases are associated with bilateral adrenal hyperplasia. The treatment of choice for an aldosterone-producing adenoma is surgical excision or unilateral adrenalectomy. However, in patients who are poor surgical risks, chronic spironolactone therapy has been effective in controlling the hypertension and hypokalemia.[1,2] In patients with primary aldosteronism without evidence of an adenoma, subtotal adrenalectomy may be tried (bilateral adrenalectomy is unacceptable because of the resultant adrenal insufficiency), but if this fails, chronic spironolactone therapy is indicated and has been found usually effective.[1,2] Sometimes additional antihypertensive drugs are required.[3] Also, short-term treatment with spironolactone has been used successfully in the pre-operative management of these patients.[4] A recent study by

---

TABLE I
GENERAL GUIDELINES FOR THE USE OF POTASSIUM-SPARING DIURETICS

- Do not administer a potassium-sparing diuretic to patients receiving supplemental potassium, either as medication or in their diet (e.g., salt substitutes and high-potassium foods). This combination is associated with a high incidence of hyperkalemia.

- Do not give more than one potassium-sparing diuretic simultaneously or in close succession, since this frequently causes hyperkalemia due to the synergistic effect of the drugs.

- Do not administer these drugs to patients with poor renal function, as they are prone to the development of hyperkalemia.

- The serum potassium, sodium, creatinine (or blood urea nitrogen) should be periodically monitored in patients receiving these drugs as these values may be adversely affected. High-risk patients, such as the elderly, should have these values checked frequently, especially when initiating therapy.

Griffing et al suggests that amiloride can reverse hypokalemia and decrease blood pressure in patients with primary aldosteronism more so than in patients with essential hypertension.[5] These results are consistent with those of other investigators.[1,2,6] However, larger doses of amiloride than normally used in essential hypertension are needed and additional drugs are generally required to maintain normal pressure. Since chronic spironolactone therapy cannot be tolerated by many patients due to the adverse reactions (e.g., decreased libido, gynecomastia, menstrual irregularities, etc.), amiloride may well serve as a useful alternative drug in these patients.

AMILORIDE (Midamor®)
Introductory years:
1969 (Europe)
1981 (U. S.)

INTRODUCTION:

Amiloride, a pyrazine carbonylguanidine (Figure 1), is a potassium-retaining agent with mild diuretic, natriuretic and antihypertensive properties. Its main clinical use is in the concomitant administration with a thiazide diuretic as Moduretic® to prevent hypokalemia while also lowering blood pressure. The diuretic and antihypertensive action of amiloride can significantly potentiate that of the thiazide agent. It exerts a direct action on the distal renal tubule where it blocks the sodium–potassium ion exchange. This blockade produces an increase in sodium excretion and a decrease in potassium and hydrogen ion excretion independent of aldosterone. The drug is not metabolized in the liver nor elsewhere and does not accumulate in the body provided renal function is adequate. Amiloride does not significantly alter glomerular filtration rate or renal blood flow.[7] Side effects appear to be

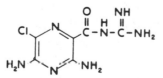

Figure 1: Structure of amiloride.

less serious than those encountered with the other potassium-sparing diuretics, spironolactone and triamterene. The principal risk of amiloride is hyperkalemia, which may be avoided by observing the contraindications and precautions and by keeping the dosage under 20 mg/day.

Amiloride has two popular uses:

1. As a potassium-retaining drug in patients who develop hypokalemia due to chronic diuretic therapy for hypertension:

The combination of amiloride plus hydrochlorothiazide provides not only the potassium retention desired, but also an additional mild antihypertensive benefit. Amiloride is often superior to oral potassium supplements in reversing hypokalemia.[8-13] Use of potassium-sparing agents also results in better patient compliance than seen with supplementation.

2. For the prevention of hypokalemia:

Amiloride can be used for patients on chronic diuretic therapy who are at an increased risk for hypokalemia because of the concurrent presence of diarrhea, diabetes mellitus, use of digitalis or corticosteroids, etc.

Amiloride has consistently been shown to have a mild antihypertensive effect when used alone.[4,14-16] However, its most worthwhile clinical use is in combination with thiazide diuretics such as in Moduretic®. It counters the kaliuresis and hydrogen ion loss produced by the thiazides and thus minimizes the risks of developing hypokalemia and/or metabolic alkalosis. Several studies have shown the combination of amiloride with a thiazide maintains serum potassium levels within normal limits much better than otherwise.[8,12,14-19] Also, the addition of amiloride reverses the hypokalemia in patients treated with thiazides.

Mantell, Walker et al[14] reported the results of a randomized double-blind multicenter study in 179 patients with mild to moderate essential hypertension. Patients were treated either with amiloride 5 mg, amiloride/hydrochlorothiazide 5/50 mg (Moduretic®) or with hydrochlorothiazide 50 mg for a total of 12 weeks. The results are shown in Table II. It will be noted that blood pressure declined 13/8 mm Hg with amiloride alone, confirming the clear antihypertensive efficacy of this drug. Blood pressures declined in the expected range with hydrochlorothiazide (21/12 mm Hg) and the combination product reduced

TABLE II
MULTICENTER STUDY IN PATIENTS WITH
MILD TO MODERATE HYPERTENSION
(179 PATIENTS FOR 12 WEEKS)

Treatment	Δ Blood Pressure (mm Hg)	Δ K+ (mEq/L)	ΔK < 3.0 (%)
Amiloride	13/8	(+) 0.23	0
Amiloride/HCTZ	23/11	(−) 0.38	2
HCTZ	21/12	(−) 0.59	23

HCTZ – hydrochlorothiazide
(From Mantell, Walker, et al[14])

blood pressure 23/11 mm Hg. The significant findings from this study, however, concern the serum potassium values. Twenty-three percent of patients (14 of 62) who were treated with hydrochlorothiazide alone had serum potassium levels less than 3.0 mEq/L. This compared with 0% of those on amiloride alone and 2% (1 of 57 patients) who received Moduretic®. No patient became hyperkalemic in excess of 5.5 mEq/L during this entire study, regardless of mode of treatment. No drug-related toxicity or clinically significant side effects occurred. It is evident in this study that the combination of drugs in Moduretic® significantly reduced systolic as well as diastolic blood pressure, while at the same time preserved for virtually all patients a normokalemic state.

Amiloride has a mild diuretic effect which enhances the diuresis and nutriuresis of thiazides. A recent study by the Multicenter Diuretic Cooperative Study Group has demonstrated an additive hypotensive effect for the combination therapy versus thiazide alone; however, other investigators have failed to substantiate these claims.[3,18,19] It appears that the addition of amiloride is likely to produce a further hypotensive effect if: 1) the dose of the thiazide is low, or 2) the patient is concurrently on a nonspecific beta-blocker. The latter observation has been noted by Castenfors,[20,21] who attributed it to suppression of the renin-angiotensin-aldosterone system by the beta-blocker timolol. This explanation is plausible, as it is well known that amiloride activates this system, increasing aldosterone levels. While increased aldosterone levels could suppress the effects of amiloride, this response is inhibited by a non-selective beta-blocker.

Indications for Amiloride

— Edema- forming states, such as congestive heart failure and hepatic cirrhosis, where diuretic therapy carries the risk of potassium depletion
— Essential hypertension
— Primary aldosteronism

Formulation

Tablets .... 5 mg

Dose in Hypertension

Amiloride is usually given at a dosage of 5 or 10 mg/day (one or two tablets), together with the usual antihypertensive dose of thiazide (or, e.g., as Moduretic®, a fixed combination of amiloride 5 mg and hydrochlorothiazide 50 mg) concurrently employed. A few patients may require more than 10 mg/day of amiloride to achieve the desired response. However, not more than 20 mg/day (four tablets) of amiloride should be given. The entire dosage of amiloride can be given as a single dose. Half-strength doses of amiloride (2.5 mg) are being studied with favorable results.

Mechanism of Action

Amiloride is structurally related to triamterene and has a similar mechanism of action. However, amiloride is a more potent compound than triamterene and may also have a greater maximal effect. Both compounds act selectively on the luminal membrane of the cells of the cortical collecting tubule and probably the cells of the medullary collecting duct as well. These cells are the same as those acted on by aldosterone. Both amiloride and triamterene block sodium–potassium ion exchange across the membrane, leading to increased natriuresis and retention of potassium and hydrogen ions. Unlike spironolactone, this activity is due to a direct effect on the renal tubule and not due to competitive antagonism of aldosterone. Thus, amiloride has a rapid onset of action, whereas that seen with spironolactone is delayed. The renal tubule appears to be the sole site of action of amiloride, and the drug has no effect on serum potassium levels in nephrectomized animals.[22]

Drug Interactions

1. Plus *Potassium Supplements:*
Potassium supplements, either as medication or as a potassium-rich diet, should not be used with amiloride due to the risk of hyperkalemia.

2. Plus *Other Diuretics or Antihypertensive Agents:*

Amiloride is a mild diuretic and antihypertensive drug, and an additive effect may occur when it is combined with other antihypertensive drugs. Amiloride should never be given in combination with other potassium-sparing diuretics.

3. Plus *Lithium:*

Diuretics, including amiloride, reduce the renal clearance of lithium and increase the risk of lithium toxicity.

Contraindications

- *Hyperkalemla*

Elevated serum potassium levels (over 5.5 mEq/l) are a contraindication to the use of amiloride.

- *Potassium Supplements or Other Potassium-conserving Therapy*

Potassium supplements or other potassium-sparing agents are contraindicated in patients taking amiloride. Such combination therapy is frequently associated with rapid increases in the serum potassium level.

- *Impaired Renal Function*

Anuria, acute renal failure, severe progressive renal disease and diabetic nephropathy are contraindications to the use of amiloride. Patients with BUN levels greater than 30 mg/dl or serum creatinine levels greater than 1.5 mg/dl should not receive amiloride without frequent monitoring of serum electrolytes and BUN or creatinine levels, especially when starting the drug. Potassium-sparing agents accentuate the potassium retention associated with renal insufficiency and may lead to rapid development of hyperkalemia.

- *Known Sensitivity to Amiloride*

As with all drugs, prior sensitization is a contraindication to the use of amiloride.

- *In Children*

The safety of amiloride in children has not been established. Therefore, amiloride is not recommended in the pediatric age group.

Use in Pregnancy

Because clinical experience is limited, amiloride is not recommended for use during pregnancy. The potential benefits of the drug must be weighed against possible hazards to the fetus if amiloride is given to a woman of child-bearing potential.

Precautions

● *Elderly Patients*

Elderly patients on amiloride appear to be particularly susceptible to hyperkalemia. It is well known that the glomerular filtration rate decreases with age. Thus renal function studies are necessary before starting amiloride therapy in elderly patients, as is careful monitoring of serum electrolytes. Doses of 2.5–5.0 mg/day are preferred.

● *Diabetes Mellitus*

Diabetic patients, especially those taking insulin, are at increased risk of developing hyperkalemia on amiloride, even more so if their renal function is compromised. The status of renal function should be determined before starting amiloride therapy in a diabetic patient, and the serum potassium level should be closely followed.

● *Metabolic or Respiratory Acidosis*

Acidosis causes a shift of potassium ions from the intracellular to the extracellular space and predisposes to hyperkalemia. Potassium-conserving therapy should be used only with extreme caution in severely ill patients in whom metabolic or respiratory acidosis may occur, such as those with shock, severe heart failure, chronic obstructive pulmonary disease and decompensated diabetes.

● *Dehydration*

The diuretic activity of amiloride can be additive to that of other concurrently administered diuretics. Excessive diuresis leading to dehydration carries substantial risk in certain patients. In patients with hepatic cirrhosis and ascites, dehydration can precipitate hepatic encephalopathy. Dehydration in patients with heart failure or moderately impaired renal function can easily lead to further azotemia and may cause acute renal failure.

Management of Overdosage or Exaggerated Response

If overdosage occurs, emesis should be induced or gastric lavage performed. Treatment is symptomatic and supportive. There is no specific antidote.

Hyperkalemia, defined as serum potassium levels over 5.5 mEq/L, is the principal risk of amiloride therapy and can be fatal. If it occurs, the drug should be discontinued immediately. The groups of patients at high risk for developing hyperkalemia include the critically ill and elderly, diabetics, those with impaired renal function and those undergoing vigorous diuresis. These patients should be monitored carefully for clinical, laboratory and electrocardiographic (ECG) evidence of hyperkalemia. Warning signs and symptoms of hyperkalemia include fatigue, muscular weakness, flaccid paralysis of the extremities, bradycardia, shock and ECG changes. The ECG in hyperkalemia shows mainly tall, peaked T waves, but also can exhibit ST depression, PR interval prolongation, widening or disappearance of the P wave, lowering of the R wave, and widening of the QRS complex, leading to a sine wave ECG.

Active measures to reduce hyperkalemia should be undertaken in patients who are symptomatic, who have significant ECG changes, or who have a serum potassium level greater than 7.5 mEq/L. These measures initially include hospitalization with intravenous calcium gluconate administration, parenteral glucose with rapid-acting insulin and/or parenteral sodium bicarbonate. To eliminate excess potassium, a cation-exchange resin such as sodium polystyrene sulfonate may be given orally or by retention enema. Dialysis may be used in patients refractory to these more conservative treatments.

Other complications of amiloride therapy, such as dehydration, electrolyte imbalance (e.g., hyponatremia), hepatic coma and acute renal failure are treated by established procedures.

Absorption, Distribution, Metabolism and Excretion

The usual dose of amiloride is 5–10 mg/day, although 2.5 mg/day is effective in many patients. This may be increased as necessary but should not exceed 20 mg/day. The drug is available only for oral administration. Approximately 50% of the total dose of amiloride is absorbed from the gastrointestinal tract; bioavailability of the drug is not dose-dependent (5 to 20 mg). Following an oral dose, the onset of action occurs about two hours later, peaking at 6–10 hours and lasting about 24 hours. Radioactive tracer studies, using a 20 mg dose, show a peak plasma level of 38–48 mg/ml at 3–4 hours.[23,24] Plasma half-life is approximately 6–9 hours. The drug is not highly bound to plasma proteins. The volume of distribution for amiloride approaches 250% of total body fluid volume, suggesting that the drug initially is widely distributed in the tissues.[24] However, fluorimetry, thin-layer chromatography and radioactive tracer studies fail to show any storage in tissues or metabolic transformation. The kidney is the sole route of excretion of amiloride. The drug has been shown to be excreted by both glomerular filtration and renal tubular secretion.[23] Fifty percent of an oral dose is excreted unchanged in the urine within 72 hours. However, peak urinary excretion occurs at about three hours, and 80% of urinary elimination is completed within 24 hours. About 40–50% of an oral dose is recovered from the stool. Since no secretion in the bile has been demonstrated, this amount is felt to represent unabsorbed drug.

As amiloride is not metabolized by the liver, it can be given to patients with hepatic dysfunction, as long as their renal function is adequate.

However, since the absorbed drug is excreted solely in the urine, good renal function is critical in preventing drug accumulation and hyperkalemia. The half-life of amiloride is greatly prolonged in patients with renal impairment.[25] Since hyperkalemia is the principal toxic effect of amiloride, and patients with renal failure are at a greatly increased risk for developing hyperkalemia anyway, amiloride is not recommended for use in patients with renal insufficiency.

TRIAMTERENE (Dyrenium®)
Introductory year: 1961

INTRODUCTION:

Triamterene, a pteridine derivative, is a potassium-sparing diuretic chemically related to folic acid (Figure 2). It is a weak diuretic when used alone, and in clinical practice it is employed solely in conjunction with more powerful diuretics, such as the thiazides (Dyazide®), for the management of edematous states and hypertension. While the mild diuretic action of triamterene may have some benefit in treating these

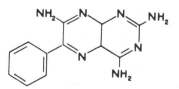

Figure 2: Structure of triamterene.

conditions, especially since it may augment the effect of other diuretics, the principal rationale for using the drug is to prevent or correct hypokalemia. Triamterene shares structural features with amiloride and has a similar mechanism of action, blocking sodium–potassium ion exchange in the distal renal tubule independent of aldosterone. It undergoes rapid metabolism in the liver and is excreted both in the urine and the bile. It has been reported to decrease slightly both glomerular filtration rate and renal blood flow. The side effects appear less marked than with the aldosterone antagonist spironolactone. As with the other potassium-sparing diuretics, hyperkalemia is the principal risk of therapy. The incidence of hyperkalemia can be minimized by observing the contraindications, precautions and dosing recommendations. In addition, there have been recent reports associating triamterene therapy with the development of kidney stones, an adverse reaction not appreciated during the early years of experience with the drug.

When should the physician consider using triamterene?
1. As a potassium-retaining drug in patients who develop hypokalemia because of chronic diuretic therapy for hypertension.
2. For prevention of hypokalemia in patients on chronic diuretic therapy for hypertension who are predisposed to hypokalemia (e.g., diarrhea) or in whom hypokalemia would entail significant risk (e.g., digitalis therapy).

Triamterene alone is not recommended as monotherapy for essential hypertension, since it produces too little reduction of blood pressure. However, it is very useful as adjunctive therapy with other diuretics, especially thiazides, as it helps prevent as well as treat hypokalemia. Serum potassium levels of patients on combination thiazide–triamterene (Dyazide®) therapy have consistently been shown to be significantly higher than those in patients on thiazides alone.

Unlike amiloride, triamterene does not appear to enhance significantly the hypotensive effect of the thiazide diuretics, although the addition of triamterene has been observed to lower blood pressure further in some patients.

Indications for Triamterene
— Edema-forming states, such as congestive heart failure, hepatic cirrhosis and nephrosis.
— Essential hypertension.

Formulation

Capsules .... 50 and 100 mg

Dose in Hypertension

Frequency: twice daily

Initial: 100 mg given twice daily after meals

Range: 100–300 mg

Usual dose: the total daily dosage should not exceed 300 mg. When combined with another diuretic, the total daily dosage of each agent should usually be lowered initially, and then adjusted to the patient's needs.

Onset of action is 2–4 hours after ingestion. Most patients will respond to triamterene during the first day of treatment. Maximal therapeutic effect, however, may not be seen for several days. Duration of diuresis depends on several factors, especially renal function, but it generally tapers off 7–9 hours after administration.

Mechanism of Action

Triamterene (like amiloride) has a unique mode of action. It inhibits the reabsorption of sodium ions in exchange for potassium and hydrogen ions at that segment of the distal tubule under the control of adrenal mineralocorticoids, especially aldosterone. This activity takes place through a direct effect on the renal tubule and not by competitive aldosterone antagonism. It is not directly related to the level of aldosterone secretion.

The fraction of filtered sodium reaching this distal tubular exchange site is relatively small, and the amount which is exchanged depends on the level of mineralocorticoid activity. Thus, the degree of natriuresis and diuresis produced by inhibition of the exchange mechanism is necessarily limited. Increasing the amount of available sodium and the level of mineralocorticoid activity by the use of more proximally acting diuretics will increase the degree of diuresis and potassium conservation. Triamterene occasionally causes increases in serum potassium which, in some instances, can result in hyperkalemia. It does not produce alkalosis because it does not cause excessive excretion of titratable acid and ammonium.

Drug Interactions

1. Plus *Other Diuretics*

Increasing the amount of available sodium and the level of mineralocorticoid activity by the use of more proximally acting diuretics will increase the degree of diuresis and potassium conservation.

Triamterene is usually not used concomitantly with spironolactone. If it is, however, the physician should frequently determine serum potassium levels, since both of these agents can cause potassium retention and, in some instances, hyperkalemia.

2. Plus *Antihypertensive Agents*

Although triamterene has not proved to be a consistent antihypertensive agent, the physician should be aware of a possible lowering of blood pressure. Concomitant use with the antihypertensive drugs may result in an additive effect.

3. Plus *Potassium Supplements*

Potassium supplements, either as medication or as a potassium-rich diet, should not be used with triamterene.

Contraindications

— Severe or progressive kidney disease or dysfunction with the possible exception of nephrosis.
— Severe hepatic disease.
— Hypersensitivity to the drug.

Triamterene has a unique mode of action. It inhibits the reabsorption of sodium ions in exchange for potassium and hydrogen ions at the distal renal tubule. It must not be given to patients with impaired renal function or azotemia. Potassium supplements, either as medications or as a potassium-rich diet, should not be used with triamterene.

Warnings

Patients should be observed closely for the possible occurrence of blood dyscrasias, liver damage, or other idiosyncratic reactions. There have been reports of blood dyscrasias in patients receiving triamterene.

Periodic BUN and serum potassium determinations should be evaluated to check kidney function, especially in patients with suspected or confirmed renal insufficiency. It is particularly important to make serum potassium determinations in elderly or diabetic patients receiving the drug; these patients should be observed carefully for possible adverse serum potassium increases.

Triamterene is usually not used concomitantly with spironolactone. If it is, however, serum potassium levels should be monitored closely, since both of these agents can cause potassium retention and, in some instances, hyperkalemia.

Use in Pregnancy

Extensive studies in animal reproduction have produced no evidence of drug-induced fetal abnormalities. However, triamterene has had only limited use in pregnancy; therefore, it should be used in pregnant patients or in women of childbearing potential only when, in the judgment of the physician, it is deemed essential to the welfare of the patient.

Precautions

Triamterene tends to conserve potassium rather than to promote its excretion as do most diuretics. Occasionally, it can cause increases in serum potassium which, in some instances, can result in hyperkalemia. In rare instances, hyperkalemia has been associated with cardiac irregularities.

Hyperkalemia will rarely occur in patients with adequate urinary output, but it is a possibility if large doses are used for considerable periods of time. If hyperkalemia is observed, triamterene should be withdrawn. Because triamterene conserves potassium, it has been theorized that, in patients who have received intensive therapy or have been given the drug for prolonged periods, a rebound kaliuresis could occur upon abrupt withdrawal. In such patients withdrawal of triamterene should be gradual.

Electrolyte imbalance, often encountered in such diseases as congestive heart failure, renal disease or cirrhosis, may be aggravated or caused independently by an effective diuretic agent which would include triamterene. The use of full doses of a diuretic when salt intake is restricted can result in a low-salt syndrome.

Triamterene can cause mild nitrogen retention which is reversible upon withdrawal of the drug and is seldom observed with intermittent (every-other-day) therapy.

By the very nature of their illness, cirrhotics with splenomegaly sometimes have marked variations in their blood picture. Since triamterene is a weak folic acid antagonist, it may contribute to the appearance of megaloblastosis in cases where folic acid stores have been depleted. Therefore, periodic blood studies in these patients are recommended.

Although triamterene has not proved to be a consistent antihypertensive agent, the physician should be aware of a possible lowering of blood pressure. Concomitant use with antihypertensive drugs may result in an additive effect.

Triamterene may cause a decreasing alkali reserve with the possibility of metabolic acidosis. Triamterene and quinidine have similar fluorescence spectra; thus, triamterene will interfere with the fluorescent measurement of quinidine.

Adverse Reactions

There have been occasional reports of diarrhea, nausea and vomiting, and other gastrointestinal disturbances. Such nausea can usually be prevented by giving the drug after meals. Weakness, headache, dry mouth, anaphylaxis, photosensitivity, and rash have also been reported. Only rarely has it been necessary to discontinue therapy because of these side effects.

It should be noted that symptoms of nausea and vomiting can also be indicative of electrolyte imbalance.

In special studies, investigators found that triamterene has little or no effect on carbohydrate metabolism; however, it has elevated uric acid, especially in persons predisposed to gouty arthritis.

Absorption, Metabolism, Excretion

Triamterene is given orally most often in combination with another diuretic. It is rapidly but incompletely absorbed from the gastrointestinal tract. This was demonstrated by Pruitt et al[1] when they showed that significant amounts of the drug were found in the feces following oral administration, but very little drug was isolated from the feces following intravenous administration. The absorption of the drug is affected by a low pH which decreases absorption.

Following the administration of triamterene, the parent compound undergoes rapid and extensive metabolism in the liver. The half-life of the drug is 90–120 minutes. The primary metabolite of the drug is 2, 4, 7-triamino 6-p-hydroxphenylpteridine. It appears in the plasma as early as 30 minutes following oral administration. The concentration of the metabolite is up to 12 times greater than that of the parent drug, reflecting its rapid rate of metabolism. Studies of the metabolite failed to demonstrate any diuretic activity.

Triamterene is excreted in the bile and the urine. Urinary excretion of the metabolite has been noted up to 15 hours following the oral dose.[2] The rate of excretion of the drug and its metabolite gradually decreases over 6–8 hours after the dose, with traces still found in the urine 12–14 hours after administration.

Doses of triamterene must be reduced in the presence of mild azotemia, and the drug should not be used in severe renal disease because of the hazard of hyperkalemia.

Since the drug is metabolized in the liver, on theoretical grounds the doses should be decreased in the presence of diffuse liver disease (e.g., acute hepatitis) and the patient carefully monitored.

The Nature of Adverse Reactions to Triamterene

Triamterene may produce gastrointestinal irritation leading to diarrhea, nausea, vomiting and other gastrointestinal complaints. The physician should carefully evaluate these symptoms since they may be due to a direct effect of the drug or may be due to an existing or drug-induced electrolyte imbalance. Other side effects include dry mouth, weakness, headache and skin rash. The most important adverse reaction is the development of hyperkalemia. Most studies have shown that fewer than 8% of the patients on triamterene must stop the drug due to noxious side effects. Table III lists the frequency of adverse reactions associated with triamterene.

TABLE III
FREQUENCY OF ADVERSE REACTIONS DUE TO TRIAMTERENE

Frequent (> 5.0%)
- nausea, hyperkalemia, hyperuricemia, weakness, leg cramps

Occasional (0.1–5.0%)
- gastrointestinal .... anorexia, gastrointestinal distress, diarrhea, constipation, vomiting
- dermatological .... rash, urticaria, pruritis without rash
- central nervous system .... dizziness, headache
- miscellaneous .... muscle pain or spasm, hyperglycemia, BUN

Rare (< 0.1%)
- megaloblastosis, bitter taste, peculiar odor to food, sore throat with coated tongue, burning skin, agitation, sedation, bradycardia, tachycardia, nocturia, dysuria, polyuria, hot and cold flashes, black spots before eyes, hypotension, paresthesias, insomnia

---

- *Hyperkalemia[3]*

Triamterene reduces potassium excretion by interfering with the exchange of potassium for sodium in the renal tubule. In some patients, particularly those with impaired renal function, this may cause severe hyperkalemia. The largest study on hyperkalemic effects of triamterene is that of Hansen and Bender.[4] They found 14% of patients (120 of 839) became hyperkalemic on triamterene alone and 7% (30 of 406) became hyperkalemic treated with a triamterene-hydrochlorothiazide combination. McDonald[5] reported that 26% (14 of 53) of diabetic patients studied developed hyperkalemia on triamterene. This figure is somewhat higher than the general population since elderly diabetics probably had significant renal disease. Heath and Freis[6] studied 32 patients on a combination of triamterene plus hydrochlorothiazide. Hyperkalemia did not develop in any of them during their one-month observation. The use of triamterene is fairly safe overall when used as indicated, but patients must be monitored since hyperkalemia may be severe and can be fatal. Drug-induced hyperkalemia was responsible for almost 50% of the "preventable" deaths reported in the Boston Collaborative Drug Study.[7]

- *Hyperuricemia[8,9]*

Spiekerman et al[8] found increases in the serum uric acid levels from a mean of 3.5 to 4.1 mg/dl following triamterene given at a dosage of 100 mg every 12 hours for two months as antihypertensive therapy. The increase in serum uric acid was found to be parallel to and additive to that produced by the thiazides. It has been estimated that the incidence of hyperuricemia in patients receiving triamterene is approximately 17%.[8] There are others who report that triamterene does not elevate serum uric acid.[9]

- *Hyperglycemia[8,10]*

Although significant increases in blood glucose have been reported during triamterene administration, it occurs much less frequently than with furosemide and thiazides. Walker et al[10] feel that the hyperglycemic effect of triamterene is seen primarily in moderate and severe diabetics but not in normals or mild diabetics.

- *Elevation in Blood Urea Nitrogen[11,12]*

Cohen[11] found that the rise in the blood urea concentration paralleled that seen with the serum potassium concentration. Other investigators have found no significant increase in the blood urea concentration[12] during triamterene therapy. The elevation of BUN seems to be readily reversible when the drug is stopped.

● *Effects on the Bone Marrow[13,14]*

Triamterene has been implicated as the cause of megaloblastosis in a few patients. The drug interferes with dihydrofolate reductase activity, thus acting as a folic acid antagonist. The enzyme is necessary to convert dihydrofolic acid to tetrahydrofolic acid, which is the one-carbon carrier essential for DNA synthesis. The production of megaloblastosis by triamterene is rare but should be considered if the drug is administered to patients with low folate stores, including pregnant women and chronic alcoholic patients.

SPIRONOLACTONE (Aldactone®)
Introductory year: 1960

INTRODUCTION:

Spironolactone (Figure 3), a 17-spirolactone steroid, is a direct competitive antagonist of the sodium-retaining and potassium-secreting steroid aldosterone.[1,2] The drug therefore prevents sodium and potassium exchange in the distal renal tubule, thereby producing potassium retention,[1-4] natriuresis and diuresis (see Figure 6, Chapter III). Spironolactone effectively lowers blood pressure in hypertension through this mechanism.[1,2,4-6]

1. In the treatment of essential hypertension:

Spironolactone alone[7] but especially combined with thiazides (as in Aldactazide®) effectively lowers blood pressure in mild and moderate

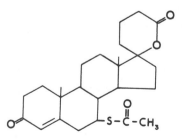

Figure 3: Structure of spironolactone.

hypertension. The drug counteracts potassium deficiency in patients who are susceptible to developing hypokalemia. (See Chapter IV, Table II for risk factors of potassium deficiency.) Spironolactone does not cause gout[1] or affect glucose metabolism.[1,8,9] It is indicated for hypertension in gouty patients prone to hyperuricemia secondary to thiazides,[10,11] and in diabetics in whom thiazides have aggravated hyperglycemia.[1,9,12]

2. In primary aldosteronism:

The drug is effective for short-term pre-operative control of blood pressure and serum potassium levels in these patients. It may also be employed as long-term maintenance therapy of aldosterone-producing adrenal adenomas and adrenal hyperplasia when surgery is not possible.

3. To prevent or treat hypokalemia in patients receiving diuretics and who are also at risk of hypokalemia because of concurrent digitalis use, excessive sweating, excessive sodium ingestion, corticosteroid use, etc.

Spironolactone effectively reduces blood pressure when used alone,[6,8-13-25] or with thiazide diuretics.[1,6,8,13,26,27] The antihypertensive effects of spironolactone and other drugs are additive when these are used in combination.[1,8,13,14,17,21] Spironolactone and thiazides equivalently lower systolic and diastolic pressures in supine and erect positions[7,8,16,20,26,28,29] and after excercise.[28] The same dosages of spironolactone or thiazide (50 mg/day of each drug[8] or 100 mg/day of each[7]) have been reported to affect blood pressure equally. Others have indicated that 400 mg/day of spironolactone is equivalent to 100 mg/day of chlorthalidone[29] or 100 mg/day of hydrochlorothiazide.[20]

The relative hypotensive and natriuretic potency of spironolactone to amiloride (each given with bendrofluazide) is 5 to 1, as reported by Ramsey et al.[30,31] In their study, the fall in systolic pressure with spironolactone was dose-related.[30]

Low plasma renin levels, characteristic of primary aldosteronism, also occur in about 25–30% of hypertensive patients.[2,29] Because of its competitive inhibition of aldosterone, spironolactone has been suggested for treatment of low renin hypertension.[15,27,32-38] There appears to be no relation of blood pressure reduction and pre-treatment renin levels,[7,8,20,26,39] although some studies indicate that spironolactone is more effective in low renin than normal renin hypertension.[15,16,22,23] It stimulates plasma renin activity, as do thiazides.[40] Data comparing spironolactone and thiazides in treating low renin hypertension are not consistent. Reports have shown spironolactone efficacy to be greater than,[16,32,34,41,] equal to,[20,22,29,39,42-45] or less than[6,30,46-48] that of thiazides. In general, spironolactone seems to be a useful alternative to thiazides for low renin hypertension.[29]

Spironolactone is more effective than potassium chloride in raising serum potassium levels.[30,47,49-54] Ramsey et al[30] found that spironolactone (100 to 200 mg/day) was more effective than any dose of KCl[30,47,49-53] and that the rise in serum potassium was related to the dosage of spironolactone. The relative potassium-retaining potency of amiloride:spironolactone was 2.8:1. Patients with more severe hypokalemia had a greater response to spironolactone than those with less serious hypokalemia.

Indications for Spironolactone

— Hypertension
— Primary hyperaldosteronism
— Hypokalemia
— Edematous conditions for patients with:
  • Congestive heart failure
  • Liver cirrhosis
  • Nephrotic syndrome

Formulation

Tablets .... 25 and 100 mg

Dose in Hypertension

Frequency: once or twice daily
Initial: 50–100 mg
Range: 20–400 mg daily
Usual dose: 50–100 mg for at least two weeks, allowing time for maximal response. Subsequent dosage is set according to patient response.

Aldactazide® is available as tablets containing 25 mg spironolactone and 25 mg hydrochlorothiazide for treatment of hypertension. Dosage is titrated for individual patients, with a recommended dosage of one tablet given one to four times daily.

Mechanism of Action

Spironolactone is a specific antagonist to aldosterone.[31,48,55,56] It competes for the aldosterone dependent sites of sodium and potassium exchange in the distal convoluted tubule and cortical collecting duct.[31,57] Spironolactone's action depends on the presence of aldosterone, although it is not related to the actual plasma aldosterone concentration.[2,30] The drug also inhibits aldosterone synthesis.[48,55,56] Spironolactone increases sodium and water elimination and potassium retention to reduce blood pressure.[7,31,58] By reducing plasma volume, spironolactone augments the efficacy of other antihypertensive drugs,[59,60] allowing lower dosages to be given with fewer side effects.[2]

Hyperaldosteronism may result from elevated renin and angiotensin II levels secondary to impaired renal blood flow in congestive heart failure, liver cirrhosis, renal disease, and from diuretic therapy.[2,7,57] Genest[61] reported high plasma aldosterone and impaired aldosterone clearance in many hypertensive patients. Potassium excretion and sodium retention in hyperaldosteronism can lead to hypokalemia and edema. Spironolactone is effective as therapy for edema, hypokalemia, and hypertension in these conditions.

Drug Interactions

1. Plus *Potassium Supplements*

Spironolactone must *not* be given with other potassium-sparing diuretics or with supplementary potassium in medications and diet, since hyperkalemia may result.

2. Plus *Other Diuretics or Antihypertensive Drugs*

The dosage of diuretics and other antihypertensive drugs, especially adrenergic-blockers, should be decreased by at least 50% when used in combination with spironolactone. The antihypertensive effects of these agents and spironolactone are additive. Long-term thiazide therapy can cause hypokalemia, diabetes mellitus[12] and gout[10] related to dosage. Treatment with spironolactone plus hydroflumethiazide has caused no gout nor change in glucose tolerance. By its potassium-sparing action, spironolactone diminishes thiazide-induced hypokalemia.[8,13,62,63] The combination of spironolactone and other diuretics can cause hyponatremia.

3. Plus *Norepinephrine*

Spironolactone reduces vascular sensitivity to norepinephrine. Anesthesia must be given with caution to patients taking spironolactone.

Contraindications

— Hyperkalemia
— Impaired renal function

— Anuria
— Acute renal insufficiency

Warnings

● *Potassium supplementation:*

Supplementary potassium should not be given with spironolactone, as hyperkalemia may result.

● *Toxicity:*

No relationship of spironolactone and tumors of endocrine organs, liver or breasts has been reported in man.[46,64,65] Chronic toxicity studies in rats have shown spironolactone to be a tumorigen at doses 25, 75 and 250 times greater than the usual human dosage (2 mg/kg). In rats, proliferative changes of endocrine organs and liver (mammary tumors in females and benign adenomas of thyroid and testes in males) were dose-related. Hepatomegaly, hyperplasiac nodules, and hepatic carcinomas occurred at the highest dosage (500 mg/day) given to rats.

Use in Pregnancy

Normal edema of pregnancy due to restriction of venous return by the expanded uterus can usually be relieved by elevation of the lower extremities and use of support hose. Diuretics should not be used to alter vascular volume, since this can endanger the mother and fetus. Edema associated with pathologic conditions may be treated with spironolactone in pregnant patients. However, spironolactone and its metabolites may cross the placenta, and the potential benefits of treatment must exceed possible harm to the fetus.

Precautions

Because of spironolactone's diuretic action, fluid and electrolyte balance must be monitored in patients. Spironolactone potentiates the effects of other antihypertensive drugs; dosages should be reduced when these are used in combination. Spironolactone plus other diuretics can cause hyponatremia and symptoms of dry mouth, thirst, lethargy and drowsiness.

Patients with renal insufficiency may develop hyperkalemia, leading to cardiac irregularities that could be fatal. Potassium supplements which increase the chance of hyperkalemia should not be given with spironolactone. Reversible hyperchloremic metabolic acidosis associated with hyperkalemia may develop in patients with decompensated hepatic cirrhosis, even though they may have normal renal function. Spironolactone may cause an elevation of creatinine of mild acidosis, especially in patients with renal dysfunction.

The metabolite canrenone is secreted in mother's breast milk; spironolactone should not be given to nursing mothers.

Management of Overdosage or Exaggerated Response
Signs and Symptoms:

Hyperkalemia is a potentially serious result of spironolactone overdosage.

Treatment:

Hyperkalemia can be temporarily diminished by giving glucose (20–50%) and insulin (0.25–0.5 units insulin per gram glucose). Spironolactone should be discontinued and potassium intake restricted.

Absorption, Distribution, Metabolism and Excretion

The bioavailability of spironolactone is over 90% after oral dosage, compared to an optimally absorbed solution of spironolactone in polyethylene glycol. Spironolactone is rapidly metabolized by the liver,[28] mostly to canrenone. Serum levels of canrenone peak two to four hours after a single oral dose. These levels decline in two phases: rapidly in the first 3–12 hours after dosage, and slowly from 12–96 hours. Spironolactone and canrenone are both over 90% bound to plasma proteins. The excretory half-life of canrenone, ranging from 13–24 hours, is about 12.5 hours with 50 mg of spironolactone given four times daily, and nearly 19 hours with 200 mg given once daily. Metabolites are excreted mainly in the urine but also in bile.

Adverse Reactions

Spironolactone is a safe drug when used appropriately (see Tables IV and V). At low doses (50 mg/day), it causes few side effects.[11] Approximately 5% of outpatients will stop taking spironolactone because of unpleasant effects.[66] The more common reactions to spironolactone include gynecomastia, lassitude, hyperkalemia, and gastrointestinal irritation. Hyperkalemia is the most serious result of spironolactone therapy. Patients who are taking supplemental potassium or who have poor renal function are more susceptible to hyperkalemia. However, spironolactone causes no hyperuricemia, hyperglycemia, or hypokalemia as do thiazide diuretics.[43] Tables IV and V summarize the nature and frequency of adverse reactions to spironolactone.

TABLE IV
NATURE OF SIDE EFFECTS OF SPIRONOLACTONE

Gastrointestinal	nausea, vomiting, cramping, diarrhea, dry mouth
Central Nervous System	drowsiness, lethargy, headache, ataxia, mental confusion
Dermatological	urticaria, maculopapular or erythematous cutaneous eruptions
Biochemical	↑ serum potassium, ↑ BUN, mild acidosis, hyponatremia
Endocrine:	
Male	gynecomastia, impotence, ↓ libido
Female	amenorrhea, irregular menses, hirsutism, postmenopausal bleeding, deepened voice

TABLE V
FREQUENCY OF ADVERSE REACTIONS DUE TO SPIRONOLACTONE

Frequent (> 5.0%)
- gastrointestinal irritation
- fatigue, lethargy
- hyperkalemia
- gynecomastia

Occasional (0.1–5.0%)
- nausea, vomiting, cramps, diarrhea, dehydration
- headache, neurological disturbances
- urticaria, maculopapular or erythematous rash
- ↑ BUN, hyponatremia
- impotence, ↓ libido (males)
- amenorrhea, menstrual irregularity, postmenopausal bleeding, deepened voice (female)

Rare (< 0.1%)
- drug fever

The Nature of Spironolactone Reactions
Pharmacological Adverse Reactions to Spironolactone:

1. Effect on Serum Potassium:

   Spironolactone usually causes an increase in plasma or serum potassium concentration.[7,28,30] Hyperkalemia may develop during therapy, particularly if this drug is misused in patients who have renal dysfunction or who are receiving supplementary potassium. Crane and Harris[16] measured a greater rise in serum potassium (by 1.4 mEq/L) in patients with primary aldosteronism, as opposed to an increase of 0.4–1.0 mEq/L in other patients. The overall incidence of hyperkalemia was 8.8% in their study. Greenblatt and Koch-Weser[67] reported a 2.8% incidence of hyperkalemia in non-azotemic patients not receiving supplementary potassium. Plasma or serum potassium levels and electrocardiograms should be monitored during dosage changes, also in unstable diabetics, and when there are signs or symptoms of hyperkalemia (paresthesias, weakness, paralysis, bradycardia, fatigue).

The hypokalemic state can be reversed by potassium repletion with spironolactone.[67]

2. Effects on the Gastrointestinal System:

Gastrointestinal irritation is the most common complaint with spironolactone, occurring in 10–20% of patients following oral spironolactone. These reactions are usually mild, although spironolactone may have to be discontinued because of nausea, vomiting, or diarrhea.

3. Effects on the Skin, Gynecomastia, and Impotency:

Skin rashes that develop usually clear upon discontinuation of spironolactone.

The incidence of gynecomastia in males appears to be related to the dosage and duration of treatment with spironolactone. Spark and Melby[34] reported gynecomastia in nearly all of their 42 patients taking 400 mg/day of spironolactone. Brown[68] reported the common occurrence of gynecomastia at doses ranging from 50–400 mg/day. Gynecomastia may be symmetrical and bilateral or present as a unilateral, painful breast nodule. The condition is benign with complete remission over several weeks or months after spironolactone is stopped. No breast cancer has been associated with spironolactone.

Impotence often occurs in males, along with gynecomastia. Spark and Melby[34] reported a 30% incidence of impotence at high doses, but only 1–2% frequency of impotence at clinical doses of spironolactone.

Female patients may experience hirsutism and deepened voice.

4. Menstrual Effects:

Amenorrhea and menstrual irregularity are uncommon but may

occur with spironolactone. Menstrual cycles return to normal within months of drug discontinuation.

5. Lethargy and Easy Fatigability:

These mild and transient conditions occur in about 20–30% of patients taking spironolactone.

6. Other Effects of Spironolactone:

Like thiazide diuretics, spironolactone elevates plasma renin[2,7,69] and angiotensin.[7,30] Increased sodium excretion and lowered plasma sodium parallel spironolactone dosage.[7,28,30] Plasma aldosterone is elevated by spironolactone.[30,31,69] Levitt[1] found that for any rise in angiotensin II, the aldosterone level was raised 20% more with amiloride than with spironolactone, since spironolactone also blocks aldosterone synthesis. By decreasing fluid volume and GFR, spironolactone elicits an increase in blood urea and slows urate clearance.[1,7, 28,30] Levitt[1] reported a rise in blood urea from 23.6 to 35.1 mg/100 ml. Plasma uric acid appears not to change,[7,30,69] although some studies report elevated serum uric acid.[1,28] Spironolactone causes no gout.[4]

REFERENCES:

Introduction and Amiloride

1. Kremer, D., Beevers, D. G., et al: Spironolactone and amiloride in the treatment of low renin hyperaldosteronism and related syndromes. *Clin. Sci. Mol. Med.*, **45**: 213S, 1973.
2. Hoefnagels, W. H. L., Drayer, J. I. M., Smals, A. G. H., and Kloppenborg, P. W. C.: Spironolactone and amiloride in hypertensive patients with and without aldosterone excess. *Clin. Pharmacol. Ther.*, **27**(3):317, 1980.
3. Biglieri, E.: Syndrome of primary aldosteronism. In M. R. Blaufox and C. Bianchi (Eds.): *Secondary Forms of Hypertension: Current Diagnosis and Management*, Grune and Stratton, New York, 1981, pp. 205–212.
4. Mobley, J. E., et al: Primary aldosteronism: Preoperative preparation with spironolactone. *JAMA*, **180**:1056, 1962.
5. Griffing, G. T., Cole, A. G., et al: Amiloride in primary hyperaldosteronism. *Clin. Pharmacol. Ther.*, **31**(1):56, 1982.
6. Kremer, D., Boddy, K., et al: Amiloride in the treatment of primary hyperaldosteronism and essential hypertension. *Clin. Endocrinol.*, **7**:151, 1977.
7. Chrysant, S. G., and Luv, T. M.: Effects of amiloride on arterial pressure and renal function. *J. Clin. Pharmacol.*, **20**(5):332, 1980.
8. Maronde, R. F., Milgrom, M., Vlachakis, N. D., and Chan, L.: Response of thiazide-induced hypokalemia to amiloride. *JAMA*, **249**(2):237, 1983.
9. Antcliff, A. C., Beevers, D. G., Hamilton, M., and Harpur, J. E.: The use of amiloride

hydrochloride in the correction of hypokalemic alkalosis induced by diuretics. *Postgrad. Med. J.*, **47**:644, 1971.

10. Carney, S., Morgan, T., Wilson, M., Matthews, G., and Roberts, R.: Sodium restriction and thiazide diuretics in the treatment of hypertension. *Med. J. Aust.*, **1**:803, 1975.

11. Croxson, M. S., Neutze, J. M., and John, M. B.: Exchangeable potassium in heart disease: Long-term effects of potassium supplements and amiloride. *Am. Heart J.*, **84**:53, 1972.

12. Kohvakka, A., Eisalo, A., and Manninen, V.: Maintenance of potassium balance during diuretic therapy. *Acta Med. Scand.*, **205**:319, 1979.

13. Nicholls, M. G., Espiner, E. A., Hughes, H., and Rogers, T.: Effect of potassium-sparing diuretics on the renin-angiotensin-aldosterone system and potassium retention in heart failure. *Br. Heart J.*, **38**:1025, 1976.

14. Multicenter Diuretic Cooperative Study Group: Multiclinic comparison of amiloride, hydrochlorothiazide, and hydrochlorothiazide plus amiloride in essential hypertension. *Arch. Intern. Med.*, **141**:482, 1981.

15. Paterson, J. W., Dollery, C. T., and Huston, R. M.: Amiloride hydrochloride in hypertensive patients. *Br. Med. J.*, **1**:422, 1968.

16. Demanet, J. C., Paduart, P., Fichefet, J. P., and Delcroix, C.: Tolerance and ionic effects in hypertensive patients of prolonged administration of an aldosterone antagonist (amiloride) as compared with a thiazide. *J. Clin. Pharmacol.*, **10**:269, 1970.

17. Magnani, B., Ambrosioni, E., Tartagni, F., Pasetti, L., and Melandri, G.: Total body potassium and long-term treatment with amiloride hydrochloride and/or hydrochlorothiazide. *Int. J. Clin. Pharmacol. Biopharm.*, **17**(10):404, 1979.

18. Fernandez, P. G., Sharma, J. N., et al: Potassium conservation with amiloride/hydrochlorothiazide ('Moduret') in thiazide-induced hypokalemia in hypertension. *Curr. Med. Res Opin.*, **8**:120, 1982.

19. Ram, C. V. S., Holland, O. B., and Kaplan, N. M.: Attenuation of diuretic-induced hypokalemia by amiloride, a potassium-sparing agent, *J. Clin. Pharmacol.*, **21**:484, 1981.

20. Castenfors, H.: Long-term treatment with a fixed combination of amiloride hydrochloride and hydrochlorothiazide. In B. Magnani (Ed.): *Diuresis, Kaliuresis and Hypertension: Long-Term Clinical Experience with a Fixed Combination of Amiloride Hydrochloride and Hydrochlorothiazide*, Futura Publishing Co., Mt. Kisco, N. Y., 1974, pp. 27–35.

21. Castenfors, H.: Long term effect of timolol and hydrochlorothiazide or hydrochlorothiazide and amiloride in essential hypertension. *Eur. J. Clin. Pharmacol.*, **12**:97, 1977.

22. Laragh, J. H.: Amiloride, a potassium conserving agent new to the U. S. A.: Mechanisms and clinical relevance. *Curr. Ther. Res.*, **32**(2):173, 1982.

23. Weiss, P., Hersey, R. M., Dujovne, C. A., and Bianchine, J. R.: The metabolism of amiloride hydrochloride in man. *Clin. Pharmacol. Ther.*, **10**:401, 1969.

24. Grayson, M. F., Smith, A. J., and Smith, R. N.: Absorption, distribution and elimination of ^{14}C-amiloride in normal human subjects. *Br. J. Pharmacol.*, **43**(2):473P, 1971.

25. George, C. F.: Amiloride handling in renal failure. *Br. J. Clin. Pharmacol.*, **9**(1):94, 1980.

Triamterene

1. Pruitt, A. W., et al: Variations in the fate of triamterene. *Clin. Pharmacol. Ther.*, **21**(5):610, 1977.

2. Cranston, W. I., et al: Effect of triamterene on elevated arterial pressure. *Am. Heart J.*, **68**:455, 1965.
3. McKenna, T. J., Donohoe, J. F., et al: Potassium sparing agents during diuretic therapy in hypertension. *Br. Med. J.*, **1**:739, 1971.
4. Hansen, K. B., and Bender, A. D.: Changes in serum potassium level occurring in patients treated with triamterene and a triamterene–hydrochlorothiazide combination. *Clin. Pharmacol. Ther.*, **8**(3):392, 1966.
5. McDonald, C. J.: Use of a computer to detect and respond to clinical events: Its effects on clinician behavior. *Ann. Intern. Med.*, **84**(2):162–167, 1976.
6. Heath, W. C., and Freis, E. D.: Triamterene with hydrochlorothiazide in the treatment of hypertension. *JAMA*, **186**:119, 1963.
7. Jick, H.: Drugs—remarkably nontoxic. *N. Engl. J. Med.*, **291**:824–828, 1974.
8. Spiekerman, R. E., et al: Potassium sparing effects of triamterene in the treatment of hypertension. *Circulation*, **34**:524, 1966.
9. Pruitt, A. W., et al: Transfer characteristics of triamterene and its analysis. *Drug Metab. Dis.*, **3**(1):30, 1975.
10. Walker, B. R., et al: Hyperkalemia after triamterene in diabetic patients. *Clin. Pharmacol. Ther.*, **13**:643, 1972.
11. Cohen, A. B.: Hyperkalemic effects of triamterene. *Ann. Intern. Med.*, **65**:521, 1966.
12. Hollander, W.: Aldosterone antagonists in arterial hypertension. *Heart Bull.*, **12**:108, 1963.
13. Lieberman, F. L., and Bateman, J. R.: Megaloblastic anemia possibly induced by triamterene in patients with alcoholic cirrhosis. *Ann. Intern. Med.*, **68**:168, 1968.
14. Corcino, J., et al: Mechanism of triamterene-induced megablastosis. *Ann. Intern. Med.*, **73**:419, 1970.

Spironolactone

1. Levitt, D.: A clinical trial of a spironolactone/thiazide combination in the treatment of hypertension in Zambian Africans. *Curr. Med. Res. Opin.*, **6**:136, 1979.
2. Goodman, L. S., and Gilman, A.: *The Pharmacological Basis of Therapeutics.* Macmillan, New York, 1980, pp. 804–805, 810, 907–908.
3. Falch, D. K., and Schreiner, A.: The effect of spironolactone on lipid, glucose, and uric acid levels in blood during long-term administration to hypertensives. *Acta. Med. Scand.*, **213**:27, 1983.
4. McMahon, F. G.: *Management of Essential Hypertension*, Futura Publishing Co., Mount Kisco, New York, 1978, pp. 132–150.
5. Tobian, L.: Why do thiazide diuretics lower blood pressure in essential hypertension? *Annu. Rev. Pharmacol.*, **7**:399, 1967.
6. Wolf, R. L., Mendolwitz, M., et al: Treatment of hypertension with spironolactone, double-blind study. *JAMA*, **198**(11):1143, 1966.
7. Walter, N. M. A., Suther, M. B., et al: A comparison between spironolactone and hydrochlorothiazide with and without alpha-methyldopa in the treatment of hypertension. *Med. J. Aust.*, **1**:509, 1978.
8. Jamil, M. A. Q.: A comparative study of spironolactone and hydroflurmethiazide alone and together in the treatment of hypertension. *Guys Hosp. Rep.*, **120**:207, 1971.
9. Gussin, R. Z.: Potassium-sparing diuretics. *J. Clin. Pharmacol.*, **17**:651, 1977.
10. Aronoff, A., and Barkum, H.: Hyperuricemia and acute gouty arthritis precipitated by thiazide diuretics. *Can. Med. Assoc. J.*, **84**:1181, 1961.

11. Bryant, J. M., et al: Hyperuricemia induced by the administration of chlorthalidone and other sulfonamide diuretics. *Am. J. Med.*, 33:408, 1962.
12. Breckenridge, A, Welborn, T. A., et al: Glucose tolerance in hypertensive patients on long-term diuretic therapy. *Lancet*, 1:61, 1967.
13. Winer, B. M., Lubbe, W. F., and Colton, T.: Antihypertensive actions of diuretics, comparative study of an aldosterone antagonist and a thiazide alone and together. *JAMA*, 204(9):775, 1968.
14. Solheim, S. B., Sunsfjord, J. A., and Giezendanner, L.: The effect of spironolactone (aldactone) and methyldopa on low and normal renin hypertension. *Acta Med. Scand.*, 197:451, 1975.
15. Carey, R. M., Douglas, J. G., et al: The syndrome of essential hypertension and suppressed plasma renin activity: Normalization of blood pressure with spirono-lactone. *Arch. Intern. Med.*, 130:849, 1972.
16. Crane, M. G., and Harris, J. J.: Effect of spironolactone in hypertensive patients. *Am. J. Med. Sci.*, 260:311, 1970.
17. Cranston, W. I., and Juel-Jensen, B. E.: The effects of spironolactone and chlor-thalidone on arterial pressure. *Lancet*, 1:1161, 1962.
18. Hollander, W., Chobanian, A. V., and Wilkins, R. W.: The role of diuretics in the management of hypertension. *Ann. NY Acad. Sci.*, 88:975, 1960.
19. Kremer, D., et al: Spironolactone and amiloride in the treatment of low renin hy-peraldosteronism and related syndromes. *Clin. Sci. Mol. Med.*, 45:213, 1973.
20. Ferguson, R. K., Turek, D. M., and Rovner, D. R.: Spironolactone and hydro-chlorothiazide in normal-renin and low-renin essential hypertension. *Clin. Phar-macol. Ther.*, 21(1):62, 1977.
21. Karlberg, B.E., et al: Controlled treatment of primary hypertension with propran-olol and spironolactone. *Am. J. Cardiol.*, 37(4):642, 1976.
22. Spark, R. F., et al: Low renin hypertension, restoration of normotension and renin responsiveness. *Arch. Intern. Med.*, 133:205, 1974.
23. Acchiardo, S., Dustan, H. P., and Tanzi, R. C.: Similar effects of hydrochloro-thiazide and spironolactone on plasma renin activity in essential hypertension. *Cleve. Clin. Q.*, 39:153, 1973.
24. Adlin, V. E., Marks, A. D., and Channick, B. J.: Spironolactone and hydrochloro-thiazide in essential hypertension. Blood pressure response and plasma renin activ-ity. *Arch. Intern. Med.*, 130:855, 1972.
25. Drayer, J. I. M., et al: Intrapatient comparison of treatment with chlorothalidone, spironolactone, and propranolol in normo-reninemic essential hypertension. *Am. J. Cardiol.*, 36:716, 1975.
26. Akbar, F. A., Boston, P. F., et al: Spironolactone and hydroflumethiazide in the treatment of hypertension. *Br. J. Clin. Pract.*, 35(9):317–321, 1981.
27. George, C. G., Breckenridge, A. M., and Dollery, C. T.: Comparison of the potas-sium-retaining effects of amiloride and spironolactone in hypertensive patients. *Lancet*, 2:1288, 1973.
28. Roberts, C. J. C., Marshall, A. J., et al: Comparison of natriuretic uricosuric, and antihypertensive properties of tienilic acid, bendrofluazide, and spironolactone. *Br. Med. J.*, 1:224, 1979.
29. Kreeft, J. H., Larochelle, P., and Ogilvie, R. I.: Comparison of chlorthalidone and spironolactone in low-renin essential hypertension. *Can. Med. Assoc. J.*, 128:31, 1983.
30. Ramsay, L. E., Hettiarachchi, J., et al: Amiloride, spironolactone, and potassium

chloride in thiazide-treated hypertensive patients. *Clin. Pharmacol. Ther.*, **27**(4): 533, 1980.

31. Bull, M. B., and Laragh, J. H.: Amiloride, a potassium-sparing natriuretic agent. *Circulation*, **37**:45, 1968.

32. Spark, R. F., and Melby, J. C.: Hypertension and low plasma renin activity: Presumptive evidence for mineralocorticoid excess. *Ann. Intern. Med.*, **75**:831, 1971.

33. Clane, M. G., Harris, J. J., and Johns, V. J.: Hyporeninemic hypertension. *Am. J. Med.*, **52**:457, 1972.

34. Spark, R. F., and Melby, J. C.: Aldosteronism in hypertension: The spironolactone response test. *Ann. Intern. Med.*, **69**:685, 1968.

35. Flanagan, M. J. et al: Primary aldosteronism: *J. Urol.*, **88**:111, 1962.

36. Mobley, J. E., et al: Primary aldosteronism: Preoperative preparation with spironolactone. *JAMA*, **180**:1056, 1962.

37. Crane, M. G., et al: Primary aldosteronism due to an adrenal carcinoma. *Ann. Intern. Med.*, **63**:494, 1965.

38. Karlberg, B. E., Kagedal, B., et al: Renin concentrations and effects of propranolol and spironolactone in patients with hypertension. *Br. Med. J.*, **1**:251, 1976.

39. Vaughan, E. D., Jr., Loragh, J. H., et al: Volume factor in low and normal renin essential hypertension. Treatment with either spironolactone or chlorthalidone. *Am. J. Cardiol.*, **32**:523, 1973.

40. Liddle, G. W.: Specific and non-specific inhibition of mineralocorticoid activity. *Metabolism*, **10**:1021, 1961.

41. Jose, A., Crout, J. R., and Kaplan, N. M.: Suppressed plasma renin activity in essential hypertension. Roles of plasma volume, blood pressure, and sympathetic nervous system. *Ann. Intern. Med.*, **72**:9, 1970.

42. Brooks, C. S., Johnson, C. A., et al: Diuretic therapies in low renin and normal renin essential hypertension. *Clin. Pharmacol. Ther.*, **22**:14, 1977.

43. Hunyor, S. N., Zweifler, A. J., et al: Effect of high dose spironolactone and chlorthalidone in essential hypertension: Relation to plasma renin activity and plasma volume. *Aust. NZ J. Med.*, **5**:17, 1975.

44. Douglas, J. G., Hollifield, J. W., and Liddle, G. W.: Treatment of low-renin essential hypertension: Comparison of spironolactone and a hydrochlorothiazide-triamterene combination. *JAMA*, **227**:518, 1974.

45. Schriver, G., and Weinberger, M. H.: Hydrochlorothiazide and spironolactone in hypertension. *Clin. Pharmacol. Ther.*, **25**:33, 1979.

46. Jick, H., and Armstrong, B.: Breast cancer and spironolactone. *Lancet*, **2**(7930):368, 1975.

47. Berg, K. J., Gisholt, K., and Wideroe, T. E.: Potassium deficiency in hypertensives treated with diuretics. Analysis of three alternative treatments by an oral test for potassium deficiency. *Eur. J. Clin. Pharmacol.*, **7**:401, 1974.

48. Erbler, H. C.: Inhibition of aldosterone production in diuretic-induced hyperaldosteronism by aldosterone antagonist canrenone in man. *Naunyn Schmiedebergs Arch. Pharmacol.*, **285**:395, 1974.

49. Antcliff, A. C., Beevers, D. G., et al: The use of amiloride hydrochloride in the correction of hypokalemic alkalosis induced by diuretics. *Postgrad. Med. J.*, **47**: 644, 1971.

50. Croxan, M. S., Neutze, J. M., and John, M. B.: Exchangeable potassium in heart disease: Long-term effects of potassium supplements and amiloride. *Am. Heart J.*, **84**:53, 1972.

51. Davidson, C., and Gillebrand, I. M.: Use of amiloride as a potassium conserving agent in severe cardiac disease. *Br. Heart J.*, **35**:456, 1973.

52. McKenna, T. J., Donahoe, J. F., et al: Potassium-sparing agents during diuretic therapy in hypertension. *Br. Med. J.*, **2**:739, 1971.

53. Nicholls, M. G., Espiner, E. A., et al: Effect of potassium-sparing diuretics on the renin-angiotensin-aldosterone system and potassium retention in heart failure. *Br. Heart J.*, **38**:1025, 1976.

54. Ibsen, H.: The effect of potassium chloride and spironolactone on thiazide-induced potassium depletion in patients with essential hypertension. *Acta Med. Scand.*, **196**:21, 1974.

55. Erbler, H. C.: The effects of saluretics and spironolactone on aldosterone production and electrolyte secretion in man. *Naunyn Schmiedebergs Arch. Pharmacol.*, **286**:145, 1974.

56. Abshagen, U., Sporl, S., et al: Competitive inhibition of 11B– and 18– hydroxylases by spironolactone. *Clin. Sci. Mol. Med.*, **51**:307s, 1976.

57. Sullivan, L. P., and Grantham, J. J.: *Physiology of the Kidney.* 2nd edition, Lea and Febiger, Philadelphia, 1982.

58. Hoffbrand, B. L., Edmonds, C. I., and Smith, T.: Spironolactone in essential hypertension: Evidence against its effect through mineralocorticoid antagonism. *Br. Med. J.*, **1**:682, 1976.

59. Gifford, R. W.: Drug combinations as rational antihypertensive therapy. *Arch. Intern. Med.*, **133**:1053, 1974.

60. Genest, J., and Nowaczynski, W.: Aldosterone and electrolyte balance in human hypertension. *J. R. Coll. Physicians Lond.*, **5**:77, 1970.

61. Dustan, H. P., Bravo, E. L., and Tarazi, R. C.: Volume dependent essential and steroid hypertension. *Am. J. Cardiol*, **31**:606, 1973.

62. Delahaye, J. P., Lieux, J. M., and Conin, A.: Anti-aldosterones and arterial hypertension—from 32 observations of hypertensive patients treated with a combination of Aldactone and a thiazide derivative. *Lyon Med.*, **216**:477, 1966.

63. Grieble, H. G., and Johnson, L. C.: Treatment of arterial hypertensive disease with diuretics. *Arch. Intern. Med.*, **110**:64, 1962.

64. O'Fallon, W., and Labarthe, D.: Rauwaolfia derivatives and breast cancer. *Lancet*, **2**(7938):773, 1975.

65. Searle, G. D., and Co.: Personal communication. May 18, 1977.

66. Beevers, D. G., Brown, J. J., et al: The use of spironolactone in the diagnosis and the treatment of hypertension associated with mineralocorticoid excess. *Am. Heart J.*, **86**:404, 1973.

67. Greenblatt, D. J., and Koch-Weser, J.: Adverse reactions to spironolactone. *JAMA*, **225**:40, 1973.

68. Brown, J. J., Davies, D. L., et al: Comparison of surgery and prolonged spironolactone therapy in patients with hypertension, aldosterone excess and low plasma renin. *Br. Med. J.*, **2**:229, 1972.

69. Roos, J. C., Boer, P., et al: Changes in intrarenal uric acid handling during chronic spironolactone treatment in patients with essential hypertension. *Nephron.*, **32**:209, 1982.

CHAPTER VI

THE CENTRALLY ACTING ALPHA₂ AGONISTS

- CLONIDINE (CATAPRES®)
- METHYLDOPA (ALDOMET®)
- GUANABENZ (WYTENSIN®)

CLONIDINE (CATAPRES®)
Introductory year (Germany): 1966
Introductory year (U. S.): 1974

INTRODUCTION:

In the ten years since its introduction on the American market, clonidine, the prototype of a new class of antihypertensive agents representing central alpha-2-adrenergic agonists, has been the subject of intensified research which, added to the insights gained through clinical experience in varied patient populations, has led to a clearer definition and a significant expansion of the indications for therapeutic use of this agent. As a result, the following attributes can now be added to the clinical profile of clonidine:

1. Clonidine can be used effectively and safely as the sole agent in the treatment of mild to moderate hypertension.

2. A low-dose clonidine–diuretic combination given once a day can provide good blood pressure control while reducing the adverse effects of higher doses of either drug given alone.

3. In moderate to severe hypertension, clonidine is a useful alternative to a beta-blocker in combined treatment with a diuretic and a vasodilator such as hydralazine or minoxidil (Step 3).

4. In refractory hypertension, the addition of low-dose clonidine

215

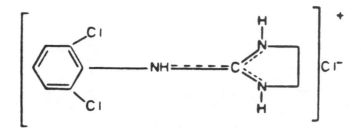

Figure 1: Structure of clonidine.

to a triple-drug regimen of diuretics, beta-blockers and vasodilators allows all of these drugs to be given in lower doses and tends to minimize or neutralize adverse effects of the individual drugs (Step 4). In advanced hypertension, clonidine may also enhance the antihypertensive effects of the calcium antagonist nifedipine or the angiotensin-converting enzyme inhibitor captopril.

5. Clonidine therapy offers important advantages in certain subgroups of hypertensive patients:

    a. Geriatrics

    b. Adolescents

    c. Patients with borderline hypertension

    d. Patients with renal impairment

    e. Diabetics.

6. Oral clonidine loading can be used successfully for rapid reduction of severely elevated blood pressure in asymptomatic patients ("hypertensive urgencies").

Mechanism of Action

Clonidine, an imidazoline compound, 2-(2,6-dichlorophenylamino)-imidazoline, was synthesized in 1962 by Stähle as an alpha-adrenoceptor stimulant which is relatively lipophilic and so easily penetrates the central nervous system; high concentrations of the drug are thus attained in the brain and the cerebrospinal fluid.[1] Clonidine has been found to have the properties of a partial alpha-adrenergic agonist in that it is bound to both presynaptic and postsynaptic alpha-adrenoceptors, showing less intrinsic activity at both receptor sites than norepinephrine.[2] Alpha-receptor stimulation leads to increased activity of hypothetical inhibitory neurons, believed to be the bulbospinal neurons, as a result of which the tone of the peripheral sympathetic nerve system is reduced with a consequent decrease in arterial blood pressure and heart rate.[1] Experimental findings suggest that the sympathetic depressant effect of clonidine is exerted at the vasomotor center of the medulla oblongata and at the hypothalamus and that the depressor baroreceptor may be activated by clonidine.[3] An effect of clonidine on the spinal neurons was suggested by studies of the effect of drugs on reflex sympathetic activity induced by stimulation of a peripheral nerve. Alpha-adrenoceptor blockers such as piperoxan and yohimbine are competitive antagonists of the central hypotensive action of clonidine.[3] It has been shown that the reduction in peripheral sympathetic tone by clonidine is associated with a lowered frequency and intensity in the discharges of the splanchnic nerve, while at the same time the plasma levels of catecholamines are also reduced.[4]

In addition to its suppression of sympathetic nervous function through action in the central nervous system, clonidine may also have an important interaction with the renin-aldosterone axis,[5] causing an initial suppression of the vasoconstrictor action of the renin-angiotensin system followed by a long-term antihypertensive effect more closely linked to suppression of aldosterone. Other investigators have disputed a relation between the antihypertensive effect of clonidine and changes in the renin-angiotensin-aldosterone system.[6] It is agreed that in chronic treatment with clonidine, neither renal blood flow nor the glomerular filtration rate is reduced.

The reduction in cardiac output, which is the predominant hemodynamic effect of clonidine in hypertensive patients—attributable mainly to decreased venous return to the right heart secondary to systemic venodilation and bradycardia[7]—manifests itself mainly at rest; cardiac output responds normally to exercise. Clonidine therapy rarely gives rise to orthostatic hypotension.[2]

Numerous studies in animals as well as humans led Kobinger[8] to the conclusion that clonidine decreases the resting tone of the sympathetic system but still permits the passage of vital reflex adjustments, apparently because it does not block the final efferent sympathetic vasomotor neurons of the medulla but exerts a modulating effect upon them. In this respect the inhibitory effect of centrally acting drugs such as clonidine differs from that of substances which block the adrenergic neurons at peripheral sites: such substances seriously interfere with pressor reflexes and can thus cause severe hypotension.

Absorption, Distribution, Metabolism, Excretion

Orally administered clonidine is almost completely absorbed from the gastrointestinal tract at a reported bioavailability of approximately 75%.[9,10] An antihypertensive effect is produced within 30–60 minutes after administration. Pharmacologically active plasma levels range from 0.2 to 2 ng/ml and have been found by some investigators to correlate positively with the decrease in mean arterial pressure.[11] Other investigators observed a strong correlation only between the individual maximum decrease in mean blood pressure and the peak plasma concentration of clonidine.[12] The plasma levels peak 1.5 to 2 hours after oral doses of 0.15 to 1.4 mg,[13-15] and the blood pressure-lowering effect of single doses of the drug usually persists for six to eight hours. Twice-daily dosing at steady state achieves adequate 24-hour blood pressure control. The plasma levels of clonidine following multiple doses or a single large dose seem to reach a plateau in 72 to 96 hours. The half-life of elimination from the plasma in patients with normal renal function varies between 7.5 and 13 hours.[11,14,16-19]

Clonidine is rapidly distributed after absorption. Kinetic analysis of plasma levels in man (doses of 75–500 mcg I. V.) suggests that the distribution can be described either by a 2-compartment or a 3-compartment model.[10,11,18-20] In human serum, clonidine is bound to proteins in a proportion of approximately 30%.[21] Autoradiographic studies and measurements of radioactivity have shown higher concentrations of clonidine in the organs than in the plasma. Clonidine itself, unlike its hydrophilic metabolites, passes through the blood–brain barrier and accumulates in the brain.[13,22,23]

The two principal routes of metabolism are cleavage of the imidazoline ring and hydroxylation of the phenyl ring. None of the metabolites has been found to have any significant pharmacologic activity.[24] Approximately 50% of the clonidine administered is excreted in human urine in unchanged form within the first 24 hours and another 5–10% appears in the second 24 hours; approximately 15–20% is excreted with the feces.[16] After oral dosage, excretion is nearly complete in 72 hours. Chronic treatment was not found to result in a changed ratio between renal and fecal excretion or in the metabolic pattern in the urine, and the likelihood of enzyme induction is therefore considered to be small.[14]

Dose in Hypertension

Frequency: usually given twice daily

Initial: 0.1 mg twice daily (a lower initial dose, viz. 0.1 mg once daily, may be preferable in elderly patients.[25] Once daily administration of 0.1 mg is also the recommended initial dose in adult dialysis patients.[26])

Range: Increase by 0.1 mg at a time, while not exceeding 2.4 mg daily, until the desired response is achieved. Studies have shown that administration twice a day with the larger portion of the daily dose taken at bedtime provides good blood pressure control and has the advantage of tending to lessen side effects such as dryness of mouth and drowsiness.[27,28]

Usual dose: 0.1 to 0.3 mg on a twice-daily schedule

When Should the Physician Consider Clonidine for Hypertension?

1. Step 1

There is growing evidence that clonidine is useful as initial monotherapy, particularly so in patients with mild to moderate hypertension and in certain subgroups of patients whom we will discuss below. Controlled studies have led investigators to the conclusion that clonidine alone can be used effectively in such cases as a viable alternative to diuretics and beta-adrenergic blocking agents. They found that blood pressure control was sustained with clonidine monotherapy for extended periods without any evidence of fluid retention, which causes the "pseudotolerance" seen with sympathetic inhibitors such as reserpine and methyldopa and with vasodilators such as hydralazine and minoxidil, necessitating addition of a diuretic to the therapeutic regimen. Clonidine monotherapy also has not been associated with any changes in cardiac output, renal blood flow, glomerular filtration rate, plasma renin activity or plasma aldosterone levels[29-35] (see Tables I and II and Figure 2).

While the Joint National Committee on Detection, Evaluation and Treatment of High Blood Pressure recommended for initial therapy of hypertension a thiazide-type diuretic,[36] the adverse effects of diuretic therapy, such as hypokalemia, hyperglycemia, hyperuricemia and hyperlipidemia, are being recognized increasingly as a cause for concern

TABLE I
CARDIAC HEMODYNAMIC VARIABLES BEFORE AND AFTER
CLONIDINE MONOTHERAPY
(Mean Values ± Standard Error of the Mean)

	Control Level	1 Week	3 Months
Blood pressure (mm Hg)			
Systolic	167 ± 4	139 ± 3*	140 ± 3*
Diastolic	105 ± 2	89.0 ± 2*	90 ± 2*
Heart rate (beats/min)	84 ± 2	67 ± 2*	69 ± 2*
Cardiac output (ml/min)	5248 ± 184	5160 ± 145	5180 ± 210
Stroke volume (ml/beat)	63.0 ± 2.3	78.2 ± 2.0*	76.4 ± 15.0*
Peripheral vascular resistance (dynes sec cm^{-5})	1852 ± 86	1569 ± 67*	1600 ± 72*

* $p < 0.001$.
From: Thananopavarn et al,[29] with permission of *The American Journal of Cardiology.*

TABLE II
RENAL HEMODYNAMIC VARIABLES BEFORE AND AFTER
TREATMENT WITH CLONIDINE ALONE
(Mean Values ± Standard Error of the Mean)

	Control Study	1 Week	3 Months
Glomerular Filtration Rate (ml/min)	105.7 ± 7.5	99.8 ± 7.4	104.5 ± 5.8
Renal Blood Flow (ml/min)	711.0 ± 6.6	622.0 ± 6.0	652.7 ± 43.7
Blood Volume (ml)	4682.3 ± 168.7	4594.5 ± 232.0	4835.9 ± 239.8
Body Weight (kg)	80.3 ± 3.2	78.5 ± 2.5	81.3 ± 3.2
Urinary sodium (mEq/L)	88.5 ± 5.0	86.3 ± 3.7	90.5 ± 7.6

From: Thananopavarn et al,[29] with permission of *The American Journal of Cardiology.*

since they may augment the risks of cardiovascular disease. Hypokalemia may potentiate ventricular ectopic activity, hyperlipidemia may promote atherogenesis, and thrombotic complications may be induced by volume contraction and hemoconcentration.[35] The Multiple Risk Factor Intervention Trial[37] confirmed that diuretics increase plasma cholesterol levels.[38] Long-term clonidine therapy, on the other hand, has been found to cause no biochemical or hemodynamic perturbations and does not stimulate the renin-angiotensin-aldosterone axis. Clini-

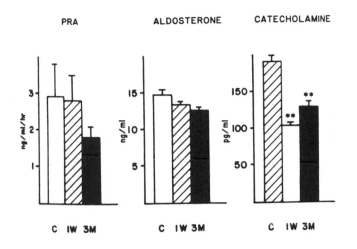

Figure 2: Effect of clonidine monotherapy on hormonal variables. ** = p < 0.001; C = control; IW = 1 week; 3M—3 months; PRA—plasma renin activity. From: Thananopavarn et a l[29] reprinted with permission of *The American Journal of Cardiology.*

cal experience has also shown that clonidine does not interfere to any significant degree with sympathetic nervous system control of posture, exercise and sexual function.[29,35] Clonidine monotherapy has been continuously and beneficially used in patients with essential hypertension for periods of four years and longer.[32]

2. Step 2

In the stepped-care regimen recommended by the Joint National Committee on Detection, Evaluation and Treatment of High Blood Pressure,[39] clonidine is among the drugs that may be added as Step-2 therapy to the initially administered diuretic. There is abundant evidence to support the conclusion that the use of thiazide-type diuretics in conjunction with clonidine not only allows the therapeutic clonidine dose to be reduced but also results in a synergistic effect in addition to minimizing adverse reactions.[40-51] Mroczek et al found clonidine with a diuretic to be effective in many cases in which treatment with guanethidine, methyldopa or hydralazine had not been successful.[44] Two years' experience with a clonidine–chlorthalidone combination in 30 hypertensive patients showed that clonidine greatly improved the blood pressure control attainable with diuretic therapy without causing any serious or prolonged side effects. The blood pressure reductions obtained as compared with chlorthalidone alone are shown in Figure 3.[45]

In three open-label studies,[52-54] once-daily administration of the

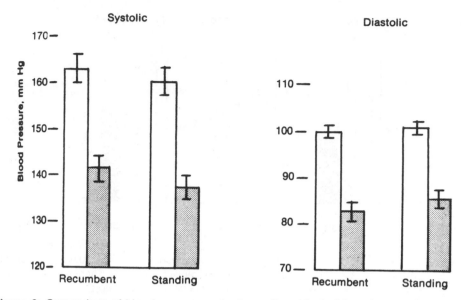

Figure 3: Comparison of blood pressure reductions after chlorthalidone (open columns) and after clonidine and chlorthalidone (shaded columns) in 30 patients (mean + SE). From Rosenman, R. H.,[45] reprinted with permission of *Archives of Internal Medicine*, 135(9):1237, 1975. "Copyright 1975, American Medical Association.

clonidine–chlorthalidone combination produced therapeutic effects that did not differ from those of twice-daily administration to any statistically significant degree, and a double-blind comparison of these two dosage schedules using the commercial tablet combining clonidine with chlorthalidone (0.1 mg + 15 mg) confirmed that once-daily doses given at bedtime produce blood pressure reductions that are clinically comparable to those obtained with twice-daily administration and are, moreover, associated with fewer side effects.[55]

3. Step 3

Clonidine has been found to be a useful alternative to beta-blockers in the Step-3 combinations, including a vasodilator and a diuretic.[51,56-59] Such triple-drug therapy has many intrinsic theoretical and practical advantages, particularly in the management of outpatients with moderate or severe hypertension. A vasodilator may tend to induce tolerance or pseudotolerance after a few weeks of treatment owing to expansion of plasma volume, and concomitant administration of a diuretic in adequate doses eliminates this problem. The reflex sympathetic tachycardia induced by the vasodilator is counteracted by the cardiac slowing effect of a beta-blocker or clonidine. Thus, the development of edema, tachycardia or pseudotolerance is generally avoided by combined administration of the three drugs.

In this triple-drug regimen, clonidine has been successfully substituted for beta-blockers in hypertensive patients with associated bronchial asthma, heart failure, or sleep disturbances.[57,59] Moreover, in the case of propranolol, the prototype of the beta-blockers, enzyme inducers such as cigarette smoking, barbiturates, diphenylhydantoin, insecticides, and alcohol ingestion will decrease plasma levels of the drug by approximately 50%, thus reducing bioavailability commensurately. The opposite effect on propranolol plasma levels is produced by concomitant administration of cimetidine.[55] Other contraindications to beta-blockers are seasonal allergic rhinitis and a history of hypoglycemic attacks.

Clonidine, like the beta-adrenergic blocking agents, can counteract the increase in adrenergic tone induced by such vasodilators as hydralazine and minoxidil. Several investigators have indeed found that addition of hydralazine to clonidine plus a diuretic results in a further lowering of standing and recumbent blood pressure without increasing the orthostatic gradient.[52,55,60,61] Mroczek and Davidov obtained significant decreases in blood pressure and heart rate at a minimal rate of side effects with a clonidine–chlorthalidone–hydralazine combination, with average supine and standing blood pressures being additionally reduced by 10% and 12%, respectively, beyond the reductions obtained with the vasodilator–diuretic combination alone.[62]

Minoxidil, a potent dilator of systemic arterioles, not only lowers the blood pressure but also activates the peripheral sympathetic nervous system, as a result of which renin release is increased, as are heart rate and cardiac output and the release of norepinephrine from sympathetic nerve endings. These secondary effects are prevented by giving minoxidil in combination with clonidine.[63] That clonidine is an effective substitute for beta-blockers in severely hypertensive patients receiving minoxidil (with or without a diuretic) has been observed by Pettinger and Mitchell, as well as by Velasco and co-workers.[57,64,65] The hemodynamic and renin effects of long-term substitution of clonidine for propranolol in patients also treated with minoxidil and a diuretic are shown in Figure 4.

4. Step 4

There have been conflicting reports about the benefits of adding

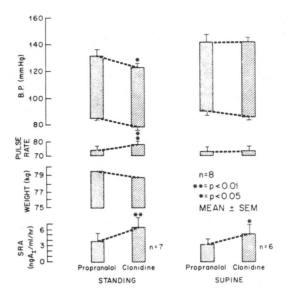

Figure 4: Hemodynamic and renin effects of long-term substitution of clonidine for propranolol in eight minoxidil–diuretic-treated patients. Hemodynamic data and weight are the averages of four consecutive clinic visits on propranolol prior to clonidine. Clonidine data are from four consecutive clinic visits on the final constant dose of clonidine. Renin assays were done once during each treatment period. From: Pettinger, W.A. et al,[57] "Clonidine and the vasodilating beta blocker antihypertensive drug interaction." *Clinical Pharmacology and Therapeutics*, 22(2):167, 1977, reprinted with permission.

guanethidine to the three-drug regimen of clonidine, a diuretic and a vasodilator.[46,51] The concomitant use of other alpha-adrenergic inhibiting agents has also been investigated with varying results. Some authors found that prazosin does not significantly enhance the antihypertensive effect of clonidine[66]; others obtained good antihypertensive responses with a three- or four-drug combination including clonidine and prazosin.[67-69] The most recent research suggests that prazosin does not bring about a further reduction of blood pressure in patients receiving high doses of clonidine.

Japanese studies have shown that concomitant administration of clonidine and furosemide enhanced the hypotensive efficacy of the angiotensin-converting enzyme inhibitor captopril in the treatment of malignant hypertension. Addition of clonidine also improved the antihypertensive effectiveness of the calcium antagonist nifedipine in such cases.[70,71]

Pettinger and associates observed that the addition of either clonidine or prazosin to maintenance therapy with minoxidil, propranolol and diuretics resulted in significant additional reduction of blood pressure in refractory patients.[57,72] The authors suggest that the effect of clonidine could be additive to that of propranolol since clonidine is believed to act principally by inhibition of sympathetic outflow from the cardiovascular control center in the brain stem.

Use of Clonidine in Special Subgroups of Hypertensive Patients

• *The Elderly*

Clonidine is especially suitable for the treatment of elevated blood pressure in the elderly in whom care must be taken to avoid interference with postural reflexes, decrease in cerebral blood flow, and metabolic disturbances. Relatively small doses of clonidine—as low as 0.05 mg twice daily—can be used effectively, with or without a diuretic, in the elderly hypertensive, and the effect is maintained in long-term therapy with no appreciable metabolic or hemodynamic changes; the symptomatic side effects of dry mouth, drowsiness and constipation tend to subside with time and with encouragement from the physician.[45,73] Combined therapy with low doses of chlorthalidone and clonidine was found effective, convenient and palatable in controlling blood pressure in elderly patients with predominantly systolic hypertension, usually by once-daily administration at bedtime[74]; it is believed that the convenience of the single daily dose, together with the general avoidance of undesired side effects, bodes well for good long-term compliance with the treatment.

Clonidine has been specifically recommended as a Step-2 drug for the elderly by the Joint National Committee.[39] Gifford favors its use as a Step-2 agent in elderly patients with isolated systolic hypertension, particularly in those with active liver disease or hypersensitivity to methyldopa, or as a Step-3 drug being added to hydralazine and a diuretic.[25] Wolf et al, in a double-blind study, obtained significant reductions in systolic blood pressure in 75% of a group of patients over 60 years of age with a total daily clonidine dose of only 0.2 mg given concomitantly with chlorthalidone.[75]

• *Adolescents*

The effectiveness and tolerability of clonidine, as compared with a diuretic, in the treatment of adolescents with essential hypertension have been intensively investigated by Falkner, Onesti and associates at the Hahnemann Medical College and Hospital.[76] The results indicate that hypertensive juveniles are more responsive to monotherapy with clonidine than with a diuretic. Using low doses of 0.1 mg clonidine b.i.d. or 25 mg hydrochlorothiazide b.i.d. for 12 weeks in 30 adolescents with fixed primary hypertension in a controlled study, these investigators achieved significant blood pressure reductions in 87% of the patients with clonidine, whereas the diuretic significantly lowered only the systolic pressure and treatment goals were attained in only 40% of the diuretic-treated group. Side effects of clonidine were minimal, but hydrochlorothiazide therapy was associated with significant increases in serum potassium and uric acid.

In this same double-blind placebo-controlled study, the investigators also compared the effects of clonidine and hydrochlorothiazide on the cardiovascular response to mental stress in these adolescents. The hyperresponsiveness to mental stress observed in adolescents with mild hypertension resembles the hyperkinetic cardiovascular state of borderline hypertension. Neither clonidine nor hydrochlorothiazide appeared to influence the systolic pressure response to mental stress, but clonidine produced a significant lessening of the diastolic pressure and heart rate responses to stress. These changes were paralleled by lower plasma catecholamine levels. In the diuretic-treated group, the heart rate response was not significantly lower, while the diastolic pressure response was somewhat higher and plasma catecholamine levels were raised.[76,77]

The same study group also found that hypertensive adolescents treated with clonidine show a hemodynamic response to exercise similar to that of untreated adolescents with borderline hypertension, and they concluded that clonidine may therefore be safely used in the physically active adolescent with primary hypertension.[78]

Another group at Harvard Medical School conducted an open-label study in 16 hypertensive children and adolescents (ages 7-18) who used daily clonidine doses of 0.15 to 1.2 mg. The results indicated that clonidine is also a useful and generally safe agent in children whose compliance can be assured.[79]

• Borderline Hypertension

Reviewing the pathophysiology and epidemiology of borderline hypertension to arrive at a basis for a rational approach to its management, Julius[80] came to the conclusion that not all patients with borderline hypertension need treatment but that treatment should be attempted in the group at highest risk for sustained hypertension and its complications. Julius and Cottier[81] conducted a randomized, double-blind, placebo-controlled crossover study of clonidine vs. propranolol in 16 patients, ages 24 to 47, with marginal elevations of blood pressure to determine whether monotherapy with either of these drugs would be feasible and effective. The patients were selected by these investigators' criterion that patients showing hypertensive readings by the home blood pressure-reading technique are candidates for treatment if the pressure can be lowered with small doses causing no side effects. Treatment with average clonidine doses of 0.24 mg/day resulted in significantly lower blood pressure values than treatment with propranolol (average daily dose 105 mg). Side effects were minor and similar in the drug-treated and placebo groups and would not have interfered with patient compliance if treatment had been prolonged.

• *Renal Failure*

Aside from the fact that clonidine therapy does not entail any decrease in renal blood flow or glomerular filtration rate, Lowenthal et al have shown in a study of the pharmacokinetics and pharmacodynamics of clonidine in patients with end-stage renal disease[82] that clonidine retains its hypotensive power even at the exaggerated plasma levels of the drug characteristic of such patients (up to 30 ng/ml). Gastric absorption of clonidine was not demonstrably impaired. Drowsiness and dry mouth were no more pronounced in these patients with very high plasma clonidine concentrations than in patients with lower concentrations of the drug. Another study,[26] designed to evaluate clonidine in patients maintained on chronic hemodialysis and the effects of renal insufficiency and dialysance on clonidine elimination, disclosed that clonidine is advantageous also because only 5% of the total body stores of the drug are removed as a result of routine dialysis. The investigators, Hulter et al, recommend initiation of clonidine treatment in the adult dialysis patient with a once-daily dose of 0.1 mg, arguing that once-daily dosage is adequate because the drug's half-life is sufficiently prolonged. They note that this dosing schedule contrasts favorably with the divided doses required with hydralazine, methyldopa or propranolol. Side effects were minimal and no rebound hypertension was observed.

Further evidence that clonidine can be used in patients with impaired renal function and that there is no deterioration in renal function as a consequence of such treatment has been furnished by an Australian study in which clonidine was given to patients with essential hypertension, renovascular hypertension, and hypertension accompanied by parenchymal renal disease. The drug proved effective in all these groups but more effective in patients with high plasma renin concentrations, possibly because the plasma renin level reflects a higher basal sympathetic drive. A diuretic increased the effect of clonidine, probably by reducing the body's sodium content.[83]

• Diabetes

Clonidine has been described as "an excellent single-entity antihypertensive agent for use in diabetic patients with hypertension."[7] Unlike thiazide diuretics and certain other hypertensive drugs, clonidine does not appreciably alter glucose tolerance in patients with diabetes mellitus. This has been demonstrated in a number of clinical studies, some of them involving long-term maintenance therapy ranging up to eight months in duration.[43,84-87]

In view of the previous finding that acute administration of clonidine can produce a significant increase in the plasma level of growth hormone, the effects of chronic administration of clonidine on growth hormone secretion were studied in hypertensive diabetics to determine whether this treatment would result in a chronic elevation of growth hormone levels, which might aggravate the course of diabetic microangiopathy. This study, involving treatment periods of at least three months, showed that at the usual antihypertensive doses of 0.15 to 0.30 mg clonidine per day, no change in growth hormone secretion resulted.[88]

Hypertensive Urgencies

Oral clonidine loading is being used as a safe and effective treatment of "hypertensive urgencies," that is, severe hypertension associated with end-organ damage requiring a relatively rapid reduction of blood pressure, in patients free of papilledema and showing no evidence of hypertensive encephalopathy or congestive heart failure. The oral therapy of hypertensive crises avoids the need for constant monitoring and the risk of hypotension that is associated with parenteral therapy. The patients are generally given 0.2 mg of clonidine orally at the outset and if the diastolic pressure has not dropped to 110 mm Hg or by at least 20 mm Hg after one hour, another 0.1 mg is given every hour until either six hours have elapsed or a maximum of 0.6 mg has been administered. In the majority of cases, the diastolic pressure will have dropped from 140–130 to 100–110 mm Hg by the 6th hour. Oral clonidine is said to have a particular advantage in that it begins to act within 30 to 60 minutes, produces its peak effect between two and four hours, and allows individualization of dosage. Freedom from orthostatic hypotension and reflex tachycardia and a high response rate have been found to make clonidine loading preferable to the use of other agents proposed for this indication, such as prazosin, labetalol, and minoxidil.[89] Use of the same drug for long-term ambulatory management facilitates individualization of the medical regimen and avoids possible adverse drug interactions. The response rate in this type of treatment ranges from 80 to 100% and the treatment becomes effective within a mean period of three hours.[89-91] The majority of patients have actually been found to respond to 0.3 mg of clonidine within two hours. Reasonable blood pressure control can be maintained thereafter without hospitalization with standard doses of clonidine and a diuretic.[91]

How Effective is Clonidine?

When used as monotherapy for mild to moderate essential hypertension (diastolic pressure: 90–115 mm Hg), clonidine reduced elevated blood pressures to normal levels in 50 to 60% of patients. A review of several studies, presented in Table III, shows that average reductions of 27/14 mm Hg were obtained at a mean maximal dose of 0.8 mg per day.

Clonidine has been found in numerous studies to reduce blood pressure in hypertension of all degrees of severity without orthostatic hypotension at rest or after exercise.[7] It remains effective in long-term maintenance treatment and, in more severe hypertension, clonidine has been added successfully, as we have shown above, to other potent antihypertensive agents. As Lawson and Keston have observed,[32] such a combined therapy allows the blood pressure to be adequately controlled with lower doses of other drugs with a greater potential for toxicity. This sparing effect allows the incidence of major side effects of such multiple-drug regimens to be reduced to a minimum. These authors found that there was a relative lack of postural and exercise hypotension even when the maximum recommended clonidine dose (0.3 mg every eight hours) was given.

The use of clonidine in conjunction with a diuretic has an additive effect on the antihypertensive properties of each drug. In several stud-

TABLE III
EFFECT OF CLONIDINE ALONE IN MILD AND MODERATE HYPERTENSION

Study (Ref. No.)	No. of Patients	Maximal Daily Dose (mm Hg)	Pre-Treatment Blood Pressure (mm Hg)	Post-Treatment Blood Pressure (mm Hg)	Decline in Blood Pressure (mm Hg)
Wilkinson et al 1977[92]	32	0.3	185/116	167/101	18/15
Karlberg et al 1977[93]	15	1.8	177/110	158/103	19/7
Kluyskens et al 1980[94]	13	0.9	172/108	143/92	29/16
Distler et al 1980[95]	16	0.9	185/114	152/98	33/16
Lauro et al 1980[96]	13	0.45	185/107	154/93	31/14
Jaattela 1980[97]	24	0.45	185/109	150/96	35/13
Walker et al 1982[98]	52	0.8	160/101	140/88	20/13
Thananopavarn et al 1982[29]	16	0.6	167/105	139/89	28/16
Mean blood pressures (mm Hg)		0.8	177/109	150/95	27/14

ies in which a fixed combination of clonidine and chlorthalidone (Combipres®) was tested in a total of 258 hypertensive patients, this treatment resulted in a mean decrease in blood pressure from 184/114 to 147/93 mm Hg at an average reduction of 37/21 mm Hg.[40,44,47,51,99] In most of these studies Combipres® treatment led to decreases of 20–25% in both systolic and diastolic blood pressure. Onesti et al[100] obtained a significant antihypertensive response with the clonidine-chlorthalidone combination at clonidine doses no higher than 0.9 mg/day in 80% of the patients treated, in both supine and standing positions.

Clonidine has been found effective in patients of all ages, even in the presence of serious vascular disease.[32]

Precautions

Patients who engage in potentially hazardous activities, such as operating machinery or driving, should be advised of the sedative effect of clonidine. The drug may intensify the CNS-depressive effect of alcohol, barbiturates and other sedatives. Like any other antihypertensive agent, clonidine should be used with caution in patients with severe coronary insufficiency, recent myocardial infarction, cerebral vascular disease or chronic renal failure. As in all hypertensive patients, periodic eye examinations should be performed also during chronic clonidine therapy. While animal studies have shown that clonidine is concentrated in the choroid of the eye in dogs and monkeys and can produce a dose-dependent increase in the incidence and severity of spontaneously occurring retinal degeneration in albino rats treated for six months or longer, no abnormal ophthalmologic findings, with the exception of some dryness of the eyes, have been reported in patients treated with clonidine for periods ranging up to several years.

Patients being treated with clonidine—or for that matter with any antihypertensive drug—should be instructed not to stop taking the medication without first consulting their physician. When discontinuing clonidine therapy, the physician should reduce the dose gradually over a period of one to two weeks to avoid a possible rapid rise in blood pressure and associated subjective symptoms such as nervousness, agitation, and headache. (Also see Post-Treatment Syndrome below.) In view of the lack of data from well-controlled studies concerning the effects of clonidine during pregnancy, use of the drug in pregnant women is not recommended.

Overdosage: Signs and symptoms of clonidine overdosage include hypotension, bradycardia, lethargy, irritability, weakness, somnolence, diminished or absent reflexes, miosis, vomiting, and hypoventilation. Reversible cardiac conduction effects or arrhythmias, apnea, seizures, and transient hypertension have been reported.[101] Recommended treatment for clonidine overdosage includes gastric lavage, fluids, administration of an analeptic and/or vasopressor, and tolazoline in intravenous doses of 10 mg every 30 minutes as needed. With proper treatment, the patient should be completely recovered within 24 hours.

Drug Interactions

1. Tricyclic Antidepressants

There have been conflicting reports regarding the effect of concomitant tricyclic antidepressant therapy on the blood pressure control obtained with clonidine. Inasmuch as clonidine rarely causes depression, the potential need for combined antihypertensive/antidepressant therapy is small. Published observations do indicate that the blood-pressure-lowering effect of clonidine may be diminished by concomitant administration of a tricyclic antidepressant such as desipramine[102] or imipramine.[103] In patients treated with such agents, caution should therefore be exercised and the clonidine dose may have to be increased.

2. CNS Depressants

The use of CNS depressants, such as barbiturates, tranquilizers and other sedatives, as well as alcoholic beverages, may cause excessive drowsiness in patients treated with clonidine, particularly at the beginning of treatment.

3. Beta-Blockers

While there have been conflicting reports as to the effectiveness of combined treatment with beta-blockers and clonidine,[41,104] the concomitant use of drugs such as propranolol, metoprolol, nadolol, and atenolol is probably best avoided and may exacerbate potential problems caused by abrupt cessation of clonidine therapy. For this reason, it is recommended that beta-blocker therapy be discontinued well in advance of the cessation of clonidine administration, bearing in mind the longer biologic activity of beta-blockers.[7]

4. Levodopa

Concomitant administration of levodopa with clonidine may lead to inhibition of the antiparkinsonian effect of the former drug and should be avoided.[105]

Post-Treatment Syndrome

It is a commonly accepted observation that patients occasionally experience symptoms of nervousness, sweating, anxiety, palpitations, nausea, abdominal cramps, and headache after abrupt discontinuation of treatment with an alpha- or beta-adrenergic blocking agent. The symptoms may be accompanied by a blood pressure rise—and, rarely, an "overshoot" of blood pressure above readings taken before the initiation of therapy—and tachyarrhythmias, especially sinus tachycardia and premature contractions.[106] This is to be distinguished from rebound hypertension, i.e., a rapid return of blood pressure to the values recorded prior to treatment, which is sometimes associated with signs and symptoms of *increased* sympathetic activity, while "overshoot" is associated with signs of *excessive* sympathetic activity. Sympathetic overactivity, in fact, is the mechanism believed to be responsible for the discontinuation syndrome.

Clonidine, as well as methyldopa, guanabenz, and guanadrel, has been associated with a post-treatment syndrome, and so have beta receptor-blocking agents, diuretics and reserpine. However, none of the retrospective studies reported to date has brought to light any incidence of "overshoot" hypertension after abrupt cessation of treatment with clonidine doses of less than 1.2 mg per day.[7] In a comprehensive review of case reports on the acute post-treatment syndrome associated with clonidine which Houston published in 1981,[107] 19 such reports involving a total of 48 patients were found and the results of 10 prospective studies covering 121 patients were analyzed. Only 26 of these 48 patients were found to have experienced symptoms after termination of treatment with clonidine alone, and in 5 of these 26 (19%), overshoot hypertension was experienced. In 4 of the 26 patients, however, propranolol treatment was continued. In the remaining 22 patients, clonidine administration was discontinued simultaneously with another antihypertensive drug so that it was difficult to assess the relative contributions of the individual agents. Eight of these 22 patients—or 36%—developed overshoot hypertension or symptoms. This finding supports the assumption that the syndrome is more likely to occur after abrupt cessation of antihypertensive combination treatment.

In the prospective studies in which treatment with either clonidine alone or with a clonidine–chlorthalidone combination was discontinued, only 2 of 121 patients (1.7%) developed overshoot hypertension and 43 (36%) experienced mild hyperadrenergic symptoms. The majority of the patients had either mild symptoms or none, while their blood pressures returned to the pre-treatment levels or below. Patients with renal insufficiency and renal artery stenosis appeared to be more predisposed to the discontinuation syndrome than patients with normal kidney function and no renovascular disorders.

Reinstitution of the previous medication, i.e., clonidine, is the most effective treatment for the syndrome. Bed rest or mild sedation may, according to Houston, be sufficient therapy for patients with generalized symptoms of sympathetic overactivity who have no severe hypertension and no other cardiovascular manifestations.

Adverse Reactions

The most commonly observed side effects of clonidine, which appear to be dose-related, are dry mouth, occurring in approximately 40% of patients; drowsiness, affecting about 33%; dizziness (16%) and constipation (10%). These reactions are generally mild and tend to diminish or disappear within two to four weeks of continued administration. Sedation and dry mouth can be reduced to a minimum by beginning treatment with small doses of 0.1 mg at night and slowly increasing the dose by 0.1 mg each week, the larger portion of the daily dose being given at bedtime.[28,60]

Less frequent adverse experiences accompanying treatment with clonidine, occurring in 0.1 to 5% of patients, are nausea and vomiting, anorexia and malaise, and mild transient abnormalities in liver function test values. Weight gain may occur in about 1% of patients. Similar percentages of patients may temporarily experience depression, headache, or a skin rash.

Loss of libido and/or impotence—disturbances associated with several types of antihypertensive therapy—have been reported in approximately 3 out of 100 patients using clonidine. A weakly positive Coombs' test has been obtained in fewer than 0.1% of all clonidine-treated patients.

Satisfactory tolerance of clonidine has been universally reported in the great majority of patients (93%). Transfer to a different antihypertensive medication was necessitated by intolerance in the remaining 7%.

METHYLDOPA (Aldomet®)
Introductory year: 1963

INTRODUCTION:

Methyldopa is still one of the most widely used antihypertensive drugs in the world. Every physician treating high blood pressure should be familiar with it. It is an aromatic amino acid (Figure 5) related to naturally occurring DOPA. Methyldopa acts chiefly by depressing sympathetic outflow from the central nervous system. It decreases peripheral vascular resistance without significantly decreasing cardiac output or heart rate. It reduces both supine and erect blood

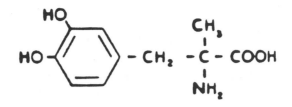

Figure 5: Structure of methyldopa.

pressure while also maintaining renal blood flow or glomerular filtration rate.

The new news about methyldopa is that doses as small as 125 to 250 mg twice daily appear to be effective in treating mild to moderate hypertension and are particularly beneficial in the elderly.

The new news about methyldopa is that doses as small as 125 to 250 mg twice daily appear to be effective in treating mild to moderate hypertension and are particularly beneficial in the elderly.[1-5] Since the development of a positive Coombs' test and other immunologic toxic reactions appear to be dose-related, utilizing daily milligram rather than gram doses offers the possibility of significantly reducing the incidence of these rare but potentially serious adverse reactions. In addition, the incidence of such minor side effects as sedation, dizziness and dry mouth appears to be diminished. Since beta-blockers have reduced efficacy and increased side effects in the elderly hypertensive, low-dose methyldopa is a most useful alternative.

Indications for Use of Methyldopa

1. Used alone as monotherapy:

Methyldopa given alone has been shown to reduce blood pressure approximately 25/15 mm Hg in patients with mild hypertension and approximately 36/21 mm Hg in moderate to severe hypertension (Tables IV and V). When methyldopa is used as the sole agent in treating hypertension, patient response to therapy ranges from 26–81%.[6-9] However, patients receiving long-term methyldopa alone may experience problems with fluid retention, weight gain, and edema.[7,10-15] Tolerance or actually a pseudotolerance frequently develops after several weeks

TABLE IV
EFFECT OF METHYLDOPA ALONE IN PATIENTS WITH MILD* HYPERTENSION

Study (Ref.)	No. of Patients	Pre-Treatment Blood Pressure (mm Hg)	Post-Treatment Blood Pressure (mm Hg)	Maximal Dose (gm/day)	Blood Pressure Decline (mm Hg)
Kirkendall et al 1962[17]	7	183/113	160/97	1.25	23/16
Putzey et al 1962[18]	12	173/106	148/97	1.5	25/9
Seedat et al 1976[19]	17	152/106	125/88	2.0	27/18
Bradley et al 1977[20]	23	161/102	155/94	3.0	6/8
Walker et al 1977[21]	19	166/111	143/98	2.0	23/13
Aranow et al 1977[22]	5	164/104	140/87	2.25	24/17
Routledge et al 1977[23]	13	196/113	156/93	2.25	40/20
Okanga et al 1978[24]	16	180/113	145/93	1.5	35/20
Louis et al 1978[25]	8	141/105	130/91	3.0	11/14
Sanders et al 1979[26]	18	181/107	153/92	1.5	28/15
Rengo et al 1980[27]	30	184/108	163/89	2.0	21/19
Rhomberg et al 1981[9]	30	180/108	149/94	0.75	31/14
Mean Values		172/108	147/93	2.0	25/15

* Diastolic $\leq$ 114 mm Hg without target organ damage.

TABLE V
EFFECT OF METHYLDOPA ALONE IN PATIENTS WITH
MODERATE OR SEVERE HYPERTENSION*

Study (Ref.)	No. of Patients	Pre-Treatment Blood Pressure (mm Hg)	Post-Treatment Blood Pressure (mm Hg)	Maximal Dose (gm/day)	Blood Pressure Decline (mm Hg)
Gillespie et al 1962[15]	9	180/116	153/99	4.0	27/17
Cannon et al 1962[28]	22	225/138	176/108	8.0	49/30
Colwill et al 1964[7]	20	180/115	158/104	3.0	22/11
Johnson et al 1966[6]	37	219/128	179/107	—	40/21
Johnson et al 1966[6]	43	202/117	172/101	—	30/16
Gibb et al 1970[29]	17	192/117	155/93	3.0	37/24
Hefferman et al 1971[30]	21	208/125	149/90	3.0	59/35
Conolly et al 1972[31]	13	201/121	156/95	10.0	45/26
Amery et al 1972[32]	23	204/125	129/84	2.5	75/41
Mroczek et al 1972[33]	41	176/116	145/96	2.5	31/20
McMahon et al 1975[16]	22	160/116	154/105	1.5	6/11
Petrie et al 1976[34]	24	189/119	164/104	0.75	25/15
Vierhapper et al 1980[35]	7	191/130	170/114	1.5	21/6
Mean Values		194/122	159/100	3.1	36/21

* Diastolic ≥ 115 mm Hg with target organ involvement.

with diminished hypotensive response due to the expanded plasma volume.[6,12]

2. With diuretics in combination therapy:

This is the principal use of this popular drug. In patients not controlled by diuretics alone, methyldopa can usually be added with good or excellent results. Combinations of methyldopa with thiazide diuretics lower pressure about 35/20 mm Hg—more than either component given alone.[6,7,11-13,16] The additive effects of the two drugs allow smaller doses to be used and result in fewer side effects from each drug. Weight gain and tolerance associated with use of methyldopa alone are eliminated when diuretics are added.[6,10,13-15,32,36] Combination therapy is excellent for patients requiring chronic therapy. In a study in which 25 hypertensive patients were followed for seven years, the mean final reduction of blood pressure was 41/20 mm Hg. The 25 patients were reported to tolerate the long-term treatment well.[37]

3. In the management of hypertension associated with renal disease:

Methyldopa effectively lowers blood pressure without further compromising glomerular filtration rate or renal blood flow.[38] In 21 patients with hypertension and renal disease (average pre-treatment blood pressure of 199/129 mm Hg), Luke and Kennedy achieved excellent control in 18 (90%) (average post-treatment blood pressure was 137/88 mm Hg).[39] Methyldopa doses ranged from 0.5 to 2.0 grams/day. Seventeen of these patients who responded showed no further deterioration of renal function while taking methyldopa. Maintenance of adequate control over extended periods may require increasing doses of methyldopa or the addition of diuretics.[39] If creatinine clearance is less than 30 ml/min, thiazides should be replaced with furosemide. Often large oral doses are required (200–1000 mg) to keep urine volume above a liter a day.

4. Alone in the parenteral therapy of hypertensive crisis:

In the treatment of hypertensive crisis, methyldopate hydrochloride is available. It generally lowers pressure within three hours of administration and the effects may last 12–24 hours.[15,17,40] However, the development of more rapidly acting agents such as nitroprusside, diazoxide and hydralazine has generally replaced methyldopate for managing hypertensive emergencies.

Studies have shown that most hypertensive patients achieve good responses to methyldopa alone (average decline of 25/15 mm Hg) in short-term studies[6,7, 9,20] (Table IV). Similarly Table V reports the reduction in blood pressure observed in 299 patients with moderate to severe hypertension. In these studies the average reduction was 36/21 mm Hg with a mean daily dose of 3.1 grams. Each of the tables shows impressive falls in blood pressure, but close attention to the data shows that while individuals with moderate to severe hypertension get a considerable fall in blood pressure, those individuals with mild hypertension are generally not reduced into a normotensive range on methyldopa therapy alone, but also need diuretics.

Formulations

Tablets .... 125, 250 and 500 mg
Injectable .... 250 mg/5 ml
Oral Suspension .... 250 mg/5 ml

Dose in Hypertension

Frequency: usually given two to three times a day in the first 48 hours. Dosage is then increased or decreased, preferably at intervals of no less than two days, until an adequate response is achieved. Presently there are conflicting reports as to the effectiveness of once-a-day doses after initial treatment.[41,42]

Initial: 125 mg twice daily

Range: 125 mg to 3 g daily

Usual dose: 250–500 mg twice daily. Aldoril®* is effective once daily for many patients.

Low Dose Methyldopa

Side effects of methyldopa are surely more common and more severe when larger doses are used, e.g., > 1.0 gm/day. This is true for the "pharmacologic" side effects like sedation, drowsiness, dry mouth, edema, and sexual difficulties, as well as for the "immunologic" or allergic reactions. It therefore is very important to use the smallest effective dose in the treatment of hypertension. Corea et al[43] studied doses of 125 and 250 mg each given twice daily in 30 patients with mild–moderate hypertension (DBP 100–120 mm Hg). After two weeks on placebo, patients were given 125 mg bid or 250 mg bid in a double-blind manner for four weeks. Twenty-three of the patients subsequently agreed to 12 months' open-label study. Results are given below

---

* A combination of methyldopa with hydrochlorothiazide.

in Table VI. Other investigators have had similar beneficial experience, particularly in the elderly hypertensive.[1-5]

Mechanism of Action

The antihypertensive properties of methyldopa were first discovered when methyldopa was being introduced to treat carcinoid tumors by inhibiting the decarboxylation of 5-hydroxytryptophan to serotonin.[44] During the treatment period. Oates et al observed the hypotensive effect of methyldopa and assumed that the mechanism of action must be the result of limiting a decarboxylation reaction, in this case the decarboxylation of DOPA to dopamine which is a precursor of the vasopressor norepinephrine[15] (Figure 6). As interest in the hypotensive effects of methyldopa increased, research showed that the hypotensive effects of the drug were related to the L-isomer only.[45] This initial mechanism of action was disputed due to studies that showed no correlation between norepinephrine depletion and either decarboxylase inhibition resulting from methyldopa administration or the degree of the hypotensive response.[46]

As the decarboxylase inhibitor theory waned, a second hypothesis for the mechanism of action of methyldopa was proposed. This was based on the fact that if methyldopa was decarboxylated to the metabolite alpha-methyldopamine, this was associated with a decreased tissue norepinephrine content.[47] With this information the theory of the false transmitter evolved for methyldopa. It was shown that methyldopa could progress through the same biochemical pathway as DOPA

TABLE VI
MEAN SUPINE BLOOD PRESSURE RESPONSES TO LOW-DOSE METHYLDOPA AFTER 4 WEEKS OF DOUBLE-BLIND THERAPY IN 28 PATIENTS AND OPEN-LABEL IN 12 PATIENTS AFTER 12 MONTHS*

	Low Dose	Control Blood Pressure (mm Hg)	4th Week Blood Pressure	12th Month Blood Pressure
Group A	125 mg Bid	174.9/107.1	153.5/94.2	146.5/85.7
Group B	250 mg Bid	169.7/108.9	148.4/90.6	141.8/84.7

* From Corea, et al.[43]

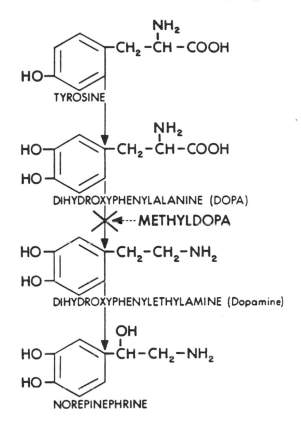

Figure 6: Hypotensive effects due to inhibition of decarboxylation of dopa with depletion of tissue norepinephrine.

and subsequently result in alpha-methyl-norepinephrine which could be stored in the nerve terminal similar to norepinephrine. This led researchers to believe that alpha-methylnorepinephrine was the active hypotensive metabolite of methyldopa with its mechanism of action being the release of methylnorepinephrine from the presynaptic nerve terminal in the place of norepinephrine, which resulted in a diluted vasopressor effect.[48,49] As with the previous mechanism, fault was found with the false transmitter theory due to the fact that methylnorepinephrine could not consistently be shown to result in a reduced sympathetic response to nerve stimulation.[50-54]

Presently methyldopa is thought to have principally a central mechanism of action. It stimulates alpha receptors in the medulla of the brain stem resulting in a decrease in sympathetic tone to the vasculature.[54] It is not clear whether the central alpha stimulation is via inhibitory alpha-2 receptors or is a variant of the false transmitter theory involving excitatory alpha-1 receptors.[55] The belief in alpha stimulation is supported by studies showing that pre-treatment with the competitive alpha blocker phentolamine prevents the hypotensive effect of methyldopa.[56] The central mechanism of action of the drug is substantiated by the fact that peripheral decarboxylase inhibitors do not inhibit the hypotensive effect of the drug.[26,57] Alpha-methylnorepinephrine is believed to be the active hypotensive metabolite for several reasons: central inhibition of dopamine-beta-hydroxylase reduces the hypotensive action of methyldopa,[58] only the active L-isomer is metabolized to methylnorepinephrine,[59] and methylnorepinephrine does not appear to cross the blood–brain barrier.[57]

Use of methyldopa for the treatment of hypertension has been shown to decrease plasma renin levels.[60] This action may contribute to methyldopa's hypotensive effect and may be an advantage when considering long-term treatment.

Whatever the mechanism of action, methyldopa's hypotensive effect results from a decrease in peripheral vascular resistance with insignificant effects on heart rate.[61-68] Cardiac output and renal blood flow and glomerular filtration rate are not affected by methyldopa.[69-71] Postural hypotension is not a common problem with methyldopa,[72-73] a great advantage in respect to exercise. Lee et al have shown that methyldopa is able to reduce myocardial oxygen demand without reducing work capacity.[74]

Benfield and Hunter report a possibly detrimental rise in triglycerides after methyldopa therapy, while Amer and Hill found a decrease in beneficial HDL-cholesterol.[75,76]

Recently there have been reports that methyldopa reduces left ventricular hypertrophy. One particular study from Cleveland shows that methyldopa reduces left ventricular hypertrophy without significant changes in the blood pressures of the patients.[77]

Drug Interactions

1. With *Diuretics or Other Antihypertensive Agents:*

The hypotensive effect of methyldopa is increased when a diuretic or a diuretic plus another agent is added.

Table VII presents the hypotensive effect obtained with methyldopa alone and in combination with diuretics. Use of these drugs in

TABLE VII
COMPARISON OF HYPOTENSIVE EFFECTS OF METHYLDOPA AND DIURETICS—
ALONE AND IN COMBINATION

Study (Ref.)	No. of Patients	Mean Pre-treatment Blood Pressure (mm Hg)	Diuretic**	Mean Blood Pressure Reduction (mm Hg)		
				After Diuretic Alone	After MD Alone	After Combination
Colwill et al 1964[7]	20	180/115	HCTZ	30/14	22/11	42/21
Wilson et al 1963[11]	15	143*	HCTZ	—	13	—
Wilson et al 1963[11]	15	147*	HCTZ	26	—	—
Wilson et al 1963[11]	15	145*	HCTZ	—	—	25
McMahon et al 1975[16]	21	170/116	HCTZ	24/10	16/11	27/21
Glazer et al 1975[87]	15	171/106	HCTZ	16/2	—	36/15
Yajnik et al 1978[88]	12	187/118	HCTZ	7/2	—	39/24
Noveck et al 1982[41]	30	164/103	HCTZ	—	—	27/15
Mroczek et al 1972[33]	31	176/116	Chlor.	13/9	—	31/20
Webster et al 1977[89]	14	181/120	Chlor.	18/9	—	38/20
Wilson et al 1977[90]	21	182/110	Chlor.	7/4	—	32/16
Smith et al 1966[13]	67	127*	Chlor.	—	15	—
Smith et al 1966[13]	60	120*	Chlor.	—	—	18
Hansen et al 1977[91]	25	190/118	Cyclo.	—	—	44/30
Van Der Merwe et al 1980[92]	10	165/106	Clorex.	6/1	—	25/13
Kristensen et al 1981[93]	48	177/111	Bendro.	2/2	—	26/12

* Mean arterial pressure = diastolic plus 1/3 pulse pressure.
** HCTZ = hydrochlorothiazide; Chlor. = chlorthalidone; Cyclo. = cyclopenthiazide, Clorex. – clorex-olone; Bendro. = bendroflumethiazide

combination produces considerably better blood pressure reduction than when used alone.[7,13]

2. With *Tricyclic Antidepressants:*

Imipramine, etc., may reduce or prevent the antihypertensive effects of methyldopa.[78-80] Blood pressure tends to rise toward pretreatment levels when the tricyclic drug is added.

3. With *Barbiturates:*

Phenobarbital reduces the efficacy of methyldopa through the induction of hepatic microsomal enzymes which increase the rate of metabolism of methyldopa and shorten its half-life.[81]

4. With *Sympathomimetic Amines:*

Amphetamines and ephedrine may interfere with the antihypertensive effects of methyldopa. Conversely, methyldopa also reduces the mydriasis produced by locally applied ephedrine.[78,79,82]

5. With *L-DOPA:*

The simultaneous administration of L-DOPA and methyldopa may interfere with the therapeutic effects of the former drug in managing parkinsonism. Potentiation of hypotension by L-DOPA should also be watched for but does not appear to be a common problem.[83-86]

6. With *Monoamine Oxidase Inhibitors:*

The hypotensive effects of methyldopa may be reduced; hypertension and CNS stimulation may occur when the two drugs are given together.[94,95]

7. With *Phenothiazines:*

The administration of trifluoperazine with methyldopa may produce a paradoxical increase in blood pressure.[96]

8. With *General Anesthesia:*

Administration of general anesthesia to patients receiving methyldopa might produce additive hypotensive effects. However, Nies reported no added risks in these people requiring surgery.[97]

9. With *Lithium:*

Symptoms of lithium toxicity may result with lithium levels within the therapeutic range when taken together with methyldopa.[98-100]

10. With *Haloperidol:*

The toxicity of haloperidol may be increased when given with methyldopa.[99]

Interference with Laboratory Tests

- *Creatinine determination:*

Determination of creatinine by the alkaline picrate method may be inaccurate in patients taking methyldopa.

- *Uric acid levels:*

Laboratory values for uric acid measurement via the phosphotungstate method may be falsely altered in patients being treated with methyldopa.

- *SGOT:*

Measurement of serum glutamic oxalocetic transaminase with colorimetric methods may be altered in patients on methyldopa therapy.

- *Urinary catecholamines:*

May be falsely elevated in patients receiving methyldopa. Methyldopa does not interfere with VMA determinations employing conversion of VMA to vanillin.

Contraindications

— Active hepatic disease, such as hepatitis and active cirrhosis.
— If previous methyldopa therapy has been associated with liver disorders.
— Hypersensitivity.

Warnings

- *In patients with a positive Coombs' test:*

With prolonged methyldopa therapy, 10 to 20% of patients develop a positive direct Coombs' test which usually occurs between 6 and 12 months of therapy. The lowest incidence is at daily doses of 1 g or less. On rare occasions, this may be associated with hemolytic anemia which could lead to potentially fatal complications. One cannot predict which patients with a positive direct Coombs' test may develop hemolytic anemia, but it is rare.

Prior existence or development of a positive direct Coombs' test is not in itself a contraindication to use of methyldopa. If a positive

Coombs' test develops during methyldopa therapy, the physician should determine whether hemolytic anemia exists or whether the positive Coombs' test may be a problem. For example, in addition to a positive direct Coombs' test, there is less often a positive indirect Coombs' test which may interfere with crossmatching of blood.

At the start of methyldopa therapy, it is desirable to do a blood count for a baseline or to establish whether there is anemia. Periodic blood counts should be done during therapy to detect hemolytic anemia. It may be useful to do a direct Coombs' test before therapy and at 6 and 12 months after the start of therapy.

If Coombs'-positive hemolytic anemia occurs, the cause may be methyldopa and the drug should be discontinued. Usually the anemia remits promptly. If not, corticosteroids may be given and other causes of anemia should be considered. If the hemolytic anemia is related to methyldopa, the drug should not be reinstituted.

When methyldopa causes Coombs' positivity, alone or with hemolytic anemia, the red cell is usually coated with gamma globulin of the IgG (gamma G) class only. The positive Coombs' test may not revert to normal until weeks or months after methyldopa is stopped.

Should a need for transfusion arise in a patient receiving methyldopa, both a direct and an indirect Coombs' test should be performed on his blood. In the absence of hemolytic anemia, usually only the direct Coombs' test will be positive. A positive direct Coombs' test alone will not interfere with typing or crossmatching. If the indirect Coombs' test is also positive, problems may arise in the major crossmatch, and the assistance of a hematologist or transfusion expert will be needed.

- *In patients with liver disorders:*

Fever occasionally occurs within the first three weeks of methyldopa therapy. The fever is associated in some cases with eosinophilia or abnormalities in one or more liver function tests, such as serum alkaline phosphatase, serum transaminases (SGOT, SGPT), bilirubin, cephalin cholesterol flocculation, prothrombin time, and bromsulphalein retention. Jaundice with or without fever may occur with onset, usually within the first two to three months of therapy. In some patients, the findings are consistent with those of cholestasis.

Rarely fatal hepatic necrosis has been reported after use of methyldopa. These hepatic changes may represent hypersensitivity reactions.

Periodic determinations of hepatic function should be done, particularly during the first 6 to 12 weeks of therapy or whenever an unexplained fever occurs. If fever, abnormalities in liver function tests, or jaundice appears, stop therapy with methyldopa. If caused by methyldopa, the temperature and the abnormalities in liver function characteristically have reverted to normal when the drug was discontinued. Methyldopa should not be reinstituted in such patients.

- *Blood dyscrasias:*
    Rarely, a reversible reduction of the white blood cell count with a primary effect on the granulocytes has been seen. The granulocyte count returned promptly to normal on discontinuance of the drug. Rare cases of granulocytopenia have been reported. In each instance, upon stopping the drug, the white cell count returned to normal. Reversible thrombocytopenia has occurred rarely.

Methyldopa and Pregnancy

While methyldopa has not been proven completely safe for treatment of hypertension associated with pregnancy, it is one of the most commonly used antihypertensives in that condition. A seven-and-one-half year study carried out by Cockburn et al found no difference in physical or mental health problems in children born to methyldopa-treated mothers as opposed to untreated hypertensive mothers.[38] Methyldopa has been shown to cross the placenta, but dosage does not appear to have any significant effect on blood pressure of the newborn.[39] Similarly, while breast feeding is contraindicated during treatment, methyldopa has been found in breast milk in such small quantities that no adverse effects have been observed.[97]

The common methyldopa treatment regimen for pregnant women includes a loading dose of 750–1000 mg followed by up to 2 gm/day initially and increasing up to 4 gm/day as needed.[101] During methyldopa control of maternal hypertension, side effects are often encountered (15%), with the most common being lack of energy and dizziness.[102]

Precautions

Methyldopa should be used with caution in patients with a history of previous liver disease or dysfunction.

Methyldopa may interfere with measurement of uric acid by the phosphotungstate method, creatinine by the alkaline picrate method, and SGOT by colorimetric methods. Interference with spectrophoto-metric methods for SGOT analysis has not been reported.

Since methyldopa causes fluorescence in urine samples at the same wave lengths as catecholamines, falsely high levels of urinary catechol-amines may be reported. This will interfere with the diagnosis of pheochromocytoma. It is important to recognize this phenomenon before a patient with a possible pheochromocytoma is subjected to surgery. Methyldopa does not interfere with measurement of VMA (vanillylmandelic acid), a test for pheochromocytoma by those meth-ods which convert VMA to vanillin. Methyldopa is not recommended for the treatment of patients with pheochromocytoma. Rarely, when urine is exposed to air after voiding, it may darken because of a break-down of methyldopa or its metabolites.

Rarely, involuntary choreoathetotic movements have been observed in patients with severe bilateral cerebrovascular disease during ther-apy with methyldopa. Should these movements occur, stop therapy.

Hypertension has recurred occasionally after dialysis in patients given methyldopa because the drug is removed in the dialysate.

Patients may require reduced doses of anesthetics when on methyl-dopa. If hypotension does occur during anesthesia, it usually can be controlled by vasopressors. The adrenergic receptors remain sensitive during treatment with methyldopa.

Absorption, Metabolism, Excretion

The absorption of methyldopa from the gastrointestinal tract var-ies between patients but averages about 50%.[103] Peak plasma levels occur two to three hours after administration. The plasma half-life of methyldopa is about two hours.[104] Since the majority of methyldopa is excreted via the kidney, a patient who has renal complications would be expected to have a longer plasma half-life. Studies dealing with the plasma levels of the drug when using oral and intravenous administra-tion indicate that methyldopa may exhibit a significant first-pass ef-fect.[105] Maximal blood pressure reduction occurs in four to six hours. Once the effective oral dose for an individual has been determined, it generally is given twice daily.

Withdrawal of methyldopa usually results in a return to pre-treat-ment blood pressure within 48 hours. Rebound hypertension occurs very rarely.[12,106-109] Tolerance or "pseudotolerance" to methyldopa treatment may occur after roughly two months of treatment. This is generally not a problem and is usually remedied by increasing the dose of methyldopa or using the same dose of methyldopa in combination with a diuretic.

Methyldopa is metabolized chiefly in the liver (and slightly in the gastrointestinal tract) to methyldopa-mono-O-sulfate. This later conjugate may be therapeutically active.[110] Patients with decreased hepatic function tend to have a decreased rate of conjugation and smaller amounts of the drug are decarboxylated. Kaldor et al showed that induction of liver enzymes with barbiturate therapy will accelerate alpha-methyldopa metabolism.[81]

Adverse Reactions

As with all hypertensive drugs, methyldopa has certain side effects that are fairly common with its use. Due to methyldopa's central mechanism of action, two frequent problems of hypertensive therapy—orthostatic hypertension and sexual dysfunction—are not as common with methyldopa as with peripheral adrenergic blocking drugs such as guanethidine. Table VIII reflects the frequency of side effects that occurred in 25 studies involving 945 patients. The most commonly mentioned problems associated with methyldopa therapy include sedation, dizziness, dry mouth, and headache. Sedation, although it appeared initially in 29% of patients taking the drug, tends to become less a problem after a week of therapy.[19,31,111] Even in the presence of side effects, on the whole, methyldopa therapy is generally well tolerated.[37] Results obtained from 18 studies showed an average of 9.3% of patients discontinued methyldopa therapy due to side effects. The occurrence of methyldopa side effects are grouped according to frequency in Table IX.

More worrisome and potentially more serious than the side effects are methyldopa's toxic reactions which fortunately are rare. Toxic reactions are believed to be the result of an autoimmune disorder and include hemolytic anemia, thrombocytopenia, leukopenia, and lupus-like syndromes. In addition, Iverson and Nordahl reported one case of retroperitoneal fibrosis accompanied by IgG, IgM, and IgA deposits on the collagen fibers in the biopsy specimen taken from a male who had received 1.4 kg of methyldopa over a five-year period.[112] Also, one case of immunoblastic lymphadenopathy was reported in a 71-year-old who had taken 250 mg of methyldopa per day for five years. Immunoblastic lymphadenopathy is believed to be a drug hypersensitivity

TABLE VIII
SIDE EFFECTS SEEN IN 25 REPORTS*
INCLUDING 945 PATIENTS

Side Effects†	Total Number of Patients Exhibiting Side Effects	% Patients Incidence
Sedation (somnolence, fatigue, etc.)	267	29.0
Dizziness (postural, exercise, etc.)	162	17.5
Dry mouth	80	9.5
Headache	71	8.6
Depression	34	4.5
Diarrhea	36	4.4
Sleep disturbance (nightmares, dreams, insomnia)	32	3.8
Nasal congestion	29	3.7
Nausea, vomiting	32	3.7
Weakness	19	2.1
Constipation	18	2.1
Dyspnea	18	2.1
Impotence	17	1.9
Weight gain	14	1.8
Edema	13	1.5
Nocturia	9	1.2
Indigestion	9	1.1
Anxiety	8	1.0
Paresthesias	6	0.8
Failure to ejaculate	5	0.7
Palpitations	5	0.6
Lactation	5	0.6
Cold extremities	5	0.6
Intermittent claudication	4	0.5
Rash	4	0.5

* Refer to reference numbers 6, 7, 11–14, 19, 20, 23, 29, 30, 32, 33, 37, 111, 114–135 at the end of this chapter.

† Other side effects from among these 945 patients include the following dermatitita (3 cases), increased sweating (3), pollakisuria (3), unpleasant taste (3), angina (3), tinnitus (2), muscle cramps (2), decreased libido (1), grippe syndrome (1), blurred vision (2), vertigo (1), nose bleed (1), sore tongue (1), pain in jaw (1).

reaction common to antibiotics which has previously not been associated with methyldopa.[113]

• *Positive Direct Coombs' Test and Hemolytic Anemia*

The correlation between methyldopa therapy and a positive direct

---

TABLE IX
FREQUENCY OF ADVERSE REACTIONS DUE TO METHYLDOPA*

FREQUENT ($> 5.0\%$)

Sedation (somnolence, fatigue), dizziness (postural, exercise), dry mouth, headache.

OCCASIONAL ($0.5-5.0\%$)

Diarrhea, sleep disturbance (nightmares, dreams, insomnia), nasal congestion, depression, nausea and vomiting, constipation, dyspnea, impotence, nocturia, anxiety, indigestion, cold extremities, failure to ejaculate, palpitations, paresthesias, weakness, weight gain, edema, rash, intermittent claudication, lactation.

RARE ($< 0.5\%$)

Dermatitis (lichenoid pruritus, eczema, lip ulcers, granulomatous lesions, hyperpigmentation). Increased diaphoresis, pollakiuria, unpleasant taste, angina, tinnitus, decreased libido, grippe syndrome, blurred vision, vertigo, nose bleed, sore tongue, pain in jaw, myocarditis, rebound hypertension after cessation of drug, sialadenitis, renal calculus, parkinsonism, forgetfulness or decreased mental activity, psychosis, galactorrhea, liver dysfunction, febrile reaction, chills, pancreatitis, impairment of AV conduction, symptomatic sinus bradycardia.

---

* Refer to reference numbers 136–138, at end of chapter.

Coombs' test (DCT), with or without production of hemolytic anemia, was cited by Carstairs et al in 1966.[139] Among 202 patients taking methyldopa, he found that 41 (20%) had positive DCT, compared with none of the 76 patients taking other antihypertensive medications.[140] Other studies place the incidence of a positive DCT in association with methyldopa therapy within a range of 10—36%.[141,142] The antibody involved is a 7S IgC warm antibody which, apart from those antibodies seen in other drug-induced anemias, shows specificity for the Rh locus on the red cell and, therefore, produces hemolysis in the absence of the drug.[143,144] Although the mechanism by which antibodies arise against the self antigen is not known, Kirtland et al postulated that methyldopa causes a persistent elevation of lymphocyte cyclic AMP which inhibits suppressor T-cell function and allows excessive antibody production.[145]

The occurrence of the positive DCT is related to dose, with 36% of patients who received over two grams daily exhibiting this trait as opposed to only 11% in patients taking less than one gram daily.[140,146] A positive DCT will revert back to negative after discontinuation of methyldopa.[147] Based on a study by Grell et al,[148] there may be evidence that the autoimmune effects of methyldopa are less prominent in black populations than in whites. The study included 137 hypertensive Jamaicans who had been taking a mean dose of 1.5 grams of methyldopa a day for an average of 36 months. The study found the incidence of a DCT to be only 0.7%.[148]

● *Hemolytic Anemia*

Hemolytic anemia occurs much less frequently than a positive DCT with studies citing an incidence of 0.1 to 0.2%. Other studies, however, have found incidences as high as 2%.[149-151] Sixty percent of the hemolytic anemias occur within 18 months of initiation of therapy while most remit within one to two months after discontinuation of therapy.[147]

Development of a positive DCT is not grounds for discontinuing methyldopa therapy,[146,152] but upon evidence of hemolysis, the drug must be withdrawn immediately. Previously, a serologic test was not available to distinguish which patients who had a positive DCT would develop hemolytic anemia and which patients would not. In a study of 11 patients with a positive DCT after methyldopa therapy, all patients who went on to hemolytic anemia had IgM antibodies and the first component of complement present in their serum while non-hemolyzing patients did not. In addition, the IgM and complement component were not present after the patients recovered from the anemia after withdrawal of the drug.[153] In the event that withdrawal of methyldopa does not return the anemia to normal or it worsens, corticosteroid therapy should be started.[149,154,155]

● *Thrombocytopenia*

Only a very few cases of thrombocytopenia associated with methyldopa therapy have been reported.[156,157] In some of these cases, platelet antibodies have been demonstrated. Removal of the drug results in disappearance of the antibodies and return of platelet counts to normal levels.

● *Leukopenia*

This is also a very rare complication of methyldopa therapy, characterized by the presence of leukopenia and by white cell antibodies that disappear with cessation of the drug.[158]

● *Non-Erythrocytic Antibodies and the Systemic Lupus Erythematosus Syndrome (SLE)*

Several studies have mentioned an apparent association between methyldopa and the development of positive antinuclear antibody (ANA), lupus erythematosus cell prep, and rheumatoid factor tests. [146,159,160] In a study of 269 patients taking methyldopa. 35 (13%) were found to have ANA while 17 of 448 patients (3.8%) treated with antihypertensive drugs other than methyldopa had ANA.[161] Some studies indicate a direct link with use of methyldopa and the development of lupus-like syndromes.[162,163] Harpey suggests that in the event patients develop a positive ANA test without clinical signs of SLE, methyldopa should be withdrawn.[164]

● *Acute Post-treatment Syndrome*

The sudden withdrawal of methyldopa has been reported to produce, very rarely, an abrupt rise in blood pressure, the so-called "rebound phenomenon."[12,106-109] A review of six published reports involving 92 patients on methyldopa therapy found that 4 of the 92 (4.4%) patients suffered from overshoot hypertension.[165] The symptoms of the rebound phenomenon and its associated hypertension are discussed more fully in Chapter XIII.

● *Hepatic Disease Associated with Methyldopa Therapy*

Hepatic dysfunction associated with methyldopa therapy was first reported in 1962 and references to it occur regularly in the literature.[166] The incidence of liver problems associated with use of methyldopa is difficult to determine, but in a review of previously published studies involving 2,604 patients, Hoyumpa and Connell found that the incidence of altered hepatic function (as represented by transient rises in transaminases, alkaline phosphatase and bilirubin) was 2.8%, and severe liver dysfunction was even less prevalent.[167] The onset of liver injury can be generally classed into short-term (< six months) or long-term (> six months). While the two groups vary in their histological presentation, patients generally experience malaise, anorexia, nausea and vomiting, and upper abdominal pain followed by jaundice and tender hepatomegaly.[168]

Biopsy specimens reveal the short-term hepatic injury consists of inflammation, parenchymatous degeneration, and focal, confluent, and massive necrosis. The long-term hepatic injury is characterized by increased fibrous trabeculae and fatty accumulation.[169]

In most patients the liver derangement is mild with complete recovery following discontinuation of therapy.[170] Some patients' laboratory values return to normal despite continuing therapy. However, in several patients, re-exposure to the drug produced similar symptoms, often occurring more rapidly and severely.[171,172] Several investigators have reported deaths associated with continued administration of the drug in the face of liver disease.[170,173-175]

The pathogenesis of these entities is apparently immunologic in nature. The disappearance of symptoms and signs following removal of the drug, and the often rapidly-occurring and more severe manifestations of hepatic injury associated with readministration of the drug, lend credence to this hypothesis.[176,177]

Patients taking methyldopa should have their liver chemistries monitored at regular intervals and the drug should be discontinued in the face of persistently elevated values. Readministration of the drug to patients in whom it has previously been discontinued due to liver toxicity is strictly inadvisable.

● *Hyperpyrexia*

Another toxic effect associated with methyldopa therapy is hyperpyrexia. It occurs in a reported 1–3% of patients taking the drug[178] and usually follows a latent period of 9 to 19 days.[179] It is often associated with constitutional symptoms and laboratory abnormalities such as eosinophilia, elevated sedimentation rate, and abnormalities of liver function. Miller speculates that one might expect to see deranged liver function following this fever whenever the patient continues to take the drug.[180] This is doubtful in light of the number of cases in which one occurs without the other. Cessation of the drug results in a return of the temperature to normal within two days. On occasion, the fever will relapse spontaneously. Rechallenging the patient after as long as 13 years off methyldopa has resulted in relapse.

Use of Methyldopa in Renal Disease

Data accumulated since the introduction of methyldopa in 1963 indicate that renal plasma flow and glomerular filtration rate are not adversely affected by the drug.[38,181] It has, therefore, been considered to be a logical choice in the treatment of patients with hypertension with renal disease. Since the kidneys are the primary route of excretion for methyldopa and its metabolites, it was suspected that patients with renal disease might exhibit enhanced or prolonged responses to regular doses of the drug. Stenback and Myhre[182] investigated this question in a group of 13 patients—six with advanced renal disease and seven with essential hypertension alone. Their data showed that despite doses and serum concentrations of the drug almost four times greater in patients with renal disease than in those with uncomplicated hypertension, the former achieved a reduction in blood pressure only 1.5 times greater than the latter group of patients.[182] Intravenous doses of the drug also produced greater reductions in supine systolic and diastolic pressures in the patients with the kidney ailments. The maximal hypotensive effects of the four doses developed somewhat later in those patients than it did in the essential hypertensives (eight hours post-injection vs. six hours). The etiology of the increased sensitivity seen in those with renal ailments may be due to higher levels of methyldopa and its metabolites and/or a heightened sensitivity.

Methyldopa is proven to be an efficacious drug when used in hypertensives with renal disease, but doses should be carefully titrated to avoid side effects secondary to the heightened sensitivity such patients exhibit for the drug.

GUANABENZ (Wytensin®)

INTRODUCTION:

Guanabenz is a new 2,6-dichlorobenzylidene derivative of aminoguanidine (Figure 7). It has been shown to possess chiefly a central agonist alpha-2 effect like clonidine but also some peripheral neuron-blocking effect similar to guanethidine.[1,2] It reduces both supine and erect blood pressures and also heart rate. It has some peripheral adrenergic effect, but dizziness and orthostatic hypotension only occasionally occur. Guanabenz shares most of the adverse effects common to

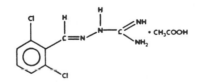

Figure 7: Structure of guanabenz acetate.

similar drugs, e.g., sedation and dry mouth, but studies have indicated that guanabenz appears to have no adverse cardiac, hepatic or metabolic effects.[3-5] Indeed, Walker et al have reported a 20% decrease in serum cholesterol with long-term use.[6] If confirmed, this is twice the response of most marketed hypolipemic agents and would represent a major advantage. While guanabenz monotherapy has been found to be effective in lowering blood pressure, it has also been shown to have increased effectiveness when used with a diuretic in combination therapy.[7]

When should the physician consider guanabenz therapy?

1. As initial monotherapy in mild hypertension:

Guanabenz is a new, centrally-acting antihypertensive drug that has been shown to reduce blood pressure in mild to moderate hypertensives an average of 19/13 mm Hg (Table X). Although thiazides, and less often, beta-blockers are clearly the most popular initial drugs given hypertensive patients, guanabenz is a viable alternative therapeutic agent as it apparently does not cause significant sodium and water retention with chronic administration. Approximately two-thirds of patients with mild to moderate hypertension who are treated will respond favorably to guanabenz alone. Of those who do not respond, some three-fourths have been shown to respond to combination treatment with hydrochlorothiazide.[6]

2. With diuretics in combination therapy:

Guanabenz given with diuretics results in a further decrease in blood pressure. Walker et al found that after an initial decline in MAP of 8 mm Hg in patients receiving a mean dose of 70 mg/day of hydrochlorothiazide, the addition of 25 mg/day of guanabenz resulted in a further reduction of supine diastolic blood pressure of 7 mm Hg.[8] In another study comparing the effectiveness of guanabenz as opposed to a combination of guanabenz and hydrochlorothiazide, there was only a slight improvement in the supine diastolic pressure of 4 mm Hg upon addition of the diuretic. Significant increases in the response to treatment were observed with 78% responding to combination treatment as opposed to 66% on guanabenz alone at the end of six months of therapy. Also at the end of six months of treatment, the incidence of adverse effects was 10% for the guanabenz group and 9% for the group receiving combination treatment. After 23 months of treatment, the

TABLE X
EFFECT OF GUANABENZ ALONE IN PATIENTS WITH MILD* HYPERTENSION

Study (Ref.)	No. of Patients	Maximum Dose (mg/day)	Pre-treatment Blood Pressure (mm Hg)	Post-treatment Blood Pressure (mm Hg) Months				Maximum Blood Pressure Decline (mm Hg)
				0.5	1.0	2.0	6.0	
McMahon et al 1976[9]	24	32	127**	112	114	—	—	15
Shah et al 1976[10]	17	48	172/104	—	158/95	—	—	14/9
Walker et al[3]	17	64	162/103	154/99	154/99	—	157/97	11/11
Walker et al[11]	131	64	164/102	144/89	144/88	—	148/91	20/14
Walker et al 1980[12]	77	48	167/104	148/92	149/92	—	—	19/12
Kluyskens et al 1980[13]	14	48	189/112	—	—	152/93	—	37/19
Hirvonen et al 1980[14]	10	64	157/99	143/92	139/89	139/89	—	18/11
Walker et al 1981[15]	39	64	156/103	—	—	—	142/88	14/15
Walker et al 1981[15]	78	64	157/102	139/91	—	—	147/91	18/11
Walker et al 1982[8]	48	64	161/103	142/89	—	—	139/88	22/15
Walker et al 1982[7]	70	48	159/98	138/86	—	—	138/85	21/13
Mean Values		55	164/103	144/91	150/92	146/91	145/90	19/13

* Diastolic ≤114 mm Hg without target organ damage.

** Mean arterial pressure = diastolic plus 1/3 of pulse pressure.

frequency of adverse effects for the guanabenz group remained at 10% while the incidence rose to 13% in the combination treatment group.[14]

Guanabenz has been shown to be effective in lowering blood pressure in two-thirds of patients with mild to moderate hypertension. Results from several studies summarized in Table X point out that a mean maximum dose of 55 mg/day of guanabenz results in an average decline in supine blood pressure of 19/13 mm Hg. According to Walker et al, concomitant use of guanabenz and hydrochlorothiazide has been shown to result in only slight further decreases in blood pressure of 4 mm Hg but is associated with a significant increase in patient response to treatment (78% vs. 66%).[7,8]

Indication for Guanabenz

Guanabenz is indicated for the treatment of hypertension. It may be used alone or in combination with a thiazide diuretic.

Formulation

Tablets .... 4 and 8 mg

Dose in Hypertension

Frequency: given twice a day. Dosage may be increased by 4 to 8 mg per day every one to two weeks depending on the patient's status. Recent studies have indicated that a once-a-day regimen of guanabenz administration before bedtime may be as effective as a twice-a-day therapy and result in fewer side effects.[6,16]

Initial: 4 mg twice daily
Range: 8–64 mg/day
Usual Dose: 8–16 mg twice daily

Mechanism of Action

Guanabenz is an orally active antihypertensive whose primary action is via central stimulation of alpha-2 receptors. Studies by Baum and Shropshire support this mechanism.[17] Using perfused sinus node preparations and debuffered cats, these researchers found that guanabenz failed to modify carotid sinus nerve activity and was not primarily mediated by baroreceptor mechanisms. They also found that use of the alpha-adrenergic blocking agent phentolamine (10 mg/kg) greatly inhibited the antihypertensive action of guanabenz.[17] In addition to its central effect, guanabenz is believed to have a secondary guanethidine-like neuronal blocking action.[18]

The acute effect of guanabenz results in a decrease in pressure without major changes in peripheral resistance, but given on a chronic basis, the antihypertensive effect appears to result from reduced peripheral resistance. This is not associated with inhibition of normal postural mechanisms and postural hypotension is not a problem.

Oral guanabenz begins to lower blood pressure in roughly one hour with the maximal effect in two to four hours. Pressure returns to pre-treatment levels in 12 hours. While reducing pressure, guanabenz has no detrimental effects on glomerular filtration rate, renal blood flow, cardiac performance, renal sodium or potassium excretion, renal concentrating ability, body fluid volume or body weight.[3,5,19] Indeed, use of guanabenz has been associated with weight losses of one to four pounds. Although the mechanism for this weight loss is not known at present, it is postulated that guanabenz inhibits ADH and the resulting diuresis could explain the weight loss.[20]

Associated with the long-term use of guanabenz are significant decreases in serum cholesterol (20 mg%),[6] total triglycerides (with no change in the HDL fraction), plasma norepinephrine, serum dopamine beta-hydroxylase, and plasma renin activity. No changes in serum electrolytes, uric acid, blood-urea nitrogen, calcium, or glucose have been observed with long-term treatment.

Drug Interactions

Guanabenz has been given to patients in combination with digitalis, diuretics, analgesics, anxiolytics, and anti-inflammatory or anti-infective agents in clinical trials with no observable interactions.

1. With *CNS depressant drugs:*

There is a potential for increased sedation when CNS depressant drugs are taken in combination with guanabenz.

Contraindications

Guanabenz is contraindicated in patients with a known sensitivity to the drug.

Use in Pregnancy

At present there are no good studies of the effect of guanabenz on the human fetus. The best data presently available deal with skeletal abnormalities found in mice and increased fetal loss in rats and rabbits at doses three to six times the recommended maximal human dose. Reproductive studies in rats have shown decreased live birth indices, fetal survival rates, and pup body weight with similar exaggerated doses. Due to the preliminary findings in animal studies and the fact that no studies have concluded whether guanabenz crosses the placenta or gets into breast milk, guanabenz is not recommended for pregnant or nursing mothers.

Precautions

Guanabenz causes sedation or drowsiness in a large percentage of patients. Caution should be exercised when guanabenz is used in conjunction with centrally active depressants, such as phenothiazines, barbiturates, benzodiazepines and alcohol due to the additive sedation effect of these drugs.

Patients with vascular insufficiency should use guanabenz with care. Individuals with severe coronary insufficiency, recent myocardial infarction, cerebrovascular disease, or severe hepatic or renal failure should use caution when taking guanabenz.

Sudden cessation of therapy with central alpha agonists like guanabenz may occasionally result in rebound hypertension (post-treatment syndrome) and commonly produces an increase in serum catecholamines and subjective symptoms such as palpitation, anxiety, nervousness, etc.

Management of Overdosage or Exaggerated Response

There has only been limited exposure to overdose with guanabenz. Excess ingestion of guanabenz has resulted in hypotension, somnolence, lethargy, irritability, miosis and bradycardia, all of which ceased within 12 hours after gastric lavage and administration of pressor substances, fluids, and oral activated charcoal. Recommended treatment for guanabenz overdose is, therefore, primarily supportive consisting of maintenance of vital signs, body fluids, and an adequate airway should the patient need assistance with respiration. There are no available data on the dialyzability of guanabenz.

Absorption, Distribution, Metabolism and Excretion

Guanabenz undergoes substantial metabolism due to the fact that of the 75% of an orally-administered dose that is absorbed, less than 1% is present in the urine as guanabenz. The primary mechanisms are hydroxylation and glucuronidation. Guanabenz is 90% bound to plasma proteins and has been found to fit a 2-compartment model based on urinary excretion and plasma concentration. Maximum plasma concentrations occur at three hours and are undetectable at 24 hours. Recovery via both urinary and fecal elimination routes has been shown to account for 87 to 98% of the administered dose after six days.[21] The plasma half-life of guanabenz averages six hours.

Adverse Reactions

As with other centrally acting agonists, guanabenz has some characteristic adverse effects. Eight separate studies involving 694 patients were reviewed for the incidence of major adverse effects as well as the percentage of patients who were forced to discontinue treatment due to noxious adverse effects. The review found that the four most frequent complaints were: sedation (20–61%), dry mouth (12–48%), weakness (10–21%) and dizziness (4–18%).[7-12,15,22] Most studies report that side effects were most frequent initially and decreased in both occurrence and severity as treatment continued. In one study comparing the adverse effects of once-a-day as opposed to twice-a-day therapy, the frequency of adverse effects was reduced with the once-a-day therapy. The examples cited noted a decline in sedation from 20 to 12% and dry mouth from 12 to 6%.[6]

Of the 697 patients in eight studies, 65 had to discontinue guanabenz because of intolerable side effects, an incidence of 9.4%.[7-12,15,22]

Withdrawal syndromes have been reported to occur with the use of guanabenz. Following a clinical trial involving 17 patients, the drug was abruptly discontinued after 24 months of therapy. Three of the four patients taking the maximal dose of 48 mg/day experienced acute withdrawal symptoms of nervousness, diaphoresis, palpitations, and insomnia. Since this syndrome failed to occur among patients treated at lower doses, it is felt that the phenomenon is dose-related,[23] as known to be the case with other central agonists.

REFERENCES:

Clonidine

1. Timmermans, P. B., Hoefke, W., Stahle, H., and van Zwieten, P. A.: *Structure-Activity Relationships in Clonidine-like Imidazolidines and Related Compounds.* Gustav Fischer Verlag, New York, 1980, p. 1.
2. Lowenstein, J.: Clonidine. *Ann. Intern. Med.*, 92:74–77, 1980.
3. Streller, I., and Klupp, H.: Studies on the mechanism of action of clonidine: Ef-

fect on efferent sympathetic activity. In K. D. Block (Ed.): *Catapresan®*. Aulendorf, Editio Cantor, 1983, pp. 111–117.

4. van Zwieten, P. A., and Timmermans, P. B.: Pharmacology and characterization of central alpha-adrenoceptors involved in the effect of centrally acting antihypertensive drugs. *Chest*, **2**(Suppl):340–343, 1983.

5. Weber, M. D., Drayer, J. I., and Hubbell, F. A.: Effects on the renin-angiotensin system of agents acting at central and peripheral adrenergic receptors. *Chest*, **2** (Suppl):374–377, 1983.

6. Golub, M. S., et al: Hormonal and hemodynamic effects of short and long-term clonidine therapy in patients with mild to moderate hypertension. *Chest*, **2** (Suppl):377–379, 1983.

7. Houston, M. C.: Clonidine hydrochloride. *South.Med. J.*, **75**(6):713–721, 1982.

8. Kobinger, W.: Central alpha-adrenergic systems as targets for hypotensive drugs. *Rev. Physiol. Biochem. Pharmacol.*, **81**:40–100, 1978.

9. Davies, D. S., Wing, L. M. H., Dollery, C. T., et al: Pharmacokinetics and concentration-effect relationships of intravenous and oral clonidine. *Clin. Pharmacol. Ther.*, **21**(5):593, 1976.

10. Davies, D. S., Neill, E., and Reid, J. L.: Applications of deuterium labelling in pharmacokinetic and concentration-effect studies of clonidine. In T.A. Baillie (Ed.): *Stable Isotopes, Applications in Pharmacology, Toxicology and Clinical Research*. Proceedings of an International Symposium on Stable Isotopes held at the Royal Postgraduate Medical School, London, U. K. on January 3rd–4th, 1977, pp. 45–54.

11. Frisk-Holmberg, M., Edlund, P. O., and Paalzow, L.: Pharmacokinetics of clonidine and its relation to the hypotensive effect in patients. *Br. J. Clin. Pharmacol.*, **6**:227–232, 1978.

12. Velasquez, M. T., Rho, J., Maronde, R. F., and Barr, J.: Plasma clonidine levels in hypertension. *Clin. Pharmacol. Ther.*, **34**(3):341–346, 1983.

13. Darda, S.: Pharmacokinetics of clonidine. In: *Recent Advances in Hypertension*. International Symposium, Monte Carlo Principality of Monaco, April 24–26, 1975, pp. 375–388.

14. Rehbinder, D.: Biochemistry of clonidine, In: *New Aspects for the Treatment of Arterial Hypertension*. Round Table Discussion, Inst. Cardiovasc. Res., University of Milan, November, 1973. Boehringer Ingelheim, Florence. pp. 3–22.

15. Jain, A. K., Ryan, J. R., and McMahon, F. G.: A comparative study of the effectiveness of various dose regimens of clonidine. *Clin. Pharmacol. Ther.*, **19**(1):109, 1976.

16. Dollery, C. T., Davies, D. S., et al: Clinical pharmacology and pharmacokinetics of clonidine. *Clin. Pharmacol. Ther.*, **19**(1):11, 1976.

17. Davies, D. S., Baillie, T. A., Neill, E., Hughes, H., and Davies, D. L.: Applications of stable isotope labelling in studies of the pharmacokinetics and metabolism of clonidine. *Adv. Pharmacol. Ther.*, **7**:215–223, 1979.

18. Wing, L. M. H., et al: Pharmacokinetic and concentration-effect relationships of clonidine in essential hypertension. *Eur. J. Clin. Pharmacol.*, **12**:463–469, 1977.

19. Keranen, A., Nykanen, S., and Taskinen, J.: Pharmacokinetics and side-effects of clonidine. *Eur. J. Clin. Pharmacol.*, **13**:97–101, 1978.

20. Edlund, P. O., and Paalzow, L. K.: Quantitative gas-liquid chromatographic determination of clonidine in plasma. *Acta Pharmacol. et Toxicol.*, **40**:145–152, 1977.

21. Heckner, R. M.: Systematische untersuchungen zur proteinbindung biologisch wirksamer substanzen. *Pharmatherapeutica*, **2**(3):177–186, 1979.

22. Jarrot, B., and Spector, S.: Disposition of clonidine in rats as determined by radio-immunoassay. *J. Pharmacol. Exp. Ther.,* **207**:195–202, 1978.
23. Wijffels, C.: Autoradiographic study of the distribution of ^{14}C-clonidine in the squirrel monkey, especially in brain. In: *New Aspects for the Treatment of Arterial Hypertension.* Round Table Discussion. Inst. Cardiovasc. Res., University of Milan, November, 1973, pp. 45–54.
24. Darda, V. S., Forster, H. J., and Stahle, H.: Metabolisher abbau von clonidin. *Arzneim Forsch,* **28**:255–259, 1978.
25. Gifford, R. W., Jr.: Isolated systolic hypertension in the elderly. *JAMA,* **247**(6): 781–785, 1982.
26. Hulter, H. N., Licht, J. H., Ilnicki, L. P., and Singh, S.: Clinical efficacy and pharmacokinetics of clonidine in hemodialysis and renal insufficiency. *J. Lab. Clin. Med.,* **94**:223–231, 1979.
27. Lilja, M., Jounela, A. J., Juustila, H., and Marvola, M.: Antihypertensive effect of clonidine. *Clin. Pharmacol. Ther.,* **25**(6):864–869, 1979.
28. Jain, A. K., Ryan, J. R., Vargas, R., and McMahon, F. G.: Efficacy and acceptability of different dosage schedules of clonidine. *Clin. Pharmacol. Ther.,* **21**(4):382–387, 1977.
29. Thananopavarn, C., Golub, M. S., Eggena, P., Barrett, J. D., and Sambhi, M. P.: Clonidine, a centrally acting sympathetic inhibitor, as monotherapy for mild to moderate hypertension. *Am. J. Cardiol.,* **49**:153–167, 1982.
30. Cressman, M., Bravo, E. L., Olin, J., Durham, F., and Pohl, M. A.: Clonidine as monotherapy for essential hypertension: Relationship between cardiovascular responses and circulatory catecholamines. *Clin. Pharmacol. Ther.,* **2**:224, 1983.
31. Chrysant, S. G., Dillard, B. L., Smith, W. J., and Manion, C. V.: Antihypertensive effectiveness of clonidine and chlorthalidone as step 1 drugs. *Curr. Ther. Res.,* **30** (6):943–955, 1981.
32. Lawson, A. A., and Keston, M.: Clonidine in hypertension: A 6-year review. *Curr. Med. Res. Opin.,* **6**(3):168–174, 1979.
33. Kochar, M. S., Humphrey, H., Kalbfleisch, J. H., Klemm, D., and Zeller, J.: Clonidine in mild and moderate hypertension. *Curr. Ther. Res.,* **29**(6):791–798, 1981.
34. Morgan, T.: Monotherapy in the treatment of hypertension. *Chest,* **2**(Suppl):419–422, 1983.
35. Sambhi, M. P.: Clonidine monotherapy in mild hypertension. *Chest,* **2**(Suppl):427–428, 1983.
36. *Report of the Joint National Committee on Detection, Evaluation and Treatment of High Blood Pressure.* U. S. Dept. of Health, Education and Welfare. DHEW Publication No. 1980 (NIH), 77-1088.
37. Multiple Risk Factor Intervention Trial: Risk factor changes and mortality results. *JAMA,* **248**(12):1465–1477, 1982.
38. Grimm, R. H., Leon, A. S., et al: Effects of thiazide diuretics on plasma lipids and lipoproteins in mildly hypertensive patients. *Ann. Intern. Med.,* **94**:7–11, 1981.
39. The 1980 Report of the Joint National Committee on Detection, Evaluation, and Treatment of High Blood Pressure. *Arch. Intern. Med.,* **140**:1280–1285, 1980.
40. Igloe, M. C.: Antihypertensive efficacy and safety of a clonidine–chlorthalidone combination. *Curr. Ther. Res.,* **15**(8):559, 1973.
41. Saarimaa, H.: Combination of clonidine and sotalol in hypertension. *Br. Med. J.,* **1** (6013):810, 1976.
42. Lund-Johansen, P.: Hemodynamic changes in long-term therapy of essential hy-

pertension: A comparative study of diuretics, alpha-methyldopa, and clonidine. *Clin. Sci. Mol. Med.*, **45**(Suppl 1):199, 1973.

43. Sung, P. K., Samet, P., and Yeh, B. K.: Effects of clonidine and chlorthalidone on blood pressure and glucose tolerance in hypertensive patients. *Curr. Ther. Res.*, **13** (5):280, 1971.

44. Mroczek, W. J., Leibel, B. A., and Finnerty, F. A., Jr.: Comparison of clonidine and methyldopa in hypertensive patients receiving a diuretic A double-blind cross-over study. *Am. J. Cardiol.*, **29**(5):712, 1972.

45. Rosenman, R. H.: Combined clonidine-chlorthalidone therapy in hypertension. Two years' experience in 30 patients. *Arch. Intern. Med.*, **135**(9):1236–1239, 1975.

46. Yeh, B. K., Nantel, A., and Goldberg, L. I.: Antihypertensive effect of clonidine. Its use alone and in combination with hydrochlorothiazide and guanethidine in the treatment of hypertension. *Arch. Intern. Med.*, **127**:233, 1971.

47. Toubes, D. B., McIntosh, T. J., Kirkendall, W. M., and Wilson, W. R.: Hypotensive effects of clonidine and chlorthalidone. *Am. Heart J.*, **82**(3):312, 1971.

48. Gifford, R. W.: Clonidine in the management of mild hypertension in twenty-two patients. *Cleveland Clinic. Quart.*, **36**:173, 1969.

49. Onesti, G., Schwartz, A. B., et al: Antihypertensive effect of clonidine. *Circ. Res.*, **28**(5):(Suppl II)53, 1971.

50. Pitkajarvi, T., Ala-Laurila, P., et al: The use of clonidine and practolol in the treatment of hypertension. *Ann. Clin. Res.*, **8**(1):48, 1976.

51. Hoobler, S. W., and Sagastume, E.: Clonidine hydrochloride in the treatment of hypertension. *Am. J. Cardiol.*, **28**(1):67, 1971.

52. Grossman, S. H., and Gunnells, J. C.: Blood pressure response to a single daily dose of a clonidine-chlorthalidone combination. *J. Clin. Pharmacol.*, **20**(4 Pt. 1): 193–196, 1980.

53. Ram, C. V., Anderson, R. J., et al: Assessment of blood pressure control during once-a-day administration of antihypertensive drugs. *Curr. Ther. Res.*, **28**(1):88–95, 1980.

54. Noveck, R. J., McMahon, F. G., Jain, A. K., and Ryan, J. R.: Clonidine–chlorthalidone combination once and twice daily in essential hypertension. *Clin. Pharmacol. Ther.*, **28**(5):581–586, 1980.

55. McMahon, F. G.: Some new aspects of modern Catapres® therapy in the United States. In K. D. Block (Ed.): *Catapresan®*. Aulendorf: Editio Cantor, 1983.

56. Dollery, C. T.: Pharmacological basis for combination therapy of hypertension. *Annu. Rev. Pharmacol. Toxicol*, **17**:311, 1977.

57. Pettinger, W., et al. Clonidine and the vasodilating beta blocker antihypertensive drug interaction. *Clin. Pharmacol. Ther.*, **22**(2):164, 1977.

58. Pitkajarvi, T., Ala-Laurila, P., Ruosteenoja, R., Torsti, P., and Masar, S. E.: Treatment of hypertension successively with a diuretic, clonidine, or a beta-blocking agent and hydralazine. *Eur. J. Clin. Pharmacol.*, **12**:161–165, 1977.

59. Velasco, M., et al: Cardiovascular hemodynamic interactions between clonidine and minoxidil in hypertensive patients. *Chest*, **2**:360–364, 1983.

60. Pettinger, W. A.: Clonidine, a new antihypertensive drug. *N. Engl. J. Med.*, **293** (23):1179–1180, 1975.

61. Onesti, G., Schwartz, A. B., Kim, K. E., Paz-Martinez, V., and Swartz, C.: Antihypertensive effect of clonidine. *Circ. Res.*, **XXVII** and **XXIX**(Suppl II):II-53–II-70, 1971.

62. Mroczek, W. J., and Davidov, M. E.: A randomized clinical trial of clonidine and

propranolol in hypertensive patients receiving a diuretic and a vasodilator. *Curr. Ther. Res.*, **23**(3):294–299, 1978.

63. Pettinger, W. A.: Minoxidil and the treatment of severe hypertension. *N. Engl. J. Med.*, **303**(16):922–926, 1980.

64. Mitchell, M. C., and Pettinger, W. A.: Long-term treatment of refractory hypertensive patients with minoxidil. *JAMA*, **239**:2131–2138, 1978.

65. Velasco, M., Morillo, J., Hernandez-Pieretti, O., and Angeli-Greaves, M.: Cardiovascular hemodynamic interactions between clonidine and minoxidil in hypertensive patients. *Chest*, **2**(Suppl):360–364, 1983.

66. Drayer, J., and Weber, M. A.: Antihypertensive agents which inhibit sympathetic activity: Potentially adverse effects of combination treatment. *Am. Heart J.*, **104** (3):660–664, 1982.

67. Kuokkanen, K., and Mattila, M. J.: Antihypertensive effect of prazosin in combination with methyldopa, clonidine, or propranolol. *Ann. Clin. Res.*, **11**:18–24, 1979.

68. Curtis, J. R., and Bateman, F. J. A.: Use of prazosin in management of hypertension in patients with chronic renal failure and in renal transplant recipients. *Br. Med. J.*, **4**:432–434, 1975.

69. Pitkajarvi, T., Kyostila, S., Kontro, J., and Mattila, M. J.: Antihypertensive drug combinations: Prazosin, hydrochlorothiazide and clonidine. *Ann. Clin. Res.*, **9**:296–300, 1977.

70. Abe, K.: Treatment of advanced hypertension: Choice of the effective antihypertensive drugs using angiotensin II antagonist. *Jpn. Circ. J.*, **45**:844–851, 1981.

71. Imai, Y., Abe, K., et al: Management of severe hypertension with nifedipine in combination with clonidine or propranolol. *Drug Res.*, **30**(1):674–678, 1980.

72. Mitchell, H. C., and Pettinger, W. A.: Clonidine and prazosin effects in hypernoradrenergic vasodilator-treated and beta-blocker-treated patients. *Clin. Pharmacol. Ther.*, **30**(3):297–302, 1981.

73. Thananopavarn, C., Golub, M. S., and Sambhi, M. P.: Clonidine in the elderly hypertensive. *Chest*, **2**(Suppl):410–411, 1983.

74. Weber, M. A., Drayer, J. I., and Gray, D. R.: Combined diuretic and sympatholytic therapy in elderly patients with predominant systolic hypertension. *Chest*, **2**(Suppl):416–418, 1983.

75. Wolf, R. L., Ji, C., Craft, R., and Kaplan, M.: The use of clonidine in the treatment of systolic hypertension in the elderly. *Physiologist*, **26**(4)A-101, 1983.

76. Falkner, B., Onesti, G., Lowenthal, D. T., and Affrime, M. B.: The use of clonidine monotherapy in adolescent hypertension. *Chest*, **2**(Suppl):425–427, 1983.

77. Falkner, B., Onesti, G., Affrime, M. B., and Lowenthal, D. T.: Effects of clonidine and hydrochlorothiazide on the cardiovascular response to mental stress in adolescent hypertension. *Clin. Sci.*, **63**(Suppl 8):455s–458s, 1982.

78. Falkner, B., Lowenthal, D. T., and Onesti, G.: Dynamic exercise response in hypertensive adolescent on clonidine therapy: Clonidine therapy in adolescent hypertension. *Pediatr. Pharmacol.*, **1**:121–128, 1980.

79. Ingelfinger, J. R., and Grupe, W. E.: Clonidine for hypertension in children and adolescents. *Pediatr. Res.*, **12**:542, 1973.

80. Julius, S.: Borderline hypertension: An overview. *Med. Clin. North Am.*, **61**(3): 495–511, 1977.

81. Cottier, C., and Julius, S.: Use of clonidine and propranolol as monotherapy in borderline hypertension. *Chest*, **2**(Suppl):422–425, 1983.

82. Lowenthal, D. T., et al: Pharmacokinetics and pharmacodynamics of clonidine in varying states of renal function. *Chest*, 2:386–390, 1983.
83. Morgan, T.: The use of centrally acting antihypertensive drugs in patients with renal disease. *Chest*, 2(Suppl):383–386, 1983.
84. Raftos, J., Bauer, G. E., et al: Clonidine in the treatment of severe hypertension. *Med. J. Aust.*, 1(16):786, 1973.
85. Mroczek, W. J., Davidov, M., and Finnerty, F. A., Jr.: Prolonged treatment with clonidine: Comparative antihypertensive effects alone and with a diuretic agent. *Am. J. Cardiol.*, 30:536–541, 1972.
86. Bhandarkar, S. D., and Vernekar, K. S.: Clonidine as an antihypertensive drug in diabetics. *J. Postgrad, Med.*, 24(3):182–185, 1978.
87. Kramer, D., Krause, W., and Renner, H.: Report on a long-term trial of 2-(2,6-dichlorophenylamino)-2-imidazoline hydrochloride with special consideration of the effect on blood pressure and on carbohydrate metabolism. *Arzneimittel-Forsch*, 20(4):519–521, 1970.
88. Passa, P., Leblanc, H., Gauville, C., Tabuteau, F., and Canivet, J.: Effects of long-term administration of clonidine on growth hormone secretion in hypertensive diabetics. *Diabete & Metabolisme* (Paris), 8:295–298, 1982.
89. Anderson, R. J., Hart, G. R., Crumpler, C. P., Reed, W. G., and Mathews, C. A.: Oral clonidine loading in hypertensive urgencies. *JAMA*, 246(8):848–850, 1981.
90. Cohen, I. M., and Katz, M. A.: Oral clonidine loading for rapid control of hypertension. *Clin. Pharmacol. Ther.*, 24(1):11–15, 1978.
91. Spitalewitz, S., Porush, J. G., and Oguagha, C.: Use of oral clondine for rapid titration of blood pressure in severe hypertension. *Chest*, 2:404–407, 1983.
92. Wilkinson, P. R., and Raftery, E. B.: A comparative trial of clonidine, propranolol and placebo in the treatment of moderate hypertension. *Br. J. Clin. Pharmacol.*, 4:289–294, 1977.
93. Karlberg, B. E., Nilsson, O., and Tolagen, K.: Clonidine in primary hypertension: Effects on blood pressure, plasma renin activity, plasma and urinary aldosterone. *Curr. Ther. Res.*, 21(1):10–20, 1977.
94. Kluyskens, Y., and Snoeck, J.: Comparison of guanabenz and clonidine in hypertensive patients. *Curr. Med. Res. Opin.*, 6(9):638–643, 1980.
95. Distler, A., Kirch, W., and Luth, B.: Antihypertensive effects of guanfacine: A double-blind, crossover trial compared with clonidine. *Br. J. Clin. Pharmacol.*, 10:49S–53S, 1980.
96. Lauro, R., Reda, G., Spallone, L., and Beretta-Anguissola, A.: Hypotensive effect of guanfacine in essential hypertension: A comparison with clonidine. *Br. J. Clin. Pharmacol.*, 10:81S–82S, 1980.
97. Jaattela, A.: Comparison of guanfacine and clonidine as antihypertensive agents. *Br. J. Clin. Pharmacol.*, 10:67S–70S, 1980.
98. Walker, B. R., Hare, L. E., and Deitch. M. W.: Comparative antihypertensive effects of guanabenz and clonidine. *J. Int. Med. Res.*, 10(1):6–14, 1982.
99. Putzeys, M. R., and Hoobler, S. W.: Comparison of clonidine and methyldopa on blood pressure and side effects in hypertensive patients. *Am. Heart J.*, 83:464, 1972.
100. Onesti, G., Schwartz, A. B., Kim, K. E., Paz-Martinez, V., and Swartz, C.: Antihypertensive effect of clonidine. *Circ. Res.*, 28(Suppl 2):53–69, 1971.
101. Conner, C. S., and Watanabe, A. S.: Clonidine overdose: A review. *Am. J. Hosp. Pharm.*, 36:906–911, 1979.

102. Briant, R. H., Reid, J. L., and Dollery, C. T.: Interaction between clonidine and desipramine in man. *Br. Med. J.*, 1:522, 1973.
103. Hui, K. K.: Hypertensive crisis induced by interaction of clonidine with imipramine. *J. Am. Geriatr. Soc.*, 31(3):164–165, 1983.
104. Lilja, M., Jounela, A. J., Juustila, H., and Mattila, M. J.: Interaction of clonidine and beta-blockers. *Acta Med. Scand.*, 207:173–176, 1980.
105. Rosenberg, J. M.: Clonidine and methyldopa. *RN*, 45(11):66–68, 1982.
106. Peters, R. W., Hamilton, B. P., Hamilton, J., Kuzbida, G., and Pavlis, R.: Cardiac arrhythmias after abrupt clonidine withdrawal. *Clin. Pharmacol. Ther.*, 34:435–439, 1983.
107. Houston, M. C.: Abrupt cessation of treatment: Consideration of clinical features, mechanisms, prevention and management of the discontinuation syndrome. *Am. Heart. J.*, 102(3):415–430, 1981.

Methyldopa

1. Anderson, R. J., Reed, G., and Kirk, L. M.: Therapeutic consideration for elderly hypertensives. *Clin. Ther.*, 5:25–38, 1982.
2. Tarazi, R. C.: Should you treat systolic hypertension in elderly patients? *Geriatrics*, 33(11):25–29, 1978.
3. Ramsay, L. E.: The use of methyldopa in the elderly. *J. R. Coll. Physicians*, 15(4):239–244, 1981.
4. Kennedy, R. D.: Drug therapy for cardiovascular disease in the aged. *J. Am. Geriatr. Soc.*, 23(3):113–120, 1975.
5. Gifford, R. W., Jr.: Isolated systolic hypertension in the elderly: Some controversial issues. *JAMA*, 247(6):781–785, 1982.
6. Johnson, P., Kitchin, A. A., et al: Treatment of hypertension with methyldopa. *Br. Med. J.*, 1:133, 1966.
7. Colwill, J. M., Dutton, A. M., Morrissey, J., and Yu, P. N.: Alpha methyldopa and hydrochlorothiazide. *N. Engl. J. Med.*, 271(14):696, 1964.
8. Bradley, W. F., Hoffman, F. G., et al: Comparison of prazosin and methyldopa in mild to moderate hypertension, a multicenter cooperative study. *Curr. Ther. Res.*, 21(1):28, 1977.
9. Rhomberg, F., and Wilder, J.: Guanfacin versus alpha-methyldopa bei benigner essentieller hypertonie. *Schweiz Med. Wschr.*, 111:1967–1968, 1981.
10. Bayliss, R. I. S., and Harvey-Smith, E. A.; Methyldopa in treatment of hypertension. *Lancet*, April:763, 1962.
11. Wilson, W. R., and Okun, R.: Methyldopa and hydrochlorothiazide in primary hypertension. *JAMA*, 185(II):819, 1963.
12. Horwitz, D., and Pettinger, W. A.: Effects of methyldopa in fifty hypertensive patients. *Clin. Pharmacol. Ther.*, 8(2):224, 1967.
13. Smith, W. M., Bachman, B., et al: Cooperative clinical trial of alpha methyldopa. *Ann. Intern. Med.*, 65(4):657, 1966.
14. Dollery, C. T., and Harrington, M.: Methyldopa in hypertension, clinical, and pharmacological studies. *Lancet*, April:759, 1962.
15. Gillespie, L., Oates, J. A., et al: Clinical and chemical studies with alpha methyldopa in patients with hypertension. *Circulation*, 25:181, 1962.
16. McMahon, F. G.: Efficacy of an antihypertensive agent. *JAMA*, 231(2):155, 1975.

17. Kirkendall, W. M., and Wilson, W. R.: Pharmacodynamics and clinical use of guanethidine, bretylium and methyldopa. *Am. J. Cardiol.*, **9**(1):107, 1962.
18. Putzey, M. R., and Hoobler, S. W.: Comparison of clonidine and methyldopa on blood pressure and side effects in hypertensive patients. *Am. Heart J.*, **83**(4):964, 1962.
19. Seedat, Y. K.: Methyldopa in combination with timolol in treatment of hypertension. *Curr. Ther. Res.*, **20**(1):10, 1976.
20. Bradley, W. F., Hoffman, F. G., et al: Comparison of prazosin and methyldopa in mild to moderate hypertension, a multicenter cooperative study. *Curr. Ther. Res.*, **21**(1):28, 1977.
21. Walker, B. R., Shah, R. S., Romanathan, K. B., Vanov, S. K., and Helfant, R. H.: Guanabenz and methyldopa on hypertension and cardiac performance. *Clin. Pharmacol. Ther.*, **22**(6):868–874, 1977.
22. Aronow, W. S., Tobis, J., Hughes, D., Siegel, J., and Easthope, J.: Comparison of trimazosin and methyldopa in hypertension. *Clin. Pharmacol. Ther.*, **22**(4):425–429, 1977.
23. Routledge, P. A., Zrino, L. V., et al: Dose-titrated, double-blind, cross-over comparison of a selective beta-blocker and methyldopa in the treatment of hypertension. *Eur. J. Clin. Pharmacol.*, **11**:159–162, 1977.
24. Okanga, J. B. O.: Atenolol (Tenormin) compared with methyldopa (Aldomet) in treatment of hypertension. *East. Afr. Med. J.*, **55**(9):447–452, 1978.
25. Louis, W. J., Vajda, F. T. E., McNeil, J. J., Doyle, A. E., and Jarrott, B: Combined use of L-alpha-methyldopahydrazine and methyldopa in the treatment of hypertension. *Clin. Exp. Pharmacol. Physiol.*, Suppl. 4:17–22, 1978.
26. Sanders, G. L., Davis, D. M., et al: A comparative study of methyldopa and labetalol in the treatment of hypertension. *Br. J. Clin. Pharmacol.*, **8**:1495–1515, 1979.
27. Rengo, F., Ricciardelli, B., et al: Long term comparative study of guanfacine and alpha-methyldopa in essential hypertension. *Arch. Int. Pharmacodyn.*, **224**:281–291, 1980.
28. Cannon, P. J., Whitlock, R. T., et al: Effect of alpha-methyldopa in severe and malignant hypertension. *JAMA*, **179**(9):673, 1962.
29. Gibb, W. E., Turner, P., et al: Comparison of bethanidine and methyldopa and reserpine in essential hypertension. *Lancet*, **2**(7667):275, 1970.
30. Hefferman, A., Carty, A., et al: A within-patient comparison of debrisoquin and methyldopa in hypertension. *Br. Med. J.*, **1**:75, 1971.
31. Conolly, M., Briant, R. H., et al: A crossover comparison of clonidine and methyldopa in hypertension. *Eur. J. Clin. Pharmacol.*, **4**:222, 1972.
32. Amery, A., Bossaert, H., et al: Clonidine vs methyldopa. *Acta Cardiol.*, **27**:22, 1972.
33. Mroczek, W., Leibel, B. A., and Finnerty, F. A.: Comparison of clonidine and methyldopa in hypertensive patients receiving a diuretic. *Am. J. Cardiol.*, **29**:712, 1972.
34. Petrie, J. C., Galloway, D. B., et al: Methyldopa and propranolol or practolol in moderate hypertension. *Br. Med. J.*, **2**(6028):137, 1976.
35. Vierhapper, H., Dudezak, R., and Waldhausl, W.: Penbutolol: Comparison of its antihypertensive effect with that of alpha-methyldopa in patients with primary hypertension. *Arzneim-Forsch.*, **30**(6):1008–1011, 1980.
36. Klapper, M. S., Richard, L. S., and Smith, G. H.: Methyldopa–chlorothiazide—a long term evaluation. *South. Med. J.*, **63**(1):77, 1970.

37. Goldner, F.: VII Effectiveness among patients treated for seven or more years. *J. Cardiovasc. Pharmacol.*, 3(Suppl. 2):S114–S119, 1981.

38. Brodwall, E. K., Myrhe, E., et al: The effect of methyldopa on renal function in patients with renal insufficiency. *Acta Med. Scand.*, **191**:339, 1972.

39. Luke, R. G., and Kennedy, A. C.: Methyldopa in treatment of hypertension due to chronic renal disease. *Br. Med. J.*, 1:27, 1964.

40. Dranov, J., Skyler, J. S., and Gunnells, J. C.: Malignant hypertension. *Arch. Intern. Med.*, **133**:795, 1974.

41. Noveck, R., McMahon, F. G., and Jain, A. K.: Treatment of elevated blood pressure with a simplified methyldopa–hydrochlorothiazide treatment regimen. *Curr. Ther. Res.*, **32**(6):822–833, 1982.

42. Gould, B. A., Hornung, R. S., Kieso, H. A., Cashman, P. M. M., and Raftery, E. B.: An intraarterial profile of methyldopa. *Clin. Pharmacol. Ther.*, **33**(4):438–444, 1982.

43. Corea, L., Bentivoglio, M., et al: Two low doses of methyldopa in mild to moderate hypertension: A comparative double blind study and a long-term follow-up. *Curr. Ther. Res.*, **34**(1):217–226, 1983.

44. Oates, J. A., Gillespie, L., Udenfriend, S., and Sjoerdsma, A.: Decarboxylase inhibition and blood pressure reduction by 2-methyl-3, 4-dihydroxy-DL-phenylalanine. *Science*, **131**:1890, 1960.

45. Porter, D. C., Torato, J. A., and Leiby, C. M.: Some biochemical effects of alpha-methyl-3, 4-dihydroxyphenylalanine and related compounds in mice. *J. Pharmacol. Exp. Ther.*, **134**:139–145, 1961.

46. Hess, S. M., Connamacher, R. H., et al: The effects of alpha-methyl-dopa and alpha-methyl-meta-tyrosine on the metabolism of norepinephrine and serotonin in vivo. *J. Pharmacol. Exp. Ther.*, **134**:129, 1961.

47. Weissbach, H., Lovenberg, W., and Underfriend, S.: Enzymatic decarboxylation of alphy-methyl amino acids. *Biochem. Biophys. Res. Commun.*, 3:225–227, 1960.

48. Day, M. D., and Rand, M. J.: A hypothesis for the mode of action of alpha-methyldopa in relieving hypertension. *J. Phar. Pharmacol.*, **15**:221–224, 1963.

49. Day, M. D., and Rand, M. J.: Some observations on the pharmacology of alpha-methyldopa. *Br. J. Pharmacol.*, **22**:76–82, 1964.

50. Sugarman, S. R., Margolius, H. S., et al: Effect of methyldopa on chronotropic responses to cardioaccelerator nerve stimulation in dogs. *J. Pharmacol. Exp. Ther.*, **162**:115–120, 1968.

51. Varma, D. R., and Benfey, B. G.: Antagonism of reserpine-induced sensitivity to tyramine by methyldopa. *J. Pharmacol. Exp. Ther.*, **141**:310–313, 1963.

52. Haefely, W., Hurliman, A., and Thoeneu, H.: The effect of stimulation of sympathetic nerves in the cat treated with reserpine, alpha-methyldopa, and alpha-methylmetatyrosine. *Br. J. Pharmacol.*, **26**:172–185, 1966.

53. Finch, L., and Haeusler, G.: Further evidence for a central hypotensive action of alpha-methyldopa in both the rat and cat. *Br. J. Pharmacol.*, **47**:217–228, 1973.

54. van Zwieten, P. A.: Centrally mediated action of alpha-methyldopa. In G. Onesti, M. Fernandes, and E. Kim (Eds.): *Regulation of Blood Pressure by the Central Nervous System.* Grune and Stratton, Inc., New York, 1976, p. 293.

55. Frolich, E. D.: Methyldopa, mechanisms and treatment 25 years later. *Arch. Intern. Med.*, **140**:954–959, 1980.

56. van Zwieten, P. A.: Antihypertensive drugs with central action. *Prog. Pharmacol.*, 1:1–63, 1975.
57. Heise, A., and Kroneberg, G.: Alpha-sympathetic receptor stimulation in the brain and hypotensive activity of alpha-methyldopa. *Eur. J. Pharmacol.*, 17:315–317, 1972.
58. Day, M. D., Roach, A. G., and Whiting, R. L.: The mechanisms of the antihypertensive action of alpha-methyldopa in hypertensive rats. *Eur. J. Pharmacol.*, 21:271–280, 1973.
59. Henning, M.: Studies on the mode of action of alpha-methyldopa. *Acta Physiol, Scand. Suppl.*, 322:1–37, 1969.
60. Mohammed, S., Fasola, A. F., et al: Effect of methyldopa on plasma renin activity in man. *Circ. Res.*, 25:543–548, 1969.
61. Chamberlain, D. A., and Howard, J.: Guanethidine and methyldopa. A hemodynamic study. *Br. Heart J.*, 26:528–536, 1964.
62. Wilson, W. R., Fisher, F. D., and Kirkendall, W. M.: The acute hemodynamic effects of alpha-methyldopa in man. *J. Chronic Dis.*, 15:907–913, 1962.
63. Sannerstedt, R., Vornauskas, E., and Werko, L.: Hemodynamic effects of methyldopa (Aldomet®) at rest and during exercise in patients with renal hypertension. *Acta Med. Scand.*, 171:75–82, 1962.
64. Vincent, W. A., Kashemsant, U., et al: The acute hemodynamic effects of L-alpha-methyldopa. *Am. J. Med. Sci.*, 246:558–568, 1963.
65. Dollery, C. T., Harrington, M., and Hodge, J. V.: Hemodynamic studies with methyldopa: Effects on cardiac output and response to pressor amines. *Br. Heart J.*, 25:670–676, 1963.
66. Onesti, G., Brest, A. N., Novack, P., et al: Pharmacodynamic effects of alpha-methyldopa in hypertensive subjects. *Am. Heart J.*, 67:32–38, 1964.
67. Frolich, E. D., Tarazi, R. C., Dustan, H. P., et al: The paradox of beta-adrenergic blockade in hypertension. *Circulation*, 37:417–423, 1968.
68. Onesti, G., Schwartz, A. B., et al: Pharmacodynamic effects of new antihypertensive drugs, Catapres (ST-155). *Circulation*, 39:219–228, 1969.
69. Lavy, S., Stern, S., Tzivoni, D., and Keren, A.: Effects of methyldopa on regional cerebral blood flow in hypertensive patients. *Isr. J. Med. Sci.*, 16:456–458, 1980.
70. Onesti, G., Martinex, E. W., and Fernandez, M.: Hemodynamic and clinical effects of antihypertensive agents with action on the central nervous system: Alpha-methyldopa and clonidine. *Hahneman International Symposium on Hypertension*, 5:317–350, 1979.
71. Safar, M. E., London, G. M., et al: Effect of alpha-methyldopa on cardiac output in hypertension. *Clin. Pharmacol. Ther.*, 25(3):266–272, 1979.
72. Freis, E. D., Rose, J. C., et al: The hemodynamic effects of hypotensive drugs in man: III. Hexamethonium. *J. Clin. Invest.*, 32:1285–1298, 1953.
73. Richardson, D. W., Wyso, E. M., et al: Circulatory effects of guanethidine: Clinical, renal, and cardiac responses to treatment with a novel antihypertensive drug. *Circulation*, 22:184–190, 1960.
74. Lee, W. R., Fox, L. M., and Slotkoff, L. M.: Effects of antihypertensive therapy on cardiovascular response to exercise. *Am. J. Cardiol.*, 44:325–328, 1979.
75. Benfield, G. F. A., and Hunter, K. R.: Oxprenolol, methyldopa, and lipids in diabetes mellitus. *Br. J. Clin. Pharm.*, 13:219–222, 1982.
76. Ames, R. P., and Hill, P.: Antihypertensive therapy and the risk of coronary heart disease. *J. Cardiovasc. Pharmacol.*, 4(Suppl. 2):S206–S212, 1982.

77. Faud, F. M., Nakashima, Y., Tarazi, R. C., and Salcedo, E. E.: Reversal of left ventricular hypertrophy in hypertensive patients treated with methyldopa. *Am. J. Cardiol.*, **49**:795–801, 1982.
78. Hansten, P. D.: *Drug Interactions*, Lea & Febiger, Philadelphia, 1975, p. 77.
79. Griffin, J. P., and Dorey, P. F.: *Adverse Drug Interactions*, John Wright & Sons, Bristol, 1975, p. 150.
80. White A. G.: Methyldopa and amitriptyline. *Lancet*, **2**:441, 1965.
81. Kaldor, A., et al: Enhancement of methyldopa metabolism with barbiturate. *Br. Med. J.*, **3**:518, 1971.
82. Dollery, C. T.: Physiological and pharmacological interactions of antihypertensive drugs. *Proc. R. Soc. Med.*, **58**:983, 1965.
83. Calne, D. B., and Fermaglich, J.: Gout induced by L-dopa and decarboxylase inhibitors. *Postgrad. Med. J.*, **52**:232, 1976.
84. Vardija, R. A., et al: Galactorrhea and Parkinson-like syndrome: An adverse effect of alpha-methyldopa. *Metabolism*, **19**:1069, 1970.
85. Peaston, M. J. T.: Parkinsonism associated with alpha methyldopa therapy. *Br. Med. J.*, **2**:168, 1964.
86. Sweet, R. D., et al: Methyldopa as an adjunct to levodopa treatment of Parkinson's disease. *Clin. Pharmacol. Ther.*, **13**:23, 1972.
87. Glazer, N.: Comparison of guanethidine and methyldopa in essential hypertension—a controlled study. *Curr. Ther. Res.*, **17**(3):249, 1975.
88. Yajnik, V. H., and Patel, S. C.: Double blind evaluation of indoramin and methyldopa in thiazide treated hypertensive patients. *Indian Heart J.*, **30**(1):51–56, 1978.
89. Webster, J., Jeffers, T. A., Galloway, D. B., Petrie, J. C., and Barker, N. P.: Atenolol, methyldopa, and chlorthalidone in moderate hypertension. *Br. Med. J.*, **1**:76–78, 1977.
90. Wilson, C., Scott, M. E., and Abdel-Mohsen, A.: Atenolol and methyldopa in the treatment of hypertension. *Postgrad. Med. J.*, **53**(Suppl 3):123–127, 1977.
91. Hansen, M., Hansen, O. P., and Lindholm, J.: Controlled clinical study on antihypertensive treatment with a diuretic and methyldopa compared with a beta-blocking agent and hydralazine. *Acta Med. Scand.*, **202**:385–388, 1977.
92. Van Der Merwe, C. J., and Kruger, S. A.: The antihypertensive effect of guanfacine compared with methyldopa. *S. Afr. Med. J.*, **57**:400–404, 1980.
93. Kristensen, B. O., Brons, M., et al: Antihypertensive effect of atenolol (100 mg once a day) and methyldopa (250 mg thrice a day). *Acta Med. Scand.*, **209**:267–270, 1981.
94. Van Rossum, J. M.: Potential dangers of monoamine oxidase inhibitors and alpha methyldopa. *Lancet*, **1**:950, 1963.
95. Paykel, E. S.: Hallucinosis on combined methyldopa + pargyline. *Br. Med. J.*, **1**: 805, 1966.
96. Westervelt, F. B., and Atuk, N. O.: Methyldopa induced hypertension. *JAMA*, **227** (5):557, 1974.
97. Nies, A. S.: Adverse reactions and interactions limiting the use of antihypertensive drugs. *Am. J. Med.*, **58**:493, 1975.
98. O'Regan, J. B.: Adverse interaction of lithium carbonate and methyldopa. *Can. Med. Assoc. J.*, **115**:385, 1976.
99. *Med. Lett. Drugs Ther.*, **19**:24, 1977.
100. Osanloo, E., and Deglin, J. H.: Interaction of lithium and methyldopa. *Ann. Intern. Med.*, **92**(3):433–434, 1980.

101. Redman, C. W. G.: Treatment of hypertension in pregnancy. *Kidney, Int.*, **18**:267–278, 1980.

102. Redman, C. W. G., Beilin, L. J., and Bonnar, J.: Treatment of hypertension in pregnancy with methyldopa: Blood pressure control and side effects. *Br. J. Obstet. Gynecol.*, **84**:419–426, 1977.

103. Kwan, K. C., Foltz, E. L., Breault, G. O., Baer, J. E., and Totaro, J. A.: Pharmocokinetics of methyldopa in man. *J. Pharmacol. Exp. Ther.*, **198**:264–277, 1976.

104. Barrett, A. J., Bobik, A., Carson, V., Korman, J. S., and McLean, A. J.: Pharmocokinetics of methyldopa, plasma levels following single intravenous, oral and multiple oral dosage in normotensive subjects. *Clin. Exp. Pharmacol. Physiol.*, **4**:331–339, 1977.

105. Saaverdaa, J. A., Reid, J. L., Jordan, W., Rawlins, M. D., and Dollery, C. T.: Plasma concentration of alpha-methyldopa and sulfate conjugate after oral administration of methyldopa hydrochloride ethyl ester. *Eur. J. Clin. Pharmacol.*, **8**: 381–386, 1975.

106. Frewin, D. B., and Penhall, R. K.: Rebound hypertension after sudden discontinuation of methyldopa therapy. *Med. J. Aust.*, **1**:659, 1977.

107. Goldberg, A. D., and Raftery, E. B.: Blood pressure and heart rate in withdrawal of antihypertensive drugs. *Br. Med. J.*, **1**(6071):1243, 1977.

108. Burden, A. C., and Alexander, C. P. T.: Rebound hypertension after acute methyldopa withdrawal. *Br. Med. J.*, **1**(6028):1056, 1976.

109. Scott, J. M., and McDevit, D. G.: Rebound hypertension after acute methyldopa withdrawal. *Br. Med. J.*, **2**(6031):367, 1976.

110. Au, W. Y. W., Drins, L. G., et al: The metabolism of ^{14}C-labelled alpha-methyldopa in normal and hypertensive human subjects. *Biochem. J.*, **129**: 1, 1972.

111. Vejlsgaard, V., Christensen, M., and Clausen, E.: Double blind trial of four hypotensive drugs: Methyldopa and three sympatholytic agents. *Br. Med. J.*, **2**:598, 1967.

112. Iverson, B. M., Nordahl, E., et al: Retroperitoneal fibrosis during treatment with methyldopa. *Lancet*, **2**:302, 1975.

113. Weisenburger, D. D.: Immunoblastic lymphadenopathy associated with methyldopa therapy. *Cancer*, **42**:2322–2327, 1978.

114. Holt, P. J. A., and Navaratham, A.: Lichenoid eruption due to methyldopa. *Br. Med. J.*, **3**:234, 1974.

115. Stevenson, C. J.: Lichenol eruptions due to methyldopa. *Br. J. Dermatol.*, **85** (6): 600, 1971.

116. Church, R.: Eczema provoked by methyldopa. *Br. J. Dermatol.*, **91**:373, 1974.

117. Mackie, B. S.: Drug induced ulcer of the lip. *Br. J. Dermatol.*, **91**:962, 1974.

118. Wells, J. D., Kurtay, M., Lochner, J. C., and George, W. L.: Granulomatous skin lesions and alpha methyldopa. *Ann. Intern. Med.*, **81**:701, 1974.

119. Almeyda, J., and Levantine, A.: Cutaneous reactions to cardiovascular drugs. *Br. J. Dermatol.*, **88**:313, 1973.

120. Burry, J. N., and Kirk, J.: Lichenoid drug reactions from methyldopa. *Br. J. Dermatol.*, **91**:475, 1974.

121. Mullick, F. G., and McAllister, H. A.: Myocarditis associated with methyldopa therapy. *JAMA*, **237**(16):1699, 1977.

122. Burden, A. C., and Alexander, C. P. T.: Rebound hypertension after acute methyldopa withdrawal. *Br. Med. J.*, **1**:1056, 1976.

123. Scott, J. N., and McDevitt, D. G.: Rebound hypertension after acute methyldopa withdrawal. *Br. Med. J.*, **2**:367, 1976.

124. Mardh, P. A.: Belfrange, I., and Naversten, E.: Sialadenitis following treatment with alpha-methyldopa. *Acta Med. Scand.*,**195**:333, 1974.

125. Murphy, K. J.: Bilateral renal calculi in patients receiving methyldopa. *Med. J. Aust.*, **2**:20, 1976.

126. Vaidya, R. A., Vaidya, A. B., Van Woert, M. H., and Kase, N. G.: Galactorrhea and Parkinson-like syndrome: An adverse effect of a methyldopa. *Metabolism*, **19**(12): 1068, 1970.

127. Ghosh, S. K.: Methyldopa and forgetfulness. *Lancet*, **1**(7952):202, 1976.

128. Fernandez, P. G.: Alpha-methyldopa and forgetfulness. *Ann. Intern. Med.*, **88** (1):128, 1976.

129. Adler, S.: Methyldopa induced decrease in mental activity. *J. Am. Med. Assoc.*, **230**(10):1428, 1974.

130. Becker-Christensen, F., Bang, H. O., and Ditzel, J.: Treatment of severe hypertension with Catapres. *Acta Med. Scand.*, **190**:21, 1976.

131. Amery, A., Verstraete, M., et al: Hypotensive action and side effects of clonidine-chlorthalidone and methyldopa-chlorthalidone in treatment of hypertension. *Br. Med. J.*, **4**:392, 1970.

132. Prichard, B. N. C., Jonston, A. W., et al: Bethanidine, guanethidine and methyldopa in treatment of hypertension: A within patient comparison. *Br. Med. J.*, **1**(5585):135, 1968.

133. Oates, J.A., Seligmann, A. W., et al: The relative efficacy of guanethidine, methyldopa and pargyline as antihypertensive agents. *N. Engl. J. Med.*, **273** (14): 729, 1965.

134. Schnaper, H. W., and Collins, M. A.: An assessment of adverse effects of methyldopa and propranolol. *J. Med. Assoc. State of Ala.*, Oct.:35–43, 1979.

135. Carr, A. A., Mulligan, O. F., and Sherrill, L. N.: Pindolol versus methyldopa for hypertension: Comparison of adverse reactions. *Am. Heart J.*, **104**:479–481, 1982.

136. Van Der Heide, H., Ten Haaft, M. A., and Stricker, B. H.: Pancreatitis caused by methyldopa. *Br. Med. J.*, **282**:1930–1931, 1981.

137. Cokkinos, D. V., and Vorides, E. M.: Impairment of atrioventricular conduction by methyldopa. *Chest*, **74**:697, 1978.

138. Scheinman. M. M., Strauss, H. C., et al: Adverse effects of sympatholytic agents in patients with hypertension and sinus node dysfunction. *Am. J. Med.*, **64**: 1013–1020, 1978.

139. Carstairs, K., Worlledge, S., Dollery, C. T., and Breckenridge, A.: Methyldopa and hemolytic anemia. *Lancet*, **2**:201, 1966.

140. Carstairs, K., Breckenridge, A., Dollery, C. T., and Worlledge, S.: Incidence of a positive direct Coombs' test in patients on alpha-methyldopa. *Lancet*, **2**:133, 1966.

141. Hope, J. G., and Provan, G. C.: Hematological effects of alpha-methyldopa. *Scott. Med. J.*, **12**:229, 1967.

142. Spence, J. M., and Gitlin, N.: Alpha methyldopa and hemolytic anemia. *South Afr. Med. J.*, **47**:195, 1973.

143. Beutler, E.: Drug induced anemia. *Fed. Proc.*, **31**:141, 1972.

144. Pisciotta, A. V.: Idiosyncratic hematologic reactions to drugs. *Postgrad. Med.*, **55**: 105, 1974.

145. Kirtland, H. H., Mohler, D. N., and Horwitz, D. A.: Methyldopa inhibition of suppressor—lymphocyte function. *N. Engl. J. Med.*, **302**(15):825–832, 1980.
146. Harth, M.: L. E. cells and positive direct Coombs' test induced by methyldopa. *Can. Med. Assoc. J.*, **99**:277, 1968.
147. Lundh, B., and Hasselgren, K. H.: Hematological side effects from antihypertensive drugs. *Acta Med. Scand.*, **628**:73–76, 1978.
148. Grell, G. A. C., Wilson, W. A., and James, O.: Prevalence of drug induced immunologic changes in hypertensive Jamaicans. *South. Med. J.*, **73**(8):1044–1045, 1980.
149. Lobell, M., and Woodburn, R.: Drug induced hemolytic anemia. *Minn. Med.*, **58**: 239, 1975.
150. Bottinger, L. E., and Wester-Holm, B.: Drug induced blood dyscrasias in Sweden. *Br. Med. J.*, 3:339, 1973.
151. Wortledge, S., Carstairs, K. C., and Dacie, J. V.: Autoimmune hemolytic anemia associated with alpha-methyldopa therapy. *Lancet*, **2**:135, 1966.
152. Adverse effects of methyldopa. *Med. Lett. Drugs Ther.*, **10**:22, 1968.
153. Lalezari, P., Louis, J. E., and Fadlallah, N.: Serologic profile of alpha-methyldopa induced hemolytic anemia: Correlation between cell-bound IgM and hemolysis. *Blood*, **59**(1):68, 1982.
154. Murad, F.: Immunohemolytic anemia during therapy with methyldopa. *J. Am. Med. Assoc.*, **203**:149, 1968.
155. Ewing, D. J., and Hughes, C. J.: Methyldopa-induced autoimmune hemolytic anemia: A report of two further cases. *Guys Hosp. Rep.*, **17**:111, 1968.
156. Marcus, G. J., Stevenson, M., and Brown, T.: Alpha methyldopa induced immune thrombocytopenia. *Am. J. Clin. Pathol.*, **64**:113, 1975.
157. Manohitharajah, S. M., Jenkins, W. J., Roberts, P. R., and Clarke, R. C.: Methyldopa and associated thrombocytopenia. *Br. Med. J.*, 1:474, 1971.
158. Clark, K. G. A.: Haemolysis and agranulocytosis complicating treatment with methyldopa. *Br. Med. J.*, 4:94, 1967.
159. Sherman, J. D., Love, D. E., and Harrington, J. F.: Anemia, positive lupus and rheumatical factors with methyldopa. *Arch. Intern. Med.*, **120**:321, 1967.
160. Perry, H. M., Chaplin, H., Carmody, S., Haynes, C., and Frei, C.: Immunologic findings in patients receiving methyldopa: A prospective study. *J. Lab. Clin. Med.*, **78**(6):905, 1971.
161. Wilson, J. D., Bullock, J. Y., Sutherland, D. C., Main, C., and O'Brein, K. D.: Antinuclear antibodies in patients receiving non-practolol beta-blockers. *Br. Med. J.*, 1: 14–16, 1978.
162. Dupont, A., and Six, R.: Lupus-like syndrome induced by methyldopa. *Br. Med. J.*, **285**:693–694, 1982.
163. Harrington, T. M., and Davis, D. E.: Systemic lupus-like syndrome induced by methyldopa therapy. *Chest*, **79**:696–697, 1981.
164. Harpey, J. P.: Lupus-like syndromes induced by drugs. *Ann. Allergy*, **33**:256, 1974.
165. Houston, M. C.: Abrupt cessation of treatment in hypertension: Consideration of clinical features, mechanisms, prevention and management of the discontinuation syndrome. *Am. Heart. J.*, **102**(3):415–430, 1981.
166. Tysell, J. E., and Knaver, C. M.: Hepatitis induced by methyldopa (Aldomet). *Am. J. Dig. Dis.*, **16**(9):849, 1971.
167. Hoyumpa, A. M., and Connell, A. M.: Methyldopa hepatitis. *Am. J. Dig. Dis.*, **18** (3):213, 1973.

168. Seggie, J., and Saunders, S. J.: Patterns of hepatic injury induced by methyldopa. *S. Afr. Med. J.*, **55**:75–83, 1979.
169. Arranto, A. J., and Sotaniemi, E. A.: Morphologic alterations in patients with alpha-methyldopa-induced liver disease after short- and long-term exposure. *Scand. J. Gastroenterol.*, **16**:853–863, 1981.
170. Toghill, P. J., Smith, P. G., Benton, P., Brown, R. C., and Matthews, H. L.: Methyldopa liver damage. *Br. Med. J.*, **3**:545, 1974.
171. Miller, A. C., and Reid, W. M.: Methyldopa induced granulomatous hepatitis. *JAMA*, **235**(18):2001, 1976.
172. Goldstein, G. B., Lam, K. C., and Mistilis, S. P.: Drug induced active chronic hepatitis. *Am. J. Dig. Dis.*, **18**(3):177, 1973.
173. Thomas, E., Bhuta, S., and Rosenthal, W. S.: Methyldopa induced liver injury. *Arch. Pathol. Lab. Med.*, **100**:132, 1976.
174. Rodman, J. S., Deutsch, D. J., and Gutman, S. I.: Methyldopa hepatitis. *Am. J. Med.*, **60**:941, 1976.
175. Rehman, O. V., Keith, T. A., and Gall, E. A.: Methyldopa induced submassive hepatic necrosis. *JAMA*, **224**(10):1390, 1973.
176. Elkington, S. G., Schreiber, W. B., and Conn, H. O.: Hepatic injury caused by alpha-methyldopa. *Circulation*, **40**(4):589, 1969.
177. Brouillard, R. P., and Barrett, O.: Methyldopa associated hepatitis. *JAMA*, **224**(6): 904, 1973.
178. Klein, H. O., and Kaminsky, N.: Methyldopa fever. *N. Y. State J. Med.*, **73**:448, 1973.
179. Glontz, G. E., and Saslaw, S.: Methyldopa fever. *Arch. Intern. Med.*, **122**:445, 1968.
180. Miller, J. P.: Febrile reaction to methyldopa with hepatotoxicity. *V. A. Med. Mon.*, **97**:159, 1970.
181. Mohammed, S., Hanenson, I. B., et al: The effects of alpha methyldopa on renal function in hypertensive patients. *Am. Heart J.*, **76**:21, 1968.
182. Stenbeck, O., Myhre, E. K., et al: Hypotensive effect of methyldopa in renal failure associated with hypertension. *Acta Med. Scand.*, **191**:333, 1971.

Guanabenz

1. Baum, T., and Shopshire, A. T.: Inhibition of spontaneous nerve activity by the antihypertensive agent (Wy-8687). *J. Pharmacol. Exp. Ther.*, **9**:503–506, 1970.
2. Baum, T., et al: General pharmacologic actions of the antihypertensive agent, 2,6-dichlorobenzylidene aminoguanidiol acetate (Wy-8687). *J. Pharmacol. Exp. Ther.*, **171**(2):276–287, 1970.
3. Walker, B. R., Shah, R. S., Ramanathan, K. B., Vanov, S. K., and Helfant, R. H.: Guanabenz and methyldopa on hypertension and cardiac performance. *Clin. Pharmacol. Ther.*, **22**(6):868–874, 1977.
4. McMahon, F. G., Cole, P. A., Boyles, P. W., and Vanov, S. K.: Study of a new antihypertensive (guanabenz). *Curr. Ther. Res.*, **16**(5):389–397, 1974.
5. Bosanac, P. B., Dubb, J., Walker, B., Goldberg, M., and Agus, Z. S.: Renal effects of guanabenz: A new antihypertensive. *J. Clin. Pharmacol.*, **16**:631–636, 1976.
6. Walker, B. R., Hare, L. E., and Deitch, M. W.: Comparative anti-hypertensive effects of guanabenz and clonidine. *J. Int. Med. Res.*, **10**(6):6–14, 1982.

7. Walker, B. R., Hare, L. E., Deitch, M. W., and Gold, J. A.: Comparative effects of guanabenz alone and in combination with hydrochlorothiazide as initial antihypertensive therapy. *Curr. Ther. Res.*, **31**(5):764–775, 1982.

8. Walker, B. R., Deitch, M. W., Gold, J. A., and Levy, B. A.: Evaluation of guanabenz added to hydrochlorothiazide therapy in hypertension. *J. Int. Med. Res.*, **10**:131, 1982.

9. McMahon, F. G., Ryan, J. R., Jain, A. K., Vargas, R., and Vanov, S. K.: Guanabenz in essential hypertension. *Clin. Pharmacol. Ther.*, **21**(3):272–277, 1977.

10. Shah, R. S., Walker, B. R., Vanov, S. K., and Helfant, R. H.: Guanabenz effects on blood pressure and noninvasive parameters of cardiac performance in patients with hypertension. *Clin. Pharmacol. Ther.*, **19**(6):732–737, 1976.

11. Walker, B. R., Schneider, B. E., and Gold, J. A.: A two-year evaluation of guanabenz in the treatment of hypertension. *Curr. Ther. Res.*, **27**(6):784–795, 1980.

12. Walker, B. R., Schneider, B. E., Rudnick, M. R., and Gold, J. A.: Effects of placebo versus guanabenz on hypertensive outpatients. *J. Int. Med. Res.*, **8**:303–313, 1980.

13. Kluyskens, Y., and Snoeck, J.: Comparison of guanabenz and clonidine in hypertensive patients. *Curr. Med. Res. Opin.*, **6**(9):638–642, 1980.

14. Hirvonen, P., Porsti, P., and Frick, M. H.: A comparison of guanabenz and methyldopa in hypertension. *Curr. Ther. Res.*, **27**(2):197–204, 1980.

15. Walker, B. R., Deitch, M. W., Schneider, B. E., and Hare, L. E.: Comparative antihypertensive effects of guanabenz and methyldopa. *Clin. Ther.*, **4**(4):275–283, 1981.

16. Walker, B. R., Deitch, M. W., Littman, G. S., and Gold, J. A.: Single versus twice a day dosage of guanabenz in hypertension therapy. *Clin. Res.*, **29**:834A, 1981.

17. Baum, T., and Shropshire, A. T.: Studies on the centrally mediated hypotensive activity of guanabenz. *Eur. J. Pharmacol.*, **37**:31–44, 1976.

18. Misu, Y., Fujie, K., and Kubo, T.: Presynaptic dual inhibitory actions of guanabenz on adrenergic transmission. *Eur. J. Pharmacol.*, **77**:177–181, 1982.

19. Warren, S. E., O'Connor, D. T., Cohen, I. M., and Mitas, J. A.: Renal hemodynamic changes during long-term antihypertensive therapy. *Clin. Pharmacol. Ther.*, **29**(3):310–317, 1981.

20. Strandhoy, J. W., Steg, B. R., and Buckalew, V. M.: Antagonism of the hydrosmotic effect of vasopressin by the antihypertensive, guanabenz. *Life Sci.*, **27**:2513–2518, 1980.

21. Hosotani, T., and Misu, Y.: Sodium sensitive active transport of bretylium into adrenergic neurons for the development of blockade in rabbit ileum. *Arch. Intern. Pharmacodyn.*, **226**:235, 1977.

22. Rosendorff, C.: Guanabenz versus methyldopa in the therapy of mild to moderate hypertension. *S. Afr. Med. J.*, **62**:435–437, 1982.

23. Ram, C. V. S., Holland, O. B., Fairchild, C., and Gomez-Sanchez, C. E.: Withdrawal syndrome following cessation of guanabenz therapy. *J. Clin. Pharmacol.*, **19**:148–150, 1979.

CHAPTER VII

BETA-ADRENERGIC BLOCKING DRUGS AND ALPHA-BETA BLOCKERS

- ATENOLOL (TENORMIN®)
- METOPROLOL (LOPRESSOR®)
- NADOLOL (CORGARD®)
- PINDOLOL (VISKEN®)
- PROPRANOLOL (INDERAL®)
- TIMOLOL (BLOCADREN®)

- LABETALOL (NORMODYNE®)

INTRODUCTORY YEAR: 1964 (in U. K.)
Vs. Hypertension: 1976 (in U. S. A.)

INTRODUCTION:

The single most important development in cardiovascular therapeutics in the past 15 years has been the beta-adrenergic blocking drugs.

The single most important development in cardiovascular therapeutics in the past 15 years has been the beta-adrenergic blocking drugs. They reduce cardiac output and therefore hypertension; they slow the heart rate and therefore are useful in the management of several tachyarrhythmias; they prevent recurrent myocardial infarction; they reduce cardiac work and myocardial oxygen consumption and so benefit anginal patients; they may decrease myocardial infarction size; and they may even prevent some instances of primary myocardial infarction.

Beta-blocking agents were first noted by Pritchard and Gillman in 1964 to decrease the blood pressure of hypertensive patients.[1] Propranolol, the prototype, was the first beta-blocking drug to be approved and widely used in the United States. Five additional beta-blockers are now available, including atenolol, metoprolol, nadolol, pindolol and timolol (Figure 1). Today, they assume a paramount role in the treatment of hypertension and a variety of other cardiovascular diseases (see Table I).

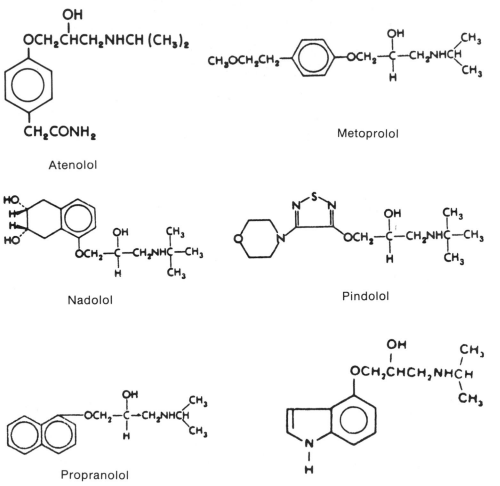

Figure 1: Structural formulas of the U. S. approved beta-blockers.

TABLE I
INDICATIONS FOR APPROVED BETA-BLOCKERS

	Atenolol	Metoprolol	Nadolol	Pindolol	Propranolol†	Timolol
Arrhythmias	*	*	*	*	X	*
Angina Pectoris	*	*	X	*	X	*
Prevention of recurrence of myocardial infarction	*	*	*	*	X	X
Hypertension	X	X	X	X	X	X

* Although current data do not permit verification, it is likely that each of the six U. S. approved beta-blocking agents is effective in the treatment of arrhythmias and angina pectoris and probably in the prevention of recurrence of myocardial infarction.
† Also indicated for prophylaxis of migraine, treatment of hypertrophic subaortic stenosis and, after alpha-blockers have been begun, as adjunctive treatment of pheochromocytoma.

1. As sole initial therapy, in "hyperkinetic" hypertension. These are chiefly younger white patients, in whom norepinephrine levels are often elevated as are heart rate and cardiac output.

Not infrequently in very early essential hypertension and particularly in so-called labile hypertension, the elevated blood pressure is actually due to increased cardiac output with an associated elevation in norepinephrine levels.[2-4] These patients are frequently young and often complain of palpitations and have rapid heart rates; their hearts are over-active or "hyperkinetic." Beta-blockers are usually ideal therapy in these individuals because their cardiac beta-1 blocking activity slows the heart and reduces the forcefulness of contractions. Thus, beta-blockers rest "hyperkinetic" hearts while also lowering blood pressure.[5,6]

Some racial trends exist among hypertensives with respect to drug responsiveness. Data recently provided by a Veterans Administration Cooperative Study Group indicate that as monotherapy for hypertension, 62% of whites achieved normal blood pressures within ten weeks on beta blockers vs. 53% of blacks. Thiazides were substantially more effective in blacks (71 vs. 55%).[7] (See Table II.) In spite of this, it should be stressed that beta-blockers can be considered as an alternative to thiazides in black patients, and numerous studies have indeed demonstrated the successful use of beta-blockers in black populations.

While thiazide diuretics are most often preferred for initial therapy of hypertension, some clinicians prefer beta-blockers on the basis that while both offer essentially equal blood pressure control, beta-blockers produce fewer subtle biochemical abnormalities (rise in cholesterol, triglycerides, glucose and uric acid) which, in the long haul, might vitiate the benefit produced by lowering blood pressue. However, beta-blockers also raise triglycerides and reduce HDL-cholesterol, factors also worth pondering when launching long-term therapy. The U. S. Joint National Committee on Detection, Evaluation, and Treatment of High Blood Pressure recommended (1980) thiazide-diuretics as initial treatment because *they cost less, they offer greater ease of dosage titration, and they produce few subjective symptoms.*[8] When choosing a drug for initial therapy, the individual patient profile and potential adverse drug effects should be carefully evaluated. Again, beta-blockers should be considered as an alternative to thiazide-diuretics, especially in younger white patients with tachycardia and with recent onset of hypertension.

Beta-Adrenergic and Alpha-Beta Blockers • 281

TABLE II
RESULTS OF VETERANS ADMINISTRATION:
PROPRANOLOL VS. HYDROCHLOROTHIAZIDE IN MONOTHERAPY††
(The decrease in blood pressure in mm Hg†)

	Phase A 10-Week Titration Period		Phase B 12-Month Chronic Therapy Period	
	Prop.	HCTZ	Prop.	HCTZ
All patients	10/11*	18/12*	8/11	8/13
White	13/13	15/11	11/12	15/12
Black	8/10*	20/13*	6/11*	20/14*
% Achieving Goal Blood Pressure**				
All patients	57	64	—	—
White	62	55	—	—
Black	53*	71*	—	—
% Maintaining Goal Blood Pressure**				
All patients	—	—	53*	66*
White	—	—	52	61
Black	—	—	55*	70*
% Requiring Additional Dosage Titration				
All patients	—	—	38*	21*
White	—	—	30*	5*
Black	—	—	35*	14*

Abbreviations: Prop. = propranolol; HCTZ = hydrochlorothiazide.
 * Statistically significant.
 ** Diastolic less than 90 mm Hg.
 † As measured from pre-titration levels.
 †† Data from Veterans Administration Cooperation Study Group on Antihypertensive Agents,[7] reprinted with permission.

2. In addition to thiazides, when the latter fail to provide sufficient blood pressure reduction.

When thiazide diuretics fail to reduce blood pressure adequately (pressure less than 140/90 mm Hg for most adults), usually a second drug needs to be added. Today, beta-blockers are the class of drugs most often selected by clinicians for combination with thiazides.[9] This drug combination is highly effective in lowering blood pressure with approximately 85% of hypertensive patients expected to achieve goal blood pressure on this drug combination.[10]

3. As a part of "triple therapy" with a vasodilator and a thiazide diuretic.

"Triple therapy," consisting of a vasodilator together with a thiazide diuretic and a beta-blocker, is often employed in patients with moderate or severe hypertension and/or in patients refractory to Step-2 therapy.[11,12] This combination is extremely effective and the rationale for its employment is attractive:

- Virtually all hypertensive patients have increased peripheral vascular resistance as their fundamental hemodynamic abnormality in their hypertension.
- Therefore, specific therapy should involve a vasodilator drug.
- The two chief problems with vasodilators are:
    1) Reflex tachycardia with possible precipitation or aggravation of angina pectoris—but this can be offset by the co-administration of a beta-blocker; and
    2) Edema—but this can be controlled by the co-administration of a diuretic.

4. In hyperreninemic hypertension, e.g., malignant or accelerated hypertension and in renovascular hypertension (when inoperable).

Malignant or accelerated hypertensive states are generally characterized biochemically by hyperreninemia and secondary hyperaldosteronism. The administration of beta-blockers clearly reduces plasma renin and aldosterone levels in these patients, thereby correcting their abnormal physiology while also lowering blood pressure.[13] It should be pointed out, however, that reduction of blood pressure remains the primary therapeutic objective and that the addition of other drugs may be necessary for adequate control. In the majority of hypertensive clinics, the oral management of patients with malignant hypertension consists of multiple drug therapy, i.e., a vasodilator such as hydralazine, together with a thiazide diuretic and a beta-blocker. A more potent drug regimen, although associated with a higher incidence of side effects, consists of the addition of either clonidine or methyldopa to the "triple therapy" regimen or the use of minoxidil as the vasodilator.

5. *In hypertensives who have a second disease for which beta-blockers are also effective, e.g., ischemic heart disease, tachyarrhythmias or previous myocardial infarction.*

The employment of beta-blockers in such patients may prove to be doubly beneficial as the dual therapeutic action may eliminate the need for multiple drug therapy and reduce the risk of side effects and adverse drug interactions.

Timolol has been shown to reduce the mortality and incidence of reinfarction in patients surviving a first myocardial infarction.[14] Propranolol also appears to have the same benefit.[15] Some authorities feel that all beta-blocking drugs probably possess this protective effect. Owing to their cardioprotective properties (their reduction in heart rate and blood pressure during exercise has a salutory effect on myocardial oxygen consumption), it is possible that beta-blockers *may also reduce the risk of a first myocardial infarction* and given early with the acute infarction, *they may reduce infarct size.* Therefore, beta-blockers should be strongly considered in hypertensive patients with a history of myocardial infarction or in patients with symptoms of ischemic heart disease. An additional benefit of beta-blockers in ischemic heart disease is that they are important components in the treatment of angina pectoris.

Beta-blockers are also useful in the management of certain arrhythmias, hypertrophic subaortic stenosis, migraine headaches, and pheochromocytoma (see Indications for Beta-blockers). Again, beta-blockers should be strongly considered in hypertensives who also have one of the aforementioned diseases.

Beta-blockers are effective as initial monotherapy for essential hypertension. The question is how does their effectiveness compare with that of thiazide diuretics, the drugs most often used in initial therapy? The Veterans Administration Cooperative Study Group compared propranolol and hydrochlorothiazide for monotherapy in the treatment of mild to moderate essential hypertension in a multi-center, double-blind, controlled clinical trial.[7] (See Table II.) Observations were made over a short-term titration period of ten weeks, and then over a long-term chronic therapy period of twelve months.

In the short-term titration phase, 683 male subjects (with diastolic pressures ranging from 94 to 115 mm Hg) were randomly allocated either propranolol or hydrochlorothiazide. Doses were titrated upward over the ten-week period until goal blood pressure (diastolic, less than

90 mm Hg) was achieved. Propranolol doses were adjusted from a low of 40 mg twice daily, to 80, 160 and 320 mg twice daily and hydrochlorothiazide doses were adjusted from a low of 25 mg twice daily to 50 and 100 mg twice daily. The following results were obtained:

— Both drugs effectively lowered systolic and diastolic pressure;
— In the total study population, hydrochlorothiazide was more effective than propranolol in lowering blood pressure;
— In white patients, no statistically significant differences were found between the two drugs with respect to lowering of systolic or diastolic pressure or percentage of patients achieving goal blood pressure;
— In black patients, hydrochlorothiazide, as compared to propranolol, resulted in significantly greater reductions in systolic and diastolic pressure, and in a significantly greater percentage of patients achieving goal blood pressure.

The chronic treatment phase involved 394 patients whose diastolic pressure was stabilized at less than 90 mm Hg in the acute titration phase. Additional titration was allowed over the 12-month period if diastolic pressure rose above 90 or problematic side effects occurred. The following results were obtained (see Table II):

— In the total study population, hydrochlorothiazide was more effective than propranolol in maintaining patients at goal blood pressure.
— In white patients, no statistically significant differences were found between the two drugs with respect to lowering of systolic or diastolic blood pressure or percentage of patients maintained at goal blood pressure.
— In black patients, hydrochlorothiazide, as compared to propranolol, resulted in significantly greater reductions in systolic and diastolic blood pressure and in a significantly greater percentage of patients maintained at goal blood pressure.
— In both whites and blacks, a significantly greater percentage of patients required additional titration for maintenance of goal blood pressure with propranolol than with hydrochlorothiazide.

The study indicates that propranolol is generally as effective as hydrochlorothiazide in whites, but that the latter is substantially more effective in blacks. In both whites and blacks, dosage titration was required more often with propranolol than with hydrochlorothiazide.

Formulations and Dosages for Beta-Blockers Approved in U. S.

Beta-Blocker	Formulations	Dosages
Atenolol (TENORMIN®)	Tablets...50 and 100 mg	Frequency: once daily Initial: 50 mg once daily Range: 25–100 mg/day Usual dose: 50 mg/day
Betaxolol		Not available yet in U. S. Usual dose: 10–20 mg once daily
Metoprolol	Tablets...50 and 100 mg	Frequency: usually given twice daily, but once-to-three times daily therapy may be satisfactory or required Initial: 50 mg twice daily Range: 100–450 mg/day Usual dose: 200 mg once daily or 100 mg twice daily
Nadolol (CORGARD®)	Tablets...40, 80, 120, and 160 mg	Frequency: once daily Initial: 40 mg once daily Range: 40–640 mg/day Usual dose: 80–480 mg once daily
Pindolol VISKEN®)	Tablets...5 and 10 mg	Frequency: twice daily Initial: 10 mg twice daily is recommended, but many patients will respond to 5 mg three times daily Range: 15–60 mg/day Usual dose: 20 mg/day
Propranolol (INDERAL®)	Tablets...10, 20, 40, 60, 80 mg Injectable...1 mg/ml ampule for IV usage reserved for life-threatening arrhythmias or those occurring under anesthesia	Frequency: usually given twice daily, but three times daily therapy may be required for adequate control Initial: 40 mg twice daily Range: 80–640 mg/day Usual dose: 80–240 mg/day
Long acting Propranolol* (INDERAL® LA)	Capsules...80, 120, 160 mg	Frequency: once daily Initial: 80 mg once daily Range: 80–640 mg/day Usual dose: 80–160 mg/day
Timolol (BLOCADREN®)	Tablets...10 and 20 mg	Frequency: twice daily Initial: 10 mg twice daily Range: 20–60 mg/day Usual dose: 10–20 mg twice daily

- Dosages must be titrated individually. Since there is wide variation in levels of sympathetic activity, it should not be assumed that beta-blocking activity directly correlates with dosage or plasma concentration. Objective clinical parameters, such as heart rate and blood pressure, should be used for titration.
- May be used alone or with other antihypertensive agents.
- Combinations with other antihypertensive agents are available in fixed preparations.
- Current data are inadequate to permit directions for pediatric use.
* The long-acting capsule formulation of propranolol should not be considered a simple mg for mg substitute for the regular formulation. Upward titration may be necessary to maintain the desired therapeutic effect over a full 24-hour period.

Notably, these results may apply to beta-blockers in general since current research indicates that all of the approved beta-blockers are similar in effectiveness and compared favorably with thiazide-diuretics in the initial treatment of hypertension.[10]

Beta-blockers are also highly effective when used in multiple drug therapy. Indeed, it can be expected that the combination of a beta-blocker and a thiazide diuretic will be successful in approximately 85% of hypertensive patients. Also, good results may be expected when beta-blockers are combined with vasodilator-antihypertensive agents such as hydralazine, nifedipine, diltiazem and others.

Beta-Receptor Blockage

Beta-blockers specifically bind to beta-adrenergic receptors and inhibit the ability of neurotransmitters and other sympathomimetic amines to interact effectively with their receptor sites[16] (Figure 2). The resultant beta-blockade inhibits physiologic responses to incoming sympathetic stimuli in various organs which fall under autonomic regulation by the sympathetic nervous system. This beta-blockade is competitive and reversible in nature, so that if the concentration of the sympathomimetic agonist (such as isoproterenol) is increased, then the block can be overcome. Beta-adrenergic receptors have been character-

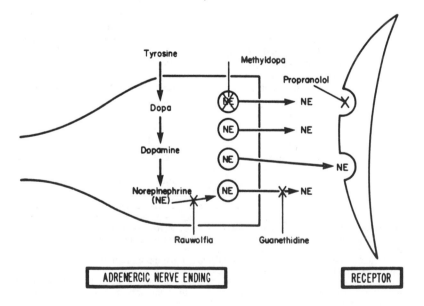

Figure 2: Simplified scheme of sympathetic neurotransmission and site of action of beta-blocking agents.

ized as either beta-1 or beta-2; beta-1 receptors predominate in cardiac tissue, and beta-2 receptors reside primarily in smooth muscle and gland cells[17] (Figure 2). Accordingly, beta-blockers should be expected to produce the effects shown in Table III.[18,19]

Some beta-blocking agents (e.g., atenolol and metoprolol) preferentially bind to beta-1 receptors and are termed "beta-1-specific" or "cardioselective." However, "beta-1-specific" blocking agents also

TABLE III
SOME MAJOR EFFECTS OF BETA-RECEPTOR BLOCKADE

Site	Primary Receptor Type*	Beta-Blocking Effects
Heart		
S-A Node	beta-1	Decrease in heart rate, often to 50–60/min
Atria	beta-1	Decrease in contractility and conduction velocity
A-V Node	beta-1	Decrease in automaticity and conduction velocity
His-Purkinie System	beta-1	Decrease in automaticity and conduction velocity
Ventricles	beta-1	Decrease in contractility, conduction velocity, automaticity, and rate of ectopic pacemakers
Arterioles		
Coronary	beta-2	Vasoconstriction
Skeletal muscle	beta-2	Vasoconstriction
Pulmonary	beta-2	Vasoconstriction
Visceral, renal	beta-2	Vasoconstriction
Lung		
Bronchial Muscle	beta-2	Bronchoconstriction
Gastrointestinal	beta-1	Increase in motility and tone
Kidney		
JG Aparatus	beta-1	Decrease in renin secretion
Liver	beta-2	Decrease in glycogenolysis and gluconeogenesis
Skeletal muscle	beta-2	Decrease in glycogenolysis and gluconeogenesis
Pancreas		
Islets (Beta cells)	beta-2	Decrease in insulin secretion
Fat Cells	beta-1	Decrease in lipolysis of FFA release

* There is evidence that both receptor subtypes can coexist in a single organ and may subserve the same physiologic response.

block beta-2 receptors, especially at larger doses, such as may be employed in hypertension therapy.

Mechanism of Action

Despite extensive research, the precise mechanism(s) of the antihypertensive action of beta-blockers has not been established and has stimulated much research. In view of the multiple physiologic effects of beta-blockers (see Table III), it is likely that a variety of mechanisms contribute to a greater or lesser extent, depending upon the pathophysiology of the patient's hypertension. One or more of the following mechanisms may be involved:

1. Cardiac Mechanism

Without question, the fall in cardiac output resulting from the negative chronotropic and inotropic effects of beta-blockers (Figure 3)

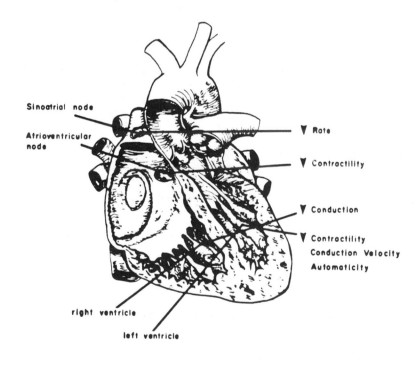

A. Effect of beta-1 blockade on the heart.

Kidney JC aparatus: lung bronchi: arterioles:
↓ renin secretion   bronchoconstriction   vasoconstriction

B. Effect of beta-2 blockade on the kidneys, lungs, and arterioles.

Figure 3: Physiologic effects of beta-blocking agents.

contributes, at least in part, to the fall in blood pressure. Following the administration of beta-blockers, however, there is considerable lag time between the fall in cardiac output and the fall in blood pressure. One study has shown that both the time course and magnitude of the fall in cardiac output indicate that the fall in blood pressure may be primarily related to changes in total peripheral resistance instead of output.[20] Also, it should be noted that not all of the beta-blockers are associated with a fall in resting cardiac output (e.g., pindolol). These facts suggest that other mechanisms are also involved in the action of beta-blockers.

2. Cardiovascular Mechanism

This mechanism involves the possibility that the various cardiodynamic effects of beta-1 blockade, such as decreased cardiac output and contractility, may elicit adaptive changes in peripheral circulation which, in turn, may lower peripheral resistance. It has been proposed that a reduction in cardiac output leads to chronic tissue underperfusion which may enact locally mediated vasodilation. Indeed, animal studies have demonstrated autoregulation in the peripheral vasculature.[21] Alternatively, it has been proposed that decreased contractility leads to more subtle circulatory changes which are antihypertensive in nature.

The administration of beta-blockers is followed initially by a fall in cardiac output, a rise in peripheral vascular resistance and little change in blood pressure. Later, there is a fall in blood pressure, peripheral vascular resistance returns to pre-treatment levels, and cardiac output remains depressed. The cardiovascular mechanism might explain this sequence of cardiovascular effects.

3. Renin Mechanism

All beta-blockers suppress renin levels, but this is probably unrelated to *how* they reduce blood pressure. Buhler and Laragh[22] first presented evidence linking the antihypertensive action of beta-blockers to the suppression of renin release from the kidney. While it is likely that the lowering of plasma renin contributes in some fashion to the lowering of blood pressure, there is strong evidence that the proposed "renin mechanism" plays only a minor role in the antihypertensive action of beta-blockers. Several studies have demonstrated no direct correlation between decreases in plasma renin and decreases in blood pressure.[23,24] Although patients with high renin profiles tend to exhibit greater responses to beta-blockers, a recent large-scale study by the Veterans Administration Cooperative Study Group found that the responses to beta-blocking therapy are not predictable from pre-treatment renin profiles.[25] The fact that diuretics effectively lower blood pressure while raising plasma renin also suggests a dissociation between plasma renin and blood pressure.

4. Central Nervous System Mechanism

Several sites of centrally located systems of adrenergic neurons appear to be concerned with blood pressure regulation, including the hypothalamus, midbrain, medulla and spinal cord.[26,27] It has been proposed that beta-blockers lower blood pressure by entering the central nervous system and interfering with sympathetic outflow to the cardiovascular system. Although direct evidence in man is lacking, animal studies have demonstrated that the administration of beta-blockers directly into the brain produces a hypotensive response.[28] Entry into the central nervous system, which is dependent upon such properties as lipid solubility, varies widely with the different beta-blockers, yet they all reduce blood pressure similarly. This fact suggests that this is probably not a major mechanism of action.

5. Baroreceptor Mechanism

Beta-blockers reduce sympathetic activity of the heart. They therefore reduce the transient rises in systolic and diastolic blood pressure, as well as cardiac output, which occur in hypertensives in response to stimuli such as dynamic exercise. It has been proposed that the baroreceptors are gradually reconditioned to regulate blood pressure at a lower level. In other words, the reduction in peak levels of sympathetic activity on the heart may recondition the baroreceptors to produce their vasomotor inhibitory impulses at lower levels of blood pressure.[29] This gradual sensitization of the baroreflex might explain the delayed onset of the full hypertensive action of beta-blockers, as well as the absence of orthostatic hypotension.

6. Pre-synaptic Receptor Mechanism

Several studies have demonstrated an important pressor effect of administered epinephrine.[30,31] It appears that circulating epinephrine promotes neurotransmitter release from adrenergic neurons by stimulating pre-synaptic beta-adrenoceptors. It has been proposed that beta-blocking activity at these pre-synaptic beta-receptors may inhibit the pressor effects of circulating endogenous epinephrine and, hence, lower blood pressure.[32]

7. Afferent Input Mechanism

It has been proposed that beta-blockers may cause a dampening of peripheral autonomic afferent input to the central nervous system resulting in a reduction in sympathetic cardiovascular tone.[33] This would involve a diminution of the continuous barrage of sensory input from the heart and great vessels, from the baroreceptors, and from the oscillations of the renin-angiotensin system. This proposal is attractive from the standpoint that it involves a multi-system mechanism partially encompassing the cardiovascular, renin, central nervous system and baroreceptor pathways.

Absorption, Metabolism, Excretion[19,34-36]

There is a great deal of person-to-person and within-individual variation in the pharmacokinetic parameters of beta-blockers. There is also a great deal of drug-to-drug variation in the kinetic properties of the various beta-blockers (see Tables IV and V). For this reason, relevant laboratory data provide only rough estimates to guide the physician in dosing (Table IV). The six FDA approved beta-blockers are rapidly absorbed and, with the exceptions of atenolol and nadolol, this absorption is almost complete. Again, plasma levels achieved are variable and may be inconsistent. This may be attributed in part to protein binding.

Propranolol, metoprolol, pindolol, and timolol undergo rapid hepatic uptake and metabolism and, with the exception of pindolol, they have a significant first-pass effect. This rapid biotransformation of these four drugs necessitates at least two doses per day. The therapeutic action of the various liver metabolites is assumed neglible.

Long-acting propranolol capsules are formulated for slower absorption and sustained release, allowing once-daily dosing.

Atenolol and nadolol undergo little or no hepatic metabolism, resulting in longer plasma half-lives which permit once-daily dosing. These two drugs are therefore safe to use in the presence of liver disease.

Most of the beta-blockers are excreted primarily by the kidney and, therefore, should be used with caution in renal failure. Atenolol and nadolol are eliminated basically unchanged by the kidney. Because of this, the half-lives of atenolol and nadolol increase with moderate

TABLE IV
PHARMACOKINETICS OF THE BETA-BLOCKERS

	Peak Plasma Levels (hrs)	Plasma Half-life (hrs)	Gut Absorption (%)	First-pass Metabolism (%)	Protein Binding (%)	Liver Metabolism (%)	Active Metabolite
Atenolol	2–4	6–7	50	0*	6–16	0*	None
Betaxolol	2–6	16–22	90	10	50	95	None
Metoprolol	1½	3–4	100*	50	12	90	None
Nadolol	3–4	20–24	30	0*	30	0*	None
Pindolol	1	3–4	95	13	40	60–65	None
Propranolol	1–1½	2–3	100*	66	90–95	100*	4-OH-P
Timolol	1–2	4	90	50	10–60	80	None

* Indicates that actual values approach but do not equal these numbers.

TABLE V
COMPARATIVE PHARMACOLOGY OF BETA-BLOCKING AGENTS

	Beta-Blocking Activity		Intrinsic* Sympathomimetic Activity (partial agonist)	Membrane Stabilizing Activity	Distribution Coefficients** (Lipid Solubility)
	B-1	B-2			
Atenolol	+	0	0	+	0.015
Betaxolol	+	0	+	+	1.0–20
Metoprolol	+	0	0	−	0.98
Nadolol	+	+	0	+	0.666
Pindolol	+	+	+	−	0.82
Propranolol	+	+	0	***	20.2
Timolol	+	+	0	−	1.16

* Presence of ISA in pindolol makes it the preferable drug in patients with pre-existing bradycardia.

** Distribution coefficients in N-octanol/buffer at pH 7.4 and 37°C (a measure of lipid solubility). Lower lipid solubility is believed to produce fewer CNS side effects.

*** Only with the new propranolol LA formulation.

renal impairment. Therefore, doses of atenolol and nadolol must be decreased in the presence of kidney disease. On the other hand, doses of propranolol and metoprolol need not be changed in the presence of kidney disease, but these two drugs should not be given in the presence of liver disease.

Drug Interactions

1. Plus *Thiazide or Loop Diuretics*

The combination of a beta-blocker and a diuretic is more effective than either drug used alone.[37] Such a combination is effective in approximately 85% of patients having mild to moderate hypertension.[10] Furthermore, this combination therapy is synergistic in nature and carries the potential of producing enhanced antihypertensive effects at lower doses of each drug, with a consequent reduction in side effects.[38]

2. Plus *Catecholamine Depleting (e.g., reserpine) or Adrenergic Blocking (e.g., clonidine) Agents*

The concomitant administration often produces an additive hypotensive and bradycardiac effect and carries the risk of precipitating unwanted hypotensive episodes. Patients treated with this combination therapy should therefore be closely observed for evidence of hypotension and/or excessive bradycardia which may produce vertigo, syncope, or postural hypotension.

3. Plus *Atropine*

Atropine is recommended as an antidote to overcome cardiac beta-1-blockade should excessive bradycardia occur (e.g., syncope from a rate of less than 40/min).

4. Plus *General Anesthetics*

Beta-blockade impairs the ability of the heart to respond to reflex adrenergic stimuli, a mechanism that may be required for maintenance of adequate cardiac function with the use of cardiodepressive anesthetic agents (see Warnings).

5. Plus *Digitalis*

Beta-blockers and digitalis, in combination, produce an additive depression of AV-nodal conduction; also, the positive inotropic action of digitalis is partially counteracted by the negative inotropic action of beta-blockers.[39]

6. Plus *Insulin or Oral Hypoglycemic Agents*

In diabetics, beta-blockers may potentiate acute hypoglycemia induced by insulin, sulfonylureas or phenformin. The hypoglycemia may then produce severe hypertension as well as convulsions. The hypertension is more severe with the nonspecific beta-blockers than with beta-1 blocking drugs.[40]

7. Plus *Prostaglandin Inhibitors (e.g., indomethacin)*

Prostaglandins are important in hormonal regulation. Prostaglandin inhibitors such as indomethacin decrease the insulin response to elevations in blood sugar. The combination of a beta-blocker with inhibitors of prostaglandin synthesis should be used with great care in diabetic patients who are more sensitive to alterations in glucose metabolism.[41]

8. With *Cimetidine:*

Cimetidine decreases hepatic blood flow and therefore raises blood levels of those beta-blockers which have a high lipid solubility and first-pass extraction, such as propranolol, metoprolol and labetalol. Therefore, concurrent administration of cimetidine with one of these beta-blockers will potentiate the antihypertensive, anti-anginal, antiarrhythmic and pulse-slowing effects of these agents. One would *not* expect this interaction with atenolol or nadolol, which have very low hepatic uptakes.

9. With *Vasodilators:*

The reflex sympathetic tachycardia from vasodilators is attenuated by concurrent beta-blocker administration. The hypotensive effects are additive.

10. With *Calcium Channel Blockers:*

Those calcium channel blockers which are verapamil-like and cardiodepressant are to be used very cautiously with beta-blockers because of the additive depressant effects on conductivity and contractility. Asystole and severe AV blockade have been reported (see Chapter X). The other calcium blockers which are not depressant (nifedipine-like) are more safely given with beta-blockers. The antihypertensive effects are additive.

11. With *Alcohol Use:*

The effect of a drinking party 6 to 12 hours before giving propranolol or sotolol to otherwise healthy volunteers was reported by Sotankmi, et al.[42] Propranolol levels were significantly reduced (and consequently, bioactivity was diminished), but not those of sotolol. The mechanism is felt to be via microsomal enzyme induction by ethanol. Therefore, one should expect reduced plasma levels of other beta-blockers, which are largely metabolized by the liver, e.g., metoprolol, labetalol, and timolol. Alcohol should not affect levels of nadolol or atenolol.

12. *Cigarette Smokers:*

Cigarette smoking induces liver microsomal enzymes and therefore increases hepatic removal of drugs highly metabolized by the liver, such as propranolol and metoprolol. Little or no effect would be expected with smoking on atenolol or nadolol.

13. With *Food:*

Simultaneous food ingestion with propranolol has been reported to decrease hepatic extraction and increase blood levels.[43]

14. *Hepatic Uptake in the Aged:*

Propranolol and metoprolol, being lipid soluble and subject to first-pass hepatic extraction, demonstrate decreased hepatic extraction and augmented plasma levels among older patients. At the same time geriatric patients show reduced responsiveness to beta-blockers, perhaps due to fewer beta-receptors. Regardless of the reason, elderly patients have more side effects and respond less well to beta-blocker therapy than do younger individuals.[44-46]

Warnings

● *In Patients with Cardiac Failure:*

Sympathetic stimulation is a vital component in supporting circulatory function in congestive heart failure, and its inhibition by beta-blockade may precipitate more severe failure. Beta-blockers are contraindicated in overt cardiac failure, but, when necessary, they can be used cautiously in patients with a history of cardiac failure who are well-compensated, usually receiving digitalis and diuretics. The negative inotropic action of beta-blockers can be expected to reduce, but not abolish, the positive inotropic action (i.e., that of supporting the strength of myocardial contractions) of digitalis. Also, the effects of beta-blockers and digitalis are additive in depressing AV-nodal conduction. Do not use them if there is more than first degree AV block.

● *In Patients without a History of Cardiac Failure:*

Continued depression of the myocardium with beta-blocking agents over a period of time can, in some cases, lead to cardiac failure. This is of particular importance in patients prone to developing cardiac failure. In rare instances, such occurrences have been observed during propranolol therapy. Therefore, at the first sign or symptom of impending cardiac failure, patients should be fully digitalized and/or treated with diuretics, and the response observed closely:

— if cardiac failure continues, beta-blocking therapy must be withdrawn, gradually if possible;

— if the patient appears to be compensating well and tachycardia is being controlled, patients can be maintained on combined therapy and closely followed until the threat of cardiac failure is over.

● *In Patients with Coronary Artery Disease and/or Angina Pectoris:*

Hypersensitivity to catecholamines has been reported in patients following abrupt withdrawal from beta-blocking therapy. Exacerbation of angina and, in some cases, precipitation of acute myocardial infarction have occurred. When discontinuation of chronically-administered beta-blockers is planned, the dosage should be gradually reduced over a period of two or more weeks and the patient should be carefully monitored. Because ischemic heart disease is common and may go unrecognized, it would be prudent to follow the above advice in all patients considered at risk.

- *In Patients with Bronchial Asthma or Other Chronic Obstructive Pulmonary Disease (COPD):*

Non-selective beta-blockers are contraindicated since they may block bronchodilatation produced by endogenous or exogenous catecholamine stimulation of beta-2 receptors located in bronchial smooth muscle. Because of their relative cardioselectivity, atenolol and metoprolol may be administered, though with caution.

- *In Patients with Diabetes Mellitus and/or Susceptibility to Hypoglycemia:*

Because of their beta-adrenergic blocking activity, beta-blockers may mask the appearance of certain premonitory signs and symptoms (tachycardia, rise in blood pressure, dizziness, sweating, and anxiety) of acute hypoglycemia. This is especially important in labile diabetics. When Ryan et al[40] induced hypoglycemia in diabetics pre-treated with either placebo, atenolol (a beta-1 specific) or propranolol (non-specific blocker), they found:

(a) signs and symptoms were *not* masked by either type of beta-blocker;

(b) hypoglycemic-induced hypertension was more frequent and more severe in patients on propranolol than those receiving atenolol.

Severe hypoglycemia has occurred in non-diabetic children without the expected tachycardia. The opposing actions of beta-blockade on blood glucose levels deserve special attention with regard to diabetics:

  — beta-blockers may potentiate insulin-induced hypoglycemia and then mask the associated signs and symptoms;

  — beta-blockers may inhibit the release of insulin in response to hyperglycemia and, therefore, necessitate dose adjustment of anti-diabetic drugs.

  — severe hypertension may occur following hypoglycemia in diabetics receiving non-specific beta-blockers.

- *In Patients Undergoing Major Surgery:*

Beta-blocking activity impairs the ability of the heart to respond to reflex adrenergic stimuli and may therefore augment the risk of protracted hypotension or low cardiac output during general anesthesia and surgical procedures. It has previously been recommended that beta-blocking therapy be withdrawn 48 hours prior to surgery, but today many authorities prefer to continue the beta-blocker, especially in patients with coronary artery disease, in whom abrupt withdrawal might precipitate myocardial infarction. If discontinued, however, they should be restarted promptly post-operatively. Beta-blockade effects can be reversed by the cautious administration of such agonists, e.g., isoproterenol or terbutaline.

- *In Patients during Anesthesia:*

With cardiodepressive anesthetic agents that require catecholamine release for maintenance of adequate cardiac function, beta-blockade will impair the desired inotropic effect. Therefore, beta-blockers should be titrated carefully when administered for arrhythmias which occur during anesthesia.

- *In Patients with Thyrotoxicosis:*

Beta-blockade may ameliorate the signs and symptoms of developing or continuing hyperthyroidism (e.g., tachycardia, tremor) or complications and give a false impression of improvement. They may reduce serum T_3 levels by 20% among hyperthyroid patients.[47] Therefore, abrupt withdrawal of beta-blockers should be avoided since this may be followed by an exacerbation of the symptoms of hyperthyroidism, including thyroid storm. Special attention should be given to the beta-blocking agents' potential for aggravating congestive heart failure.

- *In Patients with Wolff-Parkinson-White Syndrome:*

Several cases have been reported in which, after propranolol, the tachycardia was replaced by a severe bradycardia requiring a demand pacemaker. In one case this resulted after an initial dose of only 5 mg of propranolol.

Adverse Reactions

The beta-adrenergic blocking agents are immensely useful in the management of hypertension. They are generally well tolerated and compare favorably with other antihypertensive agents in terms of frequency of side effects.

A review of the literature reveals that all six of the approved beta-blockers demonstrate similarities in the frequency and nature of adverse reactions. Results from large-scale carefully controlled series suggest that 5–10% of patients placed on beta-blockers for essential hypertension will be forced to discontinue therapy due to prohibitive side effects[7,48-52] (Table VI).

Among the many beta-blockers, to date only practolol, an agent never marketed in the United States and indeed no longer available in any country, produced a very serious, bizarre, and occasionally fatal occulo-muco-cutaneous syndrome (rash, eye lesions, otitis media, sclerosing peritonitis, pleuritis, and pericarditis). This unexpected Practolol Syndrome was not detected until one million patient-years' experience had been accumulated.[53] It is prudent that all new beta-blocking agents should require careful post-marketing surveillance during the first few years.

The intravenous administration of beta-blockers is no longer indicated for the treatment of essential hypertension. In fact, only propranolol is available in intravenous form (which is restricted for use in life-threatening arrhythmias). Severe or life-threatening reactions to

TABLE VI
PERCENTAGE OF PATIENTS REQUIRING DISCONTINUATION OF BETA-BLOCKERS BECAUSE OF NOXIOUS SIDE EFFECTS

Study (Ref.)	Drug	No. of Patients Treated	Prohibitive Side Effects	%
Henningsen 1979[49]	Atenolol	104	10	10.4
Assaykeen 1982[48]	Metoprolol	703	47	6.7
Finnerty 1980[3]	Nadolol	43	3	6.9
Gonasun 1982[51]	Pindolol	323	20	6.2
V. A. Study Group 1982[2]	Propranolol	125	7	5.6
Henning 1980[50]	Timolol	44	3	6.8

propranolol were noted to be much more common with IV administration than with oral administration.[54]

With oral administration of beta-blockers, major reactions are just as likely to occur with small doses as with larger ones, and they are more apt to occur in the first few hours or days than after weeks or months of therapy.[55] These drugs shouldn't be abruptly withdrawn, but rather the doses tapered gradually over a two-week interval when one is stopping treatment, particularly in patients with underlying coronary disease.[56,57]

The Nature of Adverse Effects of Beta-Blockers

A. Pharmacological

1. The Impairment of Cardiac Function[54,55,58-72]

Tables VII and VIII list the nature of the frequency of both the pharmacological and the unpredictable or allergic reactions to beta-blockers.

All beta-blockers are cardiodepressive in nature and will produce the following pharmacologic effects: 1) reduction in heart rate and cardiac output at rest and in exercise; 2) reduction of systolic and diastolic blood pressure at rest and in exercise; 3) inhibition of isoproterenol-induced tachycardia; 4) reduction of reflex orthostatic tachycardia; 5) slowing of the sinus rate and depression of AV-nodal conduction; and 6) attenuation of aerobic exercise conditioning (see Table III). Also, several studies have demonstrated a modest (10%) increase in stroke volume at rest and in exercise. This general impairment of cardiac function may infrequently result in an array of adverse reactions.

Excessive bradycardia with lightheadedness or dizziness is the most commonly encountered cardiac side effect. Bradycardia of 50–60/min does not ordinarily produce symptoms and need not be of concern during the course of treatment. Should a patient become symptomatic at rates less than 45 or 50/min, the dose must be reduced. Symptoms generally disappear promptly.

Adverse reactions of a more serious nature, though occurring more rarely, include: severe bradycardia with hypotension, syncope, and circulatory shock; congestive heart failure involving acute pulmonary edema and shortness of breath; rhythmn disturbances and palpitations; and intensification of atrioventricular block. Also, there have been iso-

TABLE VII
NATURE OF REACTIONS TO BETA-BLOCKING DRUGS

Gastrointestinal
Nausea, vomiting, dry mouth, diarrhea, anorexia, abdominal cramps

Cardiovascular–Pulmonary
Lightheadedness, dizziness, acute pulmonary edema, congestive heart failure, bradycardia, syncope, paresthesias, cold extremities, Raynaud's phenomenon, intermittent claudication, gangrene, AV-block, hypotension, wheezing and dyspnea, palpitations, abrupt withdrawal may cause coronary insufficiency, angina pectoris or myocardial infarction in predisposed patients

Central Nervous System
Lethargy, drowsiness, fatigue, tiredness, headache, confusion, acute toxic psychosis, hallucinations, nightmares, insomnia, vivid dreams, personality changes, depression, suicide attempts, catatonia, confusion, clouded sensorium

Special Senses
Tinnitus, dizziness, vertigo, blurred vision, hypohydrosis

Dermatological
Rash, purpura, flushing

Renal
↓renal blood flow and perfusion, ↑BUN, ↑Cr.

Metabolic
Hypoglycemia, ↓serum T_3, hyperthyroidism after withdrawal or dose reduction, ↓HDL cholesterol, ↑triglycerides

Biochemical, Hematological
↓platelets, ↓white blood cells, ↓Hgb, ↓Hct, ↑eosinophils, ↑SGPT, ↑alkaline phosphatase, ↑LDH in severe coronary patients

Miscellaneous
Muscle cramps, male impotence, allergic reactions, alopecia

lated reports of complete AV-block and cerebrovascular accidents occurring with beta-blocker usage.

Although the vast majority of patients with good cardiac reserve tolerate beta-blocking therapy well, a few patients have developed life-threatening cardiac catastrophes following even small doses. Obviously, these reactions are not attributable to the usual beta-blockade but rather to the inability of a few patients with greatly impaired cardiac function to tolerate any decrease in sympathetic stimulation of the myocardium, its contractile force and its conduction system. Acute

TABLE VIII
FREQUENCY OF ADVERSE REACTIONS DUE TO PROPRANOLOL*

FREQUENT (> 5.0%)

Nausea, anorexia, fatigue, dizziness, lightheadedness, asymptomatic bradycardia

OCCASIONAL (0.1–5.0%)

GI: vomiting, abdominal cramps, dry mouth, diarrhea

CV: bradycardia, hypotension, wheezing, dyspnea, claudication, cold extremities

CNS: confusion, vivid dreams, insomnia, depression, hallucinations, nightmares, toxic psychosis, headaches

SPEC SENSE: tinnitus, blurred vision, hypohydrosis

DERM: rash, flushing

METABOLIC: hypoglycemia, hyperosmolar coma

MISC: myalgia, impotence in males, alopecia

RARE (< 0.1%)

↓platelets, ↓white blood cells

angina, suicide attempts, palpitation, ↓serum T_3 in hyperthyroid patients, purpura, mouth ulcers, fright, hyperthyroidism after withdrawal or dose-reduction, CHF, rhythmn disturbances, CVA, allergic reaction, sclerosing peritonitis

* Note: Use of propranolol where it is contraindicated, e.g., in heart failure, asthma, peripheral arterial diseases or AV-block, will cause frequent serious adverse reactions. Also, the abrupt withdrawal in patients who have prior coronary artery disease may precipitate acute coronary insufficiency or infarction.

pulmonary edema or congestive heart failure, complete atrioventricular block, bradycardia with hypotension or shock, and cardiac arrest have all been reported following small oral doses of propranolol. Fortunately, these life-threatening reactions are indeed rare, but they clearly justify the contraindication of beta-blockers in patients with 2° or 3° AV-block, in patients with previous bradycardia, or in patients who are in congestive heart failure or who may not actually be in failure but who clinically demonstrate limited cardiac reserve.

2. Effect on Peripheral Vascular System[73-80]

During the course of beta-blocker therapy, there is an initial increase in peripheral vascular resistance which is followed by, in what may be an adaptive process, a return of peripheral resistance to pretherapy levels (usually over a period of weeks). Blockade of beta-mediated vasodilation in skeletal muscle vasculature may play a role in the initial increase in peripheral resistance as well as in the potential for beta-blockers to cause exacerbation of peripheral vascular syndromes which are characterized by arteriolar vasospasm (probably from unopposed alpha-agonist activity). Indeed, the aggravation of peripheral vascular insufficiency, intermittent claudication, and Raynaud's phenomenon have been reported as rather common adverse effects after non-specific beta-blocker therapy, though they are less likely to follow beta-1 blockers.

3. Effect on Ventilatory Function[81-84]

Since blockade of beta-2 receptors in bronchial and bronchiolar smooth muscle produces increased airway resistance (one-second forced expiratory volume or FEV_1), it is not surprising that patients with chronic bronchitis, emphysema, or asthma sometimes develop severe respiratory distress and asthmatic attacks following beta-blockers. Although atenolol and metoprolol are relatively cardioselective (i.e., they possess more beta-1 than beta-2 activity), acute asthmatic attacks have also been produced by such "selective" agents. The non-selective beta-blockers are contraindicated in patients with chronic obstructive pulmonary disease while the so-called "cardioselective" beta-blockers may be used in such patients, but with caution. It should be noted that acute bronchospasm accompanied by wheezing, coughing, and dyspnea may also occur in individuals with normal healthy bronchi. Allergic rhinitis is also frequently aggravated by beta-blocking drugs, although less with the beta-1 blockers.

4. Effect on the Central Nervous System (CNS)[85-89]

Beta-blockers affect the CNS and may, in a few predisposed individuals, produce an acute organic brain syndrome or toxic psychosis or toxic encephalopathy. Patients with a history of psychiatric illness, especially severe depression, must be treated very cautiously. Depression progressing to catatonia, short-term memory loss, emotional lability with slightly clouded sensorium, anxiety, paranoia, hallucinations, and even suicide attempts have been reported. Effects on sleep may involve sleep disturbances, insomnia, vivid dreams, and nightmares. Less serious CNS effects also occur, including drowsiness, weakness, lethargy, and headache.

Entry into the CNS is primarily dependent upon lipid solubility. Propranolol, the most lipid soluble beta-blocking agent, is the most likely to produce CNS side effects. Atenolol, being the least lipid soluble, is theoretically the least likely to produce CNS side effects (see Table IX).

5. Effect on Blood Glucose[90-99]

Muscle glycogenolysis, adipose tissue lipolysis, liver glucose output, and the secretion of insulin and glucagon are all modulated by the sympathetic nervous system via beta-receptors. Thus, beta-blocking activity within these regulatory systems may result in hypoglycemia or hyperglycemia.

Since beta-blockers affect glucose metabolism at several sites, their precipitation or potentiation of hypoglycemia may involve multiple mechanisms. Whatever the mechanism, the typical hypoglycemic reaction entails increased sympathetic discharge. However, the blockade of catecholamine receptors may blunt the usual signs and symptoms of hypoglycemia, so there may be little or no tachycardia, sweating or anxiety. Furthermore, the recovery of blood glucose may be delayed due to depressed glycogenolysis. There is usually a bradycardia and an arrhythmia present. There may be grand mal seizures. Severe hypertension was reported by Ryan et al,[40] worse after the non-specific beta-blockers than after the beta-1 blocking agents. Also, myocardial infarction has been reported.

Such hypoglycemic episodes are rare but dangerous. Labile diabetics and/or diabetics receiving insulin are especially prone to these episodes. Pediatric patients, elderly patients, and fasting or malnourished patients are also susceptible. It should be noted that severe hypoglycemia may also appear, though rarely, in non-predisposed individuals. Therefore, whenever any patient on beta-blockers presents in coma, hypoglycemia must be considered.

Many authors feel that beta-blockers are contraindicated in metabolic acidosis, including diabetic acidosis, as well as in prolonged fasting because glycogenolysis is inhibited by beta-blockade.

Since beta-blockers may inhibit glycogenolysis and/or inhibit insulin secretion, anti-diabetic drug dosage requirements may either increase or decrease.

Cardioselective beta-blocking agents (e.g., atenolol and metoprolol) may decrease but not eliminate the risk of hypoglycemia.

6. Other Pharmacological Effects of Beta-blockers[100,101]

Gastrointestinal side effects are quite common, but usually mild.

TABLE IX

RELATIVE ADVANTAGES AND DISADVANTAGES AMONG THE BETA-BLOCKING AGENTS

	Atenolol	Betaxolol	Metoprolol	Nadolol	Pindolol	Propranolol	Timolol
Once daily dosing	X	X	—	X	—	—	—
Cardio-selective	X	X	X	—	—	—	—
Least bradycardia	—	X	—	—	X	—	—
Least CNS side effects	X	—	—	—	—	—	—
Most clinical experience	—	—	—	—	—	X	—
Prevents recurrent myocardial infarction	—	—	—	—	—	X	X
Safe in liver disease	X	—	—	X	—	X	—
Safe in kidney disease	—	X	—	—	—	X	X

X = indicates yes.
— = indicates no.

They consist of nausea, vomiting, dyspepsia, abdominal cramping, dry mouth, diarrhea, and constipation.

Allergic reactions occur rarely and may involve erythematous, rash, pruritis, purpura, hyperpigmentation, sore throat, fever with aching, laryngospasm, and respiratory distress. Recently, several cases of severe anaphylaxis potentiated by beta-blockers have been reported with all of the patients exhibiting angioedema, urticaria, profound shock, relative bradycardia, and a slow response to conventional therapy.

Another reported adverse effect is male impotence, which occurs less often than with guanethidine, methyldopa, and thiazide-diuretics.

Adverse effects on the special senses include blurred vision, conjunctivitis, dry eyes, otitis, tinnitus, dizziness and vertigo.

There have been rare instances of arthralgia, myalgia, systemic lupus, Peyronie's disease, exacerbation of porphyria, mesenteric arteriolar ischemic colitis, and sclerosing peritonitis (which appears to be distinctly different from the practolol-induced occulomucocutaneous syndrome).

B. Unpredictable Adverse Reactions to Beta-blockers

1. Deaths[54]

Beta-blockers, through their diffuse systemic beta-blocking activity, are capable of producing sudden death in predisposed individuals. A review of the literature on deaths associated with the use of beta-blockers reveals three important predisposing factors in life-threatening reactions:

- The intravenous use is far more hazardous than the oral drug and is not indicated in chronic antihypertensive therapy.
- Elderly patients have most of the serious reactions.
- Patients with little cardiac reserve have most of the severe reactions.

2. Hematologic Reactions

Thrombocytopenic, non-thrombocytopenic purpura, and reversible agranulocytosis have been reported, but are very rare. Slight increases in eosinophils and slight decreases in hemoglobin and hematocrit occur more frequently, but are not progressive and have not been associated with clinical manifestations.

3. Renal Physiologic Reactions[102-106]

Beta-blockers reduce cardiac output and also regional blood flow.

It is believed that the reduced renal blood flow is also due to the blockade of beta-2-mediated vasodilatation and the resulting state of alpha-adrenergic stimulation. As such, reductions in renal blood flow may be less with atenolol and metoprolol because of their relative beta-1 specificity.

Reductions of 15% in calculated renal blood flow have occurred during chronic beta-blocker therapy and have persisted after the withdrawal of therapy. Yet, generally there are no significant changes in glomerular filtration rate and no significant changes in renal function as indicated by urine osmolality, free water clearance, sodium clearance, and fractional sodium excretion (although there are slight elevations in blood urea nitrogen, creatinine, potassium, and uric acid levels). Despite the reduction in renal blood flow, levels of renin, angiotensin, and aldosterone are often depressed rather than elevated. This depression results from blockade of beta-1 receptors in the glomerular apparatus, causing decreased secretion of renin. Also, there are no significant changes in plasma volume, extracellular fluid volume, or total body water. Thus, beta-blockers are neither anti-diuretic nor anti-natiuretic and present no side effects of weight gain, fluid retention, or associated edema.

Essential hypertensives usually present with increased peripheral vascular resistance and with decreased renal blood flow. As such, it is believed that reduced renal blood flow may play a role in the genesis of the hypertensive process. It is theorized that reductions in renal blood flow produced by beta-blockers may be an important consideration in the long-term treatment of essential hypertension. Also, this may be of concern in elderly patients who generally exhibit reduced renal blood flow from aging per se. However, the usual biochemical indices of renal function remain normal with chronic beta-blocker therapy, and the clinical significance of this adverse effect has not yet been determined.

4. Lipid Effects[107-110]

Beta-blockers generally have been found to reduce HDL-cholesterol by 5–15% and to increase triglycerides 10–30% and therefore may have long-term adverse effects on cardiovascular disease in spite of the benefit from blood pressure reduction. There often is, however, a slight reduction in free fatty acid and no significant change in total cholesterol levels. Long-term epidemiologic studies need to be done, but for the present, it is felt that the reduction of blood pressure is probably more beneficial than these minor adverse effects on HDL-cholesterol and VLDL.

5. Acute Withdrawal Reactions[56,57,111-115]

Ventricular and supraventricular arrhythmias, exacerbation of angina pectoris, myocardial infarction, and sudden death have occurred in a few patients following the abrupt discontinuation of beta-blocker therapy. This "acute withdrawal syndrome" resembles a hyperadrenergic state and may involve the additional symptoms of sweating, tremor, tachycardia, and rebound hypertension. Severity is usually greatest around the sixth day after withdrawal. The incidence of this syndrome is extremely low and occurs primarily in patients with underlying ischemic heart disease or angina pectoris. Most patients do not exhibit such a clinical picture, but it is important to be aware that all or a portion of the syndrome might occur after abrupt discontinuance of beta-blocking drugs.

The most likely mechanism involved is an adaptive increase in the number of catecholamine receptors and/or an increase in catecholamine sensitivity caused by diffuse adrenergic blocking activity during the course of beta-blocker therapy. It is also theorized that these rare cases are simply the result of the progression of ischemic heart disease which is masked during beta-blocker therapy. Additionally, it is noteworthy that this syndrome resembles thyrotoxicosis and that increases in free triodothyronine (T_3) levels have been detected in some patients after beta-blocker withdrawal. In view of the potential life-threatening consequences of this syndrome, it seems prudent always to taper patients off beta-blockers over a two-week period and to advise coronary patients to restrict their physical exercise upon the discontinuation of beta-blockers.

In view of the potential life-threatening consequences of the post-treatment syndrome, it seems prudent to taper patients off beta-blockers over a two-week period and to advise coronary patients to restrict their physical exercise upon the discontinuation of beta-blockers. In surgical emergencies, most patients should be maintained on their beta-blockers.

Use in Pregnancy

Although encouraging clinical experience is accumulating, the safe use of beta-blockers in pregnancy has not yet been clearly established. It is known that beta-blocking drugs cross the placental barrier and are likely to affect fetal hemodynamics. Animal studies have demonstrated embryo and fetotoxicity at five to ten times the recommended maximum human dose. However, there are no adequately controlled studies in pregnant women. A number of controlled trials have indicated that in comparison to methyldopa, the antihypertensive drug of choice in pregnancy, beta-blockers are equally effective and appear safe for mother and fetus.[116] However, there is evidence linking the use of beta-blockers with increased uterine tone (although this apparently poses no practical obstetrical problems), intra-uterine growth retardation, neonatal bradycardia, and neonatal hypoglycemia.[14,19,34-36,49-71,116-120,123] The presence of beta-blockers in the fetal circulation may be particularly hazardous with placental insufficiency.[120] Since beta-blockers inhibit the cardiac response to reflex adrenergic stimuli, the ability of the fetal heart to respond to hypoxia may be impaired, entailing harmful fetal effects. Indeed, several case reports have described growth retardation and poor fetal response to the stresses of labor in cardiac patients treated with beta-blockers throughout pregnancy. As with any drug, the use of beta-blockers in pregnancy or in women of child-bearing potential requires thoughtful risk–benefit analysis and clinical judgment.

Beta-blockers are excreted in human milk. Therefore, nursing should not be undertaken by mothers receiving beta-blockers.

Precautions

1. Beta-blockers should be used with caution in patients with impaired hepatic or renal function (see Table IX). Adjustment in dosing may be necessary.

2. Patients receiving a combination of a catecholamine-depleting drug (e.g., reserpine) and a beta-blocking drug should be monitored carefully. The additive effects may produce excessive reduction of the resting sympathetic nervous activity which occasionally may be manifested by hypotension, marked bradycardia, vertigo, syncopal attacks, or orthostatic hypotension.

3. Patients should be told that beta-blockers may interfere with the glaucoma screening test by causing a reduction in intraocular pressure.

4. It should be noted that beta-blocking therapy may elevate serum transaminase, alkaline phosphatase, and lactate dehydrogenase.

In patients with severe heart disease, it may also elevate blood urea levels.

5. Because safety and effectiveness have not yet been determined in children, pediatric use requires close observation.

6. The intravenous administration of beta-blockers (only propranolol is currently available in IV form) has not been adequately evaluated for use in hypertensive emergencies.

7. As with any new drug given over prolonged periods, laboratory parameters should be observed at regular intervals.

Contraindications

The proper use of beta-blocking drugs presupposes that the physician is acutely aware of those circumstances in which they must not be given (see Table X).

Management of Overdosage or Exaggerated Response

A 14-year-old boy who ingested 8,000 mg of propranolol developed sudden onset of arrhythmia, cardiac failure, and convulsions. He responded to ventilator support, transvenous pacing, and massive dosage of isoproterenol. Complete recovery occurred in seven hours.[121] This case history illustrates the relative safety of the beta-blockers with healthy hearts and no contraindications, and the potential for recovery from severe life-threatening complications of beta-blocker overdosage. Beta-blockers are readily absorbed, however, and the onset and progression of profound cardiovascular collapse may be rapid. In the event of overdosage or exaggerated response, the following measures should be employed, along with gastric lavage and general supportive therapy:

— Bradycardia: Intravenous atropine to induce vagal blockade. Although 0.25 mg to 1.0 mg of atropine has been generally recommended, therapeutic value has been reported for doses as high as 2.0 mg. If bradycardia persists, administer isoproterenol cautiously.
— Heart block (greater than first degree): Isoproterenol or a transvenous pacemaker.
— Cardiac failure: Digitalis and diuretics.
— Hypotension: Vasopressors, e.g., epinephrine or levarterenol. (There is evidence that epinephrine is the drug of choice.) If circulatory shock occurs, terbutaline may be considered.
— Bronchospasm: Aminophylline, isoproterenol, or atropine.
— Hypoglycemia: Intravenous glucose.

TABLE X
CONTRAINDICATIONS FOR BETA-BLOCKERS

	Atenolol	Betaxolol	Metoprolol	Nadolol	Pindolol	Propranolol	Timolol
Bronchial Asthma or Severe COPD	—	—	—	X	X	X	X
Overt Cardiac Failure	X	X	X	X	X	X	X
Sinus Bradycardia	X	X	X	X	X	X	X
Greater Than First Degree AV-Heart Block	X	X	X	X	X	X	X
Cardiogenic Shock	X	X	X	X	X	X	X
Allergic Rhinitis During Pollen Season	—	—	—	—	—	X	—
In Patients On Adrenergic-Augmenting Psychotropic Drugs	—	—	—	—	—	X	—

X = indicates yes.
— = indicates no.

Important Differences Among the Beta-Blockers[122,123]

The six approved beta-blockers are very similar in their clinical pharmacology and in their potential adverse effects. Controlled studies indicate that they are all essentially equal in effectiveness in the treatment of hypertension. However, there are important pharmacologic differences among the beta-blockers that entail certain advantages and disadvantages of which the physician should be aware (Table IX).

Each of the six approved beta-blocking agents and their distinguishing characteristics will be discussed below.

Atenolol (TENORMIN®)

In contrast to propranolol, atenolol is the least lipid-soluble beta-blocker and, therefore, appears to produce the fewest CNS side effects.

Atenolol is a cardioselective beta-blocking agent, requires only once daily dosing, and possesses no intrinsic sympathomimetic or membrane stabilizing activity.

Cardioselectivity means that the drug preferentially binds to cardiac beta-1 receptors over non-cardiac beta-2 receptors. This selectivity, however, is only relative—the cardioselective beta blockers, atenolol and metoprolol, do exhibit some beta-2 blocking activity, at least with doses employed in treating hypertension. Thus, the property of cardioselectivity reduces but does not eliminate the unwanted effects of beta-2 blockade (e.g., increased airway resistance, potentiation of hypoglycemia, vasoconstriction, etc.). Atenolol *may be used* in patients with medical conditions which would otherwise contraindicate beta-2 blocking activity (e.g., chronic obstructive pulmonary disease, asthma, peripheral arterial disease, diabetes, etc.).

Atenolol is not taken up or metabolized by the liver because of its low lipid solubility. It is therefore excreted unchanged by the kidneys. Lower doses should be given in renal impairment. However, this property also makes it a preferable drug in patients with diseased livers.

Metoprolol (LOPRESSOR®)

Metoprolol is cardioselective though less so than atenolol. It reduces unwanted effects of beta-2 blocking activity and it may be administered with caution in patients with medical conditions aggravated by beta-2 blockage (e.g., COPD, diabetes, Raynaud's).

Metoprolol has the additional theoretical benefit of membrane stabilizing (or quinidine-like) activity, although no clinical significance of this property has been found. It possesses no intrinsic sympathomimetic activity; it requires multiple daily dosing; it is only moderately lipid soluble.

Doses of metoprolol need to be reduced both in patients with liver disease and in those with renal disease.

Nadolol (CORGARD®)

Nadolol is a non-selective beta-blocker possessing no intrinsic sympathomimetic or membrane stabilizing activity. It carries the benefit of once-daily dosing.

Its low lipid solubility value approaches that of atenolol and can, therefore, be expected to produce relatively few CNS side effects. Also, like atenolol, its low lipid solubility prevents it from being taken up and metabolized by the liver so that dose reduction isn't required in the presence of liver disease. However, doses need to be reduced in patients with renal disease.

Pindolol (VISKEN®)

Pindolol is unique among the six approved beta-blockers in that it possesses intrinsic sympathomimetic activity (ISA), so it is the beta-blocker of choice in patients who initially have slow heart rates. In addition, it appears to have little effect on resting cardiac output while decreasing total peripheral resistance. The chemical nature of pindolol allows it to combine with and "activate" beta-receptors, thus giving it partial agonist activity. This property is manifested in man by a smaller reduction in the resting heart rate (4–8 beats min) than with other beta-blockers. However, beta-blocking activity of pindolol remains intact as it attenuates increases in heart rate, systolic blood pressure and cardiac output resulting from exercise and isoproterenol administration. It is, therefore, an effective antihypertensive agent which may carry the additional benefit of moderating troublesome bradycardia.

Like propranolol and metoprolol, pindolol has membrane stabilizing (or quinidine-like) activity. It is non-selective, moderately lipophilic, and requires multiple daily dosing. Unlike propranolol or placebo, a three pound average weight gain may occur after pindolol monotherapy.

Dosage should be decreased with liver disease and probably in the presence of significant renal disease.

Propranolol (INDERAL,® INDERAL® LA)

Propranolol, the prototype, was the first beta-blocker to be approved for use in the United States (1976). Among the beta-blockers, it has enjoyed the greatest number of patient-years of experience and has been involved in the greatest number of clinical and laboratory studies.

Propranolol is a non-selective (equal affinity for beta-1 and beta-2 receptors) beta-blocker possessing membrane stabilizing activity but no intrinsic sympathomimetic activity.

The membrane stabilizing (or quinidine-like) activity of propranolol means that it has a depressant effect on the myocardium resulting from the inhibition of transfer of sodium ions across cell membranes. Although blockade of cardiac beta-1 receptors is the major component in the anti-arrhythmic action of beta-blockers, it is believed that membrane stabilizing activity may play a contributory role, particularly in digitalis-induced arrhythmias.

Propranolol is now available in a once daily dosing form (Inderal® LA) allowing for greater patient compliance.

One major disadvantage of propranolol is that it is much more lipid soluble than the other beta-blockers (Table IX). Therefore, it more readily penetrates the blood–brain barrier and is probably more likely to produce CNS side effects such as drowsiness, fatigue, confusion, etc.

Timolol (BLOCADREN®)

In April, 1981, the *New England Journal of Medicine*[124] contained a unique medical report. A double-blind multicenter randomized study with timolol vs. placebo conducted in Norway indicated that the sudden-death rate over a 33-month interval was 13.9% in the placebo group versus 7.7% in the timolol group—a reduction of 44.6%. The cumulated reinfarction rate was 20% in the placebo group and 14.4% in the timolol group—a 28% reduction. The investigators concluded that when timolol was given at a dose of 10 mg twice daily, started between 7 to 28 days after the initial myocardial infarction and continued for periods of up to 33 months, a statistically significant and clinically important reduction in reinfarction or sudden deaths occurred. Timolol subsequently became the first beta-blocker approved by the Food and Drug Administration to reduce cardiovascular mortality in patients having sustained an initial myocardial infarction.

Timolol subsequently became the first beta-blocker
approved by the Food and Drug Administration to reduce
cardiovascular mortality in patients having sustained
an initial myocardial infarction.

Timolol is a nonselective beta-blocker with no intrinsic sympatho-mimetic or membrane stabilizing activity. Although dosage is generally given on a twice-daily basis. Wilhelmsson et al[125] reported that exercised heart rate and systolic blood pressure were significantly lowered through 24 hours after once-daily administration of the drug. Yu[126] summarized the antihypertensive results from a multicenter double-blind clinical trial involving 355 patients with mild to moderate essential hypertension (95–115 mm Hg). After 12 weeks of therapy using a dose of 10 to 30 mg twice daily, timolol reduced mean supine blood pressure from 154/103 to 145/94 compared to placebo's reducing blood pressure from 156/103 to 155/102 mm Hg. Fifty-seven percent of patients receiving timolol (compared with only 13% of those receiving placebo) had an excellent or good response. Abrupt withdrawal of timolol following treatment in these patients produced no precipitous elevation or overshoot of blood pressure. Throughout his study, side effects were mild and included bradycardia which was, however, of no clinical importance.

Alcocer et al[127] reported the cardiovascular and metabolic profile of timolol in the management of hypertensive patients to be as follows. Comparing 10 mg twice daily for six weeks in ten hypertensive patients vs. placebo therapy, statistically significant differences were as follows: systolic and diastolic blood pressures were significantly reduced by timolol, heart rate was reduced from 76 to 64, cardiac output was reduced from 6.41 to 5.42 L/min, plasma renin activity was reduced from 8.63 to 3.92 ng/ml/hr, urinary aldosterone was reduced from 4.94 to 3.73 ug/24 hr, urinary sodium was increased from 58 to 67 mEq/24 hr, and ejection fraction was increased from 44.8 to 52.1%. No statistically significant changes were noted in urinary potassium excretion, stroke volume, or peripheral vascular resistance.

Timolol reduces not only resting but also exercise blood pressure. The reduction has been shown to be due, as with other beta-blockers, to a decreased cardiac output caused by a reduction in heart rate without significant changes in stroke volume. The increase in mean pulmonary artery pressure indicates increased left ventricular filling pressure occurring in spite of the drop in systemic arterial pressure.

Tocco, Abrams, and Nancarrow[128] compared propranolol lipid solubility and the central nervous system side effects of timolol and propranolol. Propranolol is much more soluble in lipid systems than is timolol; therefore, central nervous system side effects like vivid dreams, toxic psychoses, insomnia, and depression have been found to occur much more often with propranolol and rarely with timolol.

Dosage should be reduced in patients with liver disease, but need not be modified in the presence of renal disease.

LABETALOL (Normodyne®)
Introductory year: 1984

INTRODUCTION:

Labetalol hydrochloride is the prototypical drug of a new class of antihypertensive agents that combines within the same molecule non-selective beta-adrenergic blockade with post-synaptic alpha-1 blockade. The benefits of these unique properties of labetalol are apparent in its wide applicability while thus far maintaining a low incidence of adverse reactions. Unlike the non-specific alpha blockers, labetalol does not produce the marked orthostatic hypotension or reflex tachycardia. Unlike the beta-blockers, labetalol produces less bradycardia, less reduction in blood flow (particularly during exercise), and it *decreases* peripheral vascular resistance. It may be used continuously to treat many hypertensives in heart failure or with chronic obstructive pulmonary disease or arterial insufficiency.

Since its introduction in Europe in 1975, labetalol has been shown to be efficacious in the treatment of a variety of hypertensive situations. Results from both the clinical and laboratory setting suggest the full potential of labetalol has yet to be exploited and that labetalol should augment the physician's armamentarium in the management of hypertension.

When should the physician consider labetalol for hypertension?
• Labetalol is effective as a single agent in the treatment of mild to

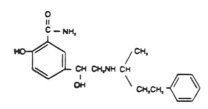

Figure 4: Structure of labetalol.

severe hypertension.[1-3] It may be used occasionally as a Step-1 or more often as a Step-2 drug. Labetalol therapy alone has been shown to be as effective as is the combined therapy of a diuretic and vasodilator.[4]

- Labetalol should be considered in the treatment of hypertensive patients with renal disease. Labetalol decreases plasma levels of renin and aldosterone, renal vascular resistance, and renal blood flow while it does not produce a significant change in the glomerular filtration rate. It lowers blood pressures in hypertensive patients with renal impairment without further deleterious effects on their renal disease.

- Parenteral labetalol should be considered in the treatment of hypertensive emergencies (see Chapter XIII). Parenteral labetalol used in the management of hypertensive emergencies produces a smooth decline in blood pressure without serious side effects.[5,6] In one recent study using labetalol to treat hypertensive emergencies, 53 of the 59 cases reached a therapeutic level with a mean decrease in blood pressure of 68/41 mm Hg.[7]

- Labetalol should be considered in the pre-operative treatment of pheochromocytoma and during abrupt withdrawal of beta-blocking or central adrenergic agonist drugs such as clonidine, guanabenz, and methyldopa. A catecholamine surge may occur and be deleterious in the pre-operative treatment of pheochromocytoma and during abrupt withdrawal of many drugs. Blockade of both alpha- and beta-adrenergic receptors during this time is desirable. Labetalol blocks both receptor types and may be the most efficacious treatment in the management of these two clinical settings.[8-11]

- Labetalol should be considered in the treatment of hypertensives with ischemic heart disease. Labetalol reduces arterial pressure and minimizes coronary spasm without changing heart rate or cardiac output. These factors reduce myocardial oxygen demand and may suggest labetalol as an ideal agent for the treatment of ischemic heart disease.

• Parenteral labetalol should be considered when a controlled decrease in blood pressure is desirable during surgery. Labetalol combined with halothane anesthesia produces a synergistic hypotensive effect that is quickly reversible when halothane is withdrawn.[12]

How Effective is Labetalol in Hypertension?

There has been considerable experience in the treatment of essential hypertension with labetalol.[13-16] When administered alone or in combination, labetalol was found to be at least as effective in lowering blood pressure as a wide range of other antihypertensives. Several investigators have reported that labetalol alone or in combination with a diuretic has often been more effective where other antihypertensive agents, including the beta-blockers, have failed.[17-22] Kane[16] reported that between 60 and 80% of severe and previously uncontrolled hypertensives with diastolic blood pressures of greater than 120 mm Hg responded satisfactorily to labetalol, as did an even larger percentage (88%) of mild to moderate hypertensives.

Many studies have shown a significant antihypertensive effect for labetalol in both fixed doses and individually titrated doses compared with placebo[23-26,51] with a corresponding dose-related fall in blood pressure during labetalol treatment.[24,27] In a majority of studies that compared the antihypertensive efficacy of labetalol and diuretics, labetalol was shown to be equivalent or superior in efficacy to the thiazides.[28,29] Figure 5[30] illustrates that the addition of labetalol to a hydrochlorothiazide regimen produces a further dose-related fall in blood pressure when compared to placebo or thiazide diuretic treatment alone.[30-32] Intravenous labetalol is very effective in the treatment of hypertensive emergencies and, once controlled, the patient can usually be easily and safely changed to oral labetalol for maintenance therapy. When maintenance therapy requires the addition of a thiazide diuretic, there is a markedly enhanced therapeutic effect such that the dose of labetalol may be reduced.

Patients with all degrees of hypertension appear to respond to labetalol administration.[33-35] Labetalol's hypotensive effects do not vary as a result of differences in race or in the underlying cause of the hypertension. Continuous monitoring of blood pressure in patients receiving labetalol twice daily has shown smooth control of pressure throughout

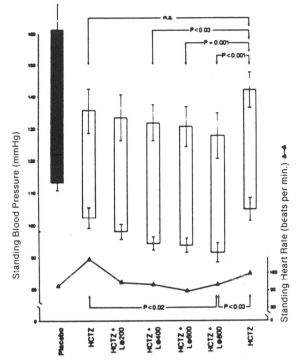

Figure 5: Standing blood pressure and heart rate responses to 50 mg/day hydrochlorothiazide (HCTZ) alone and hydrochlorothiazide plus incremental doses of labetalol in eight patients with essential hypertension.[30]

the 24-hour period.[36,37] Tolerance does not develop to the hypotensive effects of labetalol[1,38,39]; consequently, the therapeutic dosage can be relatively constant over time.

A recent clinical study[40] indicates that labetalol is equally effective in reducing arterial pressure in black as well as white patients. When compared with propranolol in the treatment of black hypertensives, labetalol required significantly fewer additions of thiazide diuretics to maintain therapeutic pressure levels.

Indications for Labetalol

— Intravenous labetalol is indicated when rapid control of blood pressure is essential in severely hypertensive patients, such as those with hypertensive encephalopathy, accelerated hypertension, and pre-eclampsia or eclampsia.
— Oral labetalol may be indicated in the treatment of hypertensive patients with renal disease, angina pectoris, and a myocardial infarction. Use in pregnant hypertensives thus far indicates efficacy and

no reports of congenital abnormalities among 91 infants.[40] Further experience is needed, however.

— More recent indications are related to the management of pre-operative pheochromocytoma, acute withdrawal of beta-blockers or central alpha-agonists, severe tetanus,[41] and when applied locally in the treatment of glaucoma.[42]

Dose in Hypertension

I. Oral:

Frequency: 2–3 times daily
Initial: 100 mg twice daily
Maintenance: 200-400 mg twice daily.

II. Parenteral (inpatient or emergency):

I.V.: initially infuse 20 mg over 2–4 minutes followed 20 minutes later by a 40 mg bolus and then subsequent 80 mg boluses until blood pressure is controlled. A maximum of 300 mg of labetalol should not be exceeded.[43] Once the hypertensive crisis is under control, an oral regimen of labetalol will provide maintenance therapy.

Mechanism of Action

In a recent review,[44] MacCarthy and Bloomfield have summarized the hemodynamic effects of labetalol when administered both intravenously and orally to hypertensive patients (Tables XI and XII). Virtually all the studies show that the major hemodynamic effects of labetalol in man are a reduction in systemic arterial blood pressure and a decrease in total peripheral vascular resistance, without significant alterations in resting heart rate or cardiac output.[45-47] Under intravenous administration of labetalol, the heart rate usually falls in the standing position or during exercise but is not significantly altered in the supine position (Table XI). Labetalol administered orally reduces blood pressure and heart rate whether at rest in the supine position, standing upright, or during exercise (Table XII). Under various conditions at rest and exercise, oral labetalol will reduce systemic vascular resistance with variable effects on both cardiac output and stroke volume.

Like intravenous labetalol, these unique hemodynamic effects of labetalol are due to its combining in the same molecule non-selective beta-adrenergic blockade with post-synaptic alpha-1 blockade.[48-53] Recent studies suggest that labetalol also possesses intrinsic sympathomi-

TABLE XI
HEMODYNAMIC EFFECTS OF INTRAVENOUS LABETALOL IN HYPERTENSIVE PATIENTS

Study (Ref.)	No. of Patients	Labetalol Dose	Position	Blood Pressure	Heart Rate	Cardiac Output	Stroke Volume	Systemic Vascular Resistance
Prichard et al[58]	12	0.5 mg/kg	Supine	↓	*	*	*	↓
Joekes et al[59]	14	0.5–1 mg/kg	Supine	↓	*	*	*	↓
Koch[46]	13	50 mg	Supine	↓	*	*	*	↓
			Upright	↓	↓	↓	↓	↓
			Exercise	↓	↓	↓	↑	↓
Bahimann et al[60]	9	0.6–1.6 mg/kg	Supine	↓	*	*	*	↓
Svendsen et al[47]	10	50 mg	Supine	↓	*	*	*	↓
			Upright	↓	↓	↓	*	↓
			Exercise	↓	↓	↓	*	*
Trap-Jensen et al[61]	8	0.75 mg/kg	Supine	↓	*	*	NR	↓
			Psychic Stress	↓	↓	↓	NR	*
Agabiti-Rosel et al[62]	18	100 mg	Supine	↓	↓	↓	*	↓
Dunn et al[63]	12	0.5–1 mg/kg	Supine	↓	*	↓	*	*
			45° tilt	↓	*	↓	↓	↑

↓ = Statistically significant reduction; ↑ = Statistically significant increase; * = No significant change; NR = Not reported.

TABLE XII
HEMODYNAMIC EFFECTS OF ORAL LABETALOL IN HYPERTENSIVE PATIENTS

Study (Ref.)	Duration (Wks)	No. of Patients	Max. Dose (g/daily)	Position	Blood Pressure	Heart Rate	Cardiac Output	Stroke Volume	Systemic Vascular Resistance	Pulmonary Vascular Resistance
Edwards et al[64]	4	11	0.8	Supine	↓	↓	*	↑	*	NR
				Exercise	↓	↓	↓	*	*	NR
Mehta et al[45]	1	6	1.6	Supine	↓	↓	*	NR	↓	NR
				Upright	↓	↓	*	NR	↓	NR
				Exercise	↓	↓	NR	NR	NR	NR
Fagard et al[50]	2.5	18	0.3–2.4	Supine	↓	↓	↓	*	*	*
				Upright	↓	↓	↓	*	↓	*
				Exercise	↓	↓	↓	↑	↓	*
Lund-Johansen et al[65]	52	15	0.2–0.8	Supine	↓	↓	*	↑	↓	NR
				Upright	↓	↓	↓	*	*	NR
				Exercise	↓	↓	↓	↑	↓	NR
Koch[46]	85	9	0.6–2.4	Supine	↓	↓	*	↑	↓	↓
				Upright	↓	↓	*	↑	↓	*
				Exercise	↓	↓	*	↑	↓	↑
Svendsen et al[47]	13	8	0.6–0.9	Supine	↓	↓	*	↑	↓	*
				Upright	↓	↓	*	*	↓	NR
				Exercise	↓	↓	↓	*	*	↑

↑ = Statistically significant increase; * = No significant change; ↓ = Statistically significant reduction; NR = Not reported.

metic activity at the beta-2 receptor.[54] Compared with propranolol and phentolamine, labetalol was approximately 1/4 as potent on a milligram basis as the beta-blocker and 1/7 as potent as the alpha-blocker, respectively. The overall ratio of alpha- to beta-blockade is approximately 1:7.

In addition to labetalol's adrenergic activity, it has been shown to decrease plasma angiotensin II and plasma aldosterone levels.[55-57] The decrease does occur much after the blood pressure response and is most notable in patients with pre-existing high levels of angiotensin II and aldosterone. Labetalol has little or no effect on plasma catecholamines.

Labetalol shares characteristics of other beta-blockers such as local anesthetic membrane stabilization and antiarrythmic properties. With respect to platelets, labetalol does not antagonize epinephrine-induced platelet aggregation. The lack of this latter effect may be due to labetalol's specific alpha-1 antagonism, while leaving the platelet alpha-2 receptor unopposed.[66]

Table XIII compares the pharmacologic properties of labetalol and

TABLE XIII
PHARMACOLOGIC PROPERTIES OF
BETA-ADRENOCEPTOR BLOCKING DRUGS

Drug	Membrane Stabilizing Activity	Intrinsic Sympathomimetic Activity	Beta$_1$-Selective blockade	Lipid Solubility
Atenolol (Tenormin®)	0	0	††	0
Metoprolol (Lopressor®)	0	0	††	†
Nadolol (Corgard®)	0	0	0	0
Pindolol (Visken®)	±	††	0	†
Propranolol (Inderal®)	††	0	0	††
Timolol (Blocadren®)	0	0	0	†
Labetalol* (Normodyne™, Trandate®)	†	0	0	††

* Labetalol also has alpha$_1$-adrenergic blocking activity, direct vasodilator activity, and intrinsic beta$_2$-sympathomimetic activity.

the pure beta-adrenoceptor blocking drugs that have been approved for clinical use by the Food and Drug Administration.[44]

Drug Interactions

— Labetalol may be used in conjunction with a loop or thiazide diuretic. The dose of labetalol should be retitrated at a lower level.
— Patients in controlled heart failure on digitalis may be given labetalol with caution.[67-69] Labetalol does not diminish the positive inotropic effects of digitalis.
— Introducing cimetidine into a regimen with labetalol should be done with caution. Cimetidine has been shown to increase the bioavailability of labetalol,[70] necessitating lower doses of labetalol.
— A synergistic antihypertensive effect has been shown between labetalol and halothane anesthesia.[71-74] Patients on labetalol receiving high concentrations of halothane (>3%) during anesthesia may experience a large reduction in cardiac output. *The anesthesiologist should be told when a patient is receiving labetalol.*
— Labetalol reduces the reflex tachycardia produced by nitroglycerin without affecting its hypotensive action.[75] When used in combination, these agents may have an additive antihypertensive effect.
— A recent article[76] reviewing the treatment of 8,573 hypertensive patients with labetalol showed no adverse drug reactions between labetalol and drugs from the classes of analgesics, anti-inflammatory agents, anti-depressants, hypnotics, tranquilizers, hormones, and hypoglycemic agents. Nevertheless, as with all new drugs, be alert for possible drug interactions.

Contraindications

• Labetalol is contraindicated in greater than first degree heart block and in cardiogenic shock. • Labetalol is contraindicated in the presurgical patient where halothane anesthesia is to be employed unless a marked hypotensive effect is desirable. • Labetalol is contraindicated in patients with asthma. • Labetalol is contraindicated in patients with uncontrolled heart failure.

Warnings

• *In patients with cardiac failure:*
   Labetalol, unlike simple beta-blockers, can be used with caution in patients with controlled heart failure. Labetalol does not abolish the positive inotropic action of digitalis.

- *In patients with ischemic heart disease:*

Exacerbation of angina pectoris has not been reported upon labetalol discontinuation.[77,78]

- *In patients with bronchospastic diseases:*

Labetalol can be used at the recommended therapeutic dosages with caution in patients with bronchospastic disease, including patients who cannot tolerate other beta-blocker antihypertensive treatment.

- *In patients with pheochromocytoma:*

While labetalol has been shown to be effective in lowering the blood pressure and relieving symptoms in patients with pheochromocytoma,[79,80] paradoxical hypertensive responses have been occasionally reported.[81,82] Use caution when administering labetalol to patients with pheochromocytoma.

Use in Pregnancy and Postpartum

In Europe labetalol has been used to treat pregnant women with hypertension. Of the 91 infants born to women treated with labetalol, none showed congenital malformations.[40] Maternal side effects ranged from minor postural hypotension to scalp tingling and skin rash.[41] Although large-scale clinical trials need to be done, early indications have shown labetalol to be very effective in the management of hypertension during pregnancy.

Labetalol is excreted in breast milk. Caution should be exercised when labetalol is administered to a nursing mother. The safety and the effectiveness of labetalol have not been determined in children.

Absorption, Metabolism, Excretion

Labetalol may be administered orally or parenterally,[83-85] Gastrointestinal absorption is rapid and complete, with peak plasma levels measured in one to two hours.[43] Once absorbed, labetalol is rapidly distributed into the tissue compartments. Thereafter, labetalol is excreted according to first-order kinetics with a serum half-life of approximately two hours. Intravenously administered labetalol exhibits an extended half-life of approximately five hours. This difference in the two half-lives suggests that labetalol is more extensively metabolized after oral administration and is quite subject to first-pass metabolism within the liver.

Eighty percent of administered labetalol is glucuronidated in the liver and excreted in the urine and via the bile into the feces. The dosage of labetalol must be reduced in patients with hepatic disease but not in patients with compromised renal function.

When compared with other antihypertensive agents, labetalol has a low partition coefficient,[86] which correlates well with low transferability across biological membranes. This feature of labetalol may make it useful in treating hypertensive women during pregnancy. Labetalol's low propensity for crossing the placenta has been confirmed with measurements of maternal and fetal labetalol levels.[87]

Overdosage

Overdosage of labetalol results in severe postural hypotension with occasional bradycardia. Patients should be treated for the shocky condition by lying supine with their legs elevated. The hypotensive episode may require the administration of a vasopressor such as norepinephrine. Excessive bradycardia may be treated with intravenous atropine.[88] Gastric lavage and hemodialysis will remove labetalol from the gastrointestinal tract and the general circulation, respectively.

Precautions

— Patients with hepatic impairment should be treated cautiously with labetalol and with small initial doses.

— Patients should be advised not to interrupt or discontinue labetalol use without a physician's advice.

— All patients should have their hepatic function periodically monitored, and labetalol therapy should be discontinued if abnormalities occur.

— Labetalol metabolites in the urine may increase the number of false positives in standard urinary catecholamine tests. High pressure liquid chromatography should be used to determine urinary catecholamines in patients treated with labetalol.

Adverse Reactions

Most adverse reactions to labetalol therapy are relatively mild and transient, but the incidence does seem to be dose-dependent.[89] Unacceptable side effects account for approximately a 10% discontinuance of the drug. For patients who remain on treatment, the incidence of unacceptable side effects diminishes rapidly.

The most commonly reported adverse reactions to labetalol therapy are dizziness, tiredness, upper gastrointestinal symptoms, and headache.[90] In a comprehensive review study of 1,061 patients treated three months with 400 mg/day or less, the incidence of side effects was 4.5%, 3.9%, 2.6% and 1.9%, respectively, for these four-symptom categories. The incidence of adverse reactions to labetalol therapy is dose-dependent; for instance, alpha adrenoceptor blockade-related postural hypotension, the most troublesome side effect reported during labetalol therapy, tends to occur more frequently in the early stages of treatment, in patients receiving labetalol with diuretic therapy and during treatment with higher doses of labetalol.[14]

In addition, there are several isolated adverse reactions to labetalol therapy that have been reported as follows: muscle cramps,[91,92] toxic myopathy, difficulty in micturation,[92] rashes,[90] reversible alopecia, and positive antinuclear factor.[92] Obviously, labetalol appears to represent an important new agent in the management of hypertension. However, more clinical experience is needed to establish its true benefit-to-risk ratio.

REFERENCES:

Beta-Adrenergic Blocking Drugs

1. Prichard, B. N. C., and Gillam, P. M. S.: The use of propranolol in the treatment of hypertension. *Br. Med. J.*, **2**(5411):725, 1964.
2. Frohlich, E. D., Kozul, V. J., and Tarazi, R. C.: Physiological comparison of labile and essential hypertension. *Circ. Res.*, **27**:55, 1970.
3. Frohlich, E. D., Tarazi, R. C., and Dustan, H. P.: Re-examination of the hemodynamics of hypertension. *Am. J. Med. Sci.*, **257**:9, 1969.
4. Rosenblum, R., and Delman, A. J.: Propranolol in the treatment of hyperkinetic heart syndrome. *Am. Heart J.*, **79**(1):134, 1970.
5. Hansson, L., and Werko, L.: Beta-adrenergic blockade in hypertension. *Am. Heart J.*, **93**(3):394, 1977.
6. Frohlich, E. D.: Pathophysiology of propranolol in hypertension. *South. Med. J.*, **70**(1):95, 1977.
7. Veterans Administration Cooperative Study Group on Antihypertensive Agents: Comparison of propranolol and hydrochlorothiazide for the initial treatment of hypertension. *JAMA*, **248**(16):1996, 1982.
8. The Joint National Committee on Detection, Evaluation, and Treatment of High Blood Pressure: The 1980 Report of the Joint National Committee on Detection, Evaluation, and Treatment of High Blood Pressure. *Arch. Intern. Med.*, **140**:1280, 1980.
9. Kaplan, N. M.: The present and future use of beta-blockers. In J. Robertson, N. Kaplan, A. Caldwell, and T. Speight (Eds.): *Drugs, Symposium on Beta-Blockers in the 1980s*, ADIS Press Australasia Pty. Limited, NSW Australia, 1982.

10. Veterans Administration Cooperative Study Group on Antihypertensive Agents: Efficacy of nadolol alone and combined with bendroflumethiazide and hydralazine for systemic hypertension. *Am. J. Cardiol.*, **52**(10):1230–1237, 1983.

11. Koch-Weser, J.: Vasodilator drugs in the treatment of hypertension. *Arch. Intern. Med.*, **133**:1017, 1974.

12. Hansson, L., and Malmcrona, R., et al: Propranolol in hypertension. *Klin. Wochenschr.*, **50**:364, 1972.

13. Buhler, F. R., Laragh, J. H., et al: The antihypertensive action of propranolol. In J. H. Laragh (Ed.): *Hypertension Manual*, Yorke Medical Books, Dunn-Donnelly Publication Corporation, New York, 1973.

14. The Norwegian Multicenter Study Group: Timolol-induced reduction in mortality and reinfarction in patients surviving acute myocardial infarction. *N. Engl. J. Med.*, **304**:801, 1981.

15. Beta-Blocker Heart Attack Trial Research Group: A randomized trial of propranolol in patients with acute myocardial infarction. *JAMA,* **247**(12):1707–1714, 1982.

16. Weiner, N.: Drugs that block adrenergic receptors. In A. G. Gilman, L. S. Goodman, and A. Gilman (Eds.): *The Pharmacological Basis of Therapeutics*, MacMillan, New York, 1980.

17. Lands, A. M., Arnold, A., et al: Differentiation of receptor systems activated by sympathomimetic amines. *Nature*, **214**:597, 1967.

18. McDevitt, D. G.: Clinical significance of Cardioselectivity. In J. Robertson, N. Kaplan, A. Caldwell, and T. Speight (Eds.): *Drugs, Symposium on Beta-Blockers in the 1980s.* ADIS Press Australasia Pty. Limited, NSW Australia, 1982, p. 219.

19. Dollery, C. T., Paterson, J. W., and Conolly, M. E.: Clinical pharmacology of beta-receptor-blocking drugs. *Clin. Pharmacol. Ther.*, **10**(6):765, 1969.

20. Tarazi, R. C., and Dustan, H. P.: Beta adrenergic blockade in hypertension: Practical and theoretical implications of long-term hemodynamic variations. *Am. J. Cardiol.*, **29**:633, 1972.

21. Guyton, A. C., Granger, H. J., and Coleman, T. G.: Autoregulation of the total systemic circulation and its relation to control of cardiac output and arterial pressure. *Circ. Res.*, **28–29**(Suppl 1):I-93, 1971.

22. Buhler, F. R., Laragh, J. H., et al: Antihypertensive action of propranolol: Specific antirenin responses in high and normal renin forms of essential, renal, renovascular and malignant hypertension. *Am. J. Cardiol.*, **32**:511, 1973.

23. Morgan, T. O., Roberts, R., Carney, S. C., Louis, W. J., and Doyle, A. E.: Beta-adrenergic receptor blocking drugs, hypertension and plasma renin. *Br. J. Clin. Pharmacol.*, **2**:159, 1975.

24. Hollifield, J. W., Sherman, K., Zwagg, R. V., and Shand, D. G.: Proposed mechanisms of propranolol's antihypertensive effect in essential hypertension. *N. Engl. J. Med.*, **295**(2):68, 1976.

25. Freis, E. D., Materson, B. J., and Flamenbaum, W.: Veterans Administration Cooperative Study Group on Antihypertensive Agents: Comparison of propranolol or hydrochlorothiazide alone for the treatment of hypertension: Evaluation of the renin-angiotensin system. From the Cooperative Studies Program, Medical Research Service of the Veterans Administration. *Am. J. Med.*, **74**:1029–1041, 1983.

26. Haeusler, G.: Cardiovascular regulation by central adrenergic mechanisms and its alteration by hypotensive drugs. *Circ. Res.*, **36-37**(Suppl I):I-223, 1975.

27. Chalmers, J. P.: Neuropharmacology of central mechanisms regulating pressure.

In D. Davies and J. Reid (Eds.): *Central Action of Drugs in Blood Pressure Regulation*, University Park Press, Baltimore, 1975, p. 36.

28. Reid, J. L., Lewis, P. J., Myers, M. G., and Dollery, C. T.: Cardiovascular effects of intracerebroventricular *d-, l-* and *dl*-propranolol in the conscious rabbit. *J. Pharmacol. Exp. Ther.,* **188**(2):394, 1974.

29. Prichard, B. N. C., and Gillam, P. M. S.: Treatment of hypertension with propranolol. *Br. Med. J.,* **1**:7, 1969.

30. Brown, M. J., and Macquin, I.: Is adrenaline the cause of essential hypertension? *Lancet,* **2**:1079, 1981.

31. Tung, L. H., Rand, M. J., and Majewski, H.: Adrenaline-induced hypertension in rats. *Clin. Sci.,* **61**:191s, 1981.

32. Langer, S. Z.: The role of alpha- and beta-presynaptic receptors in the regulation of nonadrenaline release elicited by nerve stimulation. *Clin. Sci. Mol. Med.,* **51**:423s, 1976.

33. Lewis, P.: The essential action of propranolol in hypertension. *Am. J. Med.,* **60**:837, 1976.

34. Nies, A. S., and Shand, D. G.: Clinical pharmacology of propranolol. *Circulation,* **52**(1):6, 1975.

35. Shand, D. S.: Individualization of propranolol therapy. *Med. Clin. N. Am.,* **58**(5): 1063, 1974.

36. Lowenthal, D. T., Briggs, W. A., et al: Pharmacokinetics of oral propranolol in chronic renal disease. *Clin. Pharmacol. Ther.,* **16**:761, 1974.

37. Agrawal, R. L., Alliott, R. J., et al: The treatment of hypertension with propranolol and bendrofluazide. *J. R. Coll. Gen. Pract.,* **29**:602, 1979.

38. Basson, W., and Myburgh, D. P.: Synergism of a beta-blocker and a diuretic in the once-a-day treatment of essential hypertension. *J. Clin. Pharmacol.,* **19**:571, 1979.

39. Buhler, F. R., Hulthan, U. L., Kiowski, W., and Bolli, P.: Beta-blockers and calcium antagonists. In J. Robertson, N. Kaplan, A. Caldwell, and T. Speight (Eds.): *Drugs, Symposium on Beta-Blockers in the 1980s,* ADIS Press Australasia Pty. Limited, NSW Australia, 1982, p. 50.

40. Ryan, J. R., LaCorte, W., Jain, A., and McMahon, F. G.: Response of diabetics treated with non-selective and relatively selective beta-adrenergic antagonists to insulin induced hypoglycemia. Submitted for publication.

41. Stornello, M., Di Roo, G., et al: Effects of salbutamal, indomethacin, and atenolol on insulin secretion. In J. Robertson, N. Kaplan, A. Caldwell, and T. Speight (Eds.): *Drugs, Symposium on Beta-Blockers in the 1980s,* ADIS Press Australasia Pty. Limited, NSW Australia, 1982, p. 255.

42. Sotaniemi, E. A., Anttila, M., et al: Propranolol and sotalol metabolism after a drinking party. *Clin. Pharmacol. Ther.,* **29**(6):705–710, 1981.

43. McLean, A. J., Isbister, C., Bobik, A., and Dudley, F. J.: Reduction of first-pass hepatic clearance of propranolol by food. *Clin. Pharmacol. Ther.,* **30**(1):31–34, 1981.

44. Buhler, F. R., Burkert, F., et al: Antihypertensive beta blocking action as related to renin and age: A pharmacologic tool to identify pathogenetic mechanisms in essential hypertension. *Am. J. Cardiol.,* **36**:653–669, 1975.

45. Vestal, R. E., Wood, A. J. J., and Shand, D. G.: Reduced beta-adrenoceptor sensitivity in the elderly. *Clin. Pharmacol. Ther.,* **26**(2):181–186, 1979.

46. Kaplan, N. M.: *Clinical Hypertension,* Third Edition, Williams and Adkins, Baltimore, 1982, pp. 184, 191.

47. Theilade, P., et al: Propranolol influence on serum T₃ and reserve T₃ in hyperthyroidism. *Lancet,* **II**(8033):363, 1977.
48. Finnerty, F. A., Jr.: Initial therapy of essential hypertension: Diuretic or betablocker? *J. Fam. Pract.,* **11**(2):199, 1980.
49. Assaykeen, T. A., and Michell, G.: Metoprolol in hypertension: An open evaluation. *Med. J. Aust.,* **1**:73, 1982.
50. Henningsen, N. C., and Mattiasson, I.: Long-term clinical experience with atenolol—a new selective beta-1-blocker with few side effects from the central nervous system. *Acta Med. Scand.,* **205**:61, 1979.
51. Henning, R., Karlberg, B. E., et al: Timolol and hydrochlorothiazide–amiloride in primary hypertension. *Clin. Pharmacol. Ther.,* **28**(6):707, 1980.
52. Gonasun, L. M., and Langroll, H.: Adverse reactions to pindolol administration. *Am. Heart J.,* **104**(2 part 2):374, 1982.
53. Editorial: Hazards of non-practolol beta-blockers. *Br. Med. J.,* **1**(6060):529, 1977.
54. Stephen, S. A.: Unwanted effects of propranolol. *Am. J. Cardiol.,* **18**(3):463, 1966.
55. Greenblatt, D. J., and Koch-Weser, J.: Adverse reactions to propranolol in hospitalized medical patients: A report from the Boston Collaborative Drug Surveillance Program. *Am. Heart J.,* **86**(4):478, 1973.
56. Slome, R.: Withdrawal of propranolol and myocardial infarction. *Lancet,* **1**:156, 1973.
57. Miller, R. R., Olson, H. G., et al: Propranolol-withdrawal rebound phenomena. *N. Engl. J. Med.,* **293**(9):416, 1975.
58. Sable, D. L., Brammel, H. L., et al: Attenuation of exercise conditioning by beta-adrenergic blockade. *Circulation,* **65**(4):679, 1982.
59. Zeis, P. M., Thanopoulos, B., Pierroutsakos, I. N., and Koukoutsakis, P. M.: Complete atrioventricular block associated with propranolol therapy. *J. Pediatr.,* **98**(2): 326. 1981.
60. Conway, N., Seymour, J., and Gelson, A.: Cardiac failure in patients with valvular heart disease after use of propranolol to control atrial fibrillation. *Br. Med. J.,* **2**(599):213, 1968.
61. Watt, D. A.: Sensitivity to propranolol after digoxin intoxication. *Br. Med. J.,* **2**(615):413, 1968.
62. Geyskes, G. G., Stutterheim, A., et al: Comparison of the anti-hypertensive effect of propranolol and practolol combined with chlorthalidone. *Eur. J. Clin. Pharmacol.,* **9**(2–3):85, 1975.
63. Stephen, S. A.: Cardiac failure with propranolol. *Br. Med. J.,* **2**(602):428, 1968.
64. Lewis, D. O.: Side effects of propranolol. *Br. Med. J.,* **2**(513):588, 1966.
65. Frithz, G.: Letter: Toxic effects of propranolol on the heart. *Br. Med. J.,* **1**(6012): 769, 1976.
66. Gupta, K., Lichstein, E., and Chadda, K. D.: Transient atrioventricular standstill. Etiology and management. *Jama,* **234**(10):1038, 1975.
67. Swanson, H., Beauchamp, G. D., et al: Reversible cardiogenic shock after low dose oral propranolol. *J. Kans. Med. Soc.,* **76**(11):260, 1975.
68. Aviado, D. M.: Drug action, reaction, and interaction. II. Iatrogenic cardiopathies. *J. Clin. Pharmacol.,* **15**(10):641, 1975.
69. Pettinger, W. A.: Beta-blocking therapy: Propranolol. *Postgrad. Med. J.,* **56**(5):68, 1974.
70. Abraham, A. S., and Menczel, J.: Letter: Brady-tachy syndrome with prolonged

retrograde conduction due to digitalis and propranolol intoxication. *Chest,* **67**(5): 627, 1975.

71. Gotsman, M. S.: Acute pulmonary edema from sensitivity to beta-sympathetic blockade. *S. Afr. Med. J.,* **44**(38):1097, 1970.

72. Greenblatt, D. J., and Koch-Weser, J.: Adverse reactions to beta-adrenergic receptor blocking drugs. *Drugs,* 7:118, 1974.

73. Frohlich, E. D., Tarazi, R. C., and Dustan, H. P.: Peripheral arterial insufficiency. A complication of beta-adrenergic blocking therapy. *JAMA,* **208**(13):2471, 1969.

74. Marshall, A., Barritt, D. W., and Roberts, C. J.: Letter: Raynaud's phenomenon as side effect of beta-blockers. *Br. Med. J.,* **2**(6030):301, 1976.

75. Lant, A. F., and Gibbons, D. O.: Letter: Intermittent claudication complicating beta-blockade. *Br. Med. J.,* **1**(6023):1469, 1976.

76. Marsden, C. W., and Bayliss, P. F.: Letter: Raynaud's phenomenon as side effect of beta-blockers *Br. Med. J.,* **2**(6028):176, 1976.

77. Marshall, A. J., Roberts, C. J., and Barritt, D. W.: Raynaud's phenomenon as side effect of beta-blockers in hypertension. *Br. Med. J.,* **1**(6024):1498, 1976.

78. Rodger, J. C., Sheldon, C. D., et al: Intermittent claudication complicating beta-blockade. *Br. Med. J.,* **1**(6018):1125, 1976.

79. Satya-Murti, S., et al: Possible propranolol myotonia association. *N. Engl. J. Med.,* **297**:223, 1977.

80. Shenkman, L.: Hyperthyroidism after propranolol withdrawal. *JAMA,* **238**:237, 1977.

81. Greico, M. H., and Pierson, R. N.: Mechanisms of bronchoconstriction due to beta-adrenergic blockade. Studies with practolol, propranolol and atropine. *J. Allergy Clin. Immunol.,* **48**(3):143, 1971.

82. Gaddie, J., and Skinner, L.: Risk with beta-blockers in bronchial asthma. *Br. Med. J.,* **1**(749):749, 1972.

83. Skinner, C., Gaddie, J., and Palmer, K. N.: Comparison of effects of metoprolol and propranolol on asthmatic airway obstruction. *Br. Med. J.,* **1**(6008):504, 1976.

84. Beumer, H. M.: Adverse effects of beta-adrenergic receptor blocking drugs on respiratory function. *Drugs,* **7**(1):130, 1974.

85. Hinshelwood, R. D.: Hallucinations and propranolol. *Br. Med. J.,* **2**(654):445, 1969.

86. Fitzgerald, J. D.: Propranolol-induced depression. *Br. Med. J.,* **2**(548):372, 1967.

87. Waal, H. J.: Propranolol-induced depression. *Br. Med. J.,* **2**(543):50, 1967.

88. Yorkston, N. J., Zaki, S. A., et al: Safeguards in the treatment of schizophrenia with propranolol. *Postgrad. Med. J.,* **52**(Suppl 4):175, 1976.

89. Shopsin, B., Hirsch, J., and Gershon, S.: Visual hallucinations and propranolol. *Biol. Psychiatry,* **10**(1):105, 1975.

90. Simpson, T.: Propranolol and hypoglycemia. *Lancet,* **1**(488):508, 1967.

91. Kotler, M. N., Berman, L., and Rubenstein, A. H.: Hypoglycemia precipitated by propranolol. *Lancet,* **2**(478):1389, 1966.

92. Mackintosh, T. F.: Propranolol and hypoglycemia. *Lancet,* **1**(481):104, 1967.

93. Hesse, B., and Pedersen, J. R.: Hypoglycemia after propranolol in children. *Acta Med. Scand.,* **193**:551, 1973.

94. Wray, R., and Sutcliffe, S. B. J.: Propranolol-induced hypoglycemia and myocardial infarction. *Br. Med. J.,* **2**:592, 1973.

95. Seltzer, H. S.: Drug-induced hypoglycemia: A review of 473 cases. *Diabetes,* **21**(9):955, 1972.

96. Weled, B. J., Ball, J., and Hofeldt, F. D.: The hypoglycemic hazards of propranolol in diabetic patients: Case reports. *Milit. Med.*, **145**:705, 1980.
97. Kallen, R. J., Mohler, J. H., and Lin, H. L.: Hypoglycemia: A complication of treatment of hypertension with propranolol. *Clin. Pediatr.*, **19**:567, 1980.
98. Weiner, P., Pelled, B., Alster, R., and Plavnick, L.: Propranolol-induced hypoglycemia in a non-diabetic patient during acute coronary insufficiency. *Isr. J. Med. Sci.*, **18**:725, 1982.
99. Belton, P., Carmody, M., Donohoe, J., and O'Dwyer, W. F.: Propranolol associated hypoglycaemia in non-diabetics. *J. Ir. Med. Assoc.*, **73**:173, 1980.
100. Hannaway, P. J., and Hopper, G. D. K.: Severe anaphylaxis and drug-induced beta-blockade (letter). *N. Engl. J. Med.*, **308**:1536, 1983.
101. Ahmad, S.: Sclerosing peritonitis and propranolol. *Chest,* **79**(3):361, 1981.
102. Bauer, J.: Effects of propranolol therapy on renal function and body fluid composition. *Arch. Intern. Med.*, **143**:927, 1983.
103. Falch, D. K., Odegaard, A. E., and Norman, N.: Decreased renal plasma flow during propranolol treatment in essential hypertension. *Acta Med. Scand.*, **205**:91, 1979.
104. O'Connor, D. T., Preston, R. A., and Sasso, E. H.: Renal perfusion changes during treatment of essential hypertension: Prazosin versus propranolol. *J. Cardiovasc. Pharmacol.*, **1**(Suppl):S38, 1979.
105. de Leeuw, P. W., and Birkenhager, W. H.: Renal response to propranolol treatment in hyperensive humans. *Hypertension,* **4**(1):125, 1982.
106. Wilcox, C. S., and Lewis, P. S., et al: Renal function, body fluid volumes, renin, aldosterone, and noradrenaline during treatment of hypertension with pindolol. *J. Cardiovasc. Pharmacol.*, **3**:598, 1981.
107. Schauer, I., Schauer, U., Ruhling, K., and Thielmann, K.: The effect of propranolol treatment on total cholesterol, HDL cholesterol, triglycerides, postheparin lipolytic activity and lecithin: Cholesterol acyltransferase in hypertensive individuals. *Artery,* **8**(2):146, 1980.
108. Gemma, G., Montanari, G., et al: Plasma lipid and lipoprotein changes in hypertensive patients treated with propranolol and prazosin. *J. Cardiovasc. Pharmacol.*, **4**(Suppl 2):S233, 1982.
109. Leren, P., Helgeland, A., et al: Effect of propranolol and prazosin on blood lipids: The Oslo Study. *Lancet,* **II**:4–6, 1980.
110. Johnson, B. F.: The emerging problem of plasma lipid changes during antihypertensive therapy. *J. Cardiovasc. Pharmacol.*, **4**(Suppl 2):S213–S221, 1982.
111. Kristensen, B. O., Steiness, E., and Weeke, J.: The pathogenesis of propranolol-withdrawal syndrome in essential hypertension. *Clin. Sci.*, **57**:417s, 1979.
112. Rangno, R. E., Langlois, S., and Stewart, J.: Cardiac hyper- and hyporesponsiveness after pindolol withdrawal. *Clin. Pharmacol. Ther.*, **31**(5):564, 1982.
113. Diaz, R. G., Somberg, J. C., et al: Withdrawal of propranolol and myocardial infarction. *Lancet,* **1**:1068, 1973.
114. Nellen, A.: Propranolol withdrawal and myocardial infarction. *Lancet,* **1**(7802):558, 1973.
115. Alderman, E. L., Davies, R. O., et al: Dose response effectiveness of propranolol for the treatment of angina pectoris. *Circulation,* **51**(6):964, 1975.
116. Rubin, P. C.: Beta-blockers in pregnancy. *N. Engl. J. Med.*, **305**:1323, 1982.
117. Gladstone, G. R., Hordof, A., and Gersony, W. M.: Propranolol administration during pregnancy. *J. Pediatr.*, **86**:962, 1975.

118. Habib, A., and McCarthy, J. S.: Effects on the neonate of propranolol administered during pregnancy. *J. Pediatr.*, **91**:808, 1977.

119. Cottril, C. M., McAllister, R. G., et al: Propranolol therapy during pregnancy, labor, and delivery: Evidence for transplacental drug transfer and impaired neonatal drug disposition. *J. Pediatr.*, **91**:812, 1977.

120. Lieberman, B. A., Stirrat, G. M., Cohen, S. L., Beard, R. W., and Pinker, G. D.: The possible adverse effect of propranolol on the fetus in pregnancies complicated by severe hypertension. *Br. J. Obstet. Gynaecol.*, **85**:678, 1978.

121. Tynan, R. F., Fisher, M. McD., and Ibels, L. S.: Self-poisoning with propranolol. *Med. J. Aust.*, **1**:82, 1981.

122. Shand, D. G.: Comparative pharmacology of the beta-adrenoceptor blocking drugs. In J. Robertson, N. Kaplan, A. Caldwell, and T. Speight (Eds.): *Drugs, Symposium on Beta-Blockers in the 1980s*, ADIS Press Australasia Pty Limited, NSW Australia, 1982, p. 92.

123. Cruickshank, J. M.: How safe are beta-blockers? In J. Robertson, N. Kaplan, A. Caldwell, and T. Speight (Eds.): *Drugs, Symposium on Beta-Blockers in the 1980s*, ADIS Press Australasia Pty Limited, NSW Australia, 1982, p. 331.

124. The Norwegian Multicenter Study Group: Timolol-induced reduction in mortality and reinfarction in patients surviving acute myocardial infarction. *N. Engl. J. Med.*, **304**(14):801–807, 1981.

125. Wilhelmsson, C., and Vedin, J. A.: Duration of action of different beta-blockers. In L. Hansson, S. Julius, and P. J. Richardson (Eds.): *Proceedings of the Timolol Intercontinental Symposium*, Stockholm, Sweden, October 27–28, 1979, Merck, Sharp & Dohme Int., West Point, Pa., 1981, pp. 19–25.

126. Yu, P. N.: Multicenter evaluation of timolol in the treatment of mild to moderate essential hypertension. In L. Hansson, S. Julius, and P. J. Richardson (Eds.): *Proceedings of the Timolol Intercontinental Symposium*, Stockholm, Sweden, October 27–28, 1979, Merck, Sharp & Dohme Int., West Point, Pa., 1981, pp. 329–344.

127. Alcocer, L., Arce, E., and Aspe, J.: The cardiovascular and metabolic profile of timolol maleate in the treatment of hypertension. In L. Hansson, S. Julius, and P. J. Richardson (Eds.): *Proceedings of the Timolol Intercontinental Symposium*, Stockholm, Sweden, October 27–28, 1979, Merck, Sharp & Dohme Int., West Point, Pa., 1981, pp. 175–188.

128. Tocco, D. J., Abrams, W. B., and Nancarrow, J. F.: Lipid solubility and the central nervous system effects of timolol and propranolol. In L. Hansson, S. Julius, and P. J. Richardson (Eds.): *Proceedings of the Timolol Intercontinental Symposium*, Stockholm, Sweden, October 27–28, 1979, Merck, Sharp & Dohme Int., West Point, Pa., 1981, pp. 55–65.

Labetalol

1. Koch, G.: Haemodynamic adaptation at rest and during exercise to long-term antihypertensive treatment with combined alpha- and beta-adrenoreceptor blockade by labetalol. *Br. Heart J.*, **41**:192–198, 1979.

2. McNeil, J. J., and Louis, W. J.: A double-blind crossover comparison of pindolol, metoprolol, atenolol and labetalol in mild to moderate hypertension. *Br. J. Clin. Pharmacol.*, **8**(Suppl 2):163S–166S, 1979.

3. Williams, L. C., Murphy, M. J., and Parsons, V.: Labetalol in severe and resistant hypertension. *Br. J. Clin. Pharmacol.*, **8**:143S–147S, 1979.

4. Smith, W. B., Clifton, G. G., O'Neill, W. M., et al: The use of intravenous labetalol to lower blood pressure in the patient with accelerated hypertension. *Clin. Pharmacol. Ther.*, in press.

5. Cummings, A. M. M., Brown J. J., et al: Blood pressure reduction by incremental infusion of labetalol in patients with severe hypertension. *Br. J. Clin. Pharmacol.*, 8:359–364, 1979.

6. Cummings, A. M. M., Brown J. J., et al: Treatment of severe hypertension by repeated bolus injections of labetalol. *Br. J. Clin. Pharmacol.*, 8:199S–204S, 1979.

7. Michelson, E. L., Langford, H. G., et al: *Clinical Synopsis—Labetalol: The Effects of Acute Intravenous and Subsequent Oral Labetalol Treatment in Hypertensive Patients Requiring Urgent Blood Pressure Reduction (C81-009).* Schering Corporation, Bloomfield, N. J., 1982, pp. 1–31.

8. Bailey, R. R.: Labetalol in the treatment of a patient with pheochromocytoma: A case report. *Br. J. Clin. Pharmacol.*, 8:141S–142S, 1979.

9. Agabiti, R. E., Brown J. J., et al: Treatment of pheochromocytoma and of clonidine withdrawal hypertension with labetalol. *Br. J. Clin. Pharmacol.*, Suppl:809–815, 1976.

10. Rosenthal, R., Rabinowitz, B., et al: Use of labetalol in hypertensive patients during discontinuation of clonidine therapy. *Eur. J. Clin. Pharmacol.*, 20:237–240, 1981.

11. Hurley, D. M., Vandongen, R., and Beilin, L. J.: Failure of labetalol to prevent hypertension due to clonidine withdrawal. *Br. Med. J.*, 1:1122, 1979.

12. Scott, D. B.: The use of labetalol in anaesthesia. *Br. J. Clin. Pharmacol.*, 13(Suppl 1):133S–155S, 1982.

13. Breckenridge, A., Orme, M., et al: Labetalol in essential hypertension. *Br. J. Clin. Pharmacol.*, 13(Suppl 3):37S–39S, 1982.

14. Brogden, R. N., Heel, R. C., et al: Labetalol: A review of its pharmacology and therapeutic uses in hypertension. *Drugs*, 15:251–270, 1978.

15. Prichard, B. N. C., and Richards, D. A.: Comparison of labetalol with other antihypertensive drugs. *Br. J. Clin. Pharmacol.*, 13(Suppl 1):41s–47s, 1982.

16. Kane, J. A.: Labetalol in general practice. *Br. J. Clin. Pharmacol.*, 13(Suppl 1):59s–63s, 1982.

17. Dargle, H. J., Dollery, C. T., and Daneil, J.: Labetalol in resistant hypertension. *Br. J. Clin. Pharmacol.*, 3(Suppl 3):751–755, 1976.

18. Myera, J., Morgan, T., et al: Long-term experiences with labetalol. *Med. J. Aust.*, 1:665–666, 1980.

19. Kristensen, B. O., and Peterson, E. L. C.: Effects of long-term high-dose labetalol on blood pressure in patients with severe hypertension resistant to previous therapy. *Postgrad. Med. J.*, 56(Suppl 2):57–59, 1980.

20. New Zealand Hypertension Study Group: A multicenter open trial of labetalol in New Zealand. *Br. J. Clin. Pharmacol.*, 8(Suppl 2):179s–182s, 1979.

21. Williams, L. C., Murphy, M. J., and Parsons, V.: Labetalol in severe and resistant hypertension. *Br. J. Clin. Pharmacol.*, 8(Suppl 2):143s–147s, 1979.

22. Stern, N., Telcher, A., and Rosenthal, T.: The treatment of hypertension by labetalol—a new alpha- and beta-adrenoceptor blocking agent. *Clin. Cardiol.*, 5:125–130, 1982.

23. Preziosl, P., Pisanti, N., et al: Urinary catecholamines and labetalol. *Arch. Int. Pharmacodyn.*, 236:317–319, 1978.

24. Kane, J., Gregg, I., and Richards, D. A.: A double-blind trial of labetalol. *Br. J. Clin. Pharmacol.*, 3(Suppl 3):737–741, 1976.

25. Takeda, T., Kaneko, Y., et al: The use of labetalol in Japan: Results of multicentre clinical trials. *Br. J. Clin. Pharmacol.*, **13**(Suppl 1):49s–57s, 1982.

26. Milne, B. J., and Logan, A. G.: Labetalol: Potent antihypertensive agent that blocks both alpha- and beta-adrenergic receptors. *Can. Med. Assoc. J.*, **123**:1013–1016, 1980.

27. Larochelle, P., Hamet, P., et al: Labetalol in essential hypertension. *J. Cardiovasc. Pharmacol.*, **2**:751–759, 1980.

28. Horvath, J. S., Caterson, R. J., et al: Labetalol and bendrofluazide: Comparison of their antihypertensive effects. *Med. J. Aust.*, **1**:626–628, 1979.

29. Dawson, A., Johnson, B. F., and Smith, I. K.: Comparison of the effects of labetalol, bendrofluazide and their combination in hypertension. *Br. J. Clin. Pharmacol.*, **8**:149–154, 1979.

30. Bloomfield, S., Sinkfield, A., et al: Labetalol with hydrochlorothiazide for moderate essential hypertension (abstract). *Clin. Pharmacol. Ther.*, **31**:204–205, 1982.

31. Lifshitz, A. A., McMahon, F. G., et al: Combined trichlormethiazide and labetalol therapy in moderate to severe hypertension (abstract). *Clin. Pharmacol. Ther.*, **23**:118, 1978.

32. Lechi, A., Pomarie, S., et al: Clinical evaluation of labetalol alone and combined with chlorthalidone in essential hypertension: A double-blind multicentre controlled study. *Eur. J. Clin. Pharmacol.*, **22**:289–293, 1982.

33. Prichard, B. N. C., and Richards, D. A.: Labetalol, an alpha- and beta-adrenoceptor-blocking agent: Its use in therapeutics. *Br. J. Clin. Pharmacol.*, **8**(Suppl):2395–2445, 1979.

34. Rosei, E. A., et al: Labetalol, an alpha- and beta-adrenergic blocking drug in the treatment of hypertension. *Am. Heart J.*, **93**:124–125, 1977.

35. New Zealand Hypertension Study Group: A multicentre study of labetalol in hypertension. *N. Z. Med. J.*, **93**:215–218, 1981.

36. Balasubramanian, V., et al: The effect of labetalol on continuous ambulatory blood pressure. *Br. J. Clin. Pharmacol.*, **8**(Suppl):119S–124S, 1979.

37. Sanders, G. L., et al: Interdose control of beta blockade and arterial blood pressure during chronic oral labetalol treatment. *Br. J. Clin. Pharmacol.*, **8**(Suppl):125S–128S, 1979.

38. Kane, J. et al: A long-term study of labetalol in general practice. *Br. J. Clin. Pharmacol.*, **8**(Suppl):167S–170S, 1979.

39. Prichard, B. N. C., and Boakes, A. J.: Labetalol in long-term treatment of hypertension. *Br. J. Clin. Pharmacol.*, **3**(Suppl):743–750, 1976.

40. Dustan, H., Weber, M., et al: Multicentric, double-blind parallel group, efficacy/safety comparison of labetalol and propranolol in long-term treatment of mild to moderate essential hypertension. Schering Corporation (in press).

41. Omar, M. A., Wesley, A. G., and Pather, M.: Labetalol in severe tetanus. *Br. Med. J.*, **2**:274, 1979.

42. Bonomi, L., Perfetti, S., et al: Ocular hypotensive action of labetalol in rabbit and human eyes. *Albrecht Von Graefes, Arch. Klin. Exp. Ophthalmol.*, **217**:175–181, 1981.

43. Wallin, J. D., and Oneill, W. M.: Labetalol, current research and therapeutic status. *Arch. Intern. Med.*, **143**:485–490, 1983.

44. MacCarthy, E. P., and Bloomfield, S. S.: Labetalol: A review of its pharmacology, pharmacokinetics, clinical uses and adverse effects. *Pharmacotherapy*, **3**(4):193–219, 1983.

45. Mehta, J., and Cohn, J. N.: Hemodynamic effects of labetalol, an alpha- and beta-adrenergic blocking agent, in hypertensive subjects. *Circulation*, **55**:370–375, 1977.
46. Koch, G.: Cardiovascular dynamics after acute and long-term alpha- and beta-adrenoceptor blockade at rest, supine and standing, and during exercise. *Br. J. Clin. Pharmacol.*, **8**(Suppl 2):101s–105s, 1979.
47. Svendsen, T. L., Rasmussen, S., and Hartling, O. J.: Sequential haemodynamic effects of labetalol at rest and during exercise in essential hypertension. *Postgrad. Med. J.*, **56**(Suppl 2):21–26, 1980.
48. Beilin, L. J., and Juel-Jensen, B. E.: Alpha and beta adrenergic blockade in hypertension. *Lancet*, **2**:979, 1972.
49. Dent, R., and Killaway, G. S. M.: A pilot study of labetalol (AH 5158A), a combined alpha and beta blocker in the treatment of hypertension. *N. Z. Med. J.*, **86**:213, 1977.
50. Fagard, R., Amery, A., Reybronck, T., Lijnen, P. and Billiet, L.: Response of the systemic and pulmonary circulation to alpha and beta receptor blockade (labetalol) at rest and during exercise in hypertensive patients. *Circulation*, **60**:1214, 1979.
51. Frick, M. H., and Porsti, P.: Combined alpha and beta adrenoreceptor blockade with labetalol in hypertension. *Br. Med. J.*, **1**:1046, 1976.
52. Richards, D. A., Tuckman, J., and Prichard, B. N. C.: Assessment of alpha and beta adrenoreceptor blocking actions of labetalol. *Br. J. Clin. Pharmacol.*, **3**:849, 1976.
53. Richards, D. A.: Pharmacological effects of labetalol in man. *Br. J. Clin. Pharmacol.*, (Suppl):721–723, 1976.
54. Riley, A. J.: Some further evidence for partial agonist activity of labetalol. *Br. J. Clin. Pharmacol.*, **9**:517–518, 1980.
55. Rosei, E. A., Trust, P. M., et al: Effects of intravenous labetalol on blood pressure, angiotensin II and aldosterone in hypertension: Comparison with propranolol. *Clin. Sci. Mol. Biol.*, **51**:497S–499S, 1976.
56. Trust, P. M., Rosei, E. A., et al: Effect of blood pressure, angiotensin II and aldosterone concentrations during treatment of severe hypertension with intravenous labetalol: Comparison with propranolol. *Br. J. Clin. Pharmacol.*, (Suppl.):799–803, 1976.
57. Lijnen, P. J., Amery, A. K., Fagard, R. H., et al: Effects of labetalol on plasma renin, aldosterone, and catecholamines in hypertensive patients. *J. Cardiovasc. Pharmacol.*, **1**:625–632, 1979.
58. Prichard, B. N. C., Thompson, F. O., et al: Some haemodynamic effects of compound AH 5158 compared with propranolol, propranolol plus hydralazine, and diazoxide: The use of AH 5158 in the treatment of hypertension. *Clin. Sci. Mol. Med.*, **48**:97s–100s, 1975.
59. Joekes, A. M., and Thompson, F. D: Acute hemodynamic effects of labetalol and its subsequent use as an oral hypotensive agent. *Br. J. Clin. Pharmacol.*, **3**(Suppl 3):789–793, 1976.
60. Bahlmann, J., Brod, J., et al: Effect of an alpha- and beta-adrenoceptor-blocking agent (labetalol) on haemodynamics in hypertension. *Br. J. Clin. Pharmacol.*, **8**(Suppl 2):113s–117s, 1979.
61. Trap-Jensen, J., Clausen, J. P., et al: Immediate effects of labetalol on central, splanchnic-hepatic, and forearm haemodynamics during pleasant emotional stress in hypertensive patients. *Postgrad. Med. J.*, **56**(Suppl 2):37–42, 1980.

62. Agabiti-Rosel, E., Allcandri, C. L., et al: The acute and chronic hypotensive effect of labetalol and the relationship with pre-treatment plasma noradrenaline levels. *Br. J. Clin. Pharmacol.*, **13**(Suppl 1):87s–92s, 1982.

63. Dunn, F. G., Oigman, W., et al: Hemodynamic effects of intravenous labetalol in essential hypertension. *Clin. Pharmacol. Ther.*, **33**:139–143, 1983.

64. Edwards, R. C., and Raftery, E. B.: Haemodynamic effects of long-term oral labetalol. *Br. J. Clin. Pharmacol.*, **3**(Suppl 3):733–736, 1976.

65. Lund-Johansen, P.: Comparative haemodynamic effects of labetalol, timolol, prazosin and the combination of tolamolol and prazosin. *Br. J. Clin. Pharmacol.*, **8**(Suppl 2):107s–111s, 1979.

66. Frishman, W. H., Strom, J. A., et al: Labetalol therapy in patients with systematic hypertension and angina pectoris: Effects of combined alpha- and beta-adrenoceptor blockade. *Am. J. Cardiol.*, **48**:917–928, 1981.

67. Mazzola, C., et al: Labetalol in acute management of malignant essential hypertension complicated by left ventricular failure. *Curr. Ther. Res.*, **28**:980–991, 1980.

68. Marx, P. G., and Reid, D. S.: Labetalol infusion in acute myocardial infarction with systemic hypertension. *Br. J. Clin. Pharmacol.*, **8**(Suppl):233S–238S, 1979.

69. Mazzola, C., et al: Acute antihypertensive and antiarrhythmic effects of labetalol. *Curr. Ther. Res.*, **29**:613–633, 1981.

70. Daneshmend, T. K., and Roberts, C. J. C.: Cimetidine and bioavailability of labetalol. Letter to the Editor, *Lancet*, **1**:565, 1981.

71. Hunter, J. M.: Synergism between halothane and labetalol. *Anaesthesia*, **34**:257–259, 1979.

72. Kaufman, L.: Use of labetalol during hypotensive anaesthesia and in the management of phaeochromocytoma. *Br. J. Clin. Pharmacol.*, **8**(Suppl):229S–232S, 1979.

73. Scott, D. B., et al: Circulatory effects of labetalol during halothane anaesthesia. *Anaesthesia*, **33**:145–156, 1978.

74. Scott, D. B., et al: Cardiovascular effects of labetalol during halothane anesthesia. *Br. J. Clin. Pharmacol.*, **3**(Suppl):817–821, 1976.

75. Nyberg, G., et al: Heart rate and blood pressure response to isometric exercise after sublingual nitroglycerine in hypertensive male subjects: A controlled study of propranolol and labetalol for two weeks. *Curr. Ther. Res.*, **25**:400–405, 1979.

76. Kane, J. A.: Labetalol in general practice: A review. *Br. J. Clin. Pharmacol.*, **13**(Suppl. 1):59S–63S, 1982.

77. Besterman, E. M. M., and Spencer, M.: Open evaluation of labetalol in the treatment of angina pectoris occurring in hypertensive patients. *Br. J. Clin. Pharmacol.*, **8**(Suppl):205S–209S, 1979.

78. Lubbe, W. F., and White, D. A.: Labetalol in hypertensive patients with angina pectoris—beneficial effect of combined alpha- and beta-adrenoceptor blockade. *Clin. Sci. Mol. Med.*, **55**(Suppl):283S–286S, 1978.

79. Rosei, E. A., et al: Treatment of phaeochromocytoma and of clonidine withdrawal hypertension with labetalol. *Br. J. Clin. Pharmacol.*, **3**(Suppl):809–815, 1976.

80. Reach, G., et al: Effect of labetalol on blood pressure and plasma catecholamine concentrations in patients with phaeochromocytoma. *Br. Med. J.*, **280**:1300–1301, 1980.

81. Feek, C. M., and Earnshaw, P. M.: Hypertensive response to labetalol in phaeochromocytoma. Letter to the Editor, *Br. Med. J.*, **281**:387, 1980.

82. Briggs, R. S. J., et al: Hypertensive response to labetalol in phaeochromocytoma. Letter to the Editor, *Lancet*, **4**:1045–1046, 1978.

83. Kanto, J. Allonen, H., et al: Pharmacokinetics of labetalol in healthy volunteers. *Int. J. Clin. Pharmacol. Ther. Toxicol.*, **19**:41–44, 1981.
84. Martin, L. E., Hopkins, R., and Bland, R.: Metabolism of labetalol by animals and man. *Br. J. Clin. Pharmacol.*, **3**(Suppl 3):695–710, 1976.
85. Reid, J. L., Merredith, P. A., and Elliott, H. L.: Labetalol and the management of hypertension. *J. Cardiovasc. Pharmacol.*, **3**(Suppl 1):S60–S68, 1981.
86. Truelove, J. F., VanPetten, G. R., and Willes, R. F.: Action of severe adrenoceptor blocking drugs in the pregnant sheep and fetus. *Br. J. Pharmacol.*, **47**:161–171, 1973.
87. Michael, C. A.: Use of labetalol in the treatment of severe hypertension during pregnancy. *Br. J. Clin. Pharmacol.*, **8**(Suppl 2):211–215, 1979.
88. Richards, D. A., et al: Sympathomimetic amine infusion after beta-adrenergic and parasynpathetic blockade. *Br. J. Clin. Pharmacol.*, **7**:429P (Abstract), 1979.
89. Richards, D. A., and Jackson J. L.: Postclinical surveillance of labetalol. In *Labetalol: Proceedings of a Symposium*. Florence, April 1979, European Society of Cardiology/Glaxo.
90. Lilja, M., Jounela, A. J., and Karppanen, H.: Comparison of labetalol and clonidine in hypertension. *Eur. J. Clin. Pharmacol.*, **21**:363–367, 1982.
91. Andersson, O., Berglund G., and Hansson, L.: Antihypertensive action, time of onset and effects on carbohydrate metabolism of labetalol. *Br. J. Clin. Pharmacol.*, **3**(Suppl 3):757–761, 1976.
92. Wasi-Manning, H. J., and Simpson, F. O.: Review of long-term treatment with labetalol. *Br. J. Clin. Pharmacol.*, **13**(Suppl 1):65s–73s, 1982.

CHAPTER VIII

ALPHA-ADRENERGIC BLOCKING AGENTS

- PRAZOSIN (MINIPRESS®)
- TRIMAZOSIN (CARDOVAR®)
- PHENOXYBENZAMINE HCL (DIBENZYLINE®)
- PHENTOLAMINE HCL (REGITINE®)

PRAZOSIN (Minipress®)
Introductory year: 1976

INTRODUCTION:

Prazosin, a quinazoline derivative (Figure 1) and a selective alpha-1-adrenergic antagonist, is effective in the treatment of hypertension and is often helpful in congestive heart failure. Unlike the non-selective alpha-adrenergic antagonists or the direct vasodilators, prazosin's hypotensive effect usually does not produce significant tachycardia or increase plasma renin or plasma catecholamines. Prazosin is quite versatile in that it can be used alone to treat mild to moderate hypertension or in combination to treat severe hypertension. The antihypertensive effect exceeds the plasma half-life and may be prolonged even further with chronic therapy.

As a vasodilator, prazosin is equipotent with respect to capacitance and resistance vessels, thus reducing cardiac preload and afterload. This characteristic is particularly beneficial in the treatment of patients with severe congestive heart failure. The dose of prazosin should be reduced in cardiac patients with hepatic involvement because approximately 90% of the drug is excreted via the bile into the feces.

The principle side effect of prazosin, postural dizziness, is related to the initial dose and a pre-existing hypovolemia; other side effects seldom limit therapy. The physician prescribing prazosin should be aware that the optimal hypotensive effect may not be evident for approximately six weeks.

Formulation
Capsules...1 mg (white), 2 mg (pink-white) and 5 mg (blue-white)

Dose in Hypertension
Frequency: given 2–3 times daily
Initial: 1 mg 3 times a day
Range: a) *single agent.* Dosage should be slowly titrated according to the individual patient's blood pressure response. The therapeutic range is usually between 6–15 mg/day, but a few patients may benefit from doses up to 40 mg/day.
b) *combined therapy.* Reduce dose to the initial level; then slowly retitrate.
Usual Dose: 6–15 mg in divided doses

Mechanism of Action
The hemodynamic effects of prazosin in hypertensive and congestive heart failure patients are due to its competitive blockade of vascular post-synaptic alpha-1 adrenergic receptors.[1-6] The vasodilatation produced by this selective alpha-1 block is seen in both the capacitance and resistance vessels which reduce cardiac preload and afterload. In contrast to other alpha blockers that are non-selective, prazosin does not usually increase heart rate, plasma renin or plasma norepinephrine.[7-12]

Hemodynamic studies have been carried out in man following

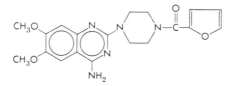

Figure 1: Structure of prazosin.

acute single-dose administration and during the course of long-term maintenance therapy. The results confirm that the therapeutic effect is a fall in blood pressure without a concomitant clinically significant change in cardiac output, heart rate, renal blood flow or glomerular filtration rate. There is no measurable negative chronotropic effect.[13]

Absorption, Metabolism, Excretion

Prazosin is readily absorbed after oral administration and reaches peak plasma levels in 2–3 hrs.[14] Ingestion of food does not appear to affect the rate of absorption or the peak levels although both parameters vary markedly among individuals.[15] Thereafter the concentration of prazosin declines according to first order kinetics with a half-life of 3–4 hrs.[16] The half-life of prazosin's antihypertensive effect appears to be considerably longer. Prazosin is 97% protein-bound and it is only during the initial period of therapy that plasma concentrations correlate well with its antihypertensive effects.[17]

Prazosin is almost exclusively metabolized in the liver by conjugation and demethylation to metabolites with minimal bioactivity. The "first pass" metabolism is significant with more than 90% of the dose being excreted via the bile into the feces. In the presence of hepatic disease, the physician should reduce the dose accordingly.

Prazosin doses need not be reduced in renal failure. Also, in mild azotemia prazosin does not decrease renal blood flow or the glomerular filtration rate so that usual dose can be utilized. Plasma renin activity (PRA) was thought to be reduced by prazosin, but more recently, PRA has been shown to increase.[18] The degree of change of PRA does not correlate with prazosin's antihypertensive effects, further substantiating prazosin's specific alpha-1 blocking activity.

When should the physician consider utilizing prazosin?

- Prazosin is effective as a single agent in the treatment of mild to moderate hypertension. It is particularly useful in patients who cannot tolerate diuretics (e.g., gout, hyperglycemia) or beta-adrenergic blockers (e.g., asthma and heart failure).
- When thiazide diuretics given alone fail to reduce blood pressure adequately, the addition of prazosin as a Step-2 drug should be considered.
- In patients who do not tolerate other Step-2 drugs (e.g., methyldopa), prazosin is frequently beneficial.
- Prazosin has its widest application as an adjunct to beta-adrenergic

342 • MANAGEMENT OF ESSENTIAL HYPERTENSION

blocking agents and thiazide diuretics.[19] This "triple therapy" is effective in moderate to severe hypertensive patients when hydralazine has failed. "Triple therapy" is particularly useful when treating severe renal hypertension.[20,21] Prazosin causes little change in glomerular filtration rate and renal blood flow and has even been shown to improve renal function.

- Prazosin has a role in the treatment of severe congestive heart failure. Prazosin is a balanced vasodilator that relaxes both the venous and arterial vasculature. Venous dilation decreases right and left heart filling pressure while relaxation of the systemic and pulmonary vasculature reduces ventricular afterload. Together these changes increase the cardiac index without increasing heart rate and are associated with marked improvement in the functional class of the congestive heart failure patient.

- Recent reports indicate prazosin may be very effective in the treatment of Raynaud's vasospasm.[22,23] In patients with vasospasm of the small digital arteries, prazosin induced and maintained a dramatic subjective and clinical improvement of digital blood flow.[22] Although this response has been confirmed in other patients, a controlled therapeutic trial is needed to define prazosin's role in this syndrome.

How effective is prazosin?

Prazosin is a versatile agent that can be used alone or in combination to control various levels of hypertension. As a single agent approximately 50% of patients with mild to moderate hypertension respond to 6 mg/day while 70% respond to 10 mg doses. As a Step-3 agent in "triple therapy" low doses of prazosin reduce the blood pressures of severe hypertensives where other antihypertensive agents may fail. Compared with other agents, one mg of prazosin is approximately equivalent to 140 mg methyldopa, 40 mg propranolol,[24] 20 mg hydralazine[25] and 0.75 mg of bendroflumethiazide.[19]

Table I displays the efficacy of prazosin alone and in combination with a diuretic. In combination the efficacy of the two agents is additive. The addition of other agents to prazosin augments the hypotensive response. Tables II and III show the results of many controlled studies, including double-blind studies comparing prazosin with methyldopa, hydralazine and in combination with methyldopa and/or a diuretic.

TABLE I
SUMMARY OF STUDIES COMPARING EFFICACY OF PRAZOSIN VS. DIURETICS:
ALONE AND IN COMBINATION

Study (Ref.)	No. of Patients	Pre-Rx Blood Pressure	Post-Rx with Prazosin	Post-Rx with Diuretics	Post-Rx with Combination
Gould et al[26]	13	164/92	157/88	—	—
Seedat et al[27]	10	186/111	166/95	154/93 (polythiazide)	145/91
Schirger et al[28]	25	178/127	140/93	—	—
	20	174/124	—	— (cyclopenthiazide)	137/95
Pitkajarvi et al[29]	14	160/101	—	137/87 (HCTZ)	—
	14	152/98	151/93	—	—
Guevara et al[30]	14	158/107	—	143/101 (polythiazide)	126/93
De La Paz et al[31]	11	122*	105	—	—
	14	136*	—	—	110*
Smith et al[32]	20	166/101	129/85	—	—
	9	178/118	—	—	141/96*
Blaufox et al[33]	20	136*	128	— (polythiazide)	112
Okun et al[34]	23	184/118	161/106	— (polythiazide)	129/89
Leren[35]	18	151/102	—	—	132/86

* Mean arterial pressure

Gould et al[26] studied prazosin given alone and with beta-blocking agents, measuring intra-arterial pressure in 20 patients after 10 months of therapy. Blood pressure declined only 7/6 mm Hg with prazosin alone and it was effective in only 30% of his patients. Only 13 completed his study, withdrawing chiefly for adverse side effects. Treatment with prazosin plus beta-blockers reduced pressure by 24/6 mm

TABLE II

SUMMARY OF FOUR-STEP CLINICAL EVALUATION OF PRAZOSIN'S EFFICACY*

Type of Study	Position	Mean Decreased Blood Pressure With Prazosin Alone (mm Hg)	Mean Decreased Blood Pressure With Thiazide Alone (mm Hg)	Mean Decreased Blood Pressure With Methyldopa Alone (mm Hg)	Mean Decreased Blood Pressure With Hydralazine (mm Hg)	Mean Decreased Blood Pressure With Prazosin, Methyldopa and Thiazide (mm Hg)
Prazosin–placebo comparison studies	supine	14/10	—	—	—	—
	erect	18/14	—	—	—	—
4 Open-label comparison studies	supine	10/8 (60)**	12/8 (65)**	—	—	—
	erect	10/11 (60)	15/10 (65)	—	—	—
1 Double-blind comparison study vs. thiazide	supine	12/8 (18)	18/5 (16)	—	—	—
	erect	11/8 (18)	20/6 (16)	—	—	—
7 Double-blind comparison studies vs. methyldopa	supine	17/11 (89)	—	21/13 (76)	—	—
	erect	20/12 (88)	—	24/14 (77)	—	—
1 Double-blind comparison study vs. hydralazine (both with thiazide)	sitting	9/9 (92)	—	—	5/8 (106)	—
	erect	10/9 (92)	—	—	7/8 (106)	—
1 Open-label randomized comparison study	sitting	—	—	—	—	20/14 (14)
	erect	—	—	—	—	25/17 (14)

* From Pitts, N. E., The clinical evaluation of prazosin hydrochloride, a new antihypertensive agent. In: *Prazosin—Evaluation of a New Antihypertensive Agent.* Amsterdam: Excerpta Medica, 1974. Reprinted with permission.

** Numbers of patients on the drug from which the means were evaluated.

TABLE III
FALL IN MEAN ARTERIAL PRESSURE (mm Hg)
WITH COMBINATION TREATMENTS

	Beta-blocker and prazosin	Beta-blocker and bendro-flumethiazide	Beta-blocker prazosin, and bendro-flumethiazide	Statistical significance (p-value)
Supine	21 ± 11	13 ± 13	30 ± 12	0.01
Standing	25 ± 10	18 ± 12	35 ± 11	0.005
Post-Exercise	26 ± 15	16 ± 12	38 ± 14	0.01

* From McMahon, F. G.[36]

Hg. Mild tachycardia and postural hypotension occurred with prazosin alone. These authors recommended using prazosin together with a beta-blocker for optimal benefit.

Drug Interactions

— Additional antihypertensive agents should be introduced into the patient's regimen with caution. When adding a diuretic or other antihypertensive agent, the dose of prazosin should be reduced to 1 mg or 2 mg three times daily and then retitrated.

— Hypotension may develop in patients given prazosin who are also receiving a beta-blocker such as propranolol.

— Increased plasma levels of low density lipoproteins (LDL) are associated with an increased risk of ischemic heart disease. Treatment of hypertensives with thiazides and/or beta-blockers has been shown to increase plasma LDL. Prazosin decreases LDL and when added to the "triple therapy" regimen, it tends to ameliorate the effects of thiazides and beta-blockers on LDL.[37-41]

Warnings

• *In patients with syncopal syndromes:*

Prazosin may cause syncope with sudden loss of consciousness. In most cases this is believed to be due to an excessive postural hypotensive effect, perhaps in a patient predisposed by sodium depletion.[41] Occasionally, the syncopal episode has been preceded by a bout of severe tachycardia with heart rates of 120–160 beats per minute. Syncopal episodes have usually occurred within 30 to 90 minutes of the initial dose of the drug; occasionally they have been reported in association with rapid dosage increases or the introduction of another antihypertensive drug into the regimen of a patient taking high doses of prazosin. The incidence of syncopal episodes is approximately 1% in patients given an initial dose of 2 mg or greater. Clinical trials conducted during the investigational phase of this drug suggest that syncopal episodes can be minimized by limiting the initial dose of the drug to 1 mg, by subsequently increasing the dosage slowly, and by introducing any additional antihypertensive drugs into the patient's regimen with caution. Many physicians give the initial 1 mg dose at bedtime to minimize the postural syncopal episode occasionally seen.

If syncope occurs, the patient should be placed in the recumbent position and treated supportively as necessary. The adverse effect is self-limiting and in most cases does not recur after the initial period of therapy or during subsequent dose titration.

Patients should always be started on 1 mg capsules of prazosin. The 2 and 5 mg capsules are not intended for initial therapy.

More common than loss of consciousness are the symptoms often associated with lowering of blood pressure, i.e., dizziness and lightheadedness. The patient should be cautioned about these possible adverse effects and advised what measures to take should they develop. The patient should also be cautioned to avoid situations where injury could result should syncope occur during the initiation of prazosin therapy.

Use in Pregnancy

Although no teratogenic effects were seen in animal testing, the safety of prazosin in pregnancy has not been established. Prazosin is not recommended during pregnancy unless the potential benefit outweighs potential risk to mother and fetus.

Management of Overdosage

Accidental ingestion of at least 50 mg of prazosin in a two-year-old child resulted in profound drowsiness and depressed reflexes. No decrease in blood pressure was noted. Recovery was uneventful.

Should overdosage lead to hypotension, support of the cardiovascular system is of primary concern. Restoration of blood pressure and normalization of heart rate may be accomplished by keeping the patient in the supine position. If this measure is inadequate, shock should first be treated with volume expanders. If necessary, vasopressors such as metaraminol should be used. Renal function should be monitored and supported as needed. Laboratory data indicate prazosin is protein bound and non-dialyzable.

Side Effects

Approximately nine percent of patients given prazosin discontinued their treatment because of intolerance to medication. Table IV shows the results from a randomized double-blind clinical trial comparing the side effects of prazosin and hydralazine.[42]

Of the three side effects with statistical differences, only postural dizziness remained significant with chronic therapy. Despite these side effects, patient compliance was similar for both drugs.[42]

It should be noted that these later studies do show an increase in the percentage of side effects, compared with those during the investi-

TABLE IV
SIDE EFFECTS[42]

Adverse Reaction	Prazosin Administration n = 92		Hydralazine Administration n = 106	
	No. of Patients	%	No. of Patients	%
Anorexia	5	5.4	5	4.7
Weakness	32	34.8	37	34.9
Orthostatic Dizziness	44	47.8††	28	26.4
Lethargy	34	37.0*	27	25.5
Headaches	37	40.2	42	39.6
Dyspnea on effort	44	47.8	44	41.5
Angina	11	12.0	9	8.5
Palpitations	26	28.3	29	27.4
Skin rash	8	8.7	11	10.4
Arthritis	23	25.0	20	18.9
Sexual Dysfunction	30	32.6†	21	19.8
Depression	13	14.1	10	9.4
Nightmares	18	19.6†	8	7.5
Ulcer symptoms	13	14.1	12	11.3
Other	49	53.3	57	53.8

From Ramirez, E. A., Comparison of prazosin with hydralazine in patients receiving hydro-chlorothiazide. *Circulation*, 64(4):776, 1981. Reprinted by permission of the American Heart Association, Inc.
Significance between regimens:
* P < 0.1
† P < 0.05
†† P < 0.01

gational period.[12] The major troublesome side effect of the first-dose phenomenon can be greatly minimized by utilizing a low initial dose and slowly titrating upward. Laboratory findings have shown no trend or suggestion of any significant hematologic, renal, liver, or other serious toxicity.

Receptor Classification
Diagram Figures 2 and 3 (proposed model)

- Vascular alpha adrenergic receptors are classified as alpha-1 and alpha-2. Originally it was thought that alpha-1 was a post-synaptic excitatory receptor while alpha-2 was a pre-synaptic inhibitory receptor. Recent work has shown that alpha-1 receptors are indeed post-synaptic and excitatory, but that alpha-2 receptors are located both pre- and post-synaptically and are both inhibitory and excitatory respectively (see Figures 2 and 3).

- Alpha-1 activation by *synaptically* released norepinephrine may cause a release of internally stored Ca^{++} ions resulting in a vasopressor response.

- Alpha-2 post-synaptic activation by non-specific *circulating* norepinephrine causes an influx of interstitial Ca^{++} resulting in a vasopressor response.

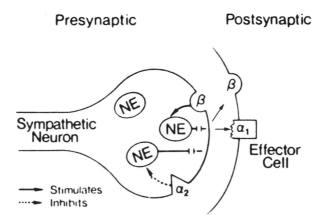

Figure 2: Adrenergic nerve ending on blood vessels. Norepinephrine (NE) is released from the adrenergic nerve terminal and interacts with specific alpha-1 and -2 end beta receptors, causing typical alpha-1 responses: vasoconstriction of the arteries and veins and increased peripheral vascular resistance. The presynaptic alpha-2 receptors mediate a reduction in catecholamine production. The beta-receptors (beta-1 and beta-2) produce an increased heart rate and force of contraction, an increased cardiac output, bronchodilation, glycogenolysis, and renin release from the kidney.

- Alpha-2 pre-synaptic activation by synaptically released norepinephrine inhibits the further release of norepinephrine resulting in vasodilation.
- Prazosin's specific action is to block peripheral alpha-1 receptors

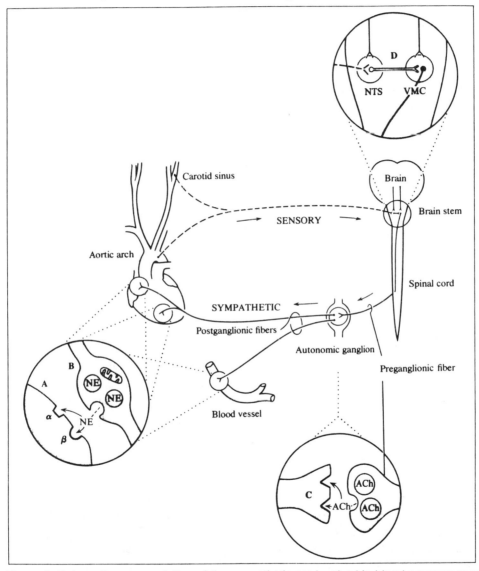

Figure 3: Schematic representation of the sympathetic arc involved in blood pressure regulation and sites where drugs may act to influence the system. (A) receptors on effector cell; (B) adrenergic varicosity; (C) nicotinic receptors (postganglionic fibers); (D) brain system nuclei. NTS = nucleus of the tractus solitarii; VMC = vasomotor center; ACh = acetylcholine; NE = norepinephrine; α = alpha-adrenoceptors; β = beta-adrenoceptors.

competitively. This attenuates the vasopressor response to synaptically released norepinephrine or to exogenously administered alpha-agonists like phenylephrine. Prazosin does not interact with alpha-2 receptors; thus it does not inhibit the negative feedback loop of the pre-synaptic receptor from decreasing norepinephrine release. These combined actions result in low levels of synaptic norepinephrine and reversal of the vasopressor effect.

- Centrally acting antihypertensive agents (e.g., clonidine, methyldopa, and guanabenz) are alpha-2 agonists. Stimulation of the alpha-2 receptors in the nucleus tractus solitarius decreases sympathetic outflow producing vasodilatation.

TRIMAZOSIN (Cardovar®)
Introductory year: 1984

Trimazosin is a new orally active antihypertensive agent derived from the quinazoline family, related chemically and pharmacologically to prazosin, but possessing several pharmacodynamic advantages over its predecessor. Unlike prazosin, no first-dose syncope has been noted, and no tolerance in the management of long-term hypertensive patients. Trimazosin exerts its hypotensive effect through arteriolar dilatation. The mechanism of action was originally thought to be direct effect,[1,2] but more recent evidence indicates it is a relatively selective alpha-1 antagonist,[3,4] with the added benefit of some direct vascular smooth muscle relaxation. The designation of alpha-1 refers to drug selectivity and not location or function of the blockade. Thus, trimazosin does not interfere with the negative-feedback regulation of norepinephrine release.

The hypotensive effect of trimazosin has been found to be dose-related. In a study of 10 hypertensive patients, McMahon et al found that low doses of trimazosin (60–150 mg per day) produced no hypotensive response but doses up to 900 mg per day were well tolerated and produced significant reductions in blood pressure.[4] Weber et al[5] studied trimazosin in 25 patients with mild to moderate hypertension using doses of 300–900 mg a day. Sixty-four percent of his patients had normalization of blood pressure (diastolic < 90 mm Hg or a fall of at least 10 mm Hg). In this 6-month study no changes were noted in plasma renin activity or urinary aldosterone excretion. When polythiazide was added to trimazosin, five of seven previously uncontrolled patients had good control. Chrysant et al[6] studied 26 patients with mild essential hypertension, 13 of whom received trimazosin and 13 received placebo. Incremental doses of 25, 50, 100, 200, and 300 mg given 3 times daily were utilized. Placebo-treated patients had no significant decrement in blood pressure, compared with good responses to trimazosin at the 600–900 mg doses. Hemodynamic studies showed a decrease in peripheral vascular resistance with no change in cardiac output. No significant effect on plasma renin activity, cholesterol, triglycerides, creatinine, glucose or uric acid were noted. No hematologic or liver function abnormalities were found. Chrysant et al,[7] studying 16 male patients at his V. A. hospital, reported a dose response with single doses of 50 mg, 100 mg, and 200 mg (p values were respectively < 0.05, < 0.01, and < 0.005). He also obtained a statistically significant and dose-related increase in pulse rates in the same patients. Furthermore, he noted trimazosin to significantly increase renal blood flow while having no effect on glomerular filtration rate or plasma renin levels. Most clinical reports have not been able to identify significant hypotensive responses to these low doses but rather require doses in the 300–900 mg per day range. Vlachakis et al[8] reported significant decrements in blood pressure in 9 essential hypertensive patients given daily doses of 300–500 mg over a period of 4 16 weeks. However, normalization of blood pressure was achieved in only 5 subjects in the recumbent position.

Several reports of excellent responses to trimazosin in the treatment of refractory heart failure have appeared in the recent literature.[9-12]

Side effects to trimazosin therapy are apparently mild and few. The reported incidence of the most common complaints, orthostatic hypotension and dizziness, varies from 0 to 10%. Other reported side effects include headache, drowsiness, excitement, restlessness, nausea, difficulty micturating, diminished hearing, chest pain, insomnia, and gastrointestinal distress.

Formulation

Tablet sizes: .... 50, 100, and 150 mg

Dose in Hypertension

Frequency: twice daily
Initial: 50 mg twice daily
Range: 100–900 mg/day total dose, but given in twice daily doses
Usual Dose: 300 mg/day given in divided doses

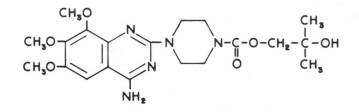

Figure 4. Molecular structure of trimazosin.

PHENOXYBENZAMINE HCL (Dibenzyline®)
PHENTOLAMINE HCL (Regitine®)

INTRODUCTION:

These two drugs are very rarely useful in the management of hypertension, but are of importance in helping understand the alpha-adrenergic mechanisms.

To reduce hypertension by inhibition of sympathetic vasoconstriction without producing untoward side effects, the blockade of alpha-adrenergic receptors with a variety of synthetic compounds has attracted medicinal chemists and pharmacologists for several decades. This approach has been ill-fated (until the discovery of prazosin) by the fact that efferent adrenergic pathways operating through alpha receptors play a critical role in the cardiovascular reflexes that permit man to ambulate. Two drugs available for many years have had limited utility in the management of hypertension: phenoxybenzamine and phentolamine (Figure 5).

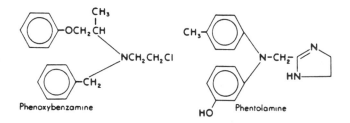

Figure 5: Structure of two clinically-useful alpha-adrenergic blockers.

Phenoxybenzamine is available in 10 mg capsules for use in early Raynaud's disease, acrocyanosis, frostbite and other vasospastic diseases. It is useful also in the management of preoperative or inoperable pheochromocytoma. It has had little success when tried as an antihypertensive agent clinically, largely because of excessive adverse side effects, particularly postural hypotension, tachycardia, impotence, miosis and nasal congestion. These side effects result from alpha-adrenergic blockade, per se, so the drug's use has been very limited as an antihypertensive.

Pharmacological tests for pheochromocytoma have been largely replaced today by more diagnostic biochemical tests. Occasionally, however, the phentolamine (Regitine®) test may be used in patients who are suspected of having pheochromocytoma. While the patient's pressure is elevated and fairly stable, a 5 mg intravenous dose of phentolamine mesylate is administered as a bolus. Blood pressure should be monitored frequently and regularly until it returns to control values. A fall of greater than 35/25 mm Hg within two minutes of injection is considered a positive test. Because of many adverse reactions and also because of an excessively high incidence of false-positive tests and many false-negative responses as well, this test has been virtually replaced by biochemical procedures. Urinary vanillymandelic acid (VMA), free catecholamines, metanephrines with normetanephrines, and, more recently, plasma catecholamine radioimmunoassays have now essentially replaced the older pharmacological test.

Phentolamine, in doses of 5 mg intravenously, is not without its adverse effects. Deaths have even occurred from arrhythmias or acute myocardial infarction. Generally, tachycardia, dizziness, hyperperistalsis, and lightheadedness are frequent side effects.

Orally, 50 mg of phentolamine hydrochloride tablets are available for use in the preoperative preparation of patients with pheochromocytoma. The usual dose is 50 mg 4 to 6 times daily. During surgery, phentolamine may need to be given intravenously to control hyper-epinephrinemia with its tachycardia, hypertension and, sometimes, convulsions.

In addition to phentolamine tests and preparative use, a third use for phentolamine is the prevention of dermal slought (add 10 ml to each liter of solution containing norepinephrine), or the treatment of burning, resulting whenever infused norepinephrine infiltrates, to help relieve symptoms and sloughing (use 5–10 ml in 10 ml saline).

REFERENCES:

Prazosin

1. Bolli, P., Wood, A. J., Phelan, E. L., et al: Prazosin: Preliminary clinical and pharmacological observations. *Clin. Sci. Mol. Med.*, 48(2):177s–179s, 1975.
2. Cavero, I., Lefevre, F.: Cardiovascular effects of prazosin in spontaneously hypertensive rats (SHR). *Clin. Exp. Pharmacol. Physiol.*, 4(3):61–64, 1977.
3. Oates, H. E., Graham, R. M., Stoker, L. M., et al: Haemodynamic effects of prazosin. *Arch. Int. Pharmacodyn. Ther.*, 224:239–247, 1976.
4. Graham, R. M., Oates, H. F., Stoker, L. M., et al: Alpha blocking action of the antihypertensive agent, prazosin. *J. Pharmacol. Exp. Ther.*, 201:747–752, 1977.
5. Oates, H. F., Graham, R. M., Stokes, G. S.: Mechanism of the hypotensive action of prazosin. *Arch. Int. Pharmacodyn. Ther.*, 227:41–48, 1977.
6. Stokes, G. S., Oates, H. F.: Prazosin: New alpha-adrenergic blocking agent in treatment of hypertension. *Cardiovasc. Med.*, 3:41–57, 1978.
7. Graham, R. M., and Pettinger, W. A.: Effects of prazosin and phentolamine on arterial pressure, heart rate, and renin activity: Evidence in the conscious rat for the functional significance of the presynaptic alpha-receptor. *J. Cardiovasc. Pharmacol.*, 1:497–502, 1979.
8. Saeed, M., Sommer, O., Holtz, J., Bassenge, E.: Alpha-adrenoceptor blockade by phentolamine causes alpha-adrenergic vasodilation by increased catecholamine release due to presynaptic alpha-blockade. *J. Cardiovasc. Pharmacol.*, 4:44–52, 1982.
9. Koshy, M. C., Mickley, D., Bougignie, J., Blaufox, M. D.: Physiologic evaluation of a new antihypertensive agent: Prazosin HCl. *Circulation*, 55:533–537, 1977.
10. DeLeeuw, P. W. Wester, A., Willemse, P. J., and Birkenhager, W. H.: Effects of prazosin on plasma noradrenaline and plasma renin concentrations in hypertensive subjects. *J. Cardiovasc. Pharmacol.*, 2(3):S361–S372, 1980.
11. Massingham, R., and Hayden, M. L.: A comparison of the effects of prazosin and hydralazine on blood pressure, heart rate and plasma renin activity in conscious renal hypertensive dogs. *Eur. J. Pharmacol.*, 30:121–124, 1975.
12. Pitts, N. E.: The clinical evaluation of prazosin hydrochloride, a new antihypertensive agent. In D. W. K. Cotton (Ed.): *Prazosin—Evaluation of a New Antihypertensive Agent*. Amsterdam: Excerpta Medica, 1974, pp. 149–163.
13. Koshy, M. C., Mickley, O., et al: Physiologic evaluation of a new antihypertensive agent: Prazosin HCl. *Circulation*, 55(3):533, 1977.
14. Wood, A. J.: Pharmacokinetics of prazosin in man. Presentation to Annual Meeting, *Aust. Soc. Clin. Exper. Pharmacol.*, Dec., 1974.
15. Verbesselt, R. M., Mullie, A., Tjandramaga, T. G., et al: The effect of food intake on the plasma kinetics and tolerance of prazosin. *Acta Therapeutica*, 2:27, 1976.
16. Wood, A. J., Bolli, P., and Simpson, F. O.: Prazosin in normal subjects: Plasma levels, blood pressure and heart rate. *Br. J. Clin. Pharmacol.*, 3:199–201, 1976.
17. Graham, R. M., Thornell, I. R., Gain, J. M., et al: Prazosin: The first-dose phenomenon. *Br. Med. J.*, 2:1293–1294, 1976.
18. Morganti, A., Sala, C., Palermo, A., Turolo, L., Zanchetti, A., and Laragh, J.: Dissociation of the effects of alpha$_1$-adrenergic blockade on blood pressure and renin release in patients with essential hypertension. *J. Cardiovasc. Pharmacol.* 4:S158–S161, 1982.

19. Marshall, A. J., Barritt, D. W., Pocock, J., et al: Evaluation of beta blockade, bendrofluazide, and prazosin in severe hypertension. *Lancet,* **1**:271–274, 1977.

20. Hayes, J. M., Graham, R. M., O'Connell, B. P., et al: Experience with prazosin in the treatment of patients with severe hypertension. *Med. J. Aust.,* **1**:562–564, 1976.

21. Curtis, J. A., and Bateman, F. J. A.: Use of prazosin in management of hypertension in patients with chronic renal failure and in renal transplant recipients. *Br. Med. J.,* **4**:432–434, 1975.

22. Waldo, R.: Prazosin relieves Raynaud's vasospasm. *JAMA,* **241**:1037, 1979.

23. Harper, F. E., and KeRoy, E. C.: Raynaud's phenomenon: An update on treatment. *J. Cardiovasc. Med.,* **7**:282–290, 1982.

24. Stokes, G. S., and Weber, M.A.: Prazosin: Preliminary report and comparative studies with other antihypertensive agents. *Br. Med. J.,* **2**:298–300, 1974.

25. Stokes, G. S., and Oates, H. F.: Prazosin: New alpha-adrenergic blocking agent in treatment of hypertension. *Cardiovasc. Med.,* **3**:41–57, 1978.

26. Gould, B. A., Hornung, R. S., Dleso, H. A., Cashman, P. M., and Raftery, E. B.: Prazosin alone and combined with beta-adrenoreceptor blockers in treatment of hypertension. *J. Cardiovasc. Pharmacol.,* **5**:678–687, 1983.

27. Seedat, Y. K., North-Coombes, D., and Rampono, J. G.: Prazosin in the treatment of hypertension. *South Afr. Med. J.,* **49**:1741, 1975.

28. Schirger, A., and Sheps, S.: Prazosin—a new hypertensive agent: A double-blind cross-over study in the treatment of hypertension. *JAMA,* **237**:989, 1977.

29. Pitkajarvi, T., Kyostila, S., et al: Antihypertensive action of drug combination: Polythiazide, prazosin and tolamolol. *Curr. Ther. Res.,* **21**(2):169, 1977.

30. Guevara, J., Collet-Velasco, H., and Velasco, M.: Antihypertensive effect of prazosin alone and its combination with polythiazide in patients with essential hypertension. *Curr. Ther. Res.,* **20**(6):751, 1976.

31. De La Paz, A. G., Reyes, A. L., De Guia, R., et al: A new quinazoline derivative in the treatment of hypertension; a cooperative study in four medical centers in the Philippines. *Philippine J. Cardiol.,* **4**:47, 1975.

32. Smith, I. S., Fernandes, M., Kim, K. E., et al: A three-phase clinical evaluation of prazosin. *Postgrad. Med. Spec. Report,* November:53, 1975.

33. Blaufox, M. D., Ross, L., Koshy, K., and Lee, Hyu-Bok: Physiologic effects of prazosin HCL: Consequences of diuretic combination therapy. *Nephron,* **29**:85–89, 1981.

34. Okun, R., and Maxwell, M.: Long-term antihypertensive therapy with prazosin plus a diuretic. *J. Cardiovasc. Pharmacol.,* **1**(Suppl):S21–S27, 1979.

35. Leren, P., Helgeland, A., Holme, I., Foss, P. O., Hjermann, I., and Lund-Larsen, P. G.: Effect of propranolol and prazosin on blood lipids. The Oslo study. *Lancet,* **2**:4–6, 1980.

36. McMahon, F. G.: *Management of Essential Hypertension.* Futura Publishing Co., Mount Kisco, N. Y., 1978, p. 284.

37. Kirkendall, W. M., Hammond, J. J., Thomas, J. C., Overturf, M. L., and Zama, A.: Prazosin and clonidine for moderately severe hypertension. *JAMA,* **240**:2553–2556, 1978.

38. Lowenstein, J., and Neusy, A. J.: The biochemical effects of antihypertensive agents and the impact on atherosclerosis. *J. Cardiovasc. Pharmacol.,* **3**(Suppl 3):S256–S260, 1981.

39. Kokubu, T., Itoh, I., Kurita, H., Ochi, T., Murata, K., and Yuba, I.: Effect of prazosin on serum lipids. *J. Cardiovasc. Pharmacol.,* **3**(Suppl 3):S199–S206, 1981.

40. Velasco, M., Silva, H., Morillo, J., Pellicer, R., Urbina-Quintana, A., and Hernandez-Pieretti, O.: Effect of prazosin on blood lipids and on thyroid function in hypertensive patients. *J. Cardiovasc. Pharmacol.*, 3(Suppl 3):S193–S198, 1981.
41. Stokes, G. S., Graham, R. M., et al: Influence of dosage and dietary sodium on the first-dose effects of prazosin. *Br. Med. J.*, 2:1507, 1977.
42. Ramirez, E. A.: Comparison of prazosin with hydralazine in patients receiving hydrochlorothiazide. *Circulation*, 64(4):772, 1981.

Trimazosin

1. DeGuia, D., Mendlowitz, M., Russo, C., Vlachakis, N., and Antram, S.: The effect of trimazosin in essential hypertension. *Curr. Ther. Res.*, 15:339–348, 1973.
2. Vlachakis, N., Mendlowitz, M., and Deguzman, D.: Treatment of essential hypertension with trimazosin, a new vasodilator agent. *Curr. Ther. Res.*, 17:564–569, 1975.
3. Singleton, W.: Postjunctional selectivity of alpha-blockade with prazosin, trimazosin, and UK-33,274 in man. *J. Cardiovasc. Pharmacol.*, 4:S145–S151, 1982.
4. Taylor, C. R., et al: Comparative pharmacology and clinical efficacy of newer agents in treatment of heart failure. *Am. Heart J.*, 102(3):515–532, 1981.
5. Weber, M. A., Brewer, D. D., et al: A vasodilator that avoids renin stimulation and fluid retention; antihypertensive treatment with trimazosin. *Clin. Pharmacol. Ther.*, 33(5):572–578, 1982.
6. Chrysant, S. G., Miller, R. F., Brown, J. L., and Danisa, K.: Long-term hemodynamic and metabolic effects of trimazosin in essential hypertension. *Clin. Pharmacol. Ther.*, 30:600–604, 1981.
7. Chrysant, S. G., Luu, T. M., Danisa, K., Kem, D. C., and Maninn, C. V.: Systemic and renal hemodynamic effects of trimazosin; a new vasodilator. *J. Cardiovasc. Pharmacol.*, 2:205–214, 1980.
8. Valchakis, N. D., Mendlowitz, M., and DeGuzman, D. D. G.: Treatment of essential hypertension with trimazosin, a new vasodilator agent. *Curr. Ther. Res.*, 17(6):564–569, 1975.
9. Taylor, D. J. E., and Bell, A. J.: Treatment of refractory heart failure with trimazosin. *Eur. Heart J.*, 2:127–133, 1981.
10. Awan, N. A., Hermanovich, J., Vera, Z., Amsterdam, E. A., and Mason, D. T.: Cardiocirculatory actions of trimazosin and sodium nitroprusside in ischemic heart disease. *Clin. Pharmacol. Ther.*, 31:290–295, 1982.
11. Taylor, C. R., et al: Comparative pharmacology and clinical efficacy of newer agents in treatment of heart failure. *Am. Heart J.*, 102(2):515–533, 1981.
12. Webber, K. T., Kinasewitz, G. T., et al: Long-term vasodilator therapy with trimazosin in chronic cardiac failure. *N. Engl. J. Med.*, 303:242–250, 1980.

CHAPTER IX

ORAL, DIRECT VASODILATORS

- HYDRALAZINE (APRESOLINE®)
- MINOXIDIL (LONITEN®)

HYDRALAZINE (Apresoline®)
Introductory year: 1951

INTRODUCTION:

Hydralazine has been available for the treatment of hypertension for over 33 years. In spite of its potential for producing serious adverse reactions, it is probably more widely used today, and indeed more helpful in managing moderate and severe hypertension than ever before. Shortly after hydralazine was introduced, it was noted that its effectiveness was limited by its adverse reactions. These reactions were the result of hydralazine being administered as the lone antihypertensive agent in large doses which were often intolerable. As a result, hydralazine fell into relative disuse. However, in recent years, hydralazine has been experiencing renewed therapeutic utilization as part of a "triple combination" therapy. As an oral vasodilator, given with a beta-blocking agent and a diuretic, hydralazine is finding good patient acceptance with few side effects at low doses. The daily dosage of hydralazine should not ordinarily exceed 200 mg.

When should a physician consider hydralazine in hypertension?
- Orally, as an adjunct to combination therapy (a diuretic plus a beta- or adrenergic-blocker) in moderate and severe hypertension. The drug decreases total peripheral resistance[1] which is the single most important and frequent hemodynamic finding in chronic hypertensive patients.

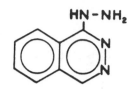

Figure 1: Structure of hydralazine.

- Orally, as an adjunct to other therapy in malignant or accelerated hypertension.[2,3]
- Orally, as an adjunct in combination therapy of essential hypertension complicated by renal insufficiency. Hydralazine is not likely to improve renal function except as a by-product of better blood pressure control; yet, neither will it worsen glomerular filtration rate nor renal blood flow, as do guanethidine, reserpine, and the thiazides.[2,4-6]
- Orally, as an adjunct in combination therapy of essential hypertension complicated by congestive heart failure characterized by lowered cardiac output, pump failure, and high ventricular impedance or preload. The drug must be used with caution as it may precipitate angina or myocardial ischemia. Hydralazine can worsen congestive heart failure by its sodium retaining effect unless administered with a diuretic. Yet, hydralazine may help reverse the failure by increasing heart rate, cardiac contractability, and cardiac output.[6,7]
- Intravenously, in hypertensive crisis. Other drugs, including nitroprusside and diazoxide, are faster acting and generally preferred for this use except in cases of acute glomerulonephritis, lupus nephritis, pre-eclampsia, or eclampsia.[2,8,9]

The principal clinical usefulness of oral hydralazine is as an adjunct to other drugs. Nevertheless, hydralazine has antihypertensive activity in its own right. Five separate studies show the drug to produce a rough, dose-related response (Table I). The reductions in the mean arterial pressure (MAP) were 8, 5, 10, 15 and 16 mm Hg, corresponding to daily total doses of 75, 100, 120, 200 and 750 mg.[4,10-13] The use of hydralazine in hypertensive crises by IV administration shows good response by dropping the MAP 10 and 15 mm Hg in a few minutes.[14,15]

Hydralazine usage has been limited by several potentially serious side effects; among them is the reflex sympathetic stimulation with a tachycardia and increased cardiac output. The increase in cardiac output can reduce the antihypertensive effect of the vasodilator by as much as 75%.[9] In the 1950s Perry, Schroeder, and Morrow, in a series of

TABLE I
EFFICACY OF HYDRALAZINE ALONE

Study (Ref.)†	Average Dose (mg/day)	No. of Patients	Duration of Therapy (wks)	Pre-Rx MAP** (mm Hg)	Post-Rx MAP (mm Hg)	Decline in MAP (mm Hg)
Persson et al[11]	75	30	3	137	129	8
West ct al[12]	100	12	6	116	111	5
Aenishanslin et al[10] ††	120	16	12	120	110	10
Silas et al[13] *	200	17	5	113	98	15
Moyer et al[4]	754	54	12	158	142	16

† See reference section to this chapter for complete information regarding sources.
†† The Aenishanslin study involved dihydralazine which is converted to hydralazine within the body. It has a similar efficacy, although it is slower in onset.
 * Drugs other than hydralazine were continued thoughout the study for ethical reasons.
** MAP = mean arterial pressure = 1/3 pulse pressure.

reports, demonstrated the effectiveness of chronic hydralazine treatment in controlling hypertension and in reducing the related morbidity and mortality.[16-21] Their reduction in diastolic blood pressure averaged as much as 45 mm Hg. Their hydralazine doses ranged as high as 470 to 590 mg/day. As a result, toxicity included 44 instances of systemic lupus-like syndromes among 316 patients. Present hydralazine therapy is generally limited to doses up to 200 mg/day and therefore side effects are considerably fewer and less severe.

Hydralazine is often given with a diuretic when the latter fails to reduce the pressure adequately. In a Veterans Administration Multi-Clinic Cooperative Study reported by Ramirez et al, 121 patients showed an additional decrease in MAP of 7 mm Hg after treatment with hydrochlorothiazide[22] (Table II). Four other separate studies, including another Veterans Administration Multi-Clinic Cooperative Study, showed the thiazide-hydralazine regimen produced a mean

TABLE II
EFFICACY OF THE COMBINATION OF
HYDRALAZINE WITH HYDROCHLOROTHIAZIDE

Study (Ref)†	Mean Doses†† (mg/day)		No. of Patients	Duration of Therapy (wks)	Pre-Rx MAP (mm Hg)	Post-Rx MAP (mm Hg)	Decline In MAP From Double Rx (mm Hg)
	H	T					
Aoki et al[23]	200	100	10	12	130	109	21
Zacest* et al[24]	182	100	23	2-5	141	133	8
Siitonen et al[25]	200	25	61	4	135	125	10
Freis[26]	200	1000**	37	12	122	110	12
Ramirez* et al[22]	116	75	121	24	112	105	7

†† H = hydralazine; T = hydrochlorothiazide.
 * Both studies by Zacest's and Ramirez's pre-therapy MAP is actually the MAP after diuretic therapy.
** The V. A. Study used chlorothiazide as the diuretic.

decrease in MAP of 11 mm Hg in mild, moderate and severe hypertension.[23-26]

The most popular current use for hydralazine is the so-called "triple therapy" regimen where hydralazine is administrated in addition to a thiazide and a beta-blocker. The net effect of these three drugs makes "triple therapy" very appealing and rational therapy for moderate or severe hypertension. Hydralazine reverses vasoconstriction, which is almost always present in established hypertension. The beta-blocker inhibits the reflex increase in heart rate and the increase in renin release, both being secondary to hydralazine administration. The diuretic compensates for the tendency of the hydralazine to retain sodium which in turn decreases the extracellular fluid compartment (Figure 2). Finally, many studies have shown that "triple therapy" permits reduced dosages of hydralazine and beta-blocker which minimize their major side effects.[27-29]

Andersson et al demonstrated that "triple therapy" administered to ten patients, after they had received no antihypertensive medication for one month, showed a decrement in MAP of 36 mm Hg[30] (Table III).

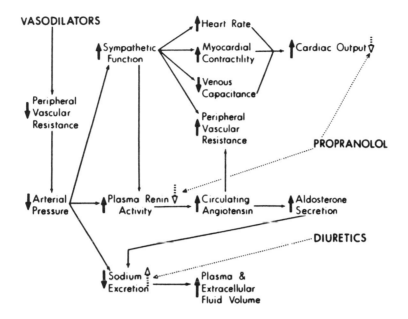

Figure 2: Primary and secondary effects of vasodilator therapy in primary hypertension and pharmacologic prevention of undesirable secondary effects. From Koch-Weser, J., *Archives of Internal Medicine*, 133:1018, 1974. Copyright 1974, American Medical Association. Reprinted with permission.

Pitkarjarvi et al, using only 75 mg/day of hydralazine in "triple therapy," reported a decrease of 27 mm Hg.[27] Forrest's studies show a decrease of 28 mm Hg in 397 patients.[31] Other studies report a more modest but significant 21 mm Hg average decrease in MAP.[28,29,32]

A combination of hydralazine and propranolol without a diuretic also produces significant lowering of blood pressure. In seven studies the mean reduction in MAP was 21 mm Hg (Table IV).[11,32,34-37] However, the addition of a thiazide diuretic to propranolol and hydralazine in the Veterans Administration Multi-Clinic Cooperative Study of 1977 showed a further decrease in the MAP of 9 mm Hg.[32]

The value of a vasodilator in the triple therapy is underscored in five studies (Table V).[25,27-29, 32] Double therapy without hydralazine gives a mean reduction in the MAP of 21 mm Hg. This is significantly less than the 26 mm Hg mean reduction obtained in MAP in the triple therapy studies (Table III).[27-32]

A Veterans Administration Multi-Clinic Cooperative Study showed a modest but significant decline in MAP after the addition of 50–200 mg/day of hydralazine to a thiazide, beta-blocker, or in triple therapy.

TABLE III
EFFICACY OF THE TRIPLE COMBINATION
(THIAZIDE + BETA-BLOCKER + HYDRALAZINE)

Study (Ref)[†]	Mean/Dose[†††] (mg/day) T	P	H	No. of Patients	Duration of Therapy (wks)	Pre-Rx MAP (mm Hg)	Post-Rx MAP (mm Hg)	Decline in MAP (mm Hg)
Freis[33][°]	5–10	80–240	50–200	19	21	117	101	16
Thomas[32]	105	120–480	105	75	24–72	120	99	21
Andersson et al[30]	50	120–160	150–225	10	48	152	116	36
Pitkajarvi* et al[27]	3	200–400	38–75	12	12	144	117	27
Aronow et al[28]	100	20–60**	40–200	15	16	132	107	25
Forrest*** et al[31]	.5	160–320	200	397	6	142	114	28
Toumilehto et al[29]	25	200††	75	24	16	125	107	18

  [†] See reference section to this chapter for complete information regarding sources.
  * Pitkajarvi used practolol and cyclothiazide and .1–.5 mg/day of clonidine.
 ** Aronow used timolol in place of propranolol.
*** Forrest used oxprenolol in place of propranolol, and cyclopenthiazide in place of hydrochloro-thiazide.
 †† Toumilento used metropolol in place of propranolol.
††† T = hydrochlorothiazide; P = propranolol; H = hydralazine.
  [°] This V. A. study used bendroflumethiazide and nadolol instead of hydrochlorothiazide and pro-pranolol.

When hydralazine was added to the bendroflumethiazide, nadolol, and their combination, the MAP was reduced 6, 7 and 7 mm Hg, respectively.[33] (See Table VI.)

In general, the vasodilator is a major and effective component of chronic antihypertensive therapy (Table VII). However, there are numerous cases when therapeutic doses (200 mg/day) of hydralazine have been too weak to be helpful optimally. In these cases, new and more potent orally-effective vasodilators, like minoxidil, are needed.[2,38]

Hydralazine, intravenously, has been used in hypertensive crisis. The onset of action is delayed 10–20 minutes. The dose, the frequency of administration, and the therapeutic effectiveness are variable.[9,15] Other vasodilators—nitroprusside and diazoxide—are preferred except in cases of acute glomerulonephritis, lupus nephritis, pre-eclampsia, or

TABLE IV
EFFICACY OF THE COMBINATION OF HYDRALAZINE WITH A BETA-ADRENERGIC BLOCKER

Study (Ref.)[†]	Mean Dose[††] (mg/day) P	Mean Dose[††] (mg/day) H	No. of Patients	Duration of Therapy (wks)	Pre-Rx MAP (mm Hg)	Post-Rx MAP (mm Hg)	Decline in MAP Double Rx (mm Hg)
Persson[11]	15	75	30	6	137	107	30
Thomas[32]	120–480	105	75	24–72	119	107	12
Barnet et al[40]	10–40*	75–150	8	8	159	131	28
Colombo et al[34]	20–40	38–75	10	12	145	126	19
Hansen et al[35]	160–240**	75–225	14	4	149	108	41
Malmberg et al[36]	160	25–225	20	12	136	114	22
Jones et al[37]	100***	75–225	9	9	134	114	20

† See reference section to this chapter for complete information regarding sources.
†† P = propranolol; H = hydralazine.
 * Pindolol is used in place of propranolol.
** Oxprenolol is used in place of propranolol.
*** Atenolol is used in place of propranolol.

TABLE V
EFFICACY OF DOUBLE THERAPY (THIAZIDE + BETA-BLOCKER)

Study (Ref.)[†]	Mean Dose[†††] (mg/day) T	Mean Dose[†††] (mg/day) P	No. of Patients	Duration Of Therapy (wks)	Pre-Rx MAP (mm Hg)	Post-Rx MAP (mm Hg)	Decline in MAP Double Rx (mm Hg)
Siitonen et al[25]	25	240*	61	4	135	123	12
Veterans[32]	105	300	77	24–72	119	103	16
Pitkajari et al[27]	3	200–400**	31	6	131	107	24
Aronow et al[28]	100	20–60***	21	10	133	115	18
Toumilehto et al[29]	50	200††	20	52	123	111	14

† See reference section to this chapter for complete information regarding sources.
 * Siitonen used oxprenolol in place of propranolol.
** Practolol was used in place of propranolol.
*** Timolol was used in place of propranolol.
†† Metoprolol was used in place of propranolol.
††† T = hydrochlorothiazide; P = propranolol

TABLE VI
EFFICACY OF HYDRALAZINE + THIAZIDE, BETA-BLOCKER,
OR BOTH IN VETERANS STUDY (1983)[33]

Variable	No. of Patients	Pre-Rx MAP (mm Hg)	Post-Rx MAP (mm Hg)	Decline in MAP (mm Hg)
Bendroflumethiazide	30	108	102	6
Nadolol	40	110	103	7
Combination	19	108	101	7

TABLE VII
SUMMARY OF EFFICACY*

Drug Regimen	Decline in MAP (mm Hg)
Hydralazine alone**	8
Hydralazine plus a thiazide diuretic	12
Hydralazine plus beta-adrenergic blocker	21
Hydralazine plus thiazide plus beta-blocker	26

* Compiled from the previous tables (Tables I through V).
** The efficacy with hydralazine alone does not include studies where the dose of hydralazine was very large or where the studies had patients on other antihypertensive drugs.

$$\frac{(\text{No. of patients/study}_1) (\text{MAP})_1 + (\text{No. patients/study}_2) (\text{MAP})_2 + —n (\text{No. of patients/study n}) (\text{MAP})}{\text{Total No. of patients } (1 + 2 + —n)}$$

eclampsia[2,8,9,39] where it is important not to impair further renal blood flow or glomerular filtration rate.

Formulations

Tablets .... 10, 25, 50 and 100 mg.
Injectable .... 1 ml ampules containing 20 mg hydralazine.

Dose in Hypertension

Frequency: For chronic hypertension, oral dosages are given initially three times daily, although twice-a-day doses appear effective for maintenance. Dosage may then be increased until blood pressure is reduced to a normal level.

Initial: Start with 10 mg two to three times daily for the first two to four days; increase to 25 mg for the balance of the first week. For the second and subsequent weeks, increase dosage to 50 mg four-times daily[8] or 100 mg twice a day. Maximal dose is usually 300 mg/day. Parenteral administration is used only in hypertensive emergencies. The usual dose is 10 to 20 or 40 mg (IV) repeated as necessary.[8] Blood pressure usually begins to fall within 10–30 minutes, and lasts three to eight hours after injection.[41] Most patients can be transferred to oral hydralazine within 24–48 hours.

Range: 40–300 mg daily, taken orally. (Children, 0.75 mg/kg of body weight daily in four doses initially to 7.5 mg/kg)[42]

Usual dose: 100–200 mg daily, orally.

One of the more recent developments related to the administration of hydralazine is the slow-release hydralazine tablets. The advantage is that the once-a-day slow-release tablets will improve patient compliance. Further, when compared to the conventional 100 mg twice daily, the slow release was shown to be just as effective.[13]

Mechanism of Action

The direct and indirect effects of hydralazine are almost entirely limited to the cardiovascular system. The drug diminishes total peripheral vascular resistance by 60% or more.[8,9,43] Early investigators attributed the peripheral hypotension to a centrally mediated inhibition of sympathetic discharge.[4,41-46] Several papers have credited hydralazine with a very limited central vasodepressor action.[47,48]

However, the predominant inducer of systemic hypotension from hydralazine is the direct relaxation of smooth muscle in the peripheral vascular beds.[43,49,50] The relaxation in vascular resistance vessels (arterioles and small arteries) is much greater than that in capacitance vessels (venules and small veins).[9,43,49,50] In addition, pulmonary artery pressure may be slightly increased.[43]

The hypotension produced by hydralazine may be reduced by as much as 75% by three counteractive properties produced by the drug (Figure 2).[8,9,51] Foremost is an increase in heart rate (Table VIII) and contractability which ultimately increases the cardiac output.[9,15,43,49]

TABLE VIII
EFFECT OF HYDRALAZINE ON HEART RATE

Study (Ref.)	Average Daily Dose (mg)	No. of Patients	Duration of Therapy (wks)	Pre-Rx Heart Rate (bpm)	Post-Rx Heart Rate (bpm)	Increase in Heart Rate (bpm)
M. Velasco et al[14]	2–10 IV	6	—	78	117	39
Tarazi et al[15]	20 IV	7	—	70	90	20
West et al[12]	100 po	12	6	72	81	9
Silas et al[13]	200 po	17	5	59	64	5
Rouleau et al[59]	100 po	10	6	90	94	4

These actions are primarily reflex in nature, although a central stimulatory component has been identified.[4,52,53] Second, hydralazine has been shown to increase plasma renin.[54-57] Propranolol has been shown to block effectively both of these mechanisms.[58] Third, hydralazine's hypotensive action is counteracted by its concomitant tendency to retain sodium and water unless a diuretic is added.[5,9,24,54]

Hydralazine's peripheral vasodilation is variable. Coronary, splanchnic, cerebral, and renal blood flow are increased, while cutaneous and muscular blood flow are usually decreased.[9,43,49]

The significant renal vasodilation, increased renal blood flow, and increased cardiac output may be useful for patients with cardiac insufficiency, chronic lung disease, or compensated hypertension.[6] Unlike the renal blood flow, hydralazine has no consistent effect on the glomerular filtration rate or other tubular transport mechanism. The filtered fraction usually decreases.[4,6,54,60,61]

Drug Interactions

1. Plus *Other Antihypertensive Agents*

When combining antihypertensive drugs, individual titration is essential to ensure the lowest possible therapeutic dose of each drug.[62,63] An additive hypotensive effect is usually obtained.

2. Plus *MAO Inhibitors*

Use MAO inhibitors with caution in patients receiving hydralazine.

3. Plus *Epinephrine*

Hydralazine may reduce the pressor responses to epinephrine.[46,64]

4. Plus *Pyridoxine*

Evidence suggests that hydralazine exerts an antipyridoxine effect. Peripheral neuritis, presenting as paresthesias, numbness, and tingling, has been observed. When symptoms develop, adding pyridoxine to the regimen is beneficial.[65,66]

Contraindications

— Hypersensitivity to hydralazine
— Coronary artery disease[4,6]
— Mitral valvular rheumatic heart disease[6,61]

Warnings

● *In patients with a clinical picture simulating systemic lupus erythematosus:*

In a few patients, hydralazine may produce a clinical picture simulating systemic lupus erythematosus. In such patients, hydralazine should be discontinued unless the benefits from the drug treatment justify the risks. Signs and symptoms usually regress when the drug is discontinued. Treatment of this hydralazine-produced syndrome sometimes requires long-term therapy with corticoids.[67-69]

● *In patients on prolonged treatment:*

Even though the patient is asymptomatic, complete blood counts, LE cell preparations, and antinuclear antibody titer determinations are indicated before and periodically during long-term treatment with hydralazine.[70] These diagnostic tests are also indicated if the patient develops arthralgia, fever, chest pain, continued malaise, or other unexplained signs or symptoms.

A positive antinuclear antibody titer and/or positive LE-cell reaction requires that the physician carefully weigh the implications of the test results against the benefits to be derived from antihypertensive therapy with hydralazine.

● *In patients using MAO inhibitors:*

Use hydralazine with caution in patients receiving MAO inhibitors.

Use in Pregnancy

Animal studies indicate that high doses of hydralazine are teratogenic in mice, possibly teratogenic in rabbits, but not in rats. There are no clinical correlations between hydralazine and teratogenecity in the human fetus. Intravenous hydralazine in combination with a diuretic and/or sympatholytic agent has successfully controlled pre-eclampsia and eclampsia.[71,72] In addition, Bott-Kanner et al[73] showed that low doses of hydralazine with propranolol are effective with no major neonatal complications. However, hydralazine should not be used during pregnancy unless the expected benefits to the mother justify the potential risk to the fetus.

Precautions

Hydralazine must be used with caution in patients with suspected coronary artery disease. Anginal attacks and electrocardiographic evidence of myocardial ischemia due to the myocardial stimulating effect of hydralazine have been reported.[4,6] The drug has been implicated in the development of myocardial infarction.[4,5,74]

The "hyperdynamic" circulation caused by hydralazine may accentuate specific cardiovascular inadequacies. For example, an increase in pulmonary artery pressure, which is common in patients treated with hydralazine, would be detrimental for those with mitral valvular disease.[6,75] Pressor response to epinephrine[46,64] and postural hypotension may result from hydralazine, although the latter is more commonly found when using ganglionic-blocking agents.[5,51] Hydralazine should be used with caution in patients with a history of cerebrovascular accident.[5]

In hypertensive patients with normal kidneys who are treated with hydralazine, there is evidence of increased renal blood flow and maintenance of glomerular filtration rate.[4,52,54,60,61,76,77] Hydralazine, as with any hypertensive agent, should be used cautiously in patients with advanced renal damage.

Management of Overdose or Exaggerated Response

The signs and symptoms of hydralazine overdose are hypotension, tachycardia, headache, and generalized skin flushing, but these are to be expected. Those symptoms that are not so frequent are myocardial ischemia, cardiac arrhythmias, and profound shock.

In treating overdosage of hydralazine, evacuate gastric contents, taking precautions against aspiration and protecting the airway. If conditions permit, instill activated charcoal slurry. However, since these manipulations may precipitate cardiac arrhythmias or increase the depth of shock, they may have to be omitted or carried out after cardiovascular status has been established.

In the management of overdose, support of the cardiovascular system is of primary importance. If possible, shock should be treated with volume expanders without resorting to the use of vasopressors. If a vasopressor is required, use one which is least likely to precipitate or aggravate cardiac arrhythmia; digitalization may be necessary. Renal function must be monitored and supported as required. No experience has been reported with extracorporeal or peritoneal dialysis.

Absorption, Distribution, Metabolism, Excretion

Hydralazine is quickly and almost totally absorbed from the gastrointestinal tract. Less than 10% of radioactive hydralazine is recovered from the feces following oral administration.[78,79] The drug is widely distributed, concentrating in the walls of muscular arteries in the kidneys, liver, spleen, heart, lung, brain and muscle.[80] Serum hydralazine is 85% albumin bound.[81]

Peak serum concentrations are between 30 minutes and two hours.[78,79,81,82] Serum concentration directly correlates with the drug's hypotensive effect which usually peaks within one hour after oral administration.[8,83] Onset of action is 10 to 20 minutes for IV and IM administration, and 20 to 30 minutes for oral administration.[8,82,84] Duration of action is approximately six hours with a range of three to eight hours.[8,84]

Plasma half-life is two to four hours with small amounts of hydralazine still detectable 24 hours after administration.[79,82] The half-life of hydralazine's antihypertensive action is much longer than its plasma half-life. Hydralazine is detectable in the muscular arterial walls long after being cleared from the blood.[81,85,86]

Ingestion of hydralazine subjects it to a biotransformation within the gut wall as well as in the liver.[81,87,88] This "first-pass mechanism" is an acetylation process and is responsible for the low bioavailability of hydralazine (26–50% of dosage) to the systemic circulation after oral administration.[78-80]

Genetically determined differences in the concentration of N-acetyltransferase account for higher plasma concentrations in "slow acetylators," and lower plasma concentrations in "fast acetylators."[80,83] Slow acetylators represent approximately 50% of the U. S. white or black populations.[5,63,89,90] Both hypotension and the incidence of toxicity are greater with the slow acetylator phenotype. Several investigators feel that patients prescribed hydralazine should be phenotyped with the sulfametamethazine test, although this is not yet routine.[74,81,82,91] While slow acetylators should be limited to 200 mg hydralazine daily, there is no such limit for fast acetylators.[5] Acetylation phenotype has little effect on plasma concentration following IV administration.[92]

The other route of hydralazine metabolism involves ring hydroxylation and conjugation with glucuronic acid.[93,94] The major portion of hydralazine and its metabolites (80%) is excreted within 48 hours, with another 10% lost through defecation.[79] Systemic accumulation of hydralazine is significant in patients with renal dysfunction; therefore, doses should be reduced.[63,79,92]

Adverse Reactions

Hydralazine has an important place as a chronic vasodilator in the management of hypertension; however, the drug also produces a high incidence of untoward reactions. The Boston Collaborative Surveillance Program found hydralazine produced an 18.5% rate of adverse reactions among hospitalized patients.[95]

Frequency of all side effects is given in Table IX. In early studies where patients were receiving over 400 mg of hydralazine daily without concomitant medication, the number of patients discontinuing hydralazine therapy (38%) was quite significant.[4,10,96,97] (For more detail, see Table X in the first edition.) The side effects necessitating

---

TABLE IX
FREQUENCY OF ADVERSE REACTIONS DUE TO HYDRALAZINE

FREQUENT (> 5.0%)
Headache, nausea, vomiting, tachycardia, palpitations, dizziness, weakness, fatigue, lethargy and postural hypotension.

OCCASIONAL (0.5–5.0%)
Diarrhea, constipation, anxiety, nightmares, sleep disturbance, angina pectoris, late toxicity syndrome (lupus-like), nasal congestion, rhinorrhea.

RARE (< 0.5%)
Dyspnea, depression, arthralgia, arthritis, myalgia, fever, drowsiness, sedation, paresthesias, flushing, conjunctivitis, acute toxic syndrome, blood-dyscrasias.

TABLE X
NATURE OF REACTIONS TO HYDRALAZINE

Gastrointestinal
  anorexia, nausea and vomiting, gastrointestinal hemorrhage, diarrhea, constipation, ileus, hepatitis

Cardiovascular/Pulmonary
  tachycardia, dizziness, angina pectoris, electrocardiographic changes of myocardial insufficiency, orthostatic hypotension, dyspnea, nasal congestion

Nervous System
  headache, dizziness, anxiety, nightmares, sleep disturbance, peripheral tingling and numbness, polyneuritis, depression, disorientation, psychosis, impotence, paresthesias

Dermatological
  flushing, sweating, skin rash, urticaria, pruritis

Metabolic
  fluid retention, weight gain

Biochemical/Hematologic
  anemia, leukopenia, thrombocytopenia, pancytopenia, purpura, agranulocytosis, eosinophilia

Miscellaneous
  fever, weakness, fatigue, lethargy, arthralgia, arthritis, myalgia, tremors, muscle cramps, acute toxic syndrome, systemic lupus erythematosus-like syndrome, malaise, lacrimation, lymphadenopathy, splenomegaly, difficulty in micturation, conjunctival ingestion, chills and fever

---

discontinuation were headache, nausea, palpitations, angina, electrocardiographic changes of myocardial ischemia, diarrhea, nervousness, and fever.[4,10,96,97] The majority of studies after 1955 involves a combination of hydralazine with other hypertensive agents. Only 4% (22 of 564) of these patients were forced to discontinue hydralazine because of noxious side effects. Interruption of therapy was caused by skin rashes, depression, chest pain, dizziness or weakness.[10,32,98] Tables X and XI describe the nature of the various hydralazine reactions and their frequency.

● *Initial Side Effects*

  Most of the adverse reactions to oral hydralazine when used alone are acute (Table XI).[4,10,95,96,99] In 436 patients using hydralazine alone, the most common adverse reactions are headache (22%), nausea or vomiting (19%), tachycardia (18%), postural hypotension (16%), and palpita-

TABLE XI
ADVERSE REACTIONS

Adverse Reactions	Hydralazine Administered Alone†		Combination Therapy* with Hydralazine††	
	No. of Patients with Adverse Reactions (of 436 Patients)	%**	No. of Patients with Adverse Reactions (of 445 Patients)	%
Headache	97	22	74	22
Nausea, vomiting	84	19	8	2
Tachycardia	73	18	2	0.4
Postural hypotension	68	16	2	0.4
Palpitations	65	15	25	6
Weakness, fatigue, lethargy	24	6	61	16
Dizziness	28	6	47	11
Diarrhea, constipation	17	4	27	6
Anxiety, nightmares, sleep disturbance	19	4	16	4
Angina pectoris	11	3	19	4
Peripheral numbness or tingling	12	3	0	0
Dyspnea	8	2	22	5
Depression	9	2	14	3
Arthralgia, myalgia	3	0.7	20	4
Fever	2	0.5	8	2
Drowsiness, sedation	1	0.2	7	2
Lupus-like syndrome	0	0	45	6
Nasal congestion	0	0	48	11

† See references 4, 10, 95–97, 99.
* Combined therapy consists of a thiazide diuretic, reserpine and/or a beta-adrenergic blocking agent with hydralazine.
†† See references 5, 10, 16, 25, 32, 54, 100–103.
** Percentages correspond to the number of patients in the various studies.

tion (15%). Other less frequent adverse reactions are dizziness (6%), weakness, fatigue or lethargy (6%), anxiety, nightmares or sleep disturbance (4%), diarrhea or constipation (4%), peripheral numbness or tingling (3%), and angina (3%). The literature includes nasal congestion, flushing, conjunctivitis, anorexia and diffuse peripheral edema as additional adverse reactions.[8,9,90,94] However, these effects were not encountered in our review of actual cases of patients treated with hydralazine as the lone antihypertensive agent.

Studies show that tachycardia, angina, flushing and, supposedly, headaches can be minimized by adding a beta-adrenergic blocking agent, such as propranolol (20–40 mg every six hours) to the hydralazine regime.[24,51] Sodium and water retention are reduced and managed with a thiazide diuretic.[8,9,67] When hydralazine is administered concomitantly with other hypertensive agents, studies show a marked decrease in side effects (a 34% drop), except headaches and angina pectoris.

Fortunately, most of the side effects are transient and tend to subside within a week with continued hydralazine administration.[4,67] Many effects can be avoided or minimized by beginning therapy at lower dosages in combination with a thiazide, with/without a beta-blocker.

- ## The Acute Hydralazine Toxicity Syndrome

The literature has few reports on toxic reactions to hydralazine which occur within the first 30 days of therapy. Perry noted toxic symptoms 7–14 days after the first administration of hydralazine.[90,104,105] In 11 cases of 371 patients the syndrome was characterized by fever (all 11 cases), arthralgia and myalgia (nine cases), rash (five cases), and lymphadenopathy (two cases). An association was made between this early, acute febrile syndrome and the late lupus-like syndrome. This association was validated when after 5 to 18 months of therapy, 6 of the 11 acutely toxic patients later developed delayed lupus-like syndromes. Although doses were rather large (400–600 mg/day), one patient was receiving only 75 mg/day. Several other cases of the syndrome have been reported after only 100 mg/day dosage.[106]

- ## The Late Toxicity Syndrome or Lupus-like Syndrome

Delayed toxicity to hydralazine was first noted in 1953—two years after the drug's introduction.[67] With over 150 cases, the etiology and manifestations are still not clearly defined. The reported incidence of the syndrome varies from 6 to 13%.[67,68,91,107-109]

Our compilations from 13 studies totaling 761 patients yield an incidence of lupus-erythematosus-like syndrome of 6% (Table XI).[10,16,24,25,32,54,98-103]

Late toxicity, upon continued hydralazine administration, has been described as a rheumatoid arthritis-like syndrome that can evolve into a full-blown systemic lupus-erythematosus syndrome.[104] However, Perry found abnormal circulating (lupus) cells and plasma proteins in a significant percentage of 138 asymptomatic patients receiving hydralazine.[70] The laboratory abnormalities he most often found were decreased hemoglobin content, decreased leukocytes, increased globulins, abnormal cephalin cholesterol flocculation and thymol turbidity, and the presence of LE cells.

• Clinical Manifestations of Delayed Toxicity

In Perry's compilations of 136 cases from 22 studies,[74,91,109-124] the major signs and symptoms are arthralgia (92%), arthritis (64%), fever (43%), malaise (31%), skin lesions (28%), chest pain (21%), asthenia (20%), hepatomegaly (20%), splenomegaly (14%), and adenopathy (8%). Other less frequent manifestations include pleuritis, pulmonary infiltration, pericarditis, and pleural and pericardial effusion.[74,108,109,114,125-127] (See Table XV of the first edition for more detail.)

• Laboratory Tests of Delayed Toxicity

Laboratory tests reveal antinuclear antibodies (ANA) (98%), abnormal cephalin-cholesterol flocculation tests (69%), positive LE cell preparations (61%), hyperglobulinemia including alpha, beta, and gamma-globulins (52%), false-positive serological tests for syphilis (23%), proteinuria (21%), and anemia, microcytic and normocytic.[74,83,91,107-109, 111-124,128] An elevated erythrocyte sedimentation[74,109,129] and an abnormal thymol turbidity test are also usually observed.[67,68,91] Other laboratory findings include gross and microscopic hematuria,[67,74,104] albuminuria,[67,91,104] leukopenia,[67,74,91,104,108,109] and, rarely, pancytopenia.[110,111] (See Table XVI of the first edition for further detail.)

Note that the presence of ANA does not indicate the inevitable development of toxicity.[90] Also, LE cells have been found in 10% of asymptomatic patients.[108] Abnormal cephalin-cholesterol flocculation and thymol turbidity tests do not imply hepatic parenchymal necrosis. Hepatic cellular damage is a rare occurrence which has been reported as transient[130] in conjunction with multiple drugs[131] and in a patient with previous obstructive jaundice.[73] Other rare individual cases have been reported.[132,133]

• Predisposing Factors to the Development of Hydralazine-Induced, Lupus-Like Syndrome (Table XII)

Various factors have been correlated with increased incidences of delayed hydralazine toxicity. (For more detail, see Table XVIII of the first edition.)

1. Duration of Exposure

In Perry's review of 136 cases,[74,91,107,134] 94% of the patients with

TABLE XII
FACTORS CORRELATED WITH AN INCREASED INCIDENCE
OF HYDRALAZINE-INDUCED, LUPUS-LIKE SYNDROME

- Slow hepatic acetylation phenotype
- Duration of treatment greater than six months
- Advanced cardiovascular–renal disease
- Summer season
- Marked early side effects
- Good control of blood pressure
- Dose over 400 mg/day

toxicity had been on hydralazine therapy for at least six months. The average length of time needed to develop this syndrome was 12 months.[67,91,107,108]

2. Slow Hepatic Acetylation Phenotype

Toxic reactions occur almost exclusively among individuals who are genetically slow acetylators of hydralazine. Slow acetylators comprise approximately 5% of Eskimos, 15% of Chinese and Japanese, 60% of Asian Indians, 60% of Europeans, 33% of Latin Americans, 65% of Jews, 64% of Finns, and 50% of American Caucasians or Blacks.[5,89,90,106] Both Perry and Alarcon-Segovia feel that toxicity can be avoided if the hydralazine dosage is determined after acetylation-phenotype determination with the sulfamethazine test.[74,82,91]

3. Advanced Cardiovascular-Renal Disease

This factor must be considered although it is less prominent in hydralazine-induced toxicity than with other drug-induced reactions.[129]

4. Time of Year

The onset of toxicity typically occurs in the summer months.[129] In one study, 10 of the 14 serious reactions occurred between May and July.[91]

5. Marked Early Toxicity

The development of an early febrile syndrome occurred in 6 to 11 toxic patients in one study and has been noted elsewhere.[67,91]

6. Good Control of Blood Pressure

Most patients with late hydralazine toxicity have been under good blood pressure control[67,91,107,129] when the syndrome appeared.

7. Average Maximal Dose Over 400 mg/day

The reported cases of toxicity involving dosages over 400 mg/day represent 67 percent of 136 toxicities (see Table XVIII of the first edition for more detail).[74,91, 107-112,114] Several fulminant cases, with the patients getting only 100 mg/day, have been reported and are well documented.[74]

- ## A Comparison of the Late Hydralazine Lupus-like Syndrome with Spontaneous Systemic Lupus Erythematosus (SLE)

Clinical presentation reveals a remarkable similarity between the late-hydralazine syndrome and spontaneous SLE. Some have postulated that they are the same disease.[74,105]

The main difference between the syndrome and the disease is the fact that the hydralazine–toxicity syndrome is reversible upon discontinuation of the drug.[67,70, 74, 90, 91,104,134] Even though clinical symptoms generally disappear within six months, rheumatoid symptoms,[74,109] antinuclear antibodies,[91,135] and LE cells have been identified years after stopping the drug.[136] Late toxicity resembling polyarteritis nodosa has remitted only when treated with corticosteroids.[115] Increased sedimentation rate, increased serum globulin, hepatosplenomegaly, skin rashes, pleuritis, fever, and leukopenia have all been observed to persist for variable periods.[74,109,136]

- ## Other Reported Toxicity of Hydralazine

1. Other Clinical Manifestations

Recurrence of exacerbation of gastrointestinal bleeding has been documented.[137,138] Difficulty in sustaining an erection[134] and acute psychosis[135] presenting as euphoria and delusions have been reported as case studies. Discontinuation of hydralazine improves both situations.

2. Anemia, Pancytopenia

Asymptomatic anemia has been ascribed to a hydralazine-induced immune hemolysis[139] and to hydralazine's affinity for iron and copper.[64] Two cases of pancytopenia with mild hypocellularity of the bone marrow have been reported with recovery following withdrawal of hydralazine.[110,111]

3. Life-threatening Reactions

Even though hydralazine has traditionally been viewed as a non-life-threatening medication, several deaths have been attributed to its use. Exacerbation of coronary insufficiency has led to acute myocardial infarction.[4,5,74] Cases of fatal pulmonary edema,[140,141] fatal renal failure,[142] and death through pulmonary, renal, splenic and muscular lesions of SLE[143] have all been reported. Wheat and Palmer et al have reported fatal hemorrhagic dissection of aortic aneurysms in hypertensive patients treated with parenteral hydralazine secondary to tachycardia.[86]

MINOXIDIL (Loniten®)
Introductory year: 1980

INTRODUCTION:

Minoxidil (Figure 3) is a valuable, potent, vasodilator antihypertensive for those severe or malignant hypertensive patients who fail to respond to other oral agents. It must be given together with a diuretic and usually a beta-blocker:

1. In the treatment of severe or accelerated hypertension after other oral drugs have been unsuccessful.
2. When other antihypertensive agents produce intolerable side effects.
3. In the azotemic hypertensive patient.

In some of the first studies with minoxidil, Gilmore et al (1970) demonstrated its effectiveness in combination with propranolol for the control of hypertension in hospitalized subjects.[1] Limas and Freis reported the effective use of minoxidil in combination with conventional antihypertensive medications in treating uncontrollable hyperetension of uremic patients on chronic hemodialysis.[2] Gottlieb et al noted the superior potency of minoxidil over hydralazine.[3] Dormois and Young reported successful management of patients with refractory

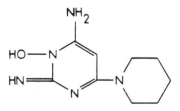

Figure 3: Structure of minoxidil.

hypertension.[4] Pettinger and Mitchell suggested minoxidil and propranolol as an alternative to nephrectomy in the treatment of refractory
hypertension.[5] Ryan, Jain and McMahon, with therapy that consisted of
minoxidil, diuretics, and propranolol, found a dose-related reduction in
both systolic and diastolic blood pressures with no postural effects
noted.[6]

In more recent studies, Devine et al reported a decline in MAP of
43 mm Hg in 44 patients who were resistant to previous treatment.[7]
Klotman et al found a significant reduction in MAP without an increase
in pulmonary hypertension or postural effects.[8] Bennett et al not only
demonstrated a 47 mm Hg decline in MAP, but also showed how
minoxidil preserves renal function despite active systemic disease.[9]
Other studies have shown minoxidil to improve renal function in many
azotemic hypertensive patients.[6,9-11] Mackay et al (1981) reported a
decline of 37 mm Hg in MAP in 87 patients with intractable hypertension who received minoxidil, a beta-blocker, and a diuretic for 27
months.[12] Hagstam et al demonstrated a significant decline in MAP and
a high level of tolerance in those patients who had side effects with
hydralazine.[13] Table XIII summarizes the efficacy of minoxidil. Note
that the studies employed minoxidil in combination with other agents.
Direct vasodilator drugs generally cause sodium and water retention;
therefore, a concurrent loop-diuretic is usually recommended. The
reflex tachycardia can be blocked with beta-blockers,[1] although central
alpha agonists like clonidine also reduce the tachycardia. Minoxidil
shares both of these properties and is usually given as part of triple
therapy, i.e., with a diuretic and a beta-adrenergic blocker.[3,14]

Formulation

Tablets .... 2.5 and 10 mg

Dose in Hypertension

Frequency: once daily. However when more rapid management is
required, give twice daily.

Initial: start with 5 mg once daily. This can be increased by 5–10
mg/day increments every two to three days up to 100
mg/day.

Range: 10–100 mg/day

Usual dose: 10–40 mg/day given as a once or twice daily dose.

TABLE XIII
EFFICACY OF MINOXIDIL IN REFRACTORY HYPERTENSION

Study (Ref.)[†]	No. of Patients	Therapy[††]	Mean Doses (mg/day)	Pre-Rx MAP[†††] (mm Hg)	Post-Rx MAP (mm Hg)	Decline in MAP (mm Hg)
Devine[7*]	44	Min.	26	158	115	43
Klotman[8]	7	Min. Prop. HCTZ	25 100 160	135	104	31
Larochelle[15]	14	Min. Prop. Fur.	24 170 120	156	119	37
Bennett[9]	10	Min. Prop. Fur.	21 120 80	164	117	47
Felts[16]	54	Min. Prop. Fur.	27 294 133	147	111	36
Mackay[12**]	87	Min. Prop. Fur.	23 440 101	155	118	37
Hagstam[13***]	19	Min. Prop.[****] Fur.	19 357 183	148	117	31

[†] See reference section to this chapter for complete information regarding sources.
[††] Min. = minoxidil; HCTZ = hydrochlorothiazide; Fur. = furosemide; Prop. = propranolol.
[†††] MAP = mean arterial pressure = diastolic + 1/3 pulse pressure.
[*] Some patients received amiloride, bethanidine, clonidine, debrisoquine, diazoxide, durosemide, guanethidine, hydralazine, labetalol, methyldopa, oxprenolol, propranolol, phenoxybenzamine, prazosin, spironolactone, and/or thiazide concomitantly.
[**] Some patients received methyldopa or bethanidine concomitantly, and a thiazide instead of furosemide.
[***] Some patients received chlorthalidone or spironolactone concomitantly.
[****] Some patients received alprenolol or metoprolol instead of propranolol.

Mechanism of Action

Minoxidil is a potent, orally-active vasodilator acting directly on the arteriolar smooth muscle by blocking calcium uptake through the cell membrane. Thereby it reduces peripheral vascular resistance without significant sympatholysis or increased venous capacitance. Minoxidil has no effect on the central nervous system nor the adrenergic nervous system.[17]

Drug Interactions

1. Plus *Other Antihypertensive Agents*
    By combining therapy an additive hypotensive effect is usually obtained.

2. Plus *Guanethidine*
    Minoxidil itself does not cause orthostatic hypotension; however, in patients already receiving guanethidine, it can result in profound orthostatic effects. If possible, guanethidine should be discontinued well before the administration of minoxidil. When this is not possible, the patient starting minoxidil therapy should be hospitalized until the orthostatic effects are no longer present or the patient has learned to avoid activities that provoke symptoms.

Contraindications

— Known or suspected pheochromocytoma
— Congestive heart failure
— Recent myocardial infarction
— Hypersensitivity

Warnings

● *Salt and water retention; congestive heart failure:*
    Minoxidil almost always requires a diuretic, usually a potent loop diuretic, to prevent fluid retention and possible congestive heart failure. Minoxidil increases plasma renin activity,[3,18] as with all vasodilators. Body weight and symptoms of heart failure should be closely monitored.

● *Tachycardia and angina:*
    Minoxidil increases the heart rate, reflexly, and may promote or worsen angina. Concomitant administration of a beta-adrenergic blocking drug or other sympathetic nervous system suppressant generally prevents the increase in heart rate and the aggravation of angina.

● *Pericardial effusion and tamponade:*
    Pericardial effusion, occasionally with tamponade, has been re-

ported in approximately 3% of treated patients not on dialysis. Patients should be observed closely for any pericardial disorder, and echocardiographic studies should be carried out if suspicion arises. More vigorous diuretic therapy, pericardiocentesis, dialysis, or surgery may be required. If the effusion persists, withdrawal of minoxidil should be considered in the context of possible other means of controlling the hypertension and the patient's general clinical status.

● *Rapid control of blood pressure:*

In patients with very severe blood pressure elevation, too rapid reduction of pressure can precipitate syncope, cerebrovascular accidents, myocardial infarction and ischemia of special sense organs. Any patient with malignant hypertension should have initial treatment with minoxidil carried out in a hospital setting to assure that blood pressure is falling and that it is not falling more rapidly than intended.

Use in Pregnancy

Minoxidil has been shown to reduce conception in rats with evidence of increased fetal resorption in rabbits when administered at five times the human dose. There is no evidence of teratogenic effects in rats and rabbits. Minoxidil should be used during pregnancy only if the potential benefit justifies the potential risk to the fetus. It is not known whether minoxidil is secreted in human milk, but as a general rule, nursing should not be undertaken while a patient is taking the drug.

Absorption, Metabolism, Excretion

Minoxidil is at least 90% absorbed, with peak plasma levels occurring within one hour. Serum half-life is four and one-half hours.[19-21] After oral administration, the hypotensive action of minoxidil develops within two hours. The full effect appears to last at least twelve hours. Minoxidil is excreted from the body primarily by biotransformation. Approximately 90% of the orally administered drug is metabolized, primarily by conjugation with glucuronic acid and excreted in the urine. The remaining 10% is filtered through the glomeruli unchanged and appears in the urine. Thus, excessive accumulation of minoxidil in hypertensive patients with renal insufficiency is unlikely. Minoxidil is not bound to plasma proteins.

Adverse Reactions

The most common side effects of minoxidil are fluid retention and edema; therefore, all patients must be monitored for edema, weight gain, and evidence of congestive heart failure. Hair growth (hypertrichosis) especially involving the face and extremities, occurs in 80% of patients after three to six weeks of therapy. Tachycardia is to be expected as is edema and should be counteracted with concurrent beta-blockers and diuretics. The cause of the abnormal body-hair growth is unknown, but it can often be controlled with depilatories and shaving. Some female patients, however, have discontinued minoxidil because of this cosmetic disturbance.[7,15] In patients with underlying coronary artery disease, angina or even myocardial infarction can be precipitated if the tachycardia is not prevented.

TABLE XIV
INCIDENCE OF SIDE EFFECTS OF MINOXIDIL

Study (Ref.)†	No. of Patients	Edema and/or Congestive Heart Failure	Weight Gain Without Congestive Heart Failure	Angina, Tachycardia	EKG Changes	Body-Hair Growth	Pericardial Effusions	Nausea
Ryan[6]	8	—	8	—	4	—	—	—
Traub[24]	11	6	—	—	—	5	—	—
Bennett[9]	10	1	††	—	—	1	2	—
Larochells[15]	14	1	††	—	3	6	—	—
Hagstam[13]	25	—	††	—	—	4	—	—
Reichgott[26]	37	—	—	—	—	—	10	—
Pedersen[27]	13	2	††	††	2	1	—	—
Cotorrulo[28]	15	2	2	3	5	13	—	2
Totals	133	12/63	10/23	3/15	14/50	30/88	12/47	2/15
Percentage		19	43	20	28	34	26	13

† See reference section to this chapter for complete information regarding sources.
†† Reported as "present."

Minoxidil studies using beagle dogs have shown an unusual lesion in the right atrium of the heart with myocyte degeneration, vascular proliferation, and fibrosis. There is no convincing evidence that the lesion is the same in man as in the beagles.[7,17,21] In a prospective study of the right atria in normotensive and hypertensive patients not treated with minoxidil, Sobota et al reported an increase in histological changes, myocardial fibrosis and hydropic vacuolization, related to age and hypertension.[23]

In contrast to hydralazine which can cause a lupus-like syndrome, minoxidil has consistently produced negative antinuclear factors and lupus erythematosus cell preparations.[3] Such side effects as orthostatic hypotension, decreased libido, and impotence which accompany other antihypertensive agents used in severe hypertension often disappear after therapy with minoxidil is initiated.[4,5,14,22,24,25] Other side effects with minoxidil include headache, nausea, conjunctivitis, electrocardiographic changes and pericardial effusion (Table XIV). Terminations due to side effects have been about 12% (14/114); over half were due to unacceptable facial hair growth.

REFERENCES:

Hydralazine

1. Bella, C., Sevey, R., and Harakal, C.: Renal and hemodynamic effects of combination therapy in hypertension. *J. Clin. Pharmacol.*, **14**:630, 1974.
2. Freis, E. D.: Hypertensive crisis. *JAMA*, **208**(2):338, 1969.
3. Dranov, J., Skyler, J. S., and Gunnelle, J. C.: Malignant hypertension, current modes of therapy. *Arch. Intern. Med.*, **133**:797, 1974.
4. Moyer, J. H.: Hydralazine (Apresoline®) hydrochloride, pharmacological observation and clinical results in the therapy of hypertension. *Arch. Intern. Med.*, **91**:419, 1953.
5. Hunyor, S. N.: Hydralazine and beta-blockade in refractory hypertension with characterization of acetylator phenotype. *Aust. N. Z. J. Med.*, **5**:530, 1975.
6. Judson, W. E., Hollander, W., and Wilkins, R. W.: The effects of intravenous Apresoline® (hydralazine) on cardiovascular and renal functions in patients with and without congestive heart failure. *Circulation*, **31**:664, 1956.
7. Franciosa, J., Pierpont, B., and Cohn, J.: Hemodynamic improvement after oral hydralazine in left ventricular failure; a comparison with nitroprusside infusion in 16 patients. *Ann. Intern. Med.*, **86**:388, 1970.

8. Koch-Weser, J.: The vasodilator antihypertensives. *Drug Ther.*, 5(5):67, 1975.
9. Koch-Weser, J.: Vasodilator drugs in the treatment of hypertension. *Arch. Intern. Med.*, 133:1017, 1974.
10. Aenishanslin, W., Pestalozzi-Kerpel, J., et al: Antihypertensive therapy with adrenergic beta-receptor blockers and vasodilators. *Eur. J. Clin. Pharmacol.*, 4:177, 1972.
11. Persson, I.: Combination therapy of essential hypertension with pindolol (Viskin®) and hydralazine. *Eur. J. Clin. Pharmacol.*, 9:91, 1975.
12. West, M. J., Wing, L. M. H., et al: Comparison of labetalol, hydralazine, and propranolol in the therapy of moderate hypertension. *Med. J. Aust.*, 1:224–225, 1980.
13. Silas, J. H., Ramsay, L. E., and Freestone, S.: Hydralazine once daily in hypertension. *Br. Med. J.*, 284:1602–1604, 1982.
14. Velasco, M., Bertoncini, H., et al: Effect of clonidine on sympathetic nervous activity in hydralazine-treated hypertensive patients. *Eur. J. Clin. Pharmacol.*, 13:317–320, 1978.
15. Tarazi, R. C., Dustan, H. P., Bravo, E. L., and Niachos, A. P.: Vasodilating drugs: Contrasting haemodynamic effects. *Clin. Sci. Mol. Med.*, 51:575s–578s, 1976.
16. Perry, H. M., Jr., Schroeder, H. A., et al: Studies on the control of hypertension. *Circulation*, 33(C):958, 1966.
17. Perry, H. M., Jr., Schroeder, H. A., and Morrow, J. D.: Studies on the control of hypertension by Hyphex: IV-Levels of the agents in urine and blood. *Am. J. Med. Sci.*, 228:405, 1954.
18. Schroeder, H. A. Morrow, J. D., and Perry, H. M., Jr.: Studies on the control of hypertension by Hyphex: I. Effects on blood pressure. *Circulation*, 8:672, 1953.
19. Perry, H., and Schroeder, H. A.: The effect of treatment on mortality rates in severe hypertension. *Arch. Intern. Med.*, 102:418, 1958.
20. Schroeder, H. A., Morrow, J. D., and Perry, H. M., Jr.: Studies on the control of hypertension by Hyphex: V. Effects on the course of the malignant stage. *Circulation*, 10:321, 1954.
21. Perry, H. M., Jr., and Schroeder, H. A.: Studies on the control of hypertension: VI. Some evidence for the reversal of the process during hexamethonium and hydralazine therapy. *Circulation*, 13:528, 1956.
22. Veterans Administration Cooperative Study Group on Antihypertensive Agents: Comparison of prazosin and hydralazine in patients receiving hydrochlorothiazide. A randomized, double-blind clinical trial. *Circulation*, 64(4):772–779, 1981.
23. Aoki, V., and Wilson, W.: Hydralazine and methyldopa in thiazide-treated hypertensive patients. *Am. Heart J.*, 79:798, 1970.
24. Zacest, R., Gilmore, E., and Koch-Weser, J.: Treatment of essential hypertension with combined vasodilation and beta-adrenergic blockade. *N. Engl. J. Med.*, 286:617, 1972.
25. Siitonen, L., Janne, J., et al: Hydralazine and beta-adrenergic blockade in the treatment of hypertension. *Ann. Clin. Res.*, 6:341, 1974.
26. Veterans Administration Multi-Clinic Cooperative Study on Antihypertensive Agents: Double blind controlled study of antihypertensive agents. III. Chlorothiazide alone and in combination with other agents; preliminary results. *Arch. Intern. Med.*, 110:230, 1962.
27. Pitkajarvi, T., Ala-Laurila, P., Ruosteenoja, R., Torsti, P., and Masar, S.: Treatment of hypertension successfully with a diuretic, clonidine, or a beta-blocking agent and hydralazine. *Eur. J. Clin. Pharmacol.*, 12:161–165, 1977.

28. Aronow, W. S., Van Herick, R., et al: Effect of timolol plus hydrochlorothiazide plus hydralazine on essential hypertension. *Circulation*, **57**(5):1017–1021, 1978.

29. Tuomilehto, J., Nissinen, A., and Honkavaara, M.: Clinical evaluation of the antihypertensive effect of metoprolol in combination with hydrochlorothiazide and hydralazine in an unselected hypertensive population. *Acta Cardiol.*, **4**:289–301, 1980.

30. Andersson, O., Hansson, L., and Sivertsson, R.: Primary hypertensive refractory to triple drug treatment: A study on central and peripheral hemodynamics. *Circulation*, **58**:4, 1978.

31. Forrest, W. A.: An open comparison between free and fixed combination of diuretic and beta-blocker in the management of essential hypertension. *J. Int. Med. Res.*, **8**(2):127–31, 1980.

32. Veterans Administration Cooperative Study Group on Antihypertensive Agents: Propranolol in the treatment of essential hypertension. *JAMA*, **237**(21):2303–2310, 1977.

33. Freis, E. D., et al: Efficacy of nadolol alone and combined with bendroflumethiazide and hydralazine with systemic hypertension. *Am. J. Cardiol.*, **52**:1230–1237, 1983.

34. Colombo, G., Fea, F., Planca, E., Savioli, G., and Pelliccioli, I.: Antihypertensive activity of labetalol and propranolol + hydralazine association in severe essential hypertension. *Ther. Res.*, **32**(6):834–843, 1982.

35. Hansen, M., Hansen, O. P., and Lindholm, J.: Controlled clinical study in antihypertensive treatment with a diuretic and methyldopa compared with a beta-blocking agent and hydralazine. *Acta Med. Scand.*, **202**:385–388, 1977.

36. Malmberg, L., Fagerberg, S., and Frithz, G.: Peripheral vasodilatation in the treatment of hypertension. Prazosin compared with hydralazine in patients not responding to beta-receptor blockade. *Acta Med. Scand.*, (Suppl), **665**:121–124, 1982.

37. Jones, J. V., and Steiner, J M · Double-blind cross-over comparison of hydralazine and prazosin in hypertensive subjects on a beta-adrenoceptor blocking agent (atenolol). *Br. J. Clin. Pharmacol.*, **10**:531–533, 1980.

38. Johnson, B. F., Black, H. R., Beckner, R., Weiner, B., and Angeletti, F.: A comparison of minoxidil and hydralazine in non-azotemic hypertensives. *J. Hyperten.*, **1**:103–107, 1983.

39. Huysman, F. T. M., Thien, R. A., and Koene, R. A.: Acute treatment of hypertension with slow infusion of diazoxide. *Arch. Intern. Med.*, **143**:882, 1983.

40. Barnett, A. J., Kalowski, S., and Guest, C.: Labetalol compared with prindolol plus hydrallazine in the treatment of hypertension. *Med. J. Aust.*, **1**:105, 1978.

41. Romanklewicz, J. A.: Pharmacology and clinical use of drugs in hypertensive emergencies. *Am. J. Hosp. Pharm.*, **34**:185–193, 1977.

42. *AMA Drug Evaluations*, 4th Ed., 1980.

43. Freis, E. D., Rose, J. C., et al: The hemodynamic effects of hypotensive drugs in man. IV. 1-hydrazinophthalazine. *Circulation*, **8**:199, 1953.

44. Moyer, J., Handley, C., and Huggins, R.: Some pharmacodynamic effects of 1-hydrazinophthalazine (C-5968) with particular reference to renal function and cardiovascular response. *J. Pharmacol.*, **103**:368, 1951.

45. Mackinnon, J.: Effect of hypotension-producing drugs in the renal circulation. *Lancet*, **2**:12, 1952.

46. Finnerty, F. J.: Relationship of an intramuscular fluid volume to the development of drug resistence in the hypertensive patient. *Am. Heart J.*, **81**:563, 1971.

47. Grimson, K. S.: *Apresoline Conference*, New York, New York, 1952 (quoted by Moyer, et al, 1953).

48. Baum, T., Shropshire, A. T., and Varner, L. L.: Contributions of the CNS to the action of several antihypertensive agents (methyldopa, hydralazine, guanethidine). *J. Pharmacol. Exp. Ther.*, **182**:135, 1972.

49. Ingenito, A., Barrett, J., and Procita, L.: Centrally mediated peripheral hypotensive effects of reserpine and hydralazine when perfused through the isolated in situ cat brain. *J. Pharmacol. Exp. Ther.*, **170**:210, 1969.

50. Craves, B., Barett, H., Cameron, H., and Yonkman, F.: The activities of 1-hydrazinophthalazine (Ba-5968), a hypotensive agent. *J. Am. Pharmacol. Assoc.* (Sci. Ed.), **40**:559, 1951.

51. Winer, N., Cholshi, D., et al: Adrenergic receptor radiation of renin secretion. *J. Clin. Endocrinol. Metab.*, **29**:1168, 1969.

52. Moyer, J. H., Huggins, R. H., and Handley, C. A.: Further cardiovascular and renal hemodynamic studies following the administration of hydrallagin (1-hydrazinophthalazine) and the effect of ganglionic blockage with hexamethonium on their response. *J. Pharmacol.*, **109**:175, 1953.

53. Barrett, W., Povalski, H., and Rutledge, R.: An hypothesis concerning the mechanism of action of hydralazine HCL. *Fed. Prac.*, **24**:712, 1965.

54. Gottlieb, T. B., Katz, F. H., and Chidsey, C. A., III: Combined therapy with vasodilator drugs and beta-adrenergic blockade in hypertension: A comparative study of minoxidil and hydralazine. *Circulation*, **45**:571, 1972.

55. Finnerty, F., Jr.: Hypertension in pregnancy. *Clin. Obstet. Gynecol.*, **18**:145, 1975.

56. Pedersen, E. B., and Kornerup, H. J.: Plasma renin concentration in essential hypertension during beta-adrenergic blockade and vasodilator therapy. *Eur. J. Clin. Pharmacol.*, **12**:93–96, 1977.

57. Siitonen, L.: Hydralazine and oxprenolol in the treatment of hypertension and the effect of these drugs on plasma renin activity. *J. Int. Med. Res.*, **8**:181–187, 1980.

58. Pettinger, W. A., and Keeton, K.: Altered renin release and propranolol potentiation of vasodilatory drug hypotension. *Clin. Invest.*, **55**:236, 1959.

59. Rouleau, J., Chatterjee, K., Benge, W., Parmley, W. W., and Hiramatsu, B.: Alterations in left ventricular function and coronary hemodynamics with captopril, hydralazine and prazosin in chronic ischemic heart failure: A comparative study. *Circulation*, **65**(4):671–678, 1982.

60. Moyer, J. H., and Head-Hadley, C. A.: Renal function and systemic blood pressure changes following the administration of hydrazinophthalazine. *J. Lab. Clin. Med.*, **36**:969, 1950.

61. Wilkinson, E., Backman, H., and Hecht, H.: Cardiovascular and renal adjustments to a hypotensive agent (1-hydrazinophthalazine: Ciba BA-5968, Apresoline®). *J. Clin. Invest.*, **31**:872, 1952.

62. The Medical Letter: Drug combinations for primary hypertension. *Med. Let. Drugs & Ther.*, **10**(9):34, Issues 243, 1968.

63. Koch-Weser, J.: Individualization of antihypertensive drug therapy. *Med. Clin. North Am.*, **258**(5):1027, 1974.

64. Merrill, D. H., and Kenyon, K.: 1-hydrazinophthalazine (Apresoline®) in the treatment of hypertensive disease — a clinical trial with control group. *Am. J. Med. Sci.*, **226**:623: 1953.

65. Kirkendall, W. M., and Page, E. B.: Polyneuritis occurring during hydralazine therapy. *JAMA*, **167**:427, 1958.

66. Raskin, N.H., and Fishman, R. A.: Pyridoxine-deficiency neuropathy due to hydralazine. *N. Engl. J. Med.*, **273**:1182, 1965.

67. Morrow, J. D., Schroeder, H. A., and Perry, H. M., Jr.: Studies in the control of hypertension by hyphex. II. Toxic reactions and side effects. *Circulation*, **8**:829, 1953.

68. Comens, P., and Schroeder, H. A.: The "LE" cell as a manifestation of delayed hydralazine intoxication. *JAMA*, **160**:1134, 1956.

69. Baer, A. N., and Pincus, T.: Occult systemic lupus erythematosus in elderly men. *JAMA*, **249**:3350, 1983.

70. Perry, H. M., Jr., Schroeder, H. A., and Conners, P.: Abnormalities of circulating cells and proteins in hydralazine patients without toxic symptoms. *Am. J. Med. Sci.*, **244**:44, 1962.

71. Martin, J.: A critical survey of drugs used in the treatment of hypertensive crises of pregnancy. *Med. J. Aust.*, **2**:252, 1974.

72. O'Malley, K., Segel, J., et al: Duration of hydralazine action in hypertension. *Clin. Pharmacol. Ther.*, **18**:581, 1975.

73. Bott-Kanner, G., Schweitzer, A., et al: Propranolol and hydralazine in the management of essential hypertension in pregnancy. *Br. Med. J. Ob. Gyn.*, **87**:110–114, 1980.

74. Alarcon-Segovia, D., Wakin, K. G., Worthington, J. W., and Wand, L. E.: Clinical and experimental studies on the hydralazine syndrome and its relationship to systemic lupus erythematosus. *Med.*, **46**:1, 1967.

75. Rogers, S., Flowers, C., and Alexander, A.: Aggressive toxemia management. *Obstet. Gynecol.*, **33**:724:1969.

76. Falch, D. K., Odegaard, A. E., and Norman, N.: Renal plasma flow and cardiac output during hydralazine and propranolol treatment in essential hypertension. *Scand. J. Clin. Lab. Invest.*, **38**:143–146, 1978.

77. Isben, H., Rasmussen, H., Jensen, A. E., and Leth, A.: Changes in glomerular filtration rate during long-term treatment with propranolol and peripheral vasodilators in patients with arterial hypertension. *Dan. Med. Bull.*, **26**:308–311, 1979.

78. Talseth, T.: Studies on hydralazine. III. Bioavailability of hydralazine in man. *Eur. J. Clin. Pharmacol.*, **10**:395, 1976.

79. Lesser, J. M., et al: Fate of hydralazine-14C in man and dog. *Clin. Pharmacol. Ther.*, **14**:140, 1973.

80. Talseth, T.: Studies on hydralazine. I. Serum concentrations of hydralazine in man after a single dose and at steady-state. *Eur. J. Clin. Pharmacol.*, **10**:183, 1976.

81. Koch-Weser, J.: Drug therapy: Hydralazine. *N. Engl. J. Med.*, **295**(6):320–323, 1976.

82. Hypotensive Agents 24:08, Hydralazine hydrochloride, USP ASHP, Formulary, C 3340, July 1977.

83. Zacest, R., and Koch-Weser, J.: Relation of hydralazine plasma concentration to dosage and hypotensive action. *Clin. Pharmacol. Ther.*, **13**:420, 1972.

84. Curre, C. L., and Hosten, A. O.: Current treatment of malignant hypertension. *JAMA*, **232**:1367, 1970.

85. Moore, J. D., and Perry, H. N. J.: Radioautographic localization of hydralazine-1-C^{14} in arterial walls. *Proc. Soc. Exp. Biol. Med.*, **122**:576, 1966.

86. Wheat, M. W., and Palmer, R.: Management of impending rupture of the aortic dissection. In G. H. Stollerman et al (Eds.): *Advances in Internal Medicine*, Vol. 17, Year Book Medical Publishers, Chicago, 1971.

87. Jenne, J. W.: Isoniazid acetylation by human liver and intestinal mucosa. *Fed. Proc.*, **22**:540, 1973.

88. Evans, D. A. P., and White, T. A.: Human acetylation polymorphism. *J. Lab. Clin. Med.*, **63**:394, 1964.

89. Evans, D. A. P.: Genetic variation in the acetylation of isoniazid and other drugs. *Ann. N. Y. Acad. Sci.*, **151**:723, 1968.

90. Perry, H. M., Jr., Tan, E. M., Carmody, S., and Sakanata, A.: Relationship of actyl transferance activity to antinuclear antibodies and toxic symptoms in hypertensive patients treated with hydralazine. *J. Lab. Clin. Med.*, **76**:114, 1970.

91. Perry, H. M., Jr.: Late toxicity to hydralazine resembling systemic lupus erythematosus or rheumatoid arthritis. *Am. J. Med.*, **54**:58, 1973.

92. Reidenberg, M. M., Drayer, D., et al: Hydralazine elimination in man. *Clin. Pharmacol. Ther.*, **14**:970, 1973.

93. Isaac, L. S. M., and Kanda, M.: The metabolism of 1-hydrazinophthalazine. *Pharmacology*, **143**:7, 1964.

94. Goodman, L. S., and Gilman, A. (Eds.): *The Pharmacological Basis of Therapeutics*, 5th edition, MacMillan, New York, 1975, pp. 705–707.

95. Kellaway, G. S. M.: Adverse drug reactions during treatment of hypertension. Symposium on Hypertension. *Drugs*, **II** (Suppl. I):91, 1976.

96. Schroeder, H. A.: The effect of 1-hydrazinophthalazine in hypertension. *Circulation*, **5**:28, 1952.

97. Schroeder, H. A.: Control of hypertension by hexamethonium and 1-hydrazinophthalazine. *Arch. Intern. Med.*, **89**:523, 1952.

98. Glazer, N.: Reserpine, hydralazine, hydrochlorothiazide combination (Ser-ap-es) in essential hypertension. *Curr. Ther. Res.*, **14**:561, 1972.

99. Hughes, W. M., Dennis, E., and Moyer, J. H.: Treatment of hypertension with oral reserpine alone and in combination with hydralazine or hexamethonium. *Am. J. Med. Sci.*, **229**:121, 1955.

100. Lee, R. E., Seligmann, A. M., et al: Reserpine-hydralazine combination therapy of hypertensive disease with hydralazine in doses generally below the "toxic range." *Ann. Intern. Med.*, **44**:456, 1956.

101. Sannerstedt, R., Stenberg, J., et al: Chronic beta adrenergic blockade in arterial hypertension: Hemodynamic influences of dihydralazine and dynamic exercise and clinical effects of combined treatment. *Am. J. Cardiol.*, **29**:718, 1972.

102. Pape, J.: The effect of alprenalol in combination with hydralazine in essential hypertension. A double-blind, crossover study and a long-term follow-up study. *Acta Med. Scand.*, (Suppl.) **554**:55, 1974.

103. Veterans Administration Multi-Clinic Cooperative Study on Antihypertensive Agents: Effects of treatment on morbidity in hypertension: Results in patients with diastolic blood pressures averaging 115 through 129 mm Hg. *JAMA*, **202**:1028, 1967.

104. Perry, H. M., Jr., and Schroeder, H. A.: Syndrome stimulating collagen disease caused by hydralazine (Apresoline®). *JAMA*, **154**:670, 1954.

105. Alarcon-Serovia, D.: Drug-induced lupus syndrome. *Mayo Clin. Proc.*, **44**:664, 1969.

106. Nasonova, V. A., et al: Disseminated vasculitis in treatment of hypertension with Apresoline®. *So. Vet. Med.*, **20**:41, 1956.

107. Dustan, H. R., Taylor, K. D., Corcoran, A. C., and Page, I. H.: Rheumatism and febrile syndrome during prolonged hydralazine treatment. *JAMA*, **154**:23, 1954.

108. Muller, J. C., Rast, C. L., Jr., Pryor, W. W., and Orgain, E. S.: Late systemic complications of hydralazine (Apresoline®) therapy. *JAMA*, **154**:894, 1955.

109. Hildreth, E. A., Biro, C. E., and McCreary, T. A.: Persistence of the "hydralazine syndrome." *JAMA*, **173**:657, 1960.

110. Kaufman, M.: Pancytopenia following use of hydralazine (Apresoline®). *JAMA*, **151**:1488, 1953.

111. McNicol, M. W., and Hutchison, H. E.: Severe toxic reaction to hydralazine. *Lancet*, **2**:1288, 1956.

112. Beelar, V. P.: Rheumatoid arthritis-like syndrome during Apresoline® therapy. *Med. Ann. DC*, **22**:651, 1953.

113. Slonium, N. B.: Arthralgia, headache, prostration and fever during hydralazine therapy. *JAMA*, **154**:1419, 1954.

114. Mantes, W. B.: Late reaction to hydralazine (Apresoline®) therapy. *N. Engl. J. Med.*, **250**:835, 1954.

115. Fedar, L. A: Febrile syndrome during prolonged hydralazine treatment of hypertension. *N. Engl. J. Med.*, **251**:273, 1954.

116. Reinhardt, D. J., and Waldron, J. M.: Lupus erythematosus-like syndrome complicating hydralazine (Apresoline®) therapy. *JAMA*, **155**:1491, 1954.

117. Shackman, N. H., Swiller, A. L., and Morrison, M.: Syndrome stimulating acute disseminated lupus crythematosus. Appearance after hydralazine (Apresoline®) therapy. *JAMA*, **155**:1492, 1954.

118. Evans, J. A., and Eisenbeir, C. H.: Hydrazinophthalazine (Apresoline®) toxicity: Report of a case of arthritis of the rheumatoid type and pancytopenia. *Lahey Clin. Foun. Bull.*, **9**:109, 1955.

119. Henn, M. J., Perkins, T. W., Hargraves, M. M., and Odel, H. M.: Acute systemic lupus erythematosus syndrome from hydralazine hydrochloride. *Arch. Intern. Med.* (Chicago), **95**:857, 1955.

120. Damin, G. W., Nora, J. R., and Reardan, J. B.: Hydralazine reaction: Case with LE cells antemortem and postmortem and pulmonary, renal, splenic, and muscular lesions of disseminated lupus erythematosus. *J. Lab. Clin. Med.*, **46**:806,1955.

121. Posey, E. L., Jr., and Stephenson, S. L., Jr.: Syndrome resembling disseminated lupus occurring during Apresoline® therapy. *Miss. Doctor*, **32**:43, 1954.

122. Grupper, M. C.: Le lupus erythemateux est-il une toxicodermie? *Bull. Soc. Franc. Derm. Syph.*, **62**:336, 1955.

123. Reynolds, H., and Caldwell, J. R.: Hydralazine syndrome — hypersensitivity or toxicity? *JAMA*, **165**:1823, 1957.

124. Siguier, F., Betourme, C., and Bonnet de la Tour, J.: Hydralazine lupus erythematosus. *Sem. Hop. Paris*, **34**:773, 1958.

125. Whitcomb, M. E.: Drug-induced lung disease. *Chest*, **63**(3):418, 1973.

126. Brettner, A. B., Heitzman, E. R., and Woodin, W. G.: Pulmonary complications of drug therapy. *Radiology*, **96**:31, 1970.

127. Ripe, E., and Nelsson, B.: Pulmonary infiltration during dihydralazine treatment in a low isonazid-inactivator. *Scand. J. Res. Dis.*, **53**:56, 1972.

128. De Jesus, J. A.: Hydralazine disease versus lupus erythematosus dissemination. *Bol. Assoc. Med. PR*, **50**:318, 1958.

129. Perry, H. M., Jr.: Multiple reactions to antihypertensive agents during treatment of malignant hypertension. *Ann. Intern. Med.*, **57**:441, 1962.

130. Jori, G. P., and Peschle, C.: Hydralazine disease associated with transient granulomas in the liver. *Gastroenterology*, **64**:1163, 1973.

131. Perry, H. M., Jr., Schroeder, H. A., Goldstein, G. S., and Meinhard, E. M.: Studies on the control of hypertension by Hyphex. III. Pharmacological and clinical observations on l-hydrazinophthalazine. *Am. J. Med. Sci.*, **228**:396, 1954.

132. Bartoli, E., Massarelli, G., Solinas, A., Faedda, R., and Chiandussi, L.: Acute hepatitis with bridging necrosis due to hydralazine intake. *Arch. Intern. Med.*, **139**:698–699, 1979.

133. Barnett, D. B., Hudson, S. A., and Golightly, P. W.: Hydralazine-induced hepatitis? *Br. Med. J.*, **280**:1165–1166, 1980.

134. Pregeon, G., and Genest, J.: Prolonged hydralazine hydrochloride administration in 132 hypertensive patients — study of toxicity. *Can. Med. Assoc. J.*, **83**:743, 1960.

135. Moser, M., Syner, J., Malitz, S., and Mattingly, T. W.: Acute psychosis as a complication of hydralazine therapy in essential hypertension. *JAMA*, **152**:1329, 1953.

136. Shulman, L. E., and Harvey, A. M.: The nature of drug-induced systemic lupus erythematosus. *Arthritis Rheum.*, **3**:414, 1960.

137. Wilkins, R. W., and Judson, D. E.: Problems arising from the use of hypotensive drugs in hypertensive patients. *Trans. Assoc. Am. Physicians*, **66**:175, 1953.

138. Reynolds, H., and Caldwell, J. R.: Hydralazine syndrome — hypersensitivity or toxicity? Its significance in understanding of collagen disease. *JAMA*, **165**:1823, 1951.

139. Orenstein, A. A., Yokulis, V., Eipe, J., and Costea, N.: Immune hemolysis due to hydralazine. *Ann. Intern. Med.*, **86**:450, 1977.

140. Cohen, B. M.: Fatal reactions to 1-hydrazinophthalazine (Apresoline®). *Am. Heart J.*, **45**:931, 1953.

141. Slonim, N. B.: Arthralgia, headache, prostration, and fever during hydralazine therapy. *JAMA*, **154**:1519, 1954.

142. White, A.: Hydralazine (Apresoline®) lupus with fatal renal failure. *J. Am. Geriatr. Soc.*, **14**:361, 1966.

143. Mandellaum, H., Brook, J., and Mandellaum, R. A.: Bleeding peptic ulcer complicating hydralazine and hexamethonium bromide therapy. *JAMA*, **155**:833, 1954.

Minoxidil

1. Gilmore, E., Weil, J. T., et al: Treatment of essential hypertension with a new vasodilator in combination with a beta-adrenergic blockade. *N. Engl. J. Med.*, **282**:521, 1970.

2. Limas, J. L., and Freis, E. D.: Minoxidil in severe hypertension with renal failure. *Am. J. Cardiol.*, **31**:355, 1973.

3. Gottlieb, T. B., Katz, F. H., et al: Combined therapy with vasodilator drugs and beta-adrenergic blockade in hypertension: A comparative study of minoxidil and hydralazine. *Circulation*, **45**:571, 1972.

4. Dormois, J. C., and Young, J. L.: Minoxidil in severe hypertension: Value when conventional drugs have failed. *Am. Heart J.*, **90**(3):360, 1975.

5. Pettinger, W. A., and Mitchell, H. C.: Minoxidil — an alternative to nephrectomy for refractory hypertension. *N. Engl. J. Med.*, **289**(4):167, 1973.

6. Ryan, J. R., Jain, A. K., and McMahon, F. G.: Minoxidil treatment of severe hypertension. *Curr. Ther. Res.*, **17**(1):68, 1975.

7. Devine, B. L., Fife, R., and Trust, P. M.: Minoxidil for severe hypertension after failure of other hypotensive drugs. *Br. Med. J.*, **2**:667–669, 1977.

8. Klotman, P. E., Grim, C. E., Weinberger, M. H., and Judson, W. E.: The effects of minoxidil on pulmonary and systemic hemodynamics in hypertensive man. *Circulation*, **55**(2):394–400, 1977.

9. Bennett, W. M., Golper, T. A., Muther, R. S., and McCarron, D. A.: Efficacy of minoxidil in the treatment of severe hypertension in systemic disorders. *J. Cardiovasc. Pharmacol.*, **2**:S142–S148, 1980.

10. Hammond, J. J., and Kirkendall, W. M.: Minoxidil therapy for refractory hypertension and chronic renal failure. *South. Med. J.*, **72**(11):1429-1432, 1979.

11. Mitchell, H. C., Graham, R. M., and Pettinger, W. A.: Renal function during long-term treatment of hypertension with minoxidil. *Ann. Intern. Med.*, **93**:676-681, 1980.

12. Mackay, A., Isles, C., Henderson, I., Fife, R., and Kennedy, A. C.: Minoxidil in the management of intractable hypertension. *Q. J. Med.*, **198**:175-190, 1981.

13. Hagstam, K. E., Lundgren, R., and Wieslander, J.: Clinical experience of long-term treatment with minoxidil in severe arterial hypertension. *Scand. J. Urol. Nephrol.*, **16**:57-63, 1982.

14. Koch-Weser, J.: The vasodilator antihypertensives. *Drug Ther. Bull.*, **5**(5):67, 1975.

15. Larochelle, P., Hamet, P., Beroniade, V., and Kuchel, O.: Minoxidil in severe hypertension. *Eur. J. Clin. Pharmacol.*, **14**:1-5, 1978.

16. Felts, J. H., and Charles, J.: Minoxidil in refractory hypertension. *J. Cardiovasc. Pharmacol.*, **2**(Suppl 2):S114-S122, 1980.

17. DuCharme, D. W., Freyburger, W. A., et al: Pharmacologic properties of minoxidil: A new hypotensive agent. *J. Pharmacol. Exp. Ther.*, **184**:662, 1973.

18. Baer, L., Radichevich, I., and Williams, G. S.: Treatment of drug-resistant hypertension with minoxidil or angiotension-converting enzyme inhibitor: Blood pressure, renin, aldosterone, and electrolyte responses. *J. Cardiovasc. Pharmacol.*, **2**:S206-S216, 1980.

19. Letendre, D. E., Chonko, A. M., and Amerson, A. B.: Managing refractory hypertension. *J. Kans. Med. Soc.*, **82**:64-68, 1981.

20. Campese, V. M.: Minoxidil: A review of its pharmacological properties and therapeutic use. *Drugs*, **22**:257-278, 1981.

21. Gottlieb, T. B., Thomas, R. C., et al: Pharmacokinetic studies of minoxidil. *J. Clin. Pharmacol.*, **13**:436, 1972.

22. Joekes, A. M., Thompson, F. D., and O'Regan, P. F. B.: Clinical use of minoxidil (Loniten). *J. R. Soc. Med.*, **74**:228-282, 1981.

23. Sobota, J. T., Martin, W. B., Carlson, R. G., and Feenstra, E. S.: Minoxidil: Right atrial cardiac pathology in animals and in man. *Circulation*, **62**:376-387, 1980.

24. Traub, Y. M., and Redmond, D. P.: Treatment of severe hypertension with minoxidil. *Isr. J. Med. Sci.*, **11**(10):991, 1975.

25. Linas, S. L., and Nies, A. S.: Minoxidil. *Ann. Intern. Med.*, **94**:61-65, 1981.

26. Reichgott, M. J.: Minoxidil and pericardial effusion: An idiosyncratic reaction. *Clin. Pharmacol. Ther.*, July, 64-70, 1981.

27. Pedersen, O. L.: Long-term experiences with minoxidil in combination treatment of severe atrial hypertension. *Acta Cardiol.*, **4**:283-293, 1977.

28. Cotorruelo, J. G., Llamazaces, C., and Florez, J.: Minoxidil in severe and moderately severe hypertension, in association with methyldopa and chlorthalidone. *J. Vasc. Diseases*, Nov., 710-719, 1982.

CHAPTER X

CALCIUM CHANNEL BLOCKERS

VERAPAMIL (ISOPTIN®, CALAN®)
NIFEDIPINE (PROCARDIA®)
DILTIAZEM (CARDIZEM®)

INTRODUCTION:

Nifedipine, verapamil and diltiazem are particularly
beneficial in elderly hypertensive patients.

Nifedipine, verapamil and diltiazem belong to a structurally and pharmacologically diverse new class of drugs known as calcium channel blockers (see Figure 1 and Table I). In 1967 and the early 1970s, Fleckenstein and others first recognized that some drugs acted as inhibitors of calcium entry into heart muscle and vascular smooth muscle cells causing a negative inotropic effect on the heart, diminished oxygen consumption of the myocardium, and dilated coronary and peripheral arteries. Thus a new class of drugs was established known as calcium ion influx inhibitors, calcium slow-channel blockers, or simply "calcium blockers."[1-5] Initially used in the treatment of variant angina and supraventricular arrhythmias, these agents are now being used effectively in the treatment of hypertension. They are particularly beneficial in elderly hypertensive patients, many of whom have low renin levels, where they may prove to be drugs of choice for initial monotherapy. Unlike other vasodilators, they do not cause reflex tachycardia or significant edema or weight gain. Like the antihypertensives hydralazine and minoxidil, calcium channel blockers are direct-acting vasodilators, but they also dilate the coronaries and improve subendo-

TABLE I
CARDIOVASCULAR EFFECTS OF CALCIUM CHANNEL BLOCKERS

Calcium Antagonist	On HR	On AV NODE Conduction	Usefulness In Treatment Supraventricular Tachyarrhythmias	On Contractility	Anti-anginal Effect Vasospastic	Classical	Decline in Blood Pressure
Verapamil	–	+++	+++	--	++	+++	+++
Nifedipine	+	±	0	–	+++	++	+++
Diltiazem	–	++	+	–	+++	+++	++

-- = moderate negative effect
– = slight negative effect
0 = no effect
+ = slight effect
++ = moderate effect
+++ = strong effect

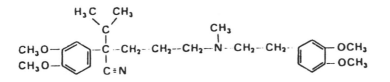

Verapamil

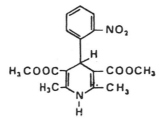

Nifedipine

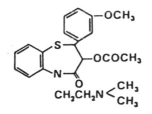

Diltiazem

Figure 1: Structures of calcium channel blockers.

cardial perfusion. Studies show that, at least over the short term, these agents do indeed have a potent antihypertensive effect when used alone or in combination with other antihypertensives. Unfortunately, long-term studies are still lacking and need to be undertaken to establish long-term efficacy and safety.

Calcium blockers can be considered to be of two pharmacological classes:

(a) *Those resembling verapamil* which therefore possess both vaso-dilating and cardiodepressing actions: verapamil, diltiazem, bepridil, gallopamil, perhexiline, tiapamil.

(b) *Those resembling nifedipine* which are vasodilating but *not* cardio-depressing: nifedipine, nicardipine, nisoldipine, felodipine, cinnarezine, flunarizine, lidoflazine, PY-108, PN-200, and nitrendipine.

1. *As a single agent in the treatment of patients with combined angina and systemic hypertension:*

Frishman et al[6] compared oral propranolol and verapamil in a placebo controlled double-blind randomized crossover trial of patients with combined angina and hypertension. They found propranolol normalized blood pressure in 7 of 12 patients as compared to 11 of 12 normalized with verapamil. The anti-anginal effect of the two was equal.

2. *As an alternative to other Step 2 drugs in stepped care approach to hypertension:[7-13]*

The calcium channel blocker, nifedipine, has been shown to be an alternative to beta-blockers in patients with asthma or chronic obstructive airways disease, conditions which can be aggravated by beta-adrenergic blockade.[8] Lewis et al[12] reported verapamil's hypotensive efficacy when substituted for beta-blockers in patients whose blood pressure was inadequately controlled using the combination of beta-blockers and thiazides.

3. *Nifedipine or verapamil as alternatives to hydralazine and other vasodilators in Step 3 of stepped-care regimens:[14-16]*

Nifedipine has been reported to have an additive hypotensive effect when combined with alpha-methyldopa,[17] beta-blockers,[9,13,14,18-25] and clonidine.[14] In addition, the calcium antagonists apparently lack the serious idiosyncratic side effects seen with other Step-3 vasodilators such as hydralazine (lupus syndrome),[26] minoxidil (hirsutism),[27] and diazoxide (diabetes).[28]

4. *Nifedipine as an alternative to other drugs in hypertensive emergencies[29-35] or severe hypertension.[13,17]*

Calcium Channel Blocker Monotherapy

Short-term nifedipine monotherapy results in a decrease of both systolic and diastolic pressure (Table II). Clinical experience with 172

TABLE II
SHORT-TERM NIFEDIPINE MONOTHERAPY

Study (Ref.)	No. Patients	Maximal Oral Dose (mg/day)	Minimal Duration of Therapy (wks)	Mean Blood Pressure Pre-treatment		Mean Blood Pressure Post-treatment		Pulse Rate (beats/min)	Decline in Blood Pressure (mm Hg)
				Supine (mm Hg)	Pulse Rate (beats/min)	Supine (mm Hg)	Pulse Rate (beats/min)		
Ekelund et al 1982[13]	14	30	4	178/99	77	158/83	82	+5	20/11
Guazzi et al 1980[17]	11	40	1	210/126	—	170/101	—	*	40/25
Eggertsen et al 1982[19]	13	30	12	157/106	—	148/96	—	—	9/10
Pedersen et al 1980[23]	13	60	3	178/112	82	153/95	89	+7	25/17
MacGregor et al 1982[36]	15	40	6	192/113	—	153/92	—	**	39/21
Hornung et al 1983[37]	15	120	8	175/98	—	141/80	—	—	34/18
Gould et al 1982[38]	9	120	6	182/106	—	148/86	—	—	34/20
Mitbo et al 1982[39]	28	40	6	149/107	67	133/93	68	+1	16/14
Murakami et al 1972[40]	7	30	1	164/98	73	138/84	76	+3	26/14
Olivari et al 1979[41]	14	20	3	190/117	—	158/97	—	*	32/20
Olivari et al 1979[41]	13	40	3	205/118	—	165/97	—	*	40/21
Klein et al 1983[42]	20	60	8	152/106	84	140/91	77	−1	12/15
TOTALS	172								27/17

* Precise values not reported; slight increase in heart rate for one hour reported.
** Significant increase in standing pulse reported; no precise values.

patients receiving nifedipine as a single agent shows an average blood pressure reduction of 27/17 mm Hg (Table II—all studies weighted equally). Note that the fall in blood pressure is related to pre-treatment blood pressure[36] and dosage given. Heart rate tends to increase with nifedipine and nifedipine-like calcium blockers,[14,17,19,35,36] in contradistinction from the verapamil-like drugs which possess cardio-depressant effects as well as vasodilatory (Table I). At least three studies reporting no significant change in heart rate used nifedipine slow-release tablets rather than capsules.[37-39]

Clinical experience with 259 mild to moderate hypertensive patients shows that short-term verapamil monotherapy results in an average decline in blood pressure of 23/17 (Table III—all studies weighted equally). Fall in blood pressure varies with pre-treatment blood pressure and dosage. Heart rate is usually decreased,[6,7,11,12,43,45] about 7%.

Four short-term diltiazem monotherapy studies found an average decline in blood pressure of 18/15 mm Hg with 153 mild to moderate hypertensive patients (Table IV).[42,46-48] Two studies reported a slight decrease (4%)[42,46] in heart rate and in two studies, heart rate was unchanged.[47,48] Since diltiazem, like verapamil, has cardio-depressant action, one can expect modest decrements in pulse rate.

Which One is Best for Hypertension?

Published double-blind studies comparing the blood pressure lowering effects of the calcium channel blockers are scarce. In an eight-week double-blind randomized study, Klein et al found diltiazem (180–270 mg/day) and nifedipine (30–60 mg/day) to be equipotent hypotensive agents.[42] Another study found that verapamil and nifedipine produced similar reductions in blood pressure, but that heart rate was lowered by verapamil and unaffected with nifedipine.[38] One investigator[39] found verapamil to have a slightly greater hypotensive effect, but admitted his results might have been influenced by the use of slow-release nifedipine tablets, resulting in insufficient drug plasma levels. Though these preliminary studies indicate hypotensive effects of these three agents are similar, more long-term double-blind studies are certainly needed.

Comparison with Beta-blocker Monotherapy

In a double-blind crossover study of 12 patients, Frishman et al reported that verapamil was slightly more effective than propranolol in reducing standing blood pressure, but that propranolol was slightly

TABLE III
SHORT-TERM VERAPAMIL MONOTHERAPY

Study (Ref.)	No. Patients	Maximal Oral Dose (mg/day)	Duration of Therapy (wks)	Mean Blood Pressure Pre-treatment Supine (mm Hg)	Pulse Rate (beats/min)	Mean Blood Pressure Post-treatment Supine (mm Hg)	Pulse Rate (beats/min)	Change in Pulse Rate (beats/min)	Decline in Blood Pressure (mm Hg)
Frishman et al 1982[6]	12	480	3	158/98	80	144/88	72	−8	24/10
Anavekar et al 1981[7]	17	360	6	172/98*	81	159/83*	80	−1	13/10
Anavekar et al 1982[8]	9	320	6	174/111*	81	154/89*	74	−7	20/22
Lewis et al 1978[11]	23	360	4	188/106*	81	161/84*	77	−4	27/22
Lewis et al 1978[11]	23	240	4	188/106*	81	173/93*	81	0	15/13
Lewis et al 1979[12]	26	480	—	201/114	81	164/87	78	−3	37/27
Gould et al 1982[38]	16	480	6	182/105	—	149/82	—	—	33/23
Buehler et al 1982[43]	43	720	6	171/108	81	152/93	74	−7	19/15
Midtbo et al 1980[44]	23	480	4	154/104	66	144/94	61	−5	10/10
Leonetti et al 1980[45]	12	480	1	177/111	79	150/96	77	−2	27/15
de Leeuw et al 1982[49]	15	480	1	170/100	72	140/81	66	−6	30/19
Leary et al 1979[50]	40	320	8	178/110	77	157/102	79	+2	21/8
TOTALS	259								22/16

* Concomitant therapy with diuretic.

TABLE IV
SHORT-TERM AND SINGLE-DOSE DILTIAZEM MONOTHERAPY

Study (Ref.)	No. Patients	Maximal Oral Dose (mg/day)	Duration of Therapy (wks)	Mean Blood Pressure Pre-treatment Supine (mm Hg)	Pulse Rate (beats/min)	Mean Blood Pressure Post-treatment Supine (mm Hg)	Pulse Rate (beats/min)	Change in Pulse Rate (beats/min)	Decline in Blood Pressure (mm Hg)
Klein et al 1984[42]	23	270	8	152/105	78	143/94	76	−2	9/11
Giesecke et al 1981[46]	80	270	6	167/106	76	137/84	72	−4	30/22
Brandt et al 1981[47]	10	360	4	152/107	—	138/91	—	—	14/16
Ikeda et al 1979[48]	40	180	6	170/102***	—	150/90***	—	—	20/12
Safar et al 1983[51]	11	*	**	179/90	69	165/81	68	−1	14/9
Levenson et al 1983[52]	16	*	**	181/90	74	157/84	70	−4	24/6
Kusaba et al 1978[53]	25	180	—	179/106***	—	163/93***	—	—	16/13

* Dose = .2 mg/kg.
** Only one administration.
*** Concomitant therapy.

more effective in reducing supine blood pressure.[6] In addition, over 90% of patients' blood pressures were normalized with verapamil whereas only about 60% of patients achieved normalization of blood pressure with propranolol.[6] Anavekar et al, in a randomized, double-blind cross-over trial of 17 hypertensive patients, found verapamil and pindolol to be equivalent in blood pressure lowering ability as well as overall responder rates.[7] Buehler et al reported that while overall hypotensive effects of verapamil and beta-blockers were similar, verapamil was more efficacious in the low renin, older patients whereas beta-blockers worked more effectively in high renin, younger patients.[43] These and other studies indicate that beta-blockers and calcium channel blockers appear similar in their overall blood pressure lowering effect.[8,12,54,55] More long-term studies are clearly needed to establish the comparative usefulness of these two classes of drugs.

Verapamil was more efficacious in the low renin,
older patients whereas beta-blockers worked more effectively in
high renin, younger patients.

Combination Therapy

There is fairly general agreement that nifedipine can be safely combined with beta blockers.[56-58] Not only does this combination have an additive hypotensive effect (Table V), but also nifedipine's side effects are greatly diminished by the addition of beta-blockers.[14,15,19,21,56,59] (See Side Effects.) One investigator reported that tolerance developed to nifedipine's antihypertensive effects during long-term treatment, but that this tolerance was not observed with combination nifedipine/beta-blocker therapy.[59]

Brennan and Blake[18] reported the addition of nifedipine to combination beta-blocker and diuretic therapy in refractory hypertension. Blood pressure was normalized (less than 140/100 mm Hg) in 17 out of 21 patients and side effects were mild. Nifedipine has also been reported to have an additive hypotensive effect when combined with alpha-methyldopa[17] and clonidine.[48] Noteworthy was Guazzi's observation that side effects and daily blood pressure fluctuations seen with nifedipine monotherapy were reduced when the drug was combined with alpha-methyldopa.[17]

Verapamil is rarely used in combination with beta-blockers due to

TABLE V

ANTIHYPERTENSIVE EFFICACY OF 20–60 MG/DAY NIFEDIPINE GIVEN WITH A BETA-BLOCKER

Study (Ref.)	No. of Patients	Minimum Duration of Therapy (wks)	Beta-Blocker Used and Dosage (mg/day)	Placebo Supine (mm Hg)	Placebo Pulse Rate (beats/min)	Nifedipine Monotherapy Supine (mm Hg)	Nifedipine Monotherapy Pulse Rate (beats/min)	Beta-Blocker Monotherapy Supine (mm Hg)	Beta-Blocker Monotherapy Pulse Rate (beats/min)	Combination Supine (mmHg)	Combination Pulse Rate (beats/min)
Eggertsen et al 1982[13]	13	12	Metoprolol 200	157/106	—	148/96	—	—	—	146/89	—
Ekelund et al 1982[14]	14	4	Metoprolol 200	178/99	77	158/88	96	156/92	60*	141/84	63*
Opie et al 1982[20]	15	4	Atenolol 100	—	—	—	—	193/120	59	155/97	64
Aoki et al 1981[21]	25	8	Propranolol 40	212/128	83	—	—	—	—	139/84	67*
Opie et al 1982[22]	15	4	Atenolol 100	—	—	—	—	165/102	*	148/94	*
Pedersen et al 1980[23]	9	4	Various	—	—	—	—	169/108	62	146/94	66
Bayley et al 1982[25]	11	2	Various	—	—	—	—	157/99	60*	138/88	63*
Husted et al 1982[59]	10	48	Various	—	—	—	—	184/115	68*	143/92	68*

* Indicates some patients treated with a diuretic in addition to other therapy.

potential additive cardio-depressant effects[60] (see Drug Interactions and Warnings). In a randomized, double-blind crossover trial, Anavekar et al reported the additive hypotensive effect of verapamil given to patients taking thiazides.[7] Lewis et al reported that the administration of verapamil to patients whose blood pressure was poorly controlled with either thiazides, alpha-methyldopa, or clonidine resulted in a further decrease in blood pressure averaging 25–30 mm Hg diastolic.[11] Leary et al reported the additive hypotensive effects of verapamil and reserpine.[50] At the present time, long-term double-blind studies are clearly lacking.

Published studies on the use of diltiazem in multi-drug regimens are scarce. Diltiazem has been reported to have an additive hypotensive effect when administered together with either thiazides[48,61] or reserpine.[48] Uncontrolled studies of 296 Japanese hypertensive patients report that diltiazem had an additive hypotensive effect when combined with various other antihypertensive medications.[62-76]

Nifedipine has been shown to be effective in hypertensive emergencies and in severe hypertension (see Table VI). A recent single-blind placebo-controlled study of 25 patients with severe hypertension by Bertel et al[29] found that after oral administration, nifedipine's antihypertensive effect was first observed after 10 minutes, was maximal after 30–40 minutes, and lasted for at least 90 minutes. Average blood pressure fell from 221/126 to 152/89 mm Hg while heart rate increased from 74 to 84 beats per minute.[29] In another study, sublingual nifedipine began to lower blood pressure in five minutes.[34]

Approved Indications for Calcium Channel Blockers
Nifedipine
— Chronic stable angina in patients who remain symptomatic despite adequate doses of beta-blockers and/or organic nitrates or who cannot tolerate these agents.
— Vasospastic angina confirmed by any of the following criteria: 1) classical pattern of angina at rest accompanied by ST segment elevation, 2) angina or coronary artery spasm provoked by ergonovine, or 3) angiographically demonstrated coronary artery spasm.

Verapamil
— Angina at rest including: 1) vasospastic (Prinzmetal's variant angina), or 2) unstable (crescendo pre-infarction angina).
— Chronic stable angina (classic effort-induced angina)

TABLE VI
NIFEDIPINE SINGLE DOSE STUDIES IN HYPERTENSIVE EMERGENCIES AND SEVERE HYPERTENSION

Study (Ref.)	No. Patients	Single Oral Dose (mg); Route of Administration	Mean Blood Pressure Pre-treatment		Mean Blood Pressure Post-treatment (30 minutes)		Pulse Rate (beats/min)	Decline in Blood Pressure (mm Hg)
			Supine (mm Hg)	Pulse Rate (beats/min)	Supine (mm Hg)	Pulse Rate (beats/min)		
Aoki et al 1978[24]	9	30;—	167/113	70	122/81	82	+12	45/32
Beer et al 1981[30]	17	10;SL	172/109	—	140/88	—	—	32/21
Beer et al 1981[30]	26	20;SL	204/128	76	160/97	89	+13	44/31
Bertel et al 1983[29]	25	20;PO	221/126	74	152/89	84	+10	69/37
Conen et al 1982[31]	18	20;PO	220/122	74	150/86	85	+11	70/36
Guazzi** et al 1977[34]	3	60;SL	307/164	—	248/112	—	—	59/52
Guazzi et al 1977[34]	17	10;PO	148*	—	112*	—	+21.6%	36*
Imai et al[14]	—	20;PO	159*	—	125*	—	—	34*
Kuwajima et al 1982[32]	6	10;PO	237/110	89	150/73	87	−2	87/34
Kuwajima et al 1982[32]	12	10;PO	205/113	72	162/92	80	+8	43/21
Polese et al 1979[37]	7	10;PO	221/120	88	177/94	96	+8	44/26

SL = sublingual; PO = oral.
* Mean arterial blood pressure.
** Results reported are 60 minutes post-treatment.

Diltiazem

— Variant or Prinzmetal's angina
— Chronic stable angina in those patients who remain symptomatic despite adequate doses of beta-blockers or nitrates or who cannot tolerate these agents.

Formulations

Verapamil (ISOPTIN®, CALAN®) . . . 80 or 120 mg tablets (sugar coated)
Nifedipine (PROCARDIA®) . . . . 10 mg gelatin capsules
Diltiazem (CARDIZEM®) . . . . 30 or 60 mg tablets

Dose in Hypertension
Diltiazem

Frequency: three or four times a day
Initial: 30 mg three or four times a day
Range: 60–240 mg/day
Usual dose: 120–240 mg/day given in divided doses

Nifedipine

Frequency: three times a day
Initial: 10 mg three times daily
Range: 10–120 mg/day
Usual dose: 10–20 mg three times daily

Verapamil

Frequency: three times a day
Initial: 80 mg three times daily
Range: 80–480 mg/day
Usual dose: 240–360 mg/day divided into three doses

Mechanism of Action

Slow channel blockers cause arteriolar dilation through a direct action on vascular smooth muscle; these drugs block or distort cell membrane calcium gates, thus interfering with the transmembrane flux of calcium ions necessary for smooth muscle contraction or impulse generation[60,77-81] (Figure 2). Although the etiology of the increased peripheral vascular resistance seen in hypertension is still controversial,[77,79,81-83] one investigator's "unified theory" closely links calcium and sodium ions to blood pressure regulation.[79,80] According to Blaustein, one cell membrane "gate" couples the inward flow of calcium ions to the outward flow of sodium ions. Thus, intracellular calcium ion concentrations are very sen-

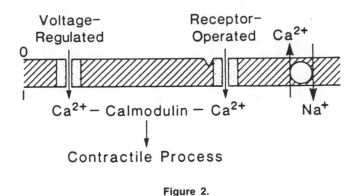

Figure 2.

sitive to changes in sodium ion concentrations.[78-80] Ingestion of a high salt load, through a complex mechanism, may increase the ratio of intracellular to extracellular sodium, resulting in an increased extrusion of sodium in exchange for calcium and, finally, an increase in peripheral vascular resistance.[79,80] Others have also suggested that calcium metabolism is abnormal in hypertension.[77,81,84] Supporting this theory of altered calcium handling in hypertensives is the finding that calcium channel blockers reduce blood pressure only minimally in normotensive patients, but cause significant blood pressure reductions in hypertensive subjects.[85] Thus, calcium channel blockers may be a more specific treatment of hypertension.[60]

The exact site of action of calcium channel blockers is not presently known. However, given their diverse chemical structures and pharmacological actions, a different site of action for each drug is a distinct possibility[43,77,86] (Table I and Figure 1).

The following mechanisms may contribute to the hemodynamic effects of calcium channel blockers:

1. Decreased peripheral vascular resistance leading to decreased afterload;
2. Decreased central venous pressure leading to reduced cardiac preload;
3. Negative inotropic, chronotropic and dromotropic effects on myocardial function;
4. Coronary vasodilation leading to increased arterial blood flow to ischemic areas of the myocardium; and
5. Inhibition of secretion of catecholamines, resulting in decreased adrenergic cardiovascular stimulation.

The calcium channel blockers, as already mentioned, can be divided into two groups based on their hemodynamic effects. Nifedipine-like Ca channel blockers decrease peripheral vascular resistance, increase heart rate and increase cardiac output.[16,17,32,34,40-42,57] In contrast to verapamil-like Ca channel blockers, the nifedipine group lacks significant depressant effects on AV nodal conduction and cardiac contractility at clinical doses.[16] Thus nifedipine-like drugs can be combined safely with beta-adrenergic blocking agents.[57,60]

Guazzi et al[34] studied the hemodynamic effects of 10 mg oral doses of nifedipine on patients with severe primary hypertension and found that 30 minutes after administration, patients showed an average decrease in supine mean arterial pressure of 24.37% (36 mm Hg), an increase in heart rate (+21.6%), stroke index (+7%), and cardiac index (+30.89) and a 42.4% reduction of total peripheral resistance. After 120 minutes, mean arterial pressure was still reduced (−19.5%) while heart rate had returned to normal.[34] They also found that magnitude of hypotensive effect was identical for both sublingual and oral administration, but that sublingual administration resulted in a faster onset time (5 to 8 minutes as compared to 20 to 25 minutes) and time of maximal effect (15 to 18 minutes as compared to 30 to 35 minutes).[34]

Hemodynamic effects of intravenously administered verapamil are more controversial.[60] While most agree that verapamil causes a significant decrease in peripheral vascular resistance and arterial pressure, heart rate and cardiac index have been reported either to increase, decrease or remain unchanged.[57,60] However, due to verapamil's negative inotropic and chronotropic effects, this drug should be very cautiously administered to patients with compromised left ventricular function.[60]

Several studies document the hemodynamic effects of diltiazem on hypertensives. All agree that diltiazem significantly lowers peripheral vascular resistance.[42,51,87,88] However, some report a decrease in cardiac output[88,89] while others report an increase in cardiac output.[42,51] Heart rate is reported to be lowered[42,88] and not significantly changed.[51,87]

Drug Interactions
Nifedipine

1. With *Beta-Adrenergic Blockade*

The rationale behind combined beta-blocker and nifedipine therapy is twofold. First, since both drugs lower blood pressure by different mechanisms, an additive antihypertensive effect is seen (Table VI). Second, and as important, many of the adverse side effects and the reflex tachycardia seen with nifedipine monotherapy are greatly diminished or completely abolished by concomitant beta-adrenergic blocker therapy.[23] Thus the dropout rate due to adverse reactions is much lower when beta-adrenergic blocking drugs are used with nifedipine.[23] Side effects reported to be reduced in these studies include palpitations, flushing and heat sensation, and headache. However, in a recent long-term trial, fluid retention or peripheral edema was a frequent adverse reaction when nifedipine was given either alone or in combination with beta-adrenergic blockade; this adverse reaction can be corrected with concomitant diuretic therapy. In addition, resistance to long-term nifedipine monotherapy was reported but not when nifedipine was combined with a beta-blocker.

Experience in over 1,400 patients in a non-comparative clinical trial has shown that concomitant administration of nifedipine and beta-adrenergic blocking agents is usually well tolerated. However, there have been occasional literature reports suggesting the combination may increase the likelihood of congestive heart failure, severe hypotension, or exacerbation of angina.

2. With *Diuretics*

Preliminary data show an additive antihypertensive effect of combined therapy.

3. With *Long-Acting Nitrates*

Nifedipine may be safely administered with nitrates, but there have been no published studies evaluating the antianginal effectiveness of this combination.

4. With *Digitalis*

Administration of nifedipine with digoxin increased digoxin levels in 9 of 12 normal volunteers. The average increase was 45%. Another investigator found no increase in digoxin levels in 13 patients with coronary artery disease. In an uncontrolled study of over 200 patients with congestive heart failure during which digitalis levels were not measured, digitalis toxicity was not observed. Since there have been isolated reports of patients with elevated digoxin levels, it is recommended that digitalis levels be monitored when initiating, adjusting or discontinuing nifedipine.

5. With *Alpha-Methyldopa*

Although large, controlled data are lacking at this time, one study of 23 subjects reported an additive hypotensive effect of these two agents. In addition, alpha-methyldopa greatly diminished the reflexive increase in heart rate seen with nifedipine monotherapy.[17]

Verapamil

1. With *Beta-Blockers*

Controlled studies in small numbers of patients suggest that the concomitant use of verapamil and beta-adrenergic blocking agents may be beneficial in patients with chronic stable angina or arterial hypertension, but available information is not sufficient to predict with confidence the effects of concomitant treatment, especially in patients with left ventricular dysfunction or cardiac conduction abnormalities. The combination of two drugs, both of which have depressant action on the SA and AV nodes, can have adverse effects on cardiac function. In one study of 15 patients treated with high doses of propranolol (median dose 480 mg/day) for severe angina, with preserved left ventricular function, the hemodynamic effects of additional therapy with verapamil were studied using invasive methods. The addition of verapamil to high dose beta-blockers induced insignificant negative inotropic and chronotropic effects which were not severe enough to limit short-term (48 hr) combination therapy in this study. However, caution is urged when using this combination. Because of the still limited experience with combination therapy, verapamil should be used alone ordinarily. If combined therapy is needed, close surveillance of vital signs and clinical status should be carried out and the need for concomitant therapy reassessed periodically. Combined therapy should usually be avoided in patients with atrioventricular conduction abnormalities and those with depressed left ventricular function.

2. With *Digitalis*

Chronic verapamil treatment increases serum digoxin levels by 50–70% during the first week of therapy and this can result in digitalis toxicity. Maintenance doses of digitalis should be reduced when verapamil is administered and the patient should be carefully monitored to avoid over- or under-digitalization. The effect of verapamil is dose-related and due to suppression of the renal and extrarenal digoxin elimination.[89]

3. With *Diuretics*

Verapamil administered concomitantly with diuretics gives an additive antihypertensive effect.

4. With *Disopyramide*

Until data on possible interactions between these drugs are obtained, disopyramide should not be administered within 48 hours before or 24 hours after verapamil administration.

5. With *Quinidine*

In a small number of patients with hypertrophic cardiomyopathy (IHSS), concomitant use of verapamil and quinidine resulted in significant hypotension. Until further data are obtained, combined therapy of verapamil and quinidine in these patients should be avoided.

6. With *Nitrates*

Verapamil has been given concomitantly with short- and long-acting nitrates without any undesirable drug interactions. The pharmacological profile of both drugs suggests beneficial interactions.

Contraindications

Nifedipine: none except known hypersensitivity reaction to drug.

Verapamil:
- a) severe left ventricular dysfunction (heart failure);
- b) hypotension (less than 90 mm Hg systolic pressure) or cardiogenic shock;
- c) sick sinus syndrome (except in patients with a functioning artificial ventricular pacemaker); and
- d) second or third degree AV block;

Diltiazem:
- a) sick sinus syndrome except in the presence of a functioning ventricular pacemaker;
- b) patients with second or third degree AV block; and
- c) patients with hypotension (less than 90 mm Hg systolic).

Warnings

1. Nifedipine:

Excessive hypotension has occurred in a few patients. These responses have usually occurred during initial titration or at the time of subsequent upward dosage adjustment and may be more likely in patients on concomitant therapy with beta-blockers. Physicians should be aware of the potential adverse reaction between nifedipine and fentanyl which results in severe hypotension and/or increased fluid volume requirements.

A few patients have developed well-documented increased frequency, duration or severity of angina on starting nifedipine or at the time of dosage increases.

Initiation of nifedipine treatment may exacerbate increased angina associated with beta-blocker withdrawal. It is important to taper beta-blockers, if possible, rather than stopping them abruptly before beginning nifedipine therapy.

Rarely, patients, usually those receiving a beta-blocker, have developed heart failure after beginning nifedipine. Patients with tight aortic stenosis are at greater risk for such an event.

2. Verapamil:

Heart Failure: Verapamil should be avoided in patients with severe left ventricular dysfunction (e.g., ejection fraction less than 37 or moderate to severe symptoms of cardiac failure) and in patients with any degree of ventricular dysfunction if they are receiving a beta-blocker. Patients with milder ventricular dysfunction should, if possible, be controlled with optimal doses of digitalis and/or diuretics before verapamil treatment.

Hypotension: Occasionally, verapamil may produce excessive hypotension. Hypotension is usually asymptomatic, orthostatic, or mild and can be controlled by a decrease in the verapamil dose.

Elevated liver enzymes: Occasional elevation of transaminases and alkaline phosphatase has been reported. The potential for hepatocellular type injury with verapamil appears to exist. Thus, patients on long-term verapamil therapy should have liver enzymes monitored periodically.

Atrial flutter/fibrillation with accessory bypass tract: Patients with atrial flutter or fibrillation with an accessory AV pathway may develop increased antegrade conduction across the aberrant pathway bypassing the AV node, producing a very rare ventricular response after receiving verapamil. Treatment is usually D. C.-cardioversion.

AV block: The effect of verapamil on AV conduction and the SA node leads to first degree AV block and transient bradycardia, sometimes accompanied by nodal escape rhythms, fairly common during the peaks of serum concentrations. Higher degrees of AV block, however, are infrequently (0.8%) observed. Marked first degree or development of second or third degree AV block requires a lowering of verapamil dosage or discontinuation of therapy and institution of appropriate therapy depending on the clinical situation.

Patients with hypertrophic cardiomyopathy treated with verapamil saw an increased incidence of severe side effects. Most adverse effects responded well to a reduction in dosage.

3. Diltiazem

Cardiac conduction: Diltiazem rarely produces bradycardia or second or third degree block (4 of 959 patients or 0.42%). Concomitant use of diltiazem with beta-blockers or digitalis may result in additive effects on cardiac conduction.

Congestive heart failure: Experience with the use of this drug in patients with impaired left ventricular function is very limited, but diltiazem's documented negative inotropic effect warrants extreme caution when using this drug in such patients.

Hypotension: Decreases in blood pressure with diltiazem may occasionally result in symptomatic hypotension.

Acute hepatic injury: There has been a single report in a patient receiving 120 mg of diltiazem t.i.d. of marked transaminase elevation (SGOT 4500, SGPT 2300), accompanied by hyperbilirubinemia (> 3 mg/dl), occurring after four days of treatment. The enzyme abnormalities resolved entirely and enzymes were nearly normal a week after cessation of treatment.

Use in Pregnancy

1. Nifedipine

The safety of nifedipine therapy during pregnancy has not been established. Nifedipine has been shown to be teratogenic in rats when given in large doses (30X normal human dose), but as of yet, there are no adequate and well-controlled studies on pregnant women. Therefore, nifedipine should be used only when potential benefits outweigh the unknown risks to the fetus.

2. Verapamil

Although animal studies have not shown this compound to be teratogenic when given in large doses, there are no adequate or well-controlled studies in pregnant women. As with nifedipine, verapamil should be administered to pregnant women only if its use is deemed essential by the physician.

3. Diltiazem

Animal studies at large doses (5–20× human dose on a mg/kg basis) have resulted in embryo and fetal lethality as well as an increased incidence of stillbirths. However, no well-controlled studies on pregnant women exist at this time. Therefore, diltiazem should only be used when potential benefits to the mother outweigh potential risk to the fetus.

Precautions

1. Nifedipine

Hypotension: Because nifedipine decreases peripheral vascular resistance, careful monitoring of blood pressure during the initial administration and titration of nifedipine is suggested. Special caution must be used in patients already taking other blood pressure lowering medication.

Peripheral edema: Mild to moderate peripheral edema, typically due to arterial dilation and not to left ventricular dysfunction, occurs in approximately one in ten patients. This edema usually occurs in the lower extremities and usually responds to diuretic therapy.

2. Verapamil

Use in patients with impaired hepatic function: Since verapamil is metabolized in the liver, it should be administered cautiously to patients with impaired hepatic function. Severe liver dysfunction prolongs the elimination half-life of verapamil to approximately 14–16 hours; hence, approximately 30% of the dose given to patients with normal liver function should be administered to these patients.

Use in patients with impaired renal function: Until further data are available, verapamil should be administered cautiously to patients with impaired renal function.

3. Diltiazem

General: Diltiazem is extensively metabolized by the liver and excreted by the kidneys and in the bile. As with any new drug given over long periods, laboratory parameters should be monitored at regular intervals and with special attention when the patient has impaired renal or hepatic function.

Management of Overdosage or Exaggerated Response

Although there is no well-documented experience with nifedipine overdosage, available data suggest that gross overdosage would result in excessive peripheral vasodilatation with subsequent marked and probably prolonged systemic hypotension. Clinically significant hypotension due to nifedipine requires active cardiovascular support, including monitoring of cardiac and respiratory function, elevation of extremities, and attention to circulating fluid volume and urine output. A vasoconstrictor (such as norepinephrine) may be helpful in restoring vascular tone and blood pressure.

Treatment of overdosage with verapamil should be supportive. Beta-adrenergic stimulation or parenteral administration of calcium solutions (calcium chloride) may increase calcium ion flux across the slow channel and has been used effectively in the treatment of deliberate overdosage with verapamil. Clinically significant hypotensive reactions or fixed high degree AV block should be treated with vasopressor agents or cardiac pacing, respectively. Asystole should be handled by the usual measures, including cardiopulmonary resuscitation.

Overdosage experience with oral diltiazem has not been reported. Single oral doses of 300 mg of diltiazem have been well tolerated by healthy volunteers. In the event of overdosage or exaggerated response, appropriate supportive measures should be employed in addition to gastric lavage. The following measures may be considered: 1) bradycardia—administer atropine (0.6 to 1.0 mg) intravenously. If there is no response to vagal blockade, administer isoproterenol cautiously; 2) high degree of AV block—treat as for bradycardia above. Fixed high-degree AV block should be treated with cardiac pacing; 3) cardiac failure—administer inotropic agents and diuretics; 4) hypotension—vasopressors (e.g., dopamine or levarterenol bitartrate).

Absorption, Metabolism, Excretion

1. Nifedipine

Following oral administration, greater than 90% of nifedipine is absorbed. The drug undergoes moderate first-pass liver metabolism (20–30% of administered dose), and the bioavailability is 65–70%. The onset of action is less than 20 minutes after oral administration and about three minutes after sublingual administration. Peak concentrations are reached in the plasma 30 minutes after oral administration. Nifedipine is extensively protein bound (90%). The drug has an initial fast half-life of 2.5 to 3 hours and a terminal slow half-life of five hours.

The drug is almost completely metabolized by the liver to a "free acid," a small fraction of which is converted to a lactone. All metabolites are pharmacologically inactive and are excreted by the kidney. A small fraction (10%) of metabolized drug appears in the feces.

2. Verapamil

Verapamil is almost completely absorbed after oral administration (90%) but undergoes extensive first-pass liver metabolism, resulting in a low bioavailability of between 20 and 35%. Peak plasma concentrations are reached between one and two hours after oral administration. Plasma half-life values range between three and seven hours. A direct relationship exists between plasma concentration and degree of prolongation of PR interval. The drug is approximately 90% protein bound.

The metabolism of verapamil is complex; 12 different metabolites have been isolated. Most metabolites have long half-lives and are either N or O de-alkylation products of verapamil itself. One matabolite, nor-verapamil, can reach steady-state plasma concentrations approaching that of the parent compound. Some metabolites may be pharmacologically active.

Excretion is primarily renal with 50% of metabolized drug passing out in the urine on the first day and 70% by the fifth day. Approximately 15% is excreted in the feces.

3. Diltiazem

About 80% of diltiazem is absorbed after oral administration and is detectable in the plasma within 30 minutes. Peak plasma levels occur within one hour with normal capsules and at three to four hours with sustained release tablets. There is extensive first-pass metabolism of this drug and consequently a bioavailability of about 40%. Diltiazem is 80% protein bound.

The primary metabolic fate is via hepatic de-acetylation. The deacetyl derivative is detectable in the plasma at concentrations of 15–30% and has about 50% the biologic activity of the parent compound.

The primary rates of excretion are hepatic (65%) and urinary (35%). Two to four percent of unmetabolized drug is found in urine. Caution should be exerted when administering diltiazem to patients with im-

TABLE VII
ADVERSE REACTIONS OF CALCIUM CHANNEL BLOCKERS* (Percent)
(BASED ON 2,100 PATIENTS STUDIED FOR ANGINA)

Side Effects Overall Incidence	Nifedipine 17.0	Verapamil 8.0	Diltiazem 4.0
Dizziness or lightheadedness	10.0	3.6	—
Peripheral edema	10.0	1.7	2.4
Headache	10.0	1.8	2.0
Flushing or heat sensation	10.0	—	—
Transient hypotension	5.0	2.9	—
Nausea	10.0	1.6	2.7
AV block (3rd degree)	—	0.8	0.4
Bradycardia	—	1.1	2.0
Palpitations	2.0	—	—
Congestive heart failure	2.0	0.9	—
Constipation	—	6.3	—
Fatigue	—	1.1	1.1
Syncope	0.5	—	—
Rash	—	—	1.8

* A blank space means the incidence is unknown, not that it is zero.

paired liver function or with drugs which interact with the liver microsomal system.

Adverse Reactions

Table VII shows the relative side effects of the three available calcium blockers. Nifedipine's side effects increase with the dosage and are usually a result of the drug's potent vasodilator properties.[58,90,91] One multi-center, double-blind placebo-controlled study[91] of the use of nifedipine monotherapy in chronic stable angina found a high incidence of the following side effects (total population size = 200): dizziness (26%), headache (20%), heat sensation (15%), palpitations (14%), flushing (14%), fatigue (12%), nausea (12%), edema (11%), and nervousness (11%). The profile of adverse reactions listed in Table VII is from a large, uncontrolled experience in over 2,100 angina patients in the United States; half of these patients were treated concomitantly with beta-adrenergic blocking agents. This above study found no significant difference in the incidence of adverse reactions in patients treated with calcium channel blocker monotherapy and those treated with a combination therapy of beta-blockers and calcium channel blockers. However, several other investigators using smaller hypertensive patient populations found nifedipine side effects, especially palpitations, flushing and headaches, to be greatly diminished in the presence of beta-adrenergic blockade.[14,21,24,56,59] Diuretic therapy was reported to help alleviate the peripheral edema often seen with nifedipine therapy.[17]

Other side effects reported occasionally or rarely have been head cloudiness,[40] dry mouth,[40] myocardial infarction,[59] premature ventricular contractions,[35,41] aggravation of cerebral ischemia,[48] ischemic EKG changes,[92] and, in combination with beta-blockers, heart failure[93] and excessive hypotension.[94] Symposium data gleaned from 8,000 angina pectoris patients show nifedipine side effects caused discontinuation of therapy in approximately 5%.[00]

GI side effects, especially constipation, are much greater with verapamil than with nifedipine (see Tables VIII and IX). Although clinical experience, including 1,166 patients with angina or arrhythmias, reports the incidence of constipation to be only 6.3%, data from ten reports including 240 hypertensive patients (Table IX) show the incidence of constipation to be 29%. Conduction defects are also more common with verapamil-type drugs. There have been several reports of asystole following verapamil therapy.[47,94-97] In the survey of 1,166 patients, the following reactions, reported in less than 0.5%, occurred

TABLE VIII
NIFEDIPINE SIDE EFFECTS SEEN IN 12 REPORTS
INCLUDING 213 HYPERTENSIVE PATIENTS*

Side Effect	Total No. of Patients Exhibiting Side Effect	Percentage Incidence
Flushing or heat sensation	36	17
Headache	30	14
Peripheral edema	20	9
Palpitations	13	6
Dizziness	8	4
Premature ventricular contraction (PVC)	—	—
Increased micturation	5	2
Constipation	4	2
Fatigue	3	1
Nausea	1	1

* Data taken collectively from the following 12 references: 14, 17, 25, 37, 39, 41, 46, 56, 99–102.

TABLE IX
VERAPAMIL SIDE EFFECTS SEEN IN 10 REPORTS
INCLUDING 240 HYPERTENSIVE PATIENTS*

Side Effect	Total No. of Patients Exhibiting Side Effect	Percentage Incidence
Constipation	70	29
Palpitations	5	2
Flushing	4	2
Burning gums or face	3	1
Increased micturation	3	1
Epigastric pain	2	1
Exanthema	2	1
Headache	2	1
AV-block	1	1
SA-block	1	1
Tremor	1	1
Fatigue	1	1

* Data taken collectively from the following 10 references: 7, 8, 11, 12, 38, 39, 44, 45, 98, 99.

under circumstances where a causal relationship is uncertain and are therefore mentioned only to alert the physician to a possible relationship: confusion, paresthesia, insomnia, somnolence, equilibrium disorder, blurred vision, syncope, muscle cramp, shakiness, claudication, hair loss, macules and spotty menstruation. In addition, more serious effects were observed, not readily distinguishable from the natural history of the disease in these patients. Of the 1,166 patients evaluated, 16 (1.4%) had myocardial infarctions.

Two studies comparing hypotensive effects of verapamil and nifedipine have reported side effects with verapamil to be much less than with nifedipine.[12,39] This is in agreement with another report indicating overall incidence of side effects with nifedipine (17%) was much greater than either verapamil (8%) or diltiazem (4%).[98]

REFERENCES:

1. Fleckenstein, A., Kammermeier, H., et al: Zum Wirkungsmechanismus neuartiger Koronardilatoren mit gleichzeitig Sauerstoff-einsparenden Myokard-Effekten. Prenylamin und Iproveratril. Z. Kreislaufforschung., **56**:716–858, 1967.

2. Fleckenstein, A.: Specific inhibitors and promoters of calcium action in the excitation-contraction coupling of heart muscle and their role in the prevention or production of myocardial lesions. In P. Harris and L. H. Opie (Eds.): *Calcium and the Heart*, Academic Press, London, 1970, pp. 135–188.

3. Brittinger, W. E., Schwarzbeck, A., et al: Klinisch-experimentelle Untersuchungen uber die blutdrucksenkende Wirkung von Verapamil. *Deutsche Med. Wschr.*, 37:1871–1877, 1970.

4. Reuter, H., Blaustein, M. P., and Hausler, G.: Na–Ca exchange and tension development in arterial smooth muscle. *Phil. Trans. R. Soc. Lond. B.*, 265:87–94, 1973.

5. Van Breemen, C., Farinas, B. R., Gerba, P., and McNaughton, E. D.: Excitation-contraction coupling in arterial smooth muscle studies by the La^{3+} method for measuring cellular calcium influx. *Circ. Res.*, 30:44–53, 1972.

6. Frishman, W. H., Klein, N. A., et al: Comparison of oral propranolol and verapamil for combined systemic hypertension and angina pectoris: A placebo-controlled double-blind randomized crossover trial. *Am. J. Cardiol.*, 50:1164–1172, 1982.

7. Anavekar, S. N., Christophidis, N., Louis, W. J., and Doyle, A. E.: Verapamil in the treatment of hypertension. *J. Cardiovasc. Pharmacol.*, 3:287–292, 1981.

8. Anavekar, S. N., Barter, C., Adam, W. R., and Doyle, A. E.: A double-blind comparison of verapamil and labetalol in hypertensive patients with coexisting obstructive airways disease. *J. Cardiovasc. Pharmacol.*, 4:S374–S377, 1982.

9. Aoki, K., Sato, K., Kawaguchi, Y., and Yamamoto, M.: Acute and long-term hypotensive effects and plasma concentrations of nifedipine in patients with essential hypertension. *Eur. J. Clin. Pharmacol.*, 23:197–201, 1982.

10. Lewis, G. R. J.: Verapamil in the management of chronic hypertension. *Clin. Invest. Med.*, 3:175–177, 1980.

11. Lewis, G. R. J., Morley, K. D., Lewis, B. M., and Bones, P. J.: The treatment of hypertension with verapamil. *N. Z. Med. J.*, 87:351–354, 1978.

12. Lewis, G. R. J., Morley, K. D., Maslowski, A. H., and Bones, P. J.: Verapamil in the management of hypertensive patients. *Aust. N. Z. J. Med.*, 9:62–64, 1979.

13. Ekelund, L. G., Ekelund, C., and Roessner, S.: Antihypertensive effects at rest and during exercise of a calcium blocker, nifedipine, alone and in combination with metoprolol. *Acta Med. Scand.*, 212:71–75, 1982.

14. Imai, B. Y., Abe, K., et al: Management of severe hypertension with nifedipine in combination with clonidine or propranolol. *Arzneimittelforschung*, 30:674–678, 1980.

15. Murphy, M. B., Scriven, A. J. I., and Dollery, C. T.: Efficacy of nifedipine as a Step 3 antihypertensive drug. *Hypertension*, 5(Suppl II):II-118–II-121, 1983.

16. Robinson, B. F., Bayley, S., et al: Long-term efficacy of calcium antagonists in resistant hypertension. *Hypertension*, 5(4)(Pt 2):II-122–II-124, 1983.

17. Guazzi, M. O., Fiorentini, C., et al: Short- and long-term efficacy of a calcium antagonistic agent (nifedipine) combined with methyldopa in treatment of severe hypertension. *Circulation*, 61:913–919, 1980.

18. Brennan, F. N., and Blake, S.: The use of nifedipine as a third-step agent in the treatment of refractory hypertension. *Ir. Med. J.*, 75:29–30, 1982.

19. Eggertsen, R., and Hansson, L.: Effect of treatment with nifedipine and metoprolol in essential hypertension. *Eur. J. Clin. Pharmacol.*, 21:389–390, 1982.

20. Opie, L. H., White, D., Lee, J., and Subbe, W. F.: Alternatives to beta-blockade in therapy of hypertension with angina pectoris: Role of nifedipine or of labetalol. *Br. J. Clin. Pharmacol.*, 13(Suppl 1):115S–122S, 1982.

21. Aoki, K., Kondo, S., et al: Hypotensive action of nifedipine (Ca^{++}-antagonist) and

propranolol in acute trials and its long-term therapy of hypertensive coronary heart disease patients. *Jpn. Heart J.*, **22**:575–584, 1981.

22. Opie, L. H., Jee, L., and White, D.: Antihypertensive effects of nifedipine combined with cardioselective beta-adrenergic receptor antagonism by atenolol. *Am. Heart J.*, **104**:606–612, 1982.

23. Pedersen, L. O., Christensen, C. K., Mikkelsen, E., and Raemsch, K. D.: Relationship between antihypertensive effect and steady-state plasma concentration of nifedipine given alone or in combination with beta-adrenoceptor blocking agent. *Eur. J. Clin. Pharmacol.*, **18**:287–293, 1980.

24. Aoki, K., Kondo, S., et al: Antihypertensive effect of cardiovascular Ca^{2+}-antagonist in hypertensive patients in the absence and presence of beta-adrenergic blockade. *Am. Heart J.*, **96**:218–226, 1978.

25. Bayley, S., Dobbs, R. J., and Robinson, B. F.: Nifedipine in the treatment of hypertension: Report of a double-blind controlled trial. *Br. J. Clin. Pharmacol.*, **14**:509–512, 1982.

26. Perry, H. M., and Schroeder, H. A.: Syndrome simulating collagen disease caused by hydrallazine (Apresoline). *JAMA*, **154**:670, 1954.

27. Dargie, H. J., Daniel, J., and Dollery, L. T.: Minoxidil in resistant hypertension. *Lancet*, **2**:515, 1977.

28. Updike, S. J., and Harrington, A. R.: Acute diabetic ketoacidosis—a complication of intravenous diazoxide treatment for refractory hypertension. *N. Engl. J. Med.*, **280**:768, 1969.

29. Bertel, O., Conen, D., et al: Nifedipine in hypertensive emergencies. *Br. Med. J.*, **286**:19–21, 1983.

30. Beer, N., Gallegos, I., et al: Efficacy of sublingual nifedipine in the acute treatment of systemic hypertension. *Chest*, **79**:571–574, 1981.

31. Conen, D., Bertel, O., and DuBach, U. C.: An oral calcium antagonist for treatment of hypertensive emergencies. *J. Cardiovasc. Pharmacol.*, **4**:S373–S382, 1982.

32. Kuwajima, I., Ueda, K., et al: A study on the effects of nifedipine in hypertensive crises and severe hypertension. *Jpn. Heart J.*, **19**(4):455–467, 1978.

33. Takekoshi, N., Murakami, E., et al: Treatment of severe hypertension and hypertensive emergency with nifedipine, a calcium-antagonistic agent. *Jpn. Circ. J.*, **45**:852–860, 1981.

34. Guazzi, M., Olivari, M., et al: Nifedipine, a new antihypertensive with rapid action. *Clin. Pharmacol. Ther.*, **22**:528–532, 1977.

35. Polese, A., Fiorentini, C., Olivari, M. T., and Guazzi, M. D.: Clinical use of a calcium antagonistic agent (nifedipine) in acute pulmonary edema. *Am. J. Med.*, **66**:825–830, 1979.

36. MacGregor, G. A., Roteuar, C., et al: Contrasting effects of nifedipine, captopril, and propranolol in normotensive and hypertensive subjects. *J. Cardiovasc. Pharmacol.*, **4**:S358–S362, 1982.

37. Hornung, R. S., Gould, M. B., et al: Nifedipine tablets for systemic hypertension: A study using continuous ambulatory intraarterial monitoring. *Am. J. Cardiol.*, **51**:1323–1327, 1983.

38. Gould, B. A., Hornung, R. S., Mann, S., Balasubramanian, V., and Raftery, E. B.: Slow channel inhibitors verapamil and nifedipine in the management of hypertension. *J. Cardiovasc. Pharmacol.*, **4**:S369–S373, 1982.

39. Midtbo, K., Hals, O., and Van Der Meer, J.: Verapamil compared with nifedipine in the treatment of essential hypertension. *J. Cardiovasc. Pharmacol.*, **4**:S363–S368, 1982.

40. Murakami, M., Murakami, E., et al: Antihypertensive effect of 4(-2-nitrophenyl)-2,

6-dimethyl-1, 4-dihydropyridine-3, 5-dicarbonic acid dimethylester (nifedipine, Bay-a 1040), a new coronary vasodilator. *Jpn. Heart J.*, **13**:128–135, 1972.

41. Olivari, M. T., Bartorelli, C., et al: Treatment of hypertension with nifedipine, a calcium antagonistic agent. *Circulation*, **59**:1056–1062, 1979.

42. Klein, W., Brandt, D., Vrecko, K., and Harringer, M.: Role of calcium antagonists in the treatment of essential hypertension. *Circ. Res.*, **52**(2):I-174–I-181, 1983.

43. Buehler, F. R., Hulthen, U. L., Kiowski, W., Mueller, F. B., and Bolli, P.: The place of the calcium antagonist verapamil in antihypertensive therapy. *J. Cardiovasc. Pharmacol.*, **4**:S350–S357, 1982.

44. Midtbo, K., and Hals, D.: Verapamil in the treatment of hypertension. *Curr. Ther. Res.*, **27**:830–838, 1980.

45. Leonetti, G., Sala, C., Bianchini, C., Terzoli, L., and Zanchetti, A.: Antihypertensive and renal effects of orally administered verapamil. *Eur. J. Clin. Pharmacol.*, **18**:375–382, 1980.

46. Giesecke, H. J., and Guckenbiehl, H. I.: Results of a multi-center study with diltiazem in hypertension (German). In F. Bender and I. Greeff (Eds.): *Calcium antagonisten zur Behandlung der Angina Pectoris, Hypertonie und Arrhythmie*, First DILZEM-Symposium, Copenhagen, June 25–27, 1981, Excerpta Medica, Amsterdam, 1982, pp. 220–226.

47. Brandt, D., and Flein, W.: Relationship between doses and effect of diltiazem in patients with essential hypertension (German). In F. Bender and I. Greeff (Eds.): *Calcium antagonisten zur Behandlung der Angina Pectoris, Hypertonie und Arrhythmie*, First DILZEM-Symposium, Copenhagen, June 25–27, 1981, Excerpta Medica, Amsterdam, 1982, pp. 202–209.

48. Ikeda, M.: Double-blind studies on diltiazem in essential hypertensive patients receiving thiazide therapy. In R. J. Bing (Ed.): *New Drug Therapy With a Calcium Antagonist*. Diltiazem Hakone Symposium, 1978. No. 487, International Congress Series, Excerpta Medica, Amsterdam, 1979, pp. 243–253.

49. De Leeuw, P. W., Smout, A. J. P. M., Willemse, P. J., and Birkenhaeger, W. H.: Effects of verapamil in hypertensive patients. In A. Zanchetti and D. M. Krikler (Eds.): *Calcium Antagonism in Cardiovascular Therapy: Experience with Verapamil*, Excerpta Medica, Amsterdam, 1981, pp. 233–237.

50. Leary, W. P., and Asmal, A. C.: Treatment of hypertension with verapamil. *Curr. Ther. Res.*, **25**:747–752, 1979.

51. Safar, M. E., Simon, A. C., Levenson, J. A., and Cazor, J. G.: Hemodynamic effects of diltiazem in hypertension. *Circ. Res.*, **52**(2):I169–I173, 1983.

52. Levenson, J. A., Safar, M. E., et al: Baroreflex response and vasodilating drugs in essential hypertension. *Chest*, **83**(2):325–327, 1983.

53. Kusaba, T.: The hypotensive effect of Herbesser® in essential hypertension. *Mod. Clin. Med.*, **20**:1859, 1978 (Japanese).

54. Leonetti, G., Pasotti, C., Ferrari, G. P., and Zanchetti, A.: Double-blind comparison of the antihypertensive effects of verapamil and propranolol. In Zanchetti and Krikler (Eds.): *Calcium Antagonism in Cardiovascular Therapy: Experience with Verapamil*. Excerpta Medica, Amsterdam-Oxford-Princeton, 1981, pp. 260–267.

55. Doyle, A. E., Anavekar, S. N., and Oliver, L. E.: A clinical trial of verapamil in the treatment of hypertension. In A. Zanchetti and D. M. Krikler (Eds.): *Calcium Antagonism in Cardiovascular Therapy: Experience with Verapamil*, Excerpta Medica, Amsterdam, 1981, pp. 252–258.

56. Henry, P. O.: Comparative pharmacology of calcium antagonists: Nifedipine, vera-pamil, and diltiazem. *Am. J. Cardiol.*, **46**:1047, 1980.
57. Stone, P. H., Antman, E. M., Muller, J. E., and Braunwald, E.: Calcium channel blocking agents in the treatment of cardiovascular disorders. Part II: Hemodynamic effects and clinical applications. *Ann. Intern. Med.*, **93**:886–904, 1980.
58. Drebs, R.: Adverse reactions with calcium antagonists. *Hypertension*, **5**(4)(Part 2):II-25–II-29, 1983.
59. Husted, S. E., Nielsen, H. K., Christensen, C. K., and Pedersen, L. O.: Long-term therapy of arterial hypertension with nifedipine given alone or in combination with beta-adrenoceptor blocking agent. *Eur. J. Clin. Pharmacol.*, **22**:101–103, 1982.
60. Spivack, C., Ocken, S., and Frishman, W. H.: Calcium antagonists: Clinical use in the treatment of systemic hypertension. *Drugs*, **25**:154–177, 1983.
61. Maeda, K., Takasugi, T., et al: Clinical study of the hypotensive effect of diltiazem hydrochloride. *Int. J. Clin. Pharmacol. Ther. Tox.*, **19**:47–55, 1981.
62. Miyazawa, K., Kanazawa, M., et al: Hemodynamic changes by oral diltiazem hydro-chloride in patients with hypertension. (Japanese) *J. Adult Dis.*, **9**:617, 1979.
63. Aoki, Y., Yamada, A., and Tanaka, N.: Use of Herbesser® in hypertension. (Japanese) *Mod. Clin. Med.*, **20**:1511–1523, 1978.
64. Abe, T.: Clinical trial of diltiazem hydrochloride in hypertension. (Japanese) *Mod. Clin. Med.*, **20**:1255–1259, 1978.
65. Aoi, W., Suzuki, S., et al: Clinical use of diltiazem hydrochloride (Herbesser®) in hypertension. (Japanese) *Clin. Rep.*, **12**:3589, 1978.
66. Kaburagi, T., Habu, I., and Yokoyama, S.: Hypotensive effect of diltiazem (Herbes-ser®). (Japanese) *Mod. Clin. Med.*, **20**:1061–1066, 1978.
67. Katsunuma, H., Koyama, T., et al: The effect of diltiazem hydrochloride (Herbesser®) on hypertension. (Japanese) *Med. Consult. New Remed.*, **14**:761, 1977.
68. Katsunuma, H., Watanabe, Y., et al: The hypotensive effect of diltiazem hydrochloride (Herbesser®) in hypertension patients with reference to renographic study. (Japanese) *Mod. Clin. Med.*, **20**:1073–1079, 1978.
69. Kawai, Y., Yamamoto, T., et al: The clinical effect of diltiazem hydrochloride on hypertension. (Japanese) *J. Adult Dis.*, **5**:1495, 1975.
70. Inagaki, K.: The effect of Herbesser® on hypertension. (Japanese) *Clin. Rep.*, **12**:982, 1978.
71. Sakai, K.: Long-term Herbesser® therapy in hypertension. (Japanese) *Mod. Clin. Med.*, **20**:1053, 1978.
72. Takemiya, T., and Yamaguchi, H.: Hypotensive effect of diltiazem hydrochloride (Herbesser®). Evaluation in 20 clinical cases. (Japanese) *Mod. Clin. Med.*, **20**:1235–1240, 1978.
73. Tsurumi, N.: Hypotensive effect of diltiazem HCl (Herbesser®). (Japanese) *Mod. Clin. Med.*, **20**:1269–1271, 1978.
74. Takahara, M.: Hypotensive effect of diltiazem hydrochloride on essential hyperten-sion. (Japanese) *Clin. Rep.*, **12**:1993, 1978.
75. Tojo, S., Shishido, H., and Yamamoto, S.: Effects of CRD-401 on blood pressure and renal function. (Japanese) *Jpn. J. Clin. Exp. Med.*, **49**:1958, 1972.
76. Yamakado, M. and Tagawa, T.: Hypotensive effect of diltiazem HCl (Herbesser®). (Japanese) *Mod. Clin. Med.*, **20**:1877–1881, 1978.
77. Cohn, J. N.: Calcium, vascular smooth muscle, and calcium entry blockers in hyperten-sion. *Ann. Intern. Med.*, **98**(Part 2):806–809, 1983.

78. Blaustein, M.P.: Sodium ions, calcium ions, blood pressure regulation and hypertension: A reassessment and a hypothesis. *Am. J. Physiol.*, **232**(3):C165–C173, 1977.

79. Blaustein, M. P., Lang, S., and James-Kracke, M.: Cellular basis of sodium-induced hypertension. In Laragh, et al (Eds). *Frontiers in Hypertension Research*, Springer-Verlag, New York, 1981, pp. 87–90.

80. Braunwald, E.: Mechanism of action of calcium-channel-blocking agents. *N. Engl. J. Med.*, **307**:1618–1627, 1982.

81. Pedersen, L. O.: Calcium blockade as a therapeutic principle in arterial hypertension. *Acta Pharmacol. Toxicol.*, **49**(2):5–29, 1981.

82. Das, U. N.: Modification of antihypertensive action of verapamil by inhibition of endogenous prostaglandin synthesis. *Prostaglandins Leukotrienes Med.*, **9**:167–169, 1982.

83. Guazzi, M. O., Polese, A., Bartorelli, A., Loaldi, A., and Fiorentini, C.: Evidence of a shared mechanism of vasoconstriction in pulmonary and systemic circulation in hypertension: A possible role of intracellular calcium. *Circulation*, **66**(4):881–886, 1982.

84. Aoki, K., Yamashita, K., and Hotta, K.: Calcium uptake by subcellular membranes from vascular smooth muscle of spontaneously hypertensive rats. *Jpn. J. Pharmacol.*, **26**:624–627, 1976.

85. Biannchetti, M. G., et al: Calcium and blood pressure regulation in normal and hypertensive subjects. *Hypertension*, **5**(Suppl II):II-57–II-65, 1983.

86. Triggle, D. J., and Swamy, V. C.: Pharmacology of agents that affect calcium. *Chest*, **78**:1, 1980.

87. Kusukawa, R., Kenoshita, M., Shimono, Y., Tomonaga, G., and Hosino, T.: Hemodynamic effects of a new antianginal drug, diltiazem hydrochloride. *Arzneim, Forsch.*, **27**:676–681, 1977.

88. Kinoshita, M., Motomura, M., Kusukawa, R., and Kawakita, S.: Comparison of the hemodynamic effects between beta-blocking agents and a new antianginal agent, diltiazem hydrochloride. *Jpn. Arc. J.*, **43**:587–598, 1979.

89. Belz, G. G., Doering, W., et al: Effect of various calcium antagonists on blood level and renal clearance of digoxin. *Circulation*, **64**(Suppl):IV-24, 1981.

90. Ebner, F., and Dunschede, H. B.: Hemodynamic, therapeutic mechanism of action and clinical finding of Adalat use based on worldwide trials. In A. D. Jateno and P. R. Lichtlen (Eds.): *Proceedings, Third International Adalat Symposium*, Excerpta Medica, Amsterdam, 1976, pp. 283–300.

91. Mueller, H. S., and Chakine, R. A.: Interim report of multicenter double-blind, placebo-controlled studies of nifedipine in chronic stable angina. *Am. J. Med.*, **71**:645–657, 1981.

92. Yagil, Y., Kobrin, I., Leibel, B., and Ben-Ishay, D.: Ischemic ECG changes with initial nifedipine therapy of severe hypertension. (Letter) *Am. Heart J.*, **103**:310–311, 1982.

93. Anastassiades, C. J.: Nifedipine and beta-blocker drugs. *Br. Med. J.*, **281**:1251–1252, 1980.

94. Opie, L. H., and White, D. A.: Adverse interaction between nifedipine and beta-blockade. *Br. Med. J.*, **281**:1462, 1980.

95. Boothby, C. B., Garrard, C. S., and Pickering, D.: Intravenous verapamil in cardiac arrhythmias. *Br. Med. J.*, **2**:349, 1972.

96. Mitchell, L. B., Schroeder, J. S., and Mason, J. W.: Comparative clinical electrophysiologic effects of diltiazem, verapamil and nifedipine: A review. *Am. J. Cardiol.*, **49**:629, 1982.

97. Balasobramanian, V., Lahiri, A., Siram, P., and Raffery, E. B.: Antiagonistic action of verapamil—A controlled study. *Am. J. Cardiol.*, **45**:389, 1980.

98. Zelis, R.: Calcium-blocker therapy for unstable angina pectoris. *N. Engl. J. Med.*, **306**(15):926–928, 1982.

99. Lewis, G. R. J., Stewart, D. J., et al: The antihypertensive effect of oral verapamil—acute and long-term administration and its effects on the high-density lipoprotein values in plasma. In Zanchetti and Krikler (Eds.): *Calcium Antagonism in Cardiovascular Therapy: Experience with Verapamil,* Excerpta Medica, Amsterdam-Oxford-Princeton, 1981, pp. 270–277.

100. Maeda, K., Tanaka, C., et al: Antihypertensive effects of the calcium antagonistic agent nifedipine. *Arzneimittelforschung,* **32**:267–271, 1982.

101. Pedersen, L. O., Mikkelsen, E., Christensen, N. J., Kornerup, H. J., and Pedersen, E. B.: Effect of nifedipine on plasma renin, aldosterone and catecholamines in arterial hypertension. *Eur. J. Clin. Pharmacol.,* **15**:235–240, 1979.

102. Giuntoli, F., Guidi, G., et al: Nifedipine as a single drug therapy in hypertension. *Curr. Ther. Res.,* **30**(4):447–452, 1981.

CHAPTER XI

CONVERTING ENZYME INHIBITORS AND ANGIOTENSIN II BLOCKERS

- CAPTOPRIL (CAPOTEN®)
- ENALAPRIL (VASORIL®)
- SARALASIN (SARENIN®)

CAPTOPRIL (Capoten®)
Introductory year: 1981

INTRODUCTION:

Captopril (Figure 1) is the first orally active antihypertensive agent that interrupts the renin-angiotensin-aldosterone pathway. Because of this mechanism, captopril appears to be particularly beneficial in patients with hyperreninemic hypertension. However, in addition to prevention of angiotensin-II formation, the drug has other mechanisms of action and, indeed, is effective in lowering blood pressure of many normoreninemic and even hyporeninemic patients with mild hypertension. It is most effective when given with a thiazide or loop diuretic. Captopril's most frequent side effects consist of skin rash and loss of taste, and occasionally, proteinuria, and rarely, acute renal failure, agranulocytosis or leukopenia. Due to the serious nature of these adverse reactions, captopril should be used only in patients who are

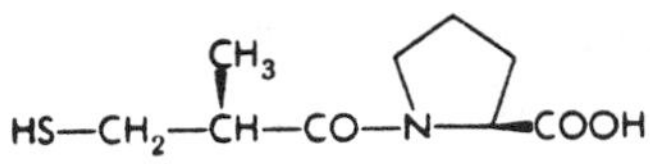

Figure 1: Structure of captopril

refractory to the usual Step-2 drugs. Captopril provides a valuable and innovative addition to the physician's array of choices in the treatment of hypertension, but its ultimate place in the management of hypertensives is not yet fully established.

When should the physician consider captopril for hypertension?

1. In patients with severe hypertension:

Captopril, usually in conjunction with a diuretic, effectively reduces blood pressure in patients with severe or refractory hypertension. This potent angiotensin-converting enzyme inhibitor is often effective when other antihypertensive drugs have failed to reduce blood pressure sufficiently. Due to captopril's adverse effects, it should only be considered when patients' blood pressures are resistant to the usual Step-2 drugs or when unacceptable side effects have developed to such regimens.

2. In patients refractory to standard triple therapy:

Captopril, often in combination with a thiazide-like diuretic or furosemide, effectively lowers blood pressure in patients who are unresponsive to standard triple therapy (which usually includes a diuretic, a beta-blocking agent and a vasodilator). Some patients with refractory hypertension who do not respond to a captopril-diuretic combination often require the addition of other agents such as a beta-blocker and vasodilator.

3. In the management of renovascular or azotemic hypertension:

In azotemic hypertensive patients or in patients with chronic renal insufficiency, captopril may be given (usually with furosemide) but only after clonidine, methyldopa, beta-blockers and vasodilators have been tried. Patients with hypertension due to end-stage renal failure, renovascular disease, or chronic maintenance hemodialysis often respond to captopril.

4. As an alternative Step-2 drug given in low doses, for the management of mild to moderate hypertension.

5. As initial monotherapy in many patients with mild hypertension.

A Veterans Administration Multiclinic Study demonstrated total daily doses of 37.5 and 75 mg effectively reduced blood pressure about 12/10 mm Hg. In addition, two daily doses of captopril were as effective as three times daily.[1]

6. Other uses for captopril:

- *Pediatric hypertension:* Captopril has been shown to be useful in neonates and children with secondary hypertension with varying degrees of renal insufficiency.[2-4] Safety and effectiveness have not been established, however, and captopril should not be used in children unless other measures prove ineffective.
- *Congestive heart failure:* In patients with cardiac failure who are refractory to digitalis, diuretics and vasodilators, captopril has proved quite effective in improving hemodynamic function and reducing disabling symptomatology.

How effective is captopril in hypertension?

Clearly, captopril is a potent and effective antihypertensive agent. When given alone to patients with mild-to-moderate essential hypertension, it will lower pressure to normal levels in the majority of patients (Table I).

Black patients respond less well to captopril than whites. A Veterans Administration Study found the blood pressure of white patients dropped 15/11 mm Hg vs. only 9/8 mm Hg in black patients. However, the addition of hydrochlorothiazide augmented these decrements and abolished these racial differences.[20] There is growing evidence that relatively small doses of 75 or even 37.5 mg/day or less are effective.[1,6,18,21]

When diuretics are also given, an additive effect leads to a further decrease in pressure. Table II summarizes many published reports which show that the addition of hydrochlorothiazide (ranging from 25–100 mg/day), or furosemide (40–1,500 mg/day) in more resistant cases, causes a significant antihypertensive effect. In severe, refractory hypertension, where patients are resistant to standard triple therapy (which usually includes a diuretic, beta-blocker and vasodilator) or double-drug therapy, large doses of captopril plus a diuretic (and occasionally a beta-blocker) result in a substantial pressure reduction (Table III).

Moreover, captopril is useful in patients who are in chronic renal failure or undergoing hemodialysis (Table IV), and in patients with renovascular hypertension (Table V). In both groups, the danger of nephrotoxicity requires that patients be carefully titrated and monitored.

Reports by Moser, a Veterans Administration study, and others have shown that black patients do not respond as well as whites to

TABLE I
SUMMARY OF 15 STUDIES EMPLOYING CAPTOPRIL ALONE IN THE TREATMENT OF HYPERTENSION

Study (Ref.)	Duration of Therapy (months)	No. of Patients	Average Dose (mg/day)	Pre-Rx Blood Pressure (mm Hg)	Post-Rx Blood Pressure (mm Hg)	Decline in Blood Pressure (mm Hg)
Weinberger 1982[5]	1.5	71	75	154/100	148/94	6/6
Vlasses et al 1982[6]	0.5	16	75	—/103	—/96	—/7
Brunner et al 1979[7]	0.25	22	200–400	174/110	144/94	30/16
MacGregor et al 1979[8]	1.0	15	450	178/112	150/97	28/15
Mizuno et al 1981[9]	8.0	13	100–200	178/107	153/93	25/14
Case et al 1981[10]	12.0	20	225–800	—/132	—/93	—/39
Gavras et al 1978[11]	6.0	12	400–1000	177/110	136/88	41/22
Friedlander 1979[12]	3.0	12	450	174/110	142/83	32/27
Ferguson et al 1982[13]	0.5	12	75	158/104	146/93	12/11
Atkinson et al 1980[14]	1.5	8	450	183/115	149/89	34/26
Aberg et al 1981[15]	3.0	15	450	165/107	143/88	22/19*
Kaneda 1982[16]	11.0	6	150	187/111	167/100	20/11
Stumpe et al 1982[17]	30.0	11	110	158/108	132/87	26/21
Lijnen et al 1980[18]	1.0	21	418	197/122	163/106	34/16
Guillevin et al 1981[19]	4.0	14	316	128**	111**	17

* 1 patient required HCTZ for blood pressure control.
** Mean arterial blood pressure.

TABLE II
BLOOD PRESSURE RESPONSE TO CAPTOPRIL PLUS DIURETIC*

Study (Ref.)	No. of Patients	Mean Dose (mg/day)	Duration of Therapy (months)	Pre-Rx Blood Pressure (mm Hg)	Post-Combination Blood Pressure (mm Hg)	Mean Decline in Blood Pressure (mm Hg)
Weinberger 1982[5]	66	75	1.5	157/103	133/88	24/15
Vlasses et al 1982[6]	16	75	1.0	— /103	— /90	— /13
Johns et al 1980[20]	6	261	0.5	170/110	140/90	30/20
Mimran et al 1982[21]	12	254	20.0	185/116	139/87	46/29
Santucci et al 1982[24]	16	75–150	6.0	202/116	151/91	51/25
Atkinson et al 1979[25]	6	450	3.0	255/116	140/90	115/26
Ferguson 1982[13]	12	75	0.5	158/104	140/87	18/17
Atkinson 1980[14]	6	450	3.0	215/116	140/90	75/26
Brunner et al 1978[26]	7	400	4.0	181/116	126/85	55/31
Stumpe et al 1982[17]	20	92	30.0	172/112	132/90	40/22
Johnston et al 1979[27]	17	75–450	8.0	182/114	142/87	40/27
Swales et al 1982[28]	15	37.5–450	40.0	224/118	184/106	30/12
Karlberg et al 1982[29]	16	246	36.0	170/109	138/90	32/19
Karlberg et al 1981[30]	24	75–450	3.0	177/110	153/95	24/15
MacGregor et al 1982[31]	16	450	1.0	182/122	138/96	44/26
Andrew et al 1982[32]	28	164	3.0	164/108	132/87	32/21
Ogihara et al 1981[33]	15	126	12.0	173/107	142/88	31/19
Maruyama et al 1980[34]	32	160	4.0	132**	121**	21**
Atkinson et al 1980[35]	11	450	6.0	225/130	155/96	70/34

* Usually HCTZ (ranging from 25–100 mg/day). Some studies used furosemide (ranging from 40–1,500 mg/day).
** Mean arterial blood pressure.

TABLE III
CAPTOPRIL MULTI-DRUG THERAPY IN SEVERE, REFRACTORY HYPERTENSION*

Study (Ref.)	No. of Patients	Mean Dose (mg/day)	Duration of Therapy	Pre-captopril Blood Pressure (mm Hg)	Post-combination Blood Pressure (mm Hg)	Mean Decline in Blood Pressure (mm Hg)
Ferguson et al 1980[36]	6	200–600	3 mos	195/116	143/85	52/31
	8	200–600	3 mos	195/116	152/94	43/22
Muskill et al 1981[37]	11	450	18 mos	225/131	182/105	43/26
Zweifler et al 1981[38]	10	405	1 mo	163/112	143/96	20/16
Havelka et al 1982[39]	36	250	30 mos	183/115	160/100	23/15
Santucci et al 1982[24]	16	75–150	6 mos	202/116	151/91	51/25
Case et al 1981[10]	10	390	35 mos	196/129	140/91	56/38
Case et al 1981[10]	10	268	35 mos	260/132	132/87	128/45
Raine et al 1982[40]	25	450	30 mos	147**	117**	30*
Havelka et al 1982[41]	30	388	18 mos	184/115	147/95	37/20
Atkinson et al 1979[25]	6	450	6 days	255/116	153/93	102/23
Bravo et al 1979[42]	17	80–1000	3 days	141**	122**	19**
Prins et al 1979[43]	17	450	4 wks	130**	114**	16**
Weinberger 1982[44]	20	600	12 mos	137**	103**	34**
Swales 1982[28]	15	37.5–450	24 mos	224/118	194/106	30/12
White 1980[45]	10	450	12 mos	220/130	140/80	80/50

* Most of these patients were refractory to standard triple therapy or double-drug therapy. Diuretics were required and, in some cases, the addition of a beta-blocker was necessary.
** Mean arterial blood pressure.

TABLE IV
BLOOD PRESSURE RESPONSE TO CAPTOPRIL IN CHRONIC RENAL FAILURE*

Study (Ref.)	No. of Patients	Mean Dose (mg/day)	Duration of Therapy (months)	Other Drugs	Pre-Captopril Blood Pressure (mm Hg)	Post-Combination Blood Pressure (mm Hg)	Mean Decline in Blood Pressure (mm Hg)
Waeber et al 1981[46]	8	50–400	6	None	194/113	151/85	43/28
Brunner et al 1979[7]	6	200–400	25	None	183/114	158/96	25/18
Harelka et al 1980[39]	18	213	30	HCTZ Furosemide Propranolol	190/115	158/94	32/21
Raine et al 1982[40]	8	450	30	Diuretic Beta-blocker	134**	108**	26**
Havelka et al 1982[41]	17	75–450	18	Diuretic Propranolol	190/114	147/93	43/21
Gassia et al 1980[47]	28	450	6	Furosemide	135**	103**	32**
Brunner et al 1978[26]	7	400	4	Furosemide	181/116	126/85	55/31
Kaneda et al 1982[16]	6	150	11	None	188/111	167/100	21/11
Wauters et al 1979[48]	8	200***	8	***	194/113	154/79	40/34

* Many patients required furosemide (ranging from 40–500 mg/day); a few patients responded well to the addition of a beta-blocker.
** Mean arterial pressure.
*** Four patients required "isovolumetric salt subtraction" for adequate blood pressure reduction.

TABLE V
BLOOD PRESSURE RESPONSE TO CAPTOPRIL IN RENOVASCULAR HYPERTENSION*

Study (Ref.)	No. of Patients	Mean Dose (mg/day)	Duration of Therapy (months)	Pre-Captopril Blood Pressure (mm Hg)	Post-Combination Blood Pressure (mm Hg)	Mean Decline in Blood Pressure (mm Hg)
Brunner et al 1979[7]	8	200–400	.25	184/11	137/89	47/21
Havelka et al 1982[39]	22	266	30.0	195/112	150/90	45/22
Gavras et al 1978[11]	6	400–1000	6.0	189/109	133/85	54/25
Havelka et al 1982[41]	20	75–450	18.0	194/112	133/85	61/27
Case et al 1982[49]	21	224	27.0	196/116	139/84	57/32
Atkinson et al 1980[14]	8	450	1.5	183/115	149/89	34/26
Bravo et al 1979[42]	7	80–1000	3 days	139*	118*	21*
Case et al 1978[50]	6	633	1.0	176/112	140/82	36/30

* Many patients required diuretics and beta-blockers.

captopril.[1,22] The Moser study yielded a drop of 22/15 mm Hg in whites vs. only 13/22 mm Hg in blacks. Doses were up to 450 mg/day in both groups.

Formulation

Tablets .... 25, 50 and 100 mg

Dose in Hypertension

Frequency: usually given three times daily, but twice daily doses appear effective for many patients

Initial: 25 mg three times daily, taken one hour before meals. Food reduces absorption by 30–40%.

Range: 37.5 to 450 mg/day. In order to avoid an acute hypotensive reaction, if the patient has been on diuretics or is sodium-depleted, the diuretic should be stopped or sodium intake be increased before commencing captopril. If 25 mg three times daily is insufficient, increase to 50 mg three times daily in one to two weeks. After one or two more weeks, if further reduction is necessary, a thiazide-type diuretic should be added and titrated upwards until its highest usual antihypertensive dose is reached. If blood pressure is still not controlled, the dose of captopril may be increased to 100 mg three times daily and then 150 mg three times daily. The maximal daily dose is 450 mg. For patients with refractory or malignant hypertension, when more rapid blood pressure control is required, the daily dose may be increased every 24 hours, under close medical supervision, until an adequate response is achieved. In patients with renal failure the initial dose should be 6.25 mg or 12.5 mg, and doses must be carefully titrated to avoid side effects secondary to the heightened sensitivity such patients exhibit to the drug.

Usual doses:
  Mild to Moderate: 25 or 50 mg two to three times daily
  Moderate to Severe: 100 mg three times daily

Mechanism of Action

Captopril is the first orally active inhibitor of angiotensin-converting enzyme which is responsible for the conversion of inactive angiotensin-I to the potent vasoconstrictor angiotensin-II (Figure 2). Inhibition of converting enzyme activity results in the reduction of plasma angiotensin-II and aldosterone levels,* with a corresponding reduction in total peripheral resistance.[51-54] There is a concomitant rise in plasma renin and angiotensin-I levels due to the removal of the negative feedback normally exerted on renin release.

Not surprisingly, captopril is most effective in high-renin hypertension. It has, nonetheless, been useful in the treatment of many low-renin and normal-renin patients. The degree to which a patient's pre-treatment renin level can predict the outcome of therapy remains controversial. Many studies have shown a significant correlation between pre-treatment renin levels and subsequent blood pressure reduction with captopril,[7,9,16,29,43,46,50] while other investigators maintain that a weak correlation, if any, exists.[6,11,18,27,38,53,57] Some workers have demonstrated that the patient's renin state relates to captopril's acute, but not chronic, antihypertensive effect.[13,19,33,34,41,56,58]

Thus, captopril's precise mechanism in patients with normal or low-renin hypertension is unclear. Converting enzyme, identical to ki-

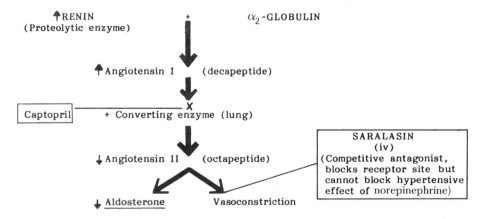

Figure 2: Mechanism of action of converting enzyme inhibitors. Decreased blood flow to the J. G. cells of the kidneys results in a rise in renin which, in turn, will produce increases in angiotensin I and II, aldosterone and blood pressure. Captopril and enalapril block the converting enzyme needed for the reaction angiotensin I → II.

* There is growing evidence for the existence of significant extra-pulmonary converting enzyme activity.[55]

ninase II, is responsible for the degradation of bradykinin, a potent vasodilator. Several investigators have related captopril administration to a significant increase in plasma and urinary kinin levels,[51,59,60] while others have been unable to demonstrate any such effect.[61] Meanwhile, there is increasing evidence that prostaglandins are an important mediator of captopril's antihypertensive effect; increased levels of plasma and urinary metabolites of prostacyclin have been detected.[52,57, 59,62-64] It has been demonstrated that captopril's antihypertensive effect is impaired by indomethacin, a prostacyclin synthetase inhibitor.[63,65]

Whatever its mechanism, captopril's hypotensive effect results in decreased peripheral resistance, while its anti-aldosterone action presumably causes natriuresis and potassium retention (and occasionally hyperkalemia in renally-compromised patients). It often counteracts the hypokalemic effects of diuretics.

Heart rate and cardiac output are essentially unaffected.

Tolerance does not develop to the drug and abrupt withdrawal does not lead to rebound hypertension.

Ferguson et al[66] and Pickering et al[67] have reported that during exercise the increase in blood pressure is unaffected by captopril, but Fazard et al have found a significant antihypertensive effect.[68,69]

Although captopril has been associated with occasional development of nephrotoxicity, including the nephrotic syndrome, neither renal blood flow nor glomerular filtration rate is diminished in patients with normal or decreased kidney function. In patients with bilateral renal arterial stenosis or in renal arterial stenosis in a solitary kidney, the administration of captopril occasionally results in an acute deterioration in the glomerular filtration rate, which is reversible if the drug is stopped.[58,70,71]

Drug Interactions

1. Plus *Diuretics*

Thiazide, thiazide-like, and "loop" diuretics have an additive antihypertensive effect when given with captopril, which counteracts the hypokalemic effects of diuretics.

2. Plus *Beta-Blockers*

In patients who are refractory to captopril-diuretic therapy, the addition of beta-blockers has an antihypertensive effect, but this is less than additive.

3. Plus *Potassium-Retaining Drugs*

Because captopril reduces aldosterone production, and elevation of serum potassium levels occasionally occurs (a few cases of hyperkalemia have been reported), potassium-sparing diuretics or potassium supplements should not be used unless the patient has hypokalemia.

4. Plus *Indomethacin*

Indomethacin, the prostacyclin synthetase inhibitor, reduces the antihypertensive effect of captopril.

5. Plus *Sodium Nitroprusside*

Nitroprusside accentuates the hypotensive effect of captopril. In patients taking chronic captopril therapy who require nitroprusside, lower starting doses of the vasodilator should be administered to avoid an acute hypotensive reaction.[72]

Interference with Laboratory Tests

- Captopril may cause a false-positive urine test for acetone.

Contraindications

— Captopril is contraindicated in patients with known sensitivity to the drug.

Warnings

An occasional but serious side effect of captopril therapy is proteinuria, which occurs in about 2% of patients treated for eight months or longer.[73] Lewis and the Captopril Collaborative Study Group report that among 4,878 patients treated between 1977 and 1981, 52 (1.1%) had proteinuria, with 0.8% having nephrotic syndrome (> 3 gm/24 hr). Sixty-five percent of these patients had pre-existing renal disease, and 27% had previous significant proteinuria. This reaction is usually, but not always, reversible. Seventy-five percent showed a disappearance or significant reduction in proteinuria when captopril was either discontinued or continued. In 17 out of 18 renal biopsies, membranous glomerulonephritis was observed. The majority of these patients were taking more than 450 mg daily, the current maximum dose, and only two were receiving less than 300 mg/day. Although it cannot be proved that the glomerulonephropathy was drug-related, there is a strong association between the occurrence of proteinuria and captopril therapy in patients with pre-existing renal disease who are taking exceptionally high doses of the drug.[74-76] Baseline renal function should be obtained on all patients prior to use. This should include urinalysis (for protein) and serum creatinine levels.

A less common but equally worrisome adverse reaction is acute, reversible renal failure. In patients with essential hypertension, where renal function is normal or decreased, there are no such reports of acute renal failure. In patients with bilateral renal artery stenosis (often the result of advanced atherosclerosis), or renal arterial stenosis in a solitary kidney, or renal transplant patients with stenosis of the transplanted renal artery, the administration of captopril occasionally results in an acute deterioration of the glomerular filtration rate, which is reversible upon discontinuation of the drug.[58,70,71,77-82] There is growing evidence that renal insufficiency results from blockade of the renin-angiotensin system in the presence of reduced kidney perfusion due to rapid blood pressure reduction. Although captopril has been shown to be efficacious in known or suspected hypertension where other drugs have failed, the risk of acute renal failure requires that the drug be administered with caution in such patients.

Rarely leukopenia and agranulocytosis have been seen.[83-85] Cooper[20] found that 44 of 6,000 patients (0.73%) developed leukopenia. Eighty-two percent of these patients had pre-existing renal impairment; two-thirds of them had serum creatinine > 2.5 mg/dl and one-third had lupus or scleroderma. In patients with normal renal function and no evidence of collagen-vascular disease, only 0.02% developed leukopenia. However, in patients whose creatinine level was 2.0 mg/dl or more, 0.40% developed leukopenia; for patients with creatinine levels of 2.0 mg/dl or more and who also had lupus or scleroderma, this figure rises to 7.20%. This reaction is usually reversible upon discontinuation of the drug within one week in 30% of patients and within three weeks in 90% of the patients. Although a causal relationship is difficult to establish, there are two cases of fatal pancytopenia associated with captopril.[86,87] Patients with normal renal function are at low risk for leukopenia, but should be instructed to contact their physician if signs of fever or infection appear. For renally-impaired patients, routine WBC counts should be measured at two-week intervals during the first three months of therapy; if lupus or scleroderma is also present, the WBC count should be monitored weekly.

Use in Pregnancy
Although no teratogenic effects were seen in animal testing, capto-

pril has been shown to be embryocidal in rabbits.[88] The safety of the drug in pregnancy has not been established,[89] and captopril is not recommended to pregnant women unless the potential benefit outweighs the potential risk.

Precautions

Upon initiation of therapy, an acute hypotensive reaction is sometimes seen. If a patient has been on diuretics or is sodium-depleted, the diuretic should be stopped or sodium intake be increased before taking captopril. If blood pressure is not controlled on 25 or 50 mg, twice to three times daily, then diuretics should be added. Because converting-enzyme inhibition is achieved with very small initial doses, if hypotension occurs, then it is recommended that sodium and water repletion, rather than dose reduction, be used to stabilize blood pressure.

In patients with impaired renal function, the initial dose should be 6.25 mg or 12.5 mg, and doses must be carefully titrated to avoid side effects secondary to the heightened sensitivity such patients exhibit for the drug.

Absorption, Metabolism, Excretion[90-92]

Captopril is rapidly absorbed after oral administration; Jarrott et al[90] have detected plasma levels at ten minutes. In patients taking captopril for the first time, peak blood levels of 0.361 ± 0.0112 mg/ml were seen at 53 minutes with a plasma half-life of 100 minutes. In patients on chronic therapy, peak blood levels of 1.08 ± 0.29 mg/ml were seen at 41 minutes, with a plasma half-life of 45 minutes. Maximal blood pressure reduction occurs 60–90 minutes after oral administration. Because food has been shown to reduce absorption significantly (30 to 40%), captopril should be given one hour before meals.

Captopril is 25 to 30% albumin bound, and significant binding to other endogenous thiol-compounds has been reported. There is decreased protein-binding in patients with decreased renal function. Animal studies indicate that it does not cross the blood–brain barrier or the placenta.

The primary route of excretion is the kidneys; in a 24-hour period, over 95% of the absorbed dose is excreted in the urine. Fifty percent of captopril is eliminated as unchanged drug; most of the remainder is excreted as the disulfide dimer and captopril-cysteine disulfide. Thus, in patients with significant renal impairment, doses need to be reduced

TABLE VI
SIDE EFFECTS OF CAPTOPRIL
(No. OF PATIENTS AND PERCENTAGES, BASED ON LITERATURE SURVEY OF 903 PATIENTS)

	Weinberger[5]	Weinberger[5]*	Waeber[46]	Karlberg[29]	Karlberg[30]*	Brunner[7]	Ferguson[36]†	MacGregor[8]	Maskill[37]†	Havelka[39]	Santucci[24]†	Case[10]*	Gavras[11]	Raine[40]†	Havelka[41]†	Case[49]†	Atkinson[14]	Case[50]*	Gassia[47]*	Aberg[15]*	Prins[43]*	Stumpe[17]*	Johnston[27]*	White[43]*	MacGregor[31]*	Andren[32]*	Maruyama[34]*	Atkinson[35]*	Luderer[99]	Totals	Percentages
No. of Patients	71	66	81	41	24	22	17	15	11	76	16	16	20	1	33	67	40	14	19	28	29	17	31	17	10	16	28	32	23	903	—
Proteinuria	—	—	4	1	1	1	—	—	—	1	—	—	3	1	1	1	4	—	2	—	1	1	—	1	—	1	—	—	—	19	2.10
Rash	4	4	20	1	2	1	5	—	3	18	—	2	—	5	4	10	—	2	9	2	2	3	1	—	3	—	3	—	7	109	12.07
Pruritis	3	—	—	—	—	—	5	—	2	9	—	1	—	—	—	—	1	—	2	1	—	—	—	—	—	—	—	1	—	24	2.66
Fever	—	—	—	1	—	—	1	—	—	—	—	—	—	2	—	5	2	2	—	—	—	1	1	1	—	—	—	—	2	15	1.66
Loss of Taste	9	1	3	—	—	2	1	2	8	2	1	—	—	1	—	4	5	2	4	2	—	1	1	1	3	1	2	—	—	56	6.20
Leukopenia or Agranulccytoses	—	1	—	—	—	—	—	—	—	1	—	—	—	—	1	—	—	—	—	—	—	—	—	—	—	—	—	—	—	3	0.33
Hypotension	—	—	—	6	2	—	1	—	—	—	—	—	—	—	—	—	1	—	—	—	—	—	—	—	—	—	—	—	—	10	1.11
Raynaud's Phenomenon	—	—	—	1	3	2	2	—	—	2	—	—	—	—	—	2	—	—	—	—	—	—	—	—	—	—	2	—	—	12	1.33
Nausea	—	—	—	—	3	—	—	—	—	—	—	—	1	4	—	—	—	—	—	1	—	—	—	—	—	—	—	—	—	9	1.00
Tachyca-dia	—	—	—	—	—	—	—	—	4	2	—	—	—	—	—	2	2	—	2	—	—	—	—	—	—	—	—	1	—	13	1.44
Dizziness	1	6	—	—	—	—	—	—	2	—	—	—	—	—	—	3	2	—	2	—	—	—	—	1	—	—	—	—	—	15	1.66
Discontinued Due to Side Effects	2	3	19	6	—	—	1	1	3	1	—	1	—	4	3	1	—	—	7	5	—	1	3	2	—	1	1	—	—	65	7.20

* Many patients required thiazide or loop diuretics.
† Many patients required diuretic and beta-blockers.

TABLE VII
FREQUENCY OF ADVERSE REACTIONS TO CAPTOPRIL

FREQUENT (> 5%)
- rash
- ageusia (loss of taste)

OCCASIONAL (0.5–5.0%)
- proteinuria
- acute renal failure
- agranulocytosis/leukopenia
- Raynaud's phenomenon
- hypotension
- diarrhea
- fatigue
- chronic, unproductive cough
- tachycardia
- dizziness
- nausea, vomiting, anorexia
- pruritis
- ↑ serum creatinine
- ↑ BUN
- ↑ serum potassium

RARE (< 0.5%)
- hyperkalemia
- myalgia
- "scalded mouth"
- hair loss
- chills
- myocardial infarction
- headache
- constipation
- muscle cramp
- pityriasis rosea
- positive Coombs' test
- ↑ ANA
- normocytic anemia
- angioedema of face, mouth, or larynx
- decreased libido
- oral ulcers
- supraventricular extra-systole
- arthralgia
- angina pectoris
- congestive heart failure
- gastric pain
- lymphadenopathy
- exfoliative dermatitis
- pemphigus
- eosinophilia
- bronchospasm
- flushing or pallor
- hepatitis

and they should be carefully titrated with smaller increments in one-to-two-week intervals.

Adverse Reactions[93-108]

Approximately 7% of patients receiving captopril discontinue their treatment because of intolerance to medication. A tabulation of these side effects is seen in Tables VI and VII. A causal relationship between some of the rare reactions and captopril has not been proven. The most serious adverse reactions are proteinuria, acute renal failure, agranulocytosis and leukopenia (see Warnings). More commonly, the usual causes of non-compliance are rashes (12%), which are usually maculopapular and are occasionally associated with pruritis and fever, and loss of taste (6%). Many investigators relate these effects to the sulfhydryl group of the molecule. Both reactions are reversible upon removal of the drug, appear more frequently at higher doses, and often do not reappear when the drug is subsequently reintroduced in lower doses. Transient hypotension, sinus tachycardia, Raynaud's phenomenon, dizziness and nausea occasionally occur, but these adverse reactions rarely affect patient compliance. Small increases in serum potassium levels frequently occur, usually in patients with impaired renal function. A few cases of hyperkalemia have been reported.

ENALAPRIL (Vasoril ®)

Enalapril maleate (Figure 3) is the newest orally active angiotensin converting enzyme inhibitor (CEI) similar in its mechanism of action to captopril, but whose side effects appear to be less severe and less frequent. It also has the advantage in that many patients can be satisfactorily controlled on once-a-day dosage. As monotherapy, enalapril controls blood pressure in about 65% of patients and, given with diuretics, it is effective in 90–95% of patients. Enalapril's molecular structure differs from captopril, particularly by the absence of the sulfhydryl group which is believed to be responsible for captopril's toxic reactions. Although more long-term studies are necessary to determine its true benefit-to-risk ratio, enalapril's side-effects profile appears to offer a major advantage. Comparative studies between enalapril and captopril in hypertensive individuals thus far favor enalapril's safety advantage.

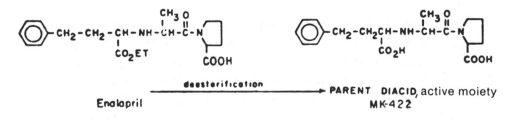

Figure 3: Structure of enalapril and its active moiety.

Davies[1] recently reported the total clinical experience of Merck, Sharp and Dohme with enalapril monotherapy in 975 patients given the drug. His results may be summarized as follows. Enalapril was significantly more effective when given alone to white patients compared with black patients. Enalapril monotherapy produced significantly greater reductions in supine diastolic pressure than did propranolol. In a total clinical experience with 2,249 patients receiving enalapril, only 0.3% had to discontinue the drug because of skin rash. Loss of taste was noted in only 0.4% of patients; only 0.66% of patients developed elevation of serum creatinine with enalapril alone. Leukopenia clearly due to the drug did not occur. Proteinurea (exceeding 1.0 g/24 hrs) was no more frequent among 915 patients given enalapril alone than in 569 control patients (0.66% versus 0.53%). Davies concluded that enalapril was effective when used alone, producing 54–66% "good-to-excellent" responses in hypertensive patients. This response rate was increased to 83-96% when used with hydrochlorothiazide. Enalapril was generally well tolerated and appeared not to be associated with the occurrence of "captopril-like" adverse effects. It was further concluded that enalapril, as with captopril, may be associated with azotemia in patients with bilateral renovascular hypertension.

Enalapril was generally well tolerated and appeared not to be associated with the occurrence of "captopril-like" adverse effects.

Many investigators report that enalapril clearly reduces pressure in patients with mild-to-moderate hypertension (Table VIII). It is most effective when given concomitantly with diuretics, usually hydrochlorothiazide 50 mg/day (Table IX). Several studies suggest that the use of thiazides leads to a synergistic, rather than an additive, reduction in pressure.[2-5]

Chrysant et al report that enalapril, like captopril, is somewhat more effective in whites than blacks.[6] Because black persons have been shown to have a higher prevalence of low-renin hypertension (and therefore low levels of angiotensin-I), their lack of response to converting enzyme inhibitors (which block the reaction: angiotensin-I → angiotensin-II) is not surprising.[16] Theoretically, CEI agents ought to be most useful in hyperreninemic, hyperangiotensinemic-II hypertension.

TABLE VIII
SUMMARY OF TEN STUDIES EMPLOYING ENALAPRIL ALONE IN TREATMENT OF HYPERTENSION

Study (Ref.)	No. of Patients	Duration of Therapy (weeks)	Average Dose (mg/day)	Pre-Rx Blood Pressure (mm Hg)	Post-Rx Blood Pressure (mm Hg)	Decline in Blood Pressure (mm Hg)
Chrysant et al[6]	11	18	10	143/94	135/88	8/6
	10	18	5†	147/96	140/90	7/6
Biollaz et al[7]	19	4	20	180/112	160/100	20/12
Gavras et al[8]	16	18	2.5-40	177/111	145/94	32/17
Hodsman et al[9]	5	12	10-40	190/101	144/83	46/18
Bergstrand et al[10]	15	4	20	161/103	148/92	13/11
	15	4	10†	164/103	149/92	15/11
Kolloch et al[11]	6	12	10-40	168/108	148/94	20/14
Guthrie et al[12]	15	4	40†	139/94	116/71	23/23
Guthrie et al[13]	14	4	10-40†	105*	94*	11*
Fitz et al[14]	7	—	40	145/97	135/89	10/8
	6	—	20†	138/95	123/86	15/9
Wilkens** et al[15]	8	12	30	146/97	144/89	2/7.5
	8	12	30	145/97	142/92	2/7.5

* Mean arterial blood pressure.
† Enalapril twice daily.
** In low-renin patients only.

TABLE IX
BLOOD PRESSURE RESPONSE TO ENALAPRIL PLUS DIURETIC*

Study (Ref.)	No. of Patients	Duration of Therapy (weeks)	Mean Dose (mg/twice day)	Pre-Rx Blood Pressure (mm Hg)	Post-Rx Blood Pressure Enalapril (mm Hg)	Post-Rx Blood Pressure Diuretic (mm Hg)	Post-Rx Blood Pressure Combination (mm Hg)	Decline in Blood Pressure (mm Hg)
Vlasses et al[2]	14	2	20	--/107	--/98	--/97	--/85	--/22
Ferguson et al[18]	8	2	5–10†	158/102	149/97	138/95	130/85	28/17
Rotmansch et al[3]	30	2	20	--/102	--/97	--/98	--/84	--/18
Nelson et al[4]	14	24	10–20	161/105	152/100	140/97	127/88	34/17
Vlasses et al[5]	14	2	20	101	98	98	86	15
Winer et al[19]	12	12	5–20	158/104	145/98	—	126/92	32/12

* Most studies used hydrochlorothiazide 50 mg/day.
† Dose given once daily.

The fact is, however, these drugs do work in many hypo- and normo-reninemic patients.

Enalapril itself is virtually inactive as a converting enzyme inhibitor, but it undergoes hepatic hydrolysis to the active diacid form (Figure 3) which is the acitve CEI. Enalapril is rapidly absorbed after oral administration, with peak serum concentrations of the inactive molecule observed at one hour, and rapid renal excretion resulting in almost complete elimination by four hours.[17] The active metabolite's peak serum concentration was seen at three to four hours while its plasma half-life is 11 hours. Seventy-two hours after drug administration, the level of active metabolite is quite low, yet converting enzyme inhibition remains significant. Thus, in addition to converting enzyme blockade, other mechanisms probably contribute to enalapril's antihypertensive effect. In comparison with captopril, enalapril is more slowly absorbed and its active metabolite has a longer half-life and duration of action. Consequently, it is usually given on a once daily basis.

Dose in Hypertension

Tablets: 10 and 20 mg
Frequency: Once or twice daily
Initial dose: 10 mg once daily
Usual dose: 10 to 40 mg/total daily dose, taken on a once- or twice-daily basis
Dose range: 10–40 mg/day

SARALASIN (Sarenin®)
Introductory year: 1982

Saralasin is a structural analogue of angiotensin-II (A-II) which specifically competes with A-II at tissue receptors, thereby blocking the vascular, renal, adrenal, cardiac, and central nervous system effects of A-II[1] (see Figure 2). Because it occupies A-II receptors, it reduces hypertension due to hyperreninemia and hyperangiotensinemia I and II. Sarcosine (N-methylglycine) at position one enhances the peptide's affinity for A-II receptors and slows hydrolysis by aminopeptidases.[2] The short half-life of saralasin (mean plasma half-life of three minutes and pharmacological half-life of eight minutes[3]) allows rapid reversal of the drug's effects.[1] Intravenous administration is necessary for continuous action. Saralasin does not penetrate the blood–brain barrier. Saralasin is available in a sterile aqueous solution, as ampules of 18 mg saralasin/30 ml saralasin acetate solution.

When Should the Physician Consider Using Saralasin?
1. In the Saralasin Test for A-II dependent hypertension
2. Occasionally in severe or malignant, high-renin hypertension.

Saralasin is useful in conjunction with other tests: plasma renin activity (PRA), intravenous pyelogram, bilateral renal vein renins and renal arteriograms to identify renovascular hypertension sometimes curable by surgery.[4-10] The drug has also been used to lower blood pressure in severe high-renin hypertension[11] and hypertensive crises of malignant hypertension.[4] It has been used safely in pediatrics.

By A-II blockade and suppression of A-II feedback on PRA levels, saralasin raises PRA[12] and diminishes peripheral vascular resistance,[5] thus lowering blood pressure.[6] The greatest fall in blood pressure with saralasin occurs in renin-dependent hypertension. In low-renin hypertension, more A-II receptor sites are vacant and available for saralasin to bind and agonistically raise blood pressure because saralasin does possess some agonist activity. The magnitude of the change in blood pressure with saralasin corresponds inversely to pre-treatment PRA levels and the change in PRA with saralasin.[7,8,13] The blood pressure response to saralasin depends ultimately upon elevated A-II levels,[8] though it is somewhat limited by saralasin's intrinsic agonist activity.

Other antihypertensive drugs can affect PRA and the blood pressure response to saralasin. All hypotensive medication should be discontinued one to two weeks before giving saralasin,[5,9] except diuretics if needed. Vasodilators such as minoxidil and hydralazine cause increased PRA, A-II-dependency of blood pressure,[14] and marked hypotension with saralasin.[15] Diuretics lower plasma volume and sodium levels,[14] which stimulate the juxtaglomerular apparatus.[6,16] The resulting rise in plasma renin and A-II will augment the saralasin-induced fall in blood pressure, diminish the saralasin agonistic pressor response, heighten saralasin antagonism of A-II, and promote angiotensin-dependency of blood pressure.[4,6,12,16,17] Diuretics do not promote a fall in blood pressure with saralasin in low-renin hypertension. Elevated sodium and plasma volume and beta-blockers lower PRA and A-II levels, inducing a pressor response to saralasin which is most pronounced in low-renin hypertension.[16-18] Under these conditions there is greater saralasin agonism,[2,5,17,19] less A-II dependency of blood pressure,[5,15] and no fall in pressure with saralasin.[6,10] Propranolol inhibits renin release, which counters the hypotensive effects of saralasin.[6,15]

Adverse reactions to saralasin are rare. Minor effects include nausea, anxiety, sweating, headache, malaise, lightheadedness, extrasystoles, and flushed skin.[20] It does not cross the placental barrier; in animal studies there has been no fetal damage at doses 550 times normal human dosage. Saralasin should be avoided during pregnancy because its effects on the human fetus are unknown. The pharmacological effects of saralasin upon blood pressure can be dangerously exaggerated. Saralasin is contraindicated in cases of hypersensitivity.

Blood pressure can be lowered by as much as 30 mm Hg in A-II-dependent hypertension, when saralasin is used with diuretics or vaso-dilators[21] or when there is excess sodium depletion during the saralasin test.[15] Patients with cerebrovascular or coronary disease are at greater risk of hypotension. This reaction can be treated by discontinuing saralasin, giving a 5% dextrose in water solution, and evaluating the lower limbs.

An immediate transient rise in blood pressure upon giving saralasin occurs in over 90% of patients.[18,22] Diastolic pressure rises by as much as 30 mm Hg. Pressure begins to increase within one minute, peaks in two to three minutes, and then falls.[8] This response can be diminished by giving saralasin as a continuous titrated infusion. A prolonged pressor response to saralasin, induced by high sodium levels or inadequate sodium depletion for the saralasin test, or by beta-blockers, is more likely in hypertension that is not A-II dependent. The rise in blood pressure may be as much as 30 mm Hg; pressure peaks within 30 minutes. Patients with severe hypertension, high pre-treatment PRA, low sodium or marked depressor response to saralasin are more likely to experience rebound hypertension one to three hours after saralasin is discontinued. This relex is probably caused by the activated renin–angiotensin system. Blood pressure in these patients should be monitored every 15 minutes for three hours after the test. Severe hypertensive reactions can be treated by readministering saralasin and then withdrawing the drug slowly.[23]

The Saralasin Test

The saralasin test is a test for A-II dependent hypertension such as with renovascular disease. It should be conducted in a hospital setting.

To enhance saralasin's effects on blood pressure, sodium is first mildly depleted by giving 80 mg furosemide p.o. the night before, 40 mg furosemide i.v. three to five hours before, or by reducing sodium intake to 10 mEq/day three to five days before the test. An i.v. solution of 5% dextrose in water is begun, and blood pressure is recorded every two minutes. Four consecutive stable readings of diastolic pressure set the control blood pressure. Saralasin is then given either at a constant rate (30 ml/20–30 min) or by increased titration to patients susceptible to an exaggerated response.[24] Titrated doses begin at 0.05 mg/kg/min and are increased at ten-minute intervals to 5.0, 10.0 and 20.0 mg/kg/min. The resulting effect of saralasin is established by the maximum consistent deviation of diastolic pressure from control levels for four consecutive readings.

Saralasin test results are interpreted by the change in the diastolic pressure. A positive result is marked by a depressor response of 7 mm Hg or more[4,6, 8-10] and a negative pressor response is indicated by a diastolic blood pressure rise of 10 mm Hg or more. Indeterminant results include changes between a 7 mm Hg fall and 10 mm Hg rise in diastolic pressure. There is a 30% frequency of false positive results[9,12] for renovascular hypertension. These may be due to high or normal renin essential hypertension with low sodium levels[7,10, 12,18,19] or PRA stimulated by vasodilator therapy,[15] or hypertension associated with coarctation of the aorta or renin-secreting tumors.[15] Renal artery stenosis or unilateral renal disease with elevated A-II levels cause true renovascular hypertension.[5] There is also a 19% frequency of false negative results. High peripheral vein PRA levels occur in only 50% of renovascular hypotension.[25] Saralasin may not depress blood pressure in normal-renin, angiotensin-dependent hypertension.

REFERENCES:

Captopril

1. Veterans Administration Cooperative Study Group on Antihypertensive Agents: Captopril: Evaluation of low doses, twice-daily doses and the addition of diuretic for the treatment of mild to moderate hypertension. *Clin. Sci.*, **63**:443s, 1982.
2. Oberfield, S., Rapaport, R., Levine, L., and New, M.: Long-term treatment of childhood hypertension with captopril. *Ped. Ann.*, **11**:614, 1982.
3. Hymes, L., and Warshaw, B.: Captopril: Long-term treatment of hypertension in a pre-term infant and in older children. *Am. J. Dis. Child.*, **137**:263, 1983.

4. Bifano, E., Post, E., Springer, J., and Williams, M.: Treatment of neonatal hypertension with captopril. *J. Pediatr.*, **100**:143, 1982.

5. Weinberger, M. H.: Comparison of captopril and hydrochlorothiazide alone and in combination in mild to moderate essential hypertension. *Br. J. Clin. Pharmacol.*, **14**:127S, 1982.

6. Vlasses, P., Rotmensch, H., Swanson, B., Mojaverian, P., and Ferguson, R.: Low-dose captopril—its use in mild to moderate hypertension unresponsive to diuretic treatment. *Arch. Intern. Med.*, **142**:1098, 1982.

7. Brunner, H. Gavras, H., et al: Oral angiotensin converting enzyme inhibitor in long-term treatment of hypertensive patients. *Ann. Intern. Med.*, **90**:19, 1979.

8. MacGregor, G. A., Markandu, N. O., Roulston, J., and Jones, J.: Essential hypertension: Effect of an oral inhibitor of angiotensin-converting enzyme. *Br. Med. J.*, **2**:1106, 1979.

9. Mizuno, K., Gotoh, M., Matsui, J., and Fukuchi, S.: Antihypertensive effect of the oral angiotensin I-converting enzyme inhibitor in long-term treatment of hypertensive patients. *Jpn. Heart J.*, **22**:903, 1981.

10. Case, D., Atlas, S., Sullivan, P., and Laragh, J.: Acute and chronic treatment of severe and malignant hypertension with the oral angiotensin-converting enzyme inhibitor captopril. *Circulation*, **64**:765, 1981.

11. Gavras, H., Brunner, H., et al: Antihypertensive effect of the oral angiotensin converting-enzyme inhibitor SQ 14225 in man. *N. Engl. J. Med.*, **298**:991, 1978.

12. Friedlander, D. H.: Captopril and propranolol in mild and moderate essential hypertension: Preliminary report. *N. Z. Med. J.*, **90**:146, 1979.

13. Ferguson, R., Vlasses, P., et al: Comparison of the effects of captopril, diuretic and their combination in low and normal-renin essential hypertension. *Life Sci.*, **30**:59, 1982.

14. Atkinson, A., Morton, J., et al: Captopril in clinical hypertension. *Br. Heart J.*, **44**:290, 1980.

15. Aberg, H., Frithz, G., and Morlin, C: Comparison of captopril with hydrochlorothiazide in the treatment of essential hypertension. *Int. J. Clin. Pharmacol. Biopharm.*, **19**:368, 1981.

16. Kaneda, H., et al: Effect of captopril on blood pressure and renin-angiotensin-aldosterone system in hypertensive patients on hemodialysis. *Tohoku J. Exp. Med.*, **137**:21, 1982.

17. Stumpe, K., Overlack, A., Kolloch, R., and Schreyer, S.: Long-term efficacy of angiotensin-converting-enzyme inhibition with captopril in mild-to-moderate essential hypertension. *Br. J. Clin. Pharmacol.*, **14**:121S, 1982.

18. Lijnen, P., Fagard, R., et al: Dose response to captopril therapy of hypertension. *Clin. Pharmacol. Ther.*, **28**:310, 1980.

19. Guillevin, L., Lardoux, M., and Corvol, P.: Effects of captopril on blood pressure, electrolytes, and certain hormones in hypertension. *Clin. Pharmacol. Ther.*, **29**:699, 1981.

20. Cooper, R. A.: Captopril-associated neutropenia—who is at risk? *Arch. Intern. Med.*, **143**:659, 1983.

21. Mimran, A., and Jover, B.: Maintenance of the antihypertensive efficacy of captopril despite consistent reduction in daily dosage. *Br. J. Clin. Pharmacol.*, **14**:81 S, 1982.

22. Moser, M., and Lunn, J.: Responses to captopril and hydrochlorothiazide in black patients with hypertension. *Clin. Pharmacol. Ther.*, **32**:307, 1982.

23. Johns, D., Baker, K., et al: Acute and chronic effect of captopril in hypertensive patients. *Hypertension*, **2**:567, 1980.

24. Santucci, A., Aguglia, F., DeMattia, G., and Balsano, F.: Long-term captopril treatment in moderate to severe hypertension. *Br. J. Clin. Pharmacol.*, **14**:77S, 1982.
25. Atkinson, A., Brown, J., et al: Captopril in hypertension with renal artery stenosis and in intractable hypertension; acute and chronic changes in circulating concentrations of renin, angiotensins I and II and aldosterone, and in body composition. *Clin. Sci.*, **57**:139s, 1979.
26. Brunner, H., Wauters, J., et al: Inappropriate renin secretion unmasked by captopril in hypertension of chronic renal failure. *Lancet*, **ii**:704, 1978.
27. Johnston, C., McGrath, B., Millar, J., and Matthews, P.: Long-term effects of captopril on blood pressure and hormone levels in essential hypertension. *Lancet*, **ii**:493, 1979.
28. Swales, J., Heagerty, A., et al: Treatment of refractory hypertension. *Lancet*, **i**:894, 1982.
29. Karlberg, B., Asplund, J., Wettre, S., Ohman, K., and Nilsson, O.: Long-term experience of captopril in the treatment of primary (essential) hypertension. *Br. J. Clin. Pharmacol.*, **14**:133S, 1982.
30. Karlberg, B., Asplund, J., Nilsson, O., Wattre, S., and Ohman, K.: Captopril, an orally active converting enzyme inhibitor, in the treatment of primary hypertension. *Acta Med. Scand.*, **209**:245, 1981.
31. MacGregor, G., Markandu, N., et al: Captopril in essential hypertension; contrasting effects of adding hydrochlorothiazide or propranolol. *Br. Med. J.*, **284**:693, 1982.
32. Andren, L., Karlberg, B., et al: Captopril and atenolol combined with hydrochlorothiazide in essential hypertension. *Br. J. Clin. Pharmacol.*, **14**:107S, 1982.
33. Ogihara, T., et al: Hormonal responses to long-term converting enzyme inhibition in hypertensive patients. *Clin. Pharmacol. Ther.*, **30**:328, 1981.
34. Maruyama, A., et al: Long-term effects of captopril in hypertension. *Clin. Pharmacol. Ther.*, **28**:316, 1980.
35. Atkinson, A., Lever, A., Brown, J., and Robertson, J.: Combined treatment of severe intractable hypertension with captopril and diuretic. *Lancet*, **ii**:105, 1980.
36. Ferguson, R., Vlasses, P., et al: Captopril in severe treatment-resistant hypertension. *Am. Heart J.*, **99**:579, 1980.
37. Maskill, M., Orme, M., MacIver, M., Serlin, M., and Breckenridge, A.: Efficacy and adverse effects of captopril in severe refractory hypertension. *J. Cardiovasc. Pharmacol.*, **3**:1287, 1981.
38. Zweifler, A., Julius, S., Nicholls, M.: Efficacy of an oral angiotensin-converting enzyme inhibitor (captopril) in severe hypertension. *Arch. Intern. Med.*, **141**:907, 1981.
39. Havelka, J., Boerlin, H., et al: Long-term experience with captopril in severe hypertension. *Br. J. Clin. Pharmacol.*, **14**:71S, 1982.
40. Raine, A., and Ledingham, J.: Clinical experience with captopril in the treatment of severe drug-resistant hypertension. *Am. J. Cardiol.*, **49**:1475, 1982.
41. Havelka, J., Vetter, H., et al: Acute and chronic effects of the angiotensin-converting enzyme inhibitor captopril in severe hypertension. *Am. J. Cardiol.*, **49**:1467, 1982.
42. Bravo, E. L., and Tarazi, R. C.: Converting enzyme inhibition with an orally active compound in hypertensive man. *Hypertension*, **1**:39, 1979.
43. Prins, E., Danker, A., et al: Treatment of moderate to severe hypertensive patients with an orally active converting-enzyme inhibitor. *Proc. Eur. Dial. Transplant Assoc.*, **16**:603, 1979.
44. Weinberger, M. H.: Role of sympathetic nervous system activity in the blood pressure response to long-term captopril therapy in severely hypertensive patients. *Am. J. Cardiol.*, **49**:1542, 1982.

45. White, N. J., Yahaya, H., Rajagopalan, B., and Ledingham, J.: Captopril and furosemide in severe drug-resistant hypertension. *Lancet*, ii:108, 1980.
46. Waeber, B., Gavras, I., Brunner, H., and Gavras, H.: Safety and efficacy of chronic therapy with captopril in hypertensive patients: An update. *J. Clin. Pharmacol.*, 21:508, 1981.
47. Gassia, J. P., Durand, D., That, H., Degroc, F., and Suc, J.: Long-term effect of captopril in hypertension with chronic renal failure. *Proc. Eur. Dial. Transplant Assoc.*, 17:719, 1980.
48. Wauters, J., Waeber, B., et al: Captopril and salt subtraction to treat "uncontrollable" hypertension in hemodialysis patients. *Proc. Eur. Dial. Transplant Assoc.*, 16:610, 1979.
49. Case, D., Atlas, S., Murion, R., and Laragh, J.: Long-term efficacy of captopril in renovascular and essential hypertension. *Am. J. Cardiol.*, 49:1440, 1982.
50. Case, D., Atlas, S., et al: Clinical experience with blockade of the renin-angiotensin-aldosterone system by an oral converting-enzyme inhibitor (SQ 14225, captopril) in hypertensive patients. *Prog. Cardiovasc. Dis.*, 21:195, 1978.
51. Mookherjee, S., Anderson, G., et al: Acute effects of captopril on cardiopulmonary hemodynamics and renin-angiotensin-aldosterone and bradykinin profile on hypertension. *Am. Heart J.*, 105:106, 1983.
52. Hornych, A., Safar, M., et al: Effects of captopril on prostaglandin and natriuresis in patients with essential hypertension. *Am. J. Cardiol.*, 49:1524, 1982.
53. Sullivan, J., Ginsburg, B., et al: Hemodynamic and antihypertensive effects of captopril, an orally active angiotensin converting enzyme inhibitor. *Hypertension*, 1:397, 1979.
54. Fouad, F., Ceimo, J., Tarazi, R., and Bravo, E.: Contrasts and similarities of acute hemodynamic responses to specific antagonism of Angiotensin II ([Sar[1], Thr[8]] AII) and to inhibition of converting enzyme (captopril). *Circulation*, 61:163, 1980.
55. Ferguson, R. K., et al: A specific orally active inhibitor of angiotensin-converting enzyme in man. *Lancet*, 1:775, 1977.
56. Lijnen, P., Staessen, J., Fagard, R., and Amery, A.: Increase in plasma aldosterone during prolonged captopril treatment. *Am. J. Cardiol.*, 49:1561, 1982.
57. Mimran, A., Targhetta, R., and Laroche, B.: The antihypertensive effect of captopril: Evidence for an influence of kinins. *Hypertension*, 2:732, 1980.
58. Blythe, W. B.: Captopril and renal autoregulation. *N. Engl. J. Med.*, 308:390, 1983.
59. Waldron, T., Antonaccio, M., and Murthy, V.: Reversal of bradykinin-induced reflex tachycardia to bradycardia by captopril: Evidence for prostacyclin involvement. *Eur. J. Pharmacol.*, 79:283, 1982.
60. Ohman, K., Karlberg, B., Nilsson, O., and Wettre, S.: Captopril in primary hypertension: Effects related to the renin-angiotensin-aldosterone and kallikrein-kinin systems. *Acta Med. Scand.*, (Suppl.), 646:98, 1981.
61. Crantz, F., Swartz, S., et al: Differences in response to the peptidyldipeptide hydrolase inhibitors SQ 20,881 and SQ 14,225 in normal-renin essential hypertension. *Hypertension*, 2:604, 1980.
62. Goldstone, R., Martin, K., Zipser, R., and Horton, R.: Evidence for a dual action of converting enzyme inhibitor on blood pressure in normal man. *Prostaglandins*, 22:587, 1981.
63. Moore, T., Crantz, F., et al: Contribution of prostaglandins to the antihypertensive action of captopril in essential hypertension. *Hypertension*, 3:168, 1981.
64. Swartz, S., Williams, G., et al: Captopril-induced changes in prostaglandin production. *J. Clin. Invest.*, 65:1257, 1980.

65. Witzgall, H., Hirsch, F., Scherer, B., and Weber, P.: Acute hemodynamic and hormonal effects of captopril are diminished by indomethacin. *Clin. Sci.*, **62**:611, 1982.
66. Ferguson, R., Vlasses, P., et al: Effect of captopril and propranolol, alone and in combination, on the responses to isometric and dynamic exercise in normotensive and hypertensive man. *Pharmacotherapy*, **3**:125, 1983.
67. Pickering, T., Case, D., Sullivan, P., and Laragh, J.: Comparison of antihypertensive and hormonal effects of captopril and propranolol at rest and during exercise. *Am. J. Cardiol.*, **49**:1566, 1982.
68. Fagard, R., Lijnen, P., and Amery, A.: Hemodynamic response to captopril at rest and during exercise in hypertensive patients. *Am. J. Cardiol.*, **49**:1569, 1982.
69. Fagard, R., Bulpitt, C., Lijnen, P., and Amery, A.: Response of the systemic and pulmonary circulation to converting-enzyme inhibition (captopril) at rest and during exercise in hypertensive patients. *Circulation*, **65**:33, 1982.
70. Hrick, O., Browning, R., et al: Captopril-induced functional renal insufficiency in patients with bilateral renal-artery stenoses or renal-artery stenosis in a solitary kidney. *N. Engl. J. Med.*, **308**:373, 1983.
71. Curtis, J., Luke, R., et al: Inhibition of angiotensin-converting enzyme in renal-transplant recipients with hypertension. *N. Engl. J. Med.*, **308**:377, 1983.
72. Jennings, G., Gelman, J., Stockigt, J., and Korner, P.: Associated hypotensive effect of sodium nitroprusside in man after captopril. *Clin. Sci.*, **61**:521, 1981.
73. Heel, R. C., Brogden, R. N., Speight, T. M., and Avery, G. S.: Captopril: A preliminary review of its pharmacological properties and therapeutic efficacy. *Drugs*, **20**:409, 1980.
74. Lewis, E. J., and the Captopril Collaborative Study Group: Proteinuria and abnormalities of the renal glomerulus in patients with hypertension. *Clin. Exp. Pharmacol. Physiol.* (Suppl.), **7**:105, 1982.
75. Captopril Collaborative Study Group: Does captopril cause renal damage in hypertensive patients? *Lancet*, **i**:988, 1982.
76. Hoorntje, S., Weening, J., et al: Immune-complex glomerulopathy in patients treated with captopril. *Lancet*, **i**:1212, 1980.
77. Farrow, P., and Wilkinson, R.: Reversible renal failure during treatment with captopril. *Br. Med. J.*, **i**:1680, 1979.
78. Grossman, A., Eckland, D., Price, P., and Edwards, C.: Captopril: Reversible renal failure with severe hyperkalemia (letter). *Lancet*, **i**:712, 1980.
79. Luderer, J., Schoolwerth, A., et al: Acute renal failure, hemolytic anemia and skin rash associated with captopril therapy. *Am. J. Med.*, **71**:493, 1981.
80. Kawamura, J., Okada, Y., Nishibuchi, S., and Yoshida, O.: Transient anuria following administration of angiotensin I-converting enzyme inhibitor (SQ 14225) in a patient with renal artery stenosis of the solitary kidney successfully treated with renal autotransplantation. *J. Urol.*, **127**:111, 1982.
81. Silas, J., Klenka, Z., Solomon, S., and Bone, J.: Captopril induced reversible renal failure: A marker of renal artery stenosis affecting a solitary kidney. *Br. Med. J.*, **286**:1702, 1983.
82. Schreiber, M., and Fang, L.: Renal failure associated with captopril (letter). *JAMA*, **250**:31, 1983.
83. *Medical Letter on Drugs and Therapeutics*, **22**:39, 1980.
84. van Brummelen, Willemze, R., Tan, W., and Thompson, J.: Captopril-associated agranulocytosis (Letter). *Lancet*, **i**:150, 1980.

85. Elijovisch, F., and Krakoff, L.: Captopril associated granulocytopenia in hypertension after renal transplantation. *Lancet*, **i**:927, 1980.

86. Gavras, I., Graff, L., et al: Fatal pancytopenia associated with the use of captopril. *Ann. Intern. Med.*, **94**:58, 1981.

87. El Matri, A., et al: Fatal bone-marrow suppression associated with captopril. *Br. Med. J.*, **283**:277, 1981.

88. Keith, I., Will, J., and Weir, E.: Captopril: Association with fetal death and pulmonary vascular changes in the rabbit. *Proc. Soc. Exp. Biol. Med.*, **170**:378, 1982.

89. Duminy, P., and Burger, P.: Fetal abnormality associated with the use of captopril during pregnancy (Letter). *S. Afr. Med. J.*, **60**:805, 1981.

90. Jarrott, B., Drummer, O., et al: Pharmacokinetic properties of captopril after acute and chronic administration to hypertensive subjects. *Am. J. Cardiol.*, **49**:1547, 1982.

91. Duchin, K., Singhvi, S., et al: Captopril kinetics. *Clin. Pharmacol. Ther.*, **31**:452, 1982.

92. Singhvi, S., McKinstry, D., et al: Effect of food on the bioavailability of captopril in healthy subjects. *J. Clin. Pharmacol.*, **22**:135, 1982.

93. Aberg, H., Morlin, C., and Frithz, G.: Captopril-associated lymphadenopathy. *Br. Med. J.*, **283**:1297, 1981.

94. Kallenberg, C., Hoorntje, S., et al: Antinuclear and antinative DNA antibodies during captopril treatment. *Acta Med. Scand.*, **211**:297, 1982.

95. Atkinson, A., Brown, J., et al: Neurological dysfunction in 2 patients receiving captopril and cimetidine (Letter). *Lancet*, **ii**:37, 1980.

96. Kayanakis, J., Giraud, P., Fauvel, J., and Bounhoure, J.: Eosinophilia during captopril treatment (Letter). *Lancet*, **ii**:923, 1980.

97. Vandenburg, M., Parfrey, P., Wright, P., and Lazda, E.: Hepatitis associated with captopril treatment (Letter). *Br. J. Clin. Pharmacol.*, **11**:105, 1981.

98. Baker, K., Johns, O., Ayers, C., and Carey, R.: Ischemic cardiovascular complications concurrent with administration of captopril. *Hypertension*, **2**:73, 1980.

99. Luderer, J., Lookingbill, D., et al: Captopril-induced skin eruptions. *J. Clin. Pharmacol.*, **22**:151, 1982.

100. Solinger, A. M.: Exfoliative dermatitis from captopril. *Cutis*, **29**:473, 1982.

101. Parfrey, P., Clement, M., Vandenburg, M., and Wright, P.: Captopril-induced pemphigus. *Br. Med. J.*, **281**:194, 1980.

102. Vlasses, P., Rotmensch, H., Ferguson, R., and Sheaffer, S.: "Scalded-mouth" caused by angiotensin-converting-enzyme inhibitors. *Br. Med. J.*, **284**:1672, 1982.

103. Seedat, Y. K.: Aphthous ulcers of mouth from captopril (Letter). *Lancet*, **ii**:1297, 1979.

104. Wilkin, J., Hammond, J., and Kirkendall, W.: The captopril-induced eruption. A possible mechanism: Cutaneous kinin potentiation. *Arch. Dermatol.*, **116**:902, 1980.

105. Wilkin, J., and Kirkendall, W.: Pityriasis rosea-like rash from captopril. *Arch. Dermatol.*, **118**:186, 1982.

106. Rado, J. P., et al: Glucose-induced hyperkalemia developing in the upright position in captopril-treated hypertensives. *Res. Commun. Chem. Pathol. Pharmacol.*, **38**:161, 1982.

107. Rado, J. P.: Glucose-induced hyperkalemia during captopril treatment (Letter). *Arch. Intern. Med.*, **143**:389, 1983.

108. Warren, S. E., and O'Connor, D. T.: Hyperkalemia resulting from captopril administration. *JAMA*, **244**:2551, 1980.

Enalapril

1. Davies, R. O.: *Symposium on Enalapril*. Anaheim, (CA,) Nov. 12, 1983.
2. Vlasses, P. H., Rotmensch, H., et al: Comparative antihypertensive effects of enala- pril maleate and hydrochlorothiazide, alone and in combination. *J. Clin. Pharmacol.*, **23**:227, 1983.
3. Rotmensch, H., Vlasses, P., Swanson, B., Mojaverian, P., and Ferguson, R.,: Captopril and enalapril: Comparative blood pressure and humoral responses in hypertensive patients. *Clin. Res.*, **30**:217A, 1982.
4. Nelson, E., Pool, J., Taylor, A., and Mitchell, J.: Long-term efficacy of enalapril plus hydrochlorothiazide in the treatment of essential hypertension. *Clin. Pharmacol. Ther.*, **33**:230, 1983.
5. Vlasses, P., Ferguson, R., et al: Synergistic antihypertensive effect of MK-421 and hydrochlorothiazide. *Am. J. Cardiol.* (Abstracts), **49**:923, 1982.
6. Chrysant, S., Brown, R., Kem, D., and Brown, J.: Antihypertensive and metabolic effects of a new converting enzyme inhibitor, enalapril. *Clin. Pharmacol. Ther.*, **33**:741, 1983.
7. Biollaz, J., Brunner, H., Gavras, I., Waeber, B., and Gavras, H.: Antihypertensive therapy with MK-421: Angiotensin II-renin relationships to evaluate efficacy of con- verting enzyme blockade. *J. Cardiovasc. Pharmacol.*, **4**:966, 1982.
8. Gavras, H., Waeber, B., et al: Antihypertensive effect of the new oral angiotensin converting enzyme inhibitor MK-421. *Lancet*, **ii**:543, 1981.
9. Hodsman, G., Brown, J., et al: Converting-enzyme inhibitor enalapril (MK-421) in treatment of hypertension with renal artery stenosis. *Br. Med. J.*, **285**:1697, 1982.
10. Bergstand, R., Johansson, S., Vendin, A., and Wihelmsson, C: Comparison of once-a- day and twice-a-day dosage regimens of enalapril (MK-421) in patients with mild hypertension. *Br. J. Clin. Pharmacol.*, **14**:136P, 1982.
11. Kolloch, R., Stumpe, K., Bahner, U., and Kryck, F.: Acute and long-term effects of the new converting enzyme inhibitor MK-421 in blood pressure and the renin angio- tensin system in hypertensive patients. *Eur. J. Clin. Invest.* (Abstracts), **12**:20, 1982.
12. Guthrie, G., Hammond, J., and Kotchen, T.: Abrupt cessation of enalapril (MK-421) in essential hypertension. *Clin. Res.*, **30**:733A, 1982.
13. Guthrie, G., and Kotchen, T.: Effects of chronic enalapril (MK-421) treatment upon the pressor and aldosterone responses to angiotensin and ACTH in essential hyper- tension. *Clin. Res.*, **30**:775A, 1982.
14. Fitz, A., Lawton, W., Reimer, J., and Nelson, G.: The effect of enalapril, a non-thiol converting enzyme inhibitor, on vasoactive factors in hypertension. *Clin. Res.*, **30**:775A, 1982.
15. Wilkins, L. H., Dustan, H. P., Walker, J. F., and Oparil, S.: Enalapril in low-renin essential hypertension. *Clin. Pharmacol. Ther.*, **9**:297–302, 1983.
16. Chrysant, S. G., Danisa, K., et al: Racial differences in pressure, volume and renin interrelationships in essential hypertension. *Hypertension*, **1**:136, 1979.
17. Biollaz, J., Schelling, J., et al: Enalapril maleate and a lysine analogue (MK-521) in normal volunteers; relationship between plasma drug levels and the renin angioten- sin system. *Br. J. Clin. Pharmacol.*, **14**:363, 1982.
18. Ferguson, R., Vlasses, P., Irvin, J., Swanson, B., and Lee, R: A comparative pilot study of enalapril, a new converting enzyme inhibitor, and hydrochlorothiazide in essential hypertension. *J. Clin. Pharmacol.*, **22**:281, 1982.

19. Winer, N., and Carter, C.: Effect of enalapril (MK-421) and metoprolol on blood pressure, converting enzyme, renin and catecholamines. *Clin. Pharmacol. Ther.*, 33:232, 1983.

Saralasin

1. Castellion, A. W., and Fulton, R. W.: Preclinical pharmacology of saralasin. *Kidney Int.*, 15:5–11, 1979.
2. Goodman and Gilman, *The Pharmacological Basis of Therapeutics*, 6th edition, Macmillan, New York, 1980, pp. 648, 656–659, 807.
3. Pettinger, W. A., Keeton, K., and Tanaka, K.: The radioimmunoassay and pharmacokinetics of saralasin (1-Sar-8-Ala-angiotensin II) in the rat and hypertensive man. *Clin. Pharmacol. Ther.*, 17:146, 1975.
4. Zawada, E. T., Jr., Stinson, J., and Ramirez, G.: Hypertension screening and treatment with angiotensin inhibitors. Saralasin and captopril. *Postgrad. Med.*, 68(4):89, 1980.
5. Use of saralasin as a diagnostic test in hypertension: Report of a Consensus Committee. *Arch. Intern. Med.*, 142:1437, 1982.
6. Parra-Carrillo, J. Z., Baer, L. and Radichevick, I.: Physiologic determinants and clinical applications of angiotensin II blockade in hypertensive disorders. *Cardiovasc. Clin.*, 9(1):183, 1978.
7. Brunner, H. R., Gavras, H., Laragh, J. H., and Keenan, R.: Angiotensin II blockade in man by 1-Sar-8-Ala-angiotensin II for understanding and treatment of high blood pressure. *Lancet*, 2:1045, 1973.
8. Corey, R. M., Vaughan, E. D., et al: The immediate pressor effect of saralasin in man. *J. Clin. Endocrinol. Metab.*, 46(1):36, 1978.
9. Saralasin for diagnosis of renovascular hypertension. *Med. Lett. Drugs Ther.*, 24(600):3, 1982.
10. Brunner, H. R., Gavras, H., et al: Hypertension in Man: Exposure of the renin and sodium components using angiotensin II blockade. *Circ. Res.*, 34,35(Suppl 1):35, 1974.
11. Zawada, E. T., Maxwell, M. H., et al: The diagnostic and therapeutic uses of saralasin in renal transplant hypertension. *J. Urol.*, 123:148, 1980.
12. Thananopavarn, C., Golub, M. S., et al: Angiotensin II, plasma renin, and sodium depletion as determinants of blood pressure response to saralasin in essential hypertension. *Circulation*, 61(5):920, 1980.
13. Marks, L. S., Maxwell, M .H., and Kaufman, J. J.: Renin, sodium, and vasodepressor response to saralasin in renovascular and essential hypertension. *Ann. Intern. Med.*, 87:176, 1977.
14. Mitchell, H. C., Keeton, T. K., and Pettinger, W. A.: Drug interactions with saralasin. *Kidney Int.*, 15:S-101, 1979.
15. Pettinger, W. A., and Mitchell, H. C.: Renin release, saralasin, and the vasodilator-beta-blocker drug interaction in man. *N. Engl. J. Med.*, 292:1214, 1975.
16. Gavras, H., et al: Reciprocal relation between renin dependency and sodium dependency in essential hypertension. *N. Engl. J. Med.*, 295:1278, 1976.
17. Case, D. B., Wallace, J. M., and Laragh, J. H.: Comparison between saralasin and converting enzyme inhibitor in hypertensive disease. *Kidney Int.*, 15:S-107, 1979.

18. Case, D. B., Wallace, J. M., et al: Usefulness and limitations of saralasin, a partial competitive agonist of angiotensin. *Am. J. Med.*, **60**:825, 1976.

19. Anderson, G. H., Dalakos, T. H., et al: Diuretic therapy and response of essential hypertension ot saralasin. *Ann. Intern. Med.*, **87**:183, 1977.

20. Horne, M. L., Conklin, V. M., et al: Angiotensin II profiling with saralasin: Summary of Eaton collaborative study. *Kidney Int.*, **15**(Suppl 9):S115, 1979.

21. Pettinger, W. A., and Keeton, K.: Altered renin release and propranolol potentiation of vasodilatory drug hypotension. *J. Clin. Invest.*, **55**:236, 1975.

22. Vaughan, E. D., Jr., Carey, R. M., et al: The renin response to diuretic therapy. A limitation of antihypertensive potential. *Circ. Res.*, **42**(3):376, 1978.

23. Keim, H. J., Drayer, J. I., et al: A role for renin in rebound hypertension of saralasin acetate (1-Sar-8-Ala-angiotensin II). *N. Engl. J. Med.*, **295**:1175, 1976.

24. Wallace, J. M., Case, D. B., et al: The immediate pressor response to saralasin: A measure of the degree of angiotensin II vascular receptor vacancy. *Trans. Assoc. Am. Physicians*, **40**:300, 1977.

25. Marks, L. S., and Maxwell, M. H.: Renal vein renin: Value and limitations in the prediction of operative results. *Urol. Clin. North Am.*, **2**:311, 1975.

CHAPTER XII

PERIPHERAL ADRENERGIC BLOCKING AGENTS

- RAUWOLFIA
- GUANADREL (HYLOREL®)
- GUANETHIDINE (ISMELIN®)
- BETHANIDINE (TENATHAN®, ESBATAL®)
- DESBRISOQUINE (DECLINAX®)

RAUWOLFIA ALKALOIDS AND DERIVATIVES
Introductory years:
1931 (INDIA)
1952 (U. S. A.)

INTRODUCTION:

Rauwolfia serpentina is a climbing shrub of the Apocynaceae family which is indigenous to India. Rauwolfia plant extracts were used in primitive Hindu medicine for snakebite, hypertension, insomnia, and insanity. Over 100 rauwolfia species exist and *R. serpentina* alone contains at least 20 alkaloids. Reserpine is the most widely used derivative of rauwolfia; other alkaloids do not differ from it pharmacologically or therapeutically.[1,2] In 1931, Sen and Bose reported the use of the whole root for treatment of psychoses and hypertension in India. Wilkins[3] first used rauwolfia serpentina for hypertension in the United States in 1952.

Reserpine is the most popular rauwolfia product used in hypertension. It blocks the transfer of norepinephrine into storage granules of the adrenergic nerve ending so that less neurotransmitter is available. Alone, it reduces blood pressure only about 3/5 mm Hg, but given with

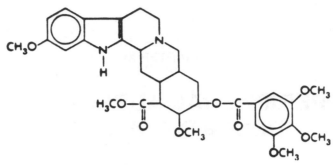

Figure 1: Structure of reserpine.

a diuretic, it reduces pressure about 14/11 mm Hg[4,5] with few side effects.

When should the physician consider rauwolfia preparation for hypertension?

1. In mild and moderate hypertension:

Reserpine is most beneficial when used as a Step-2 addition to diuretic therapy in mild or moderate hypertension.[6,7] Reserpine alone has been used for mild hypertension when diuretics are contraindicated, although the drug is less effective and causes more side effects than thiazides.[8] Fixed combination tablets of a diuretic with reserpine, and perhaps also a vasodilator, have been quite popular for use once individual drug doses are established.[7,9,10]

2. In hypertensive emergencies:

Parenterally-administered reserpine can rapidly lower blood pressure during hypertensive crises[11] associated with acute heart failure, pheochromocytoma, acute glomerular nephritis, toxemia of pregnancy, and dissecting aortic aneurysm.

How effective are rauwolfia preparations in the treatment of essential hypertension?

Reserpine effectively lowers blood pressure when used with thiazide diuretics, and it causes no more side effects than other antihypertensive drugs. The combination of reserpine and a diuretic is more effective than reserpine alone for hypertension[12-14]; reserpine alone does not control blood pressure in severe hypertension.[15] Addition of a vasodilator to the diuretic plus reserpine lowers blood pressure even more.[16,17] Blood pressure has been lowered by as much as 43/29.7 mm Hg in severe hypertension and 27.2/17.4 mm Hg in mild hypertension by the combination of hydrochlorothiazide, reserpine, and hydralazine.[16] Combination therapy allows smaller drug doses and causes fewer side effects than any of the drugs used individually.[13,14]

Indications for Reserpine

- Mild essential hypertension
- Moderate and severe hypertension, with other antihypertensive agents
- Parenterally, to lower blood pressure rapidly in hypertensive emergencies such as acute hypotensive encephalopathy

Formulation

Alkaloids isolated from rauwolfia include reserpine, rescinnamine, syrosingopine, and deserpidine. Rauwolfia fractions, alkaloids, and semisynthetic derivatives are available in various preparations as single drugs or combination tablets. Common forms of rauwolfia drugs include:

Rauwolfia serpentina (whole root) (Raudixin®)
    Tablets .... 50 and 100 mg
Reserpine (Serpasil®, Sandril®)
    Elixir .... 0.05 mg/ml
    Injection .... 2.5 mg/ml in 2 ml
                                                ampules or 10 mg vials
    Tablets .... 0.1, 0.25, 0.5, 1.0 mg
    Capsule .... 0.5 mg
Rescinnamine (Moderil®)
    Tablets .... 0.25 and 0.5 mg
Deserpidine (Harmonyl®)
    Tablets .... 0.1 and 0.25 mg

Dose in Hypertension
A. Reserpine (oral)

Frequency: once daily
Initial: 0.1 mg or 0.25 mg once daily
Range: 0.1–0.5 mg/day[18]
Usual dose: 0.1–0.25 mg/day. In children, 0.01–0.02 mg/kg/day

B. Reserpine (parenteral)

Frequency: intramuscular injection at titrated doses, for short-term therapy
Initial: 0.5–1.0 mg, followed by 2–4 mg doses at 3-hour intervals until blood pressure is effectively lowered.[18-20] If this

treatment is ineffective, other antihypertensive agents should be used.

Range: 0.5–4.0 mg

Usual dose: 2.5–4.0 mg, after an initial small dose to test patient responsiveness

Mechanism of Action

Reserpine depletes catecholamine and 5-hydroxytryptamine (5-HT) stores in brain, myocardium, blood vessels, adrenal medulla, and adrenergic nerve terminals to bring about its pharmacological effects[8,21-23] (see Figure 2, Chapter VII). The drug competitively and irreversibly blocks the ATP-Mg^{++}-dependent mechanism of dopamine uptake by chromaffin granules. Normally, dopamine enters chromaffin granules, where it is then converted to norepinephrine by dopamine beta-hydroxylase. Inhibition of dopamine uptake and, therefore, of norepinephrine synthesis may be the means of norepinephrine depletion by rauwolfia alkaloids. Dopamine beta-hydroxylase is released from chromaffin granules with norepinephrine. With reserpine, there is no release of dopamine beta-hydroxylase which would indicate the presence of released catecholamines.[24] Catecholamine depletion begins within one hour after drug administration and is maximal in 24 hours. Catecholamines are restored slowly and chronic doses of reserpine are cumulative. There is an increase of tyrosine hydroxylase activity and norepinephrine turnover with chronic use of reserpine due to a compensatory firing of adrenergic neurons. Since norepinephrine depletion also depends on nerve activity, this catecholamine loss due to reserpine is reduced in the spinal cord section or ganglionic blockade. Reserpine causes hypersensitivity to catecholamines[25] which may involve increased calcium availability in effector cells.[26] Blood pressure is maximally lowered in two to three weeks after beginning therapy.

Drug Interactions of the Rauwolfia Compounds

1. Plus *Diuretics and Other Antihypertensive Agents:*

Concomitant use of diuretics, vasodilators (hydralazine, prazosin), centrally-acting drugs (clonidine),[11] or adrenergic-blockers (guanethidine, methyldopa) with reserpine necessitates careful titration of each agent, since their antihypertensive effects are additive.

2. Plus *MAO Inhibitors:*

MAO inhibitors cause an increase in the intracellular stores of free amines. Reserpine releases norepinephrine stores and can precipitate an exaggerated hypertensive response in patients taking an MAO inhibitor. MAO inhibitors and reserpine should not be used together.

3. Plus *Digitalis, Ouabain, Quinidine:*

Use of reserpine with these drugs may cause cardiac arrhythmias that involve ectopic ventricular activity or atrial arrhythmias.[27,28] Both digitalis and reserpine release myocardial catecholamines, and their co-administration can cause arrhythmias that simulate digitalis intoxication.

4. Plus *Tricyclic Antidepressants:*

Tricyclic antidepressants antagonize the beneficial hypotensive effects of adrenergic neuron blockage by reserpine.[29] Concurrent use of reserpine and tricyclic antidepressants should be avoided, since this combination can produce a "stimulating" effect in depressed patients receiving tricyclic drugs.

5. Plus *Heparin:*

Hematemesis has developed following intra-arterial reserpine given for Raynaud's disease in patients on heparin therapy.[30]

6. Plus *CNS Depressants:*

Barbiturates added to reserpine increase the frequency of side effects from 8.5% with reserpine alone to 23% when the drugs are used together.[31] Methotrimeprazine decreases blood pressure and causes orthostatic hypotension, which makes control of blood pressure with reserpine erratic.[32]

7. Plus *L-Dopa*

Reserpine antagonizes the effect of L-dopa in the treatment of parkinsonism and can worsen transient orthostatic hypotension caused by L-dopa. Alone, reserpine can induce parkinsonism by depletion of brain dopamine. Parkinsonism patients should not be given reserpine.[29,33]

8. Plus *Anticholinergic or Adrenergic Drugs:*

Drugs including metaraminol and norepinephrine can improve adverse vagocirculatory effects of reserpine. Reserpine decreases the action of ephedrine by depleting ephedrine from adrenergic neurons.

Contraindications

— Hypersensitivity
— Mental depression: history of depressive episodes, signs suggestive

of depression,[34] suicidal tendencies
— Active peptic ulcer, ulcerative colitis
— Electro-convulsive therapy[35]
— Anticoagulation therapy: Two cases of massive hematemesis following reserpine have been reported in patients who had Raynaud's phenomenon and were taking anticoagulant therapy.

Warnings

- Extreme caution should be used in treating patients with a history of mental depression. Reserpine should be discontinued at any sign of despondency, early morning insomnia, loss of appetite, impotence, or self-deprecation. Drug-induced depression may persist for months after withdrawal of reserpine and may be severe enough to result in suicide. Reserpine should not be prescribed for a patient who appears depressed or who has had a recent bereavement. Intravenous dosage should not exceed 0.25 mg/day.
- Intravenous reserpine should not be given to patients receiving other potent antihypertensive drugs.
- MAO inhibitors should be used with extreme caution.
- Blood pressure can rapidly increase to dangerous levels upon abrupt cessation of reserpine therapy.[36,37] The rise in pressure is proportional to the severity of hypertension before treatment.
- Depletion of myocardial catecholamines can cause decreased AV conduction or heart block in patients with AV conduction deficits.[23]
- Gastrointestinal ulceration or intestinal obstruction can occur when potassium chloride is used with reserpine.[38,39]

Use in Pregnancy

Reserpine should be avoided during pregnancy and lactation. It has been used in pre-eclamptic toxemia of pregnancy but has the disadvantages of slow onset of action, greatly variable effect on blood pressure, and lack of anticonvulsant action.[40] Reserpine *does* cross the placental barrier[20] and appears in cord blood and breast milk. Nasal congestion, increased respiratory tract secretions, lethargy, thermal instability, cyanosis, and anorexia can occur in neonates and breast-fed infants of mothers taking reserpine.[20,41,42] Reserpine increases infant morbidity but does not affect fetal mortality.[43]

Precautions

Reserpine can cause depression; doses should be limited to 0.5

mg/day.[44,45] The drug should be discontinued two weeks prior to electroshock therapy.

Rauwolfia alkaloids increase gastrointestinal motility and secretion and should be taken with food to avoid gastrointestinal upset.[46] Reserpine must be used cautiously in patients with peptic ulcer, ulcerative colitis, or gallstones.

The reserpine dose should be lowered in patients with renal disease, since these patients adjust poorly to lowered blood pressure and may develop azotemia.

Use of digitalis or quinidine with reserpine may cause cardiac arrhythmias.

Patients with cerebrovascular hemorrhage are often unusually responsive to reserpine. To avoid a hypotensive response, the initial dose for such patients should be 0.25 mg.

Management of Overdosage or Exaggerated Response
Signs and Symptoms

Overdosage of reserpine inhibits the central nervous system and vasopressor reflex, which leads to mental depression and hypotension. Acute ingestion of reserpine can cause hypotension and sinus bradycardia. [47,48] Impaired consciousness ranges from drowsiness to coma; flushed skin and pupillary constriction are seen as well. Hypothermia, central respiratory depression, and diarrhea may result from overdosage.

Treatment of Overdose

Stomach contents should be evacuated with precautions against aspiration and airway obstruction, and activated charcoal slurry should be instilled. If a vasopressor is needed for hypotension, those that act directly upon vascular smooth muscle (e.g., phenylephrine, levaterenol, metaraminol) are recommended. Freis[20] has suggested intravenous infusion of 4 mg levaterenol bitartrate (one ampule) in 1,000 ml 5% dextrose solution in water. Vagal-blocking agents such as atropine can counter marked bradycardia and cardiac arrhythmia. These patients must be watched for at least 72 hours because of reserpine's long-lasting effects.

Absorption, Distribution, Metabolism, Excretion

Rauwolfia alkaloids are readily absorbed from the gastrointestinal tract and parenteral sites of injection. Reserpine is taken up by lipid-containing tissues and is uniformly distributed in the brain. The onset of reserpine's action is delayed for two to three hours following administration.[20]   Effects on behavior and catecholamine depletion persist for a time after the drug has been excreted, since it takes time for the body to replace endogenous catecholamines. The potency and toxicity[49] of reserpine are greater when this agent is given subcutaneously or intramuscularly than when given intraperitoneally. The IM route has required higher mean daily doses (1.28 mg/day) than oral administration (0.37 mg/day) to achieve similar antihypertensive effects.[31] The rate of reserpine metabolism is at least as rapid as its rate of absorption. Metabolic products are reserpic acid, syringic acid, and syringoyl-methyl-reserpine.

Adverse Reactions

The frequency of adverse reactions to reserpine is directly related to drug dosage. These effects are often corrected with dose adjustment or improved with continued therapy[50] and are reversible upon drug discontinuation. Approximately 5% of patients stop taking rauwolfia drugs because of incompatible reactions. Depression is most common, occurring at approximately a 10% frequency.[33,51,52] Nasal congestion and rhinitis are caused by the drug's cholinergic effects. Nasal occlusion is worsened by cholinesterase inhibitors and sympatholytics and improved with atropine.[53,54] There is a 13% frequency of drowsiness and sedation and a 9% frequency of lethargy and weakness in patients taking rauwolfia drugs. Increased appetite and weight gain are also common. There is no consistent association between rauwolfia use and breast cancer in hypertensive patients. Several studies, including the Boston Collaborative Drug Surveillance Program in 1974, concluded that reserpine increases the risk of breast cancer.[55-57] However, these reports seem to have been based on biased samples.[58-61] Subsequent studies have shown *no* association of reserpine with breast cancer.[62-68]

The Nature of Rauwolfia Reactions

Administration of reserpine causes peripheral vascular vasodilation, depressed myocardium,[22,23] increased gastric acid secretion and peptic ulceration.[69] Initially, reserpine potentiates the body's response to indirect-acting sympathomimetics; this reflex is later depressed with continued reserpine administration. Reserpine has been shown to diminish the pressor reflex in animal experiments. With reserpine, impaired adrenergic nerve transmission lowers peripheral resistance, and decreased venous return reduces cardiac output.[70] There is a slight de-

---

TABLE I
FREQUENCY OF ADVERSE REACTIONS TO RAUWOLFIA DRUGS

Frequent (> 5.0%)
- ↑ appetite, weight gain
- Depression, drowsiness and sedation, lethargy and weakness
- Nasal congestion

Occasional (0.1–5.0%)
- Diarrhea, nausea, vomiting, ulceration, ↑ bowel movements, biliary colic
- Fever
- Paradoxical anxiety, nightmares, dizziness and vertigo, headache, nervousness, parkinsonism, giddiness
- Hypotension, palpitation and arrhythmias, fluid retention and edema, syncope, chest pain
- Bronchospasm, wheezing, shortness of breath
- Rash, pruritis
- Arthalgia, myalgia
- ↓ libido, impotence

Rare (< 0.1%)
- Stupor, deafness, glaucoma, uveitis, optic atrophy
- Purpura
- Gynecomastia
- Epistasis, menorrhagia, metrorrhagia, thrombocytopenia

---

crease in renal blood flow and glomerular filtration rate with chronic drug use and lowered arterial blood pressure.[71] Reserpine's central nervous system effects of tranquilization and depression are caused by depletion of catecholamines and 5-hydroxytryptamine in the hypothalamus and vasomotor center.[72]

Reserpine decreases plasma renin activity slightly; when used in triple combination therapy with dihydralazine, reserpine may prevent any tachycardia or rise in PRA and plasma NE due to dihydralazine.[17]

In one study, reserpine caused a rise in prolactin levels, which may be significant in pathological conditions involving the hypophyseal-gonadal axis or the development of breast cancer.[73]

GUANADREL (Hylorel®)
Introductory year: 1983

INTRODUCTION:

Guanadrel is a new antihypertensive adrenergic blocking agent which produces no central nervous system side effects, such as drowsiness, and which effectively reduces blood pressure by decreasing peripheral vascular resistance. It is a guanidine derivative chemically and pharmacologically related to guanethidine, but differing significantly since it has a shorter half-life and rapid onset of action.

Guanadrel can effectively reduce blood pressure in cases
of mild, moderate, and severe hypertension.

When should the physician consider guanadrel for hypertension?

Guanadrel can effectively reduce blood pressure in cases of mild, moderate, and severe hypertension. Morning orthostatic hypotension, diarrhea, and male impotence appear to be less of a problem with guanadrel because of its rapid onset and its much shorter half-life than guanethidine. Because of its peripheral action, it produces no drowsiness, sedation or other central nervous system effects common to many other Step-2 drugs. Guanadrel should always be accompanied by a diuretic to decrease retained sodium and water and expanded plasma volume.[1-3] Hypotensive effects of diuretics and guanadrel are additive; diuretics reduce the dosage requirements of guanadrel.[4,5] Under these conditions, side effects are usually minimal.[2,4,6,7] As a Step-2 drug, guanadrel is generally well-tolerated in moderate or severe hypertension when a diuretic alone has failed to reduce blood pressure adequately.[4,6,8,9,10]

Howe effective is guanadrel in hypertension?

Ordinarily given with a diuretic (Tables II and III), guanadrel effectively reduces blood pressure and is suited for treatment of mild to moderate hypertension in low doses. Dunn[3] reported that an average

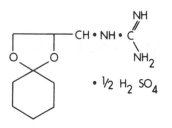

Figure 2: Structure of guanadrel.

TABLE II
BLOOD PRESSURE RESPONSE TO GUANADREL ALONE

Study (Ref.)†	No. of Patients	Duration of Treatment	Mean Dose or Range (mg/day)	Pre-treatment MAPφ (mm Hg)		Post-treatment MAPφ (mm Hg)		Decline in MAPφ (mm Hg)	
				Supine	Erect	Supine	Erect	Supine	Erect
Bloomfield et al[4]	20	17 wks	30–400 (range)	151	150	138	128	13	22
Bloomfield et al[9]	20	6–36 wks (avg. 17 wks)	275	151	151	141	134	10	17
Cangiano et al[12]	6	7–60 days*	162	141	149	124	106	18	43
Total:	46						Means:	13.7	27

† See reference section to this chapter for complete information regarding sources.
φ Mean Arterial Pressure.
* At time of maximum antihypertensive response.

TABLE III

BLOOD PRESSURE RESPONSE TO GUANADREL PLUS HYDROCHLOROTHIAZIDE

Study (Ref.)†	No. of Patients	Duration of Treatment	Mean Dose or Range (mg/day)	Pre-treatment Blood Pressure (mm Hg)		Post-treatment Blood Pressure (mm Hg)		Decline in Blood Pressure (mm Hg)	
				Supine	Erect	Supine	Erect	Supine	Erect
Chrysant et al[1]	5	52 wks	72	167/111	168/122	151/98	131/93	16/13	37/29
Dunn et al[3]	164	12 wks	58	163/99	157/103	146/91	132/86	17/8	25/17
Mroczek[10]	121	24 wks	56	161/103	161/105	147/91	140/91	14/12	21/14
Malinow[13]	7	24 wks	10–75	165/103	159/104	152/92	140/88	13/11	19/16
Totals:	466					Means:		15/11	26/19

† See reference section to this chapter for complete information regarding sources.

dose of 55 mg/day, with hydrochlorothiazide, effectively controlled supine blood pressure in 63% of the patients studied.

Guanadrel appears to be at least as effective as guanethidine in controlling blood pressure.[1,6,9,11] It reduces erect pressure more than supine pressure[2,5,8,9] and may be more effective than guanethidine in controlling erect blood pressure.[12]

Guanadrel and methyldopa, in conjunction with a diuretic, are equally effective in treating hypertension.[5,7,10] It tends to have a greater effect than methyldopa in reducing erect pressure, but on the other hand, methyldopa reduces supine pressure more than guanadrel.[5,7] Compared with propranolol, guanadrel decreases erect pressure more effectively, while propranolol reduces supine pressure more.[8]

Formulation

Tablets . . . . 10 and 25 mg

Dose in Hypertension

Frequency: twice daily; three or four times daily when large doses are needed

Initial: 5 mg twice daily

Range: 10–600 mg/day

Usual Dose: 25 mg twice daily

The dose required for good control of blood pressure must be determined for each individual because of the variability in dose response. *Erect blood pressures must always be considered before adjusting dosage.* From initial low doses, the dosage may be increased daily, weekly or monthly until the desired blood pressure is attained. A diuretic should be given with guanadrel. Tolerance to guanadrel and a need to increase the dosage for hypotensive effects can develop during long-term monotherapy. In a two-year study by Nugent et al,[7] there was a 20% increase in the mean daily dose during the second year. Pseudotolerance and elevated blood pressure caused by edema can be diminished with a diuretic.

Mechanism of Action

Guanadrel is an adrenergic-blocking agent structurally similar to guanethidine. It enters sympathetic nerve terminals by the norepinephrine pump. The drug blocks norepinephrine release from peripheral sympathetic neurons upon nerve stimulation and displaces norepinephrine from storage vesicles. As with guanethidine, there occasionally may be an initial transient pressor response due to early release of catecholamines.[9,11] Bloomfield[9] recorded an early rise in cardiac output, total peripheral resistance, and arterial blood pressure after an intravenous dose of guanadrel. This is followed by depletion of catecholamines from nerve terminals of vascular walls and myocardium. The loss of norepinephrine relaxes vascular smooth muscle, decreases peripheral resistance and venous return, and lowers arterial blood pressure.[1,6]

Drug Interactions

1. Plus *Thiazide Diuretics*

The hypotensive effects of thiazides and guanadrel are additive. Thiazides should usually be given first with guanadrel added subsequently in order to reduce sodium and water retention and to lower the required dose of guanadrel.

2. Plus *Tricyclic Antidepressants*

Tricyclic antidepressants block the action of guanadrel by competitive inhibition of its uptake at the norepinephrine pump.[14]

3. Plus *Sympathomimetics*

Indirect-acting sympathomimetic amines, often included in cold and asthma medications, block the effects of guanadrel.

4. Plus *Phenothiazines*

Phenothiazines might inhibit guanadrel action by blocking guanadrel uptake at the norepinephrine pump and displacing guanadrel from the nerve terminals.

5. Plus *Alcohol*

Alcohol causes vasodilatation and may augment guanadrel's hypotensive effect.

6. Plus *Monoamine Oxidase Inhibitors (MAOI)*

MAO inhibitors counteract guanadrel's antihypertensive effects. Use of MAO inhibitors should be discontinued at least one week before giving guanadrel.

7. *Adrenergic Blockers and Rauwolfia Drugs*

Alpha- and beta-adrenergic blockers and reserpine augment the hypotensive adrenergic response to guanadrel. This may result in excessive postural hypotension and bradycardia.

Contraindications

— Pheochromocytoma

— Frank congestive heart failure
— Use of monoamine oxidase inhibitors
— Hypersensitivity

Warnings

● *In Patients with Symptoms of Orthostatic Hypotension:*

Along with a reduction in blood pressure, guanadrel causes symptoms of orthostatic hypotension, mainly dizziness, weakness, and syncope. These signs are augmented by hot weather, alcohol, fever, exercise, standing, and upon arising quickly. Elderly patients should be taught to sit quietly on the edge of their beds for a moment or so before arising.

● *In Patients with Cerebral Insufficiency:*

These patients are susceptible to orthostatic hypotension and should not ordinarily use guanadrel.

● *In Patients with Coronary Artery Disease:*

Guanadrel should not ordinarily be used for patients with coronary insufficiency since the risk of orthostatic hypotension could lead to sudden aggravation of the coronary disease.

● *In Preoperative Hypertensive Patients:*

Guanadrel should be discontinued 48–72 hours before surgery to lessen the chance of vascular collapse during anesthesia. If medication cannot be stopped, anesthesia should be given carefully. Guanadrel increases the vasopressor response and may cause arrhythmias.

● *In Patients with Pheochromocytoma:*

Guanadrel should not be given to patients with pheochromocytoma since the drug enhances sensitivity to circulating norepinephrine by preventing norepinephrine uptake.

● *In Asthmatic Patients:*

The asthmatic condition may be irritated by depletion of catecholamines caused by guanadrel. In addition, sympathomimetic medications used for asthma interfere with the action of guanadrel.

Use in Pregnancy

Guanadrel is not recommended during pregnancy. There have been no substantial studies on the effects of guanadrel in pregnant women.

Precautions

● *Weight Gain and Edema:*

A diuretic should be used with guanadrel to diminish sodium and water retention and weight gain. Of course, dietary sodium restriction is important.

● *In Patients with Congestive Heart Failure:*

Guanadrel interferes with sympathetic compensatory reflexes of the heart and should be used carefully in patients with impaired heart function.[12]

● *In Patients with Peptic Ulcer:*

Peptic ulcers can be irritated by the relative increase in parasympathetic tone with guanadrel administration.

● *In Patients with Renal Failure:*

Guanadrel reduces glomerular filtration rate and renal blood flow in the erect position. The drug should be used cautiously in patients with existing renal damage since it can aggravate azotemia.[12]

● *In Nursing Mothers:*

Guanadrel should not be used to treat nursing mothers since it is not known if the drug is excreted in mother's milk.

Management of Overdose or Exaggerated Response

Signs and Symptoms:

An overdose of guanadrel causes excessive sympathetic blockade, which is characterized mainly by orthostatic hypotension and its symptoms of dizziness, blurred vision, and syncope.

Treatment:

The patient should remain in the supine position until symptoms dissipate. If more intense therapy is needed, a vasoconstrictor like norepinephrine or phenylephrine can be given, but *cautiously*. Guanadrel-induced hypersensitivity to vasoconstrictors can cause cardiac arrhythmias.

Absorption, Metabolism, Excretion

Guanadrel has a rapid onset and offset of activity.[3,6,11,14] Its maximal effects occur in four to six hours. The drug's half-life is about 12 hours but with much individual variability. After a single oral dose of guanadrel (12.5 or 25 mg), Pascual and Julius[11] measured an onset of effects in 30–120 minutes (average time of 77 minutes), and an offset of action in 4–14 hours (average time of nine hours). Three of their patients experienced a transient pressor response within 30–120 minutes and it lasted for 60–90 minutes. The initial release of catecholamines from nerve terminals increased blood pressure by an average of 45/22 mm Hg in the supine position, and 36/35 mm Hg erect.

Guanadrel is rapidly absorbed into the blood stream with plasma levels peaking in 1.5–2 hours.[14] About 60% of the drug is metabolized by the liver, while 40% is excreted unchanged. Approximately 85% of the drug is eliminated by the kidneys. Excretion is nearly complete 24 hours after the dose is given. Guanadrel is not lipid-soluble and does not cross the blood–brain barrier; thus, there are no effects upon the central nervous system.

Adverse Reactions

The side effects of guanadrel are results of the drug's mechanism of action. The severity of undesirable effects generally parallels the size of the dose. Because of the drug's short half-life, there is not a severe inhibition of the sympathetic nervous system, and complications are usually mild and tolerable. When medication is stopped, adverse reactions dissipate and are minimal. Complaints during guanadrel therapy are often those related to the drug's hypotensive action: weakness, lassitude, and syncope. Nausea and vomiting may occur.[4] Diarrhea and sexual dysfunction are slight,[1,3-7,9,12] and morning orthostatic hypotension is rare and less frequent than with guanethidine.[1,3-7,9-12,14] Reichgott[2] reported no significant difference in the frequency of orthostatic hypotension before and after guanadrel was added to hydrochlorothiazide therapy. Orthostasis occurred in about 10.5% of the 199 patients he studied.[2] Guanadrel has fewer side effects related to drug action than does guanethidine.[12] In addition, there is less variability in blood pressure during the day with guanadrel.[6,11]

Elderly patients should generally receive smaller doses, as they are more sensitive to the drug and orthostasis is more of a hazard in these patients.

Guanadrel and methyldopa have comparable efficacy as antihypertensive agents. Mroczek[10] noted an equivalent and low frequency of side effects with either drug in a study of 242 patients. Specific side effects are due to the different mechanism of action of the drugs.

Methyldopa acts on the central nervous system and may cause depression, fatigue, and impotence.[14] Orthostatic faintness, diarrhea, and sexual dysfunction are more frequent with guanadrel than with methyldopa,[5,10] while drowsiness and constipation are more common with methyldopa.[5,7,10] Morning hypotension and libido do not differ significantly with either drug, although guanadrel may produce slightly more morning hypotension.[5,7]

The Nature of Guanadrel Reactions

1. Sexual Dysfunction

Retrograde ejaculation is a minor side effect of guanadrel's sympathetic blocking action. With guanadrel, Reichgott[2] noted a slight increase in the percentage of patients affected by sexual dysfunction, from 2.3% of patients on hydrochlorothiazide alone to 6.3% of those taking guanadrel plus the diuretic. Some investigators have reported no sexual disturbance in patients receiving guanadrel,[1,4,9] but did note a disruption of function with guanethidine. Others observed an equally frequent but less severe sexual impairment with guanadrel than with guanethidine.[6,11] Palmer reported that the sexual impairment associated with guanadrel occurs slightly more frequently than with methyldopa and less than with guanethidine.[14]

2. Fall in Blood Pressure and Orthostasis

As with all peripherally acting adrenergic blockers, guanadrel lowers blood pressure, particularly in the erect position. Orthostatic hypotension does occur, especially when one stands up abruptly or when one exercises, climbs stairs, etc. Inhibition of vasomotor reflexes by guanadrel can cause orthostatic hypotension, but it is usually not frequent or severe.[1,5-7,10,11,14] DeQuattro[8] observed a decrease of blood pressure during exercise in guanadrel-treated subjects, with a 50% loss of plasma norepinephrine.

Guanadrel decreases systolic and diastolic blood pressures, but systolic pressure is lowered more than diastolic.[1,3,10] Blood pressure is reduced in both supine and erect positions but to a greater extent when the patient is erect[2-5,8,11,13] (Tables II and III).

Guanadrel's short duration of effect may lessen blood pressure variability throughout the day to provide smoother control of blood pressure.[6,11] The evening dose of guanadrel dissipates by morning so that orthostasis upon arising is diminished while blood pressure remains lowered.[3,5-7,9-11,14]

3. Hemodynamic Effects

Long-term treatment with guanadrel lowers blood pressure by reducing total peripheral resistance.[7,8,11,12] Guanadrel causes little or no change in cardiac output and stroke volume.[7,8,11,12] With guanadrel, heart rate is lowered by about five beats/min. It is reduced from control values in supine and erect positions[1,5,12] and during exercise.[3] Peripheral resistance does increase from supine to erect positions with guanadrel, but not as much as with a diuretic alone.[11] Upon initial drug administration or intravenous dosage, a transient pressor response has been reported.[4,9,11]

Tolerance to guanadrel may develop even when it is given with a diuretic.[7,11] Pascual and Julius[11] had to increase guanadrel dosage in five of their eight patients who developed tolerance to treatment of guanadrel plus a diuretic. Others reported no tolerance, even when guanadrel was given alone and in higher doses.[4,9] Edema formation may occur, causing resistance to guanadrel. Sosnow and McMahon[5] eliminated pseudotolerance due to fluid accumulation by giving thiazides. Bloomfield[9] added a diuretic to the guanadrel therapy in resistant patients and got a good response of lowered blood pressure.

4. Effect of Guanadrel on Renal Function

Guanadrel decreases glomerular filtration rate (GFR) and renal blood flow (RBF). Some observers have recorded no change in renal function with guanadrel therapy.[1,3,9] Cangiano and Bloomfield[12] measured renal function in six patients taking guanadrel. The decreases in RBF and GFR in the supine position were not significant. However, in the erect position, there was a significant fall of RBF below control values by 42%, from 557 to 325 ml/min, and of GFR by 30%, from 96 to 68 ml/min, when guanadrel was given.

5. Gastrointestinal Catecholamines

Intestinal norepinephrine is depleted less by guanadrel than by guanethidine. Although some studies report an equal frequency of diarrhea during guanadrel or guanethidine therapy,[1] many have recorded less frequent and less severe diarrhea bouts[6,8,11,13] or no diarrhea[2,3,9] with guanadrel.

GUANETHIDINE (Ismelin®)
Introductory year: 1959

INTRODUCTION:

Guanidine derivatives have a wide variety of medical applications. Guanethidine is a guanidine derivative synthesized by Maxwell.[1] It is an adrenergic-neuronal blocking agent used in the management of more severe hypertension.

When should the physician consider guanethidine for hypertension?
1. In the patient with severe hypertension:

Guanethidine, always in conjunction with a diuretic, is often effective in reducing blood pressures of patients with severe hypertension when other antihypertensive drugs have failed to reduce blood pressure adequately.

2. In the patient with malignant or accelerated hypertension:

Three regimens incorporate the use of guanethidine in treating the hospitalized patient with malignant or accelerated hypertension (see Chapter 1):

- guanethidine + diuretic + vasodilator
- guanethidine + triple therapy (beta blocker-diuretic-vasodilator)
- guanethidine + diuretic

3. In the patient with moderate hypertension:

Guanethidine, traditionally reserved for treatment of severe hypertension, may be acceptable therapy when used at low doses with a diuretic in patients who have moderate hypertension.[2] The drug has limited penetration of the blood–brain barrier and does not produce such central nervous system effects as depression or sedation. Serious toxicity other than that due to its sympathetic blockade is rare. The long half-life allows once-daily dosage for a sustained effect.

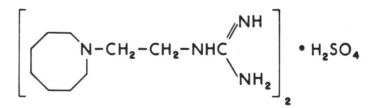

Figure 3: Structure of guanethidine sulfate.

How effective is guanethidine in hypertension?

Use of guanethidine plus a thiazide diuretic for the management of ambulatory patients with moderate or severe hypertension is supported by numerous studies. A compilation of data from many studies indicates that use of guanethidine alone (average dose 60 mg/day) effectively lowered blood pressure in 78% of a total 269 patients. There was a decrease in mean arterial blood pressure by 22 mm Hg supine and 37 mm Hg erect.[3]

Indications for Guanethidine

— Hypertension
— Dissecting aortic aneurysm
— Thyroid storm[4]

Formulation

Tablets .... 10 and 25 mg

Dose in Hypertension

Frequency: single dose daily
Initial: ambulatory—10 mg daily
            hospitalized—25–50 mg daily
Range: 10–200 mg daily
Usual dose: ambulatory—25–50 mg daily

Absorption, Metabolism, Excretion

With chronic oral administration of guanethidine, only 3–27% of the administered dose is absorbed into the systemic circulation.[5] Absorption varies considerably among patients but is fairly constant within each patient. The plasma level and rate of excretion of unchanged drug after oral administration suggest that guanethidine is continuously absorbed over a period of at least 12 hours. After absorption occurs, there is some first-pass metabolism of the drug by the liver.

Guanethidine is transported from the plasma to storage sites. This retention involves specific uptake by the norepinephrine pump into sympathetic nerve terminals and nonspecific tissue uptake. Due to its extensive tissue localization, guanethidine has a long half-life of about five days. The slow elimination from the body explains the drug's cumulative and prolonged effects after oral administration.

Approximately half the drug is excreted unchanged in the urine; the other half is metabolized into more polar, less antihypertensive metabolites that are excreted in urine and bile.[6] The ratio of metabolites to unchanged drug in the urine is larger after oral administration than after intramuscular injection in the same patient, which indicates that a significant amount of drug is metabolized by the liver.[5,7] Renal clearance of guanethidine exceeds the clearance of creatinine, reflecting the tubular secretion of this strong base.

Dose in Hypertension

• *Ambulatory patients with moderate or severe hypertension:*

Treatment begins with a small dose (10 mg) once daily, along with a thiazide diuretic. If there is no decrease in standing blood pressure from previous levels, the dose may be increased by 10 mg each week until the desired reduction in blood pressure is achieved. Due to its long duration of action, the dose should not be increased more often than every five to seven days. Dosage can be increased to the point at which the patient just begins to experience orthostasis upon arising in the morning or climbing stairs, or notices lightheadedness. If an excessive fall in orthostatic pressure, normal supine pressure or severe diarrhea occur, the dosage should be reduced. Usually the dose of guanethidine is given once a day; however, Caldwell[8] suggests that the administration be split as a precaution against overdosage. Better control of blood pressure is attained if the patient can check his own blood pressure at home.

Mechanism of Action

Guanethidine is an adrenergic-blocking agent. It has selective action at peripheral sympathetic neurons, which inhibits the response to nerve stimulation and thereby decreases arteriolar vasoconstriction. Guanethidine enters the neuron by the active transport mechanism for norepinephrine uptake into sympathetic nerve terminals. It accumulates in catecholamine storage granules, displacing norepinephrine. The released norepinephrine is inactivated by monoamine oxidase (MAO). When given intravenously, guanethidine causes a sudden large release of catecholamines that produce hypertension. This is followed by its hypotensive effects as norepinephrine is depleted. Chronic administration of the drug results in impaired release of norepinephrine from peripheral adrenergic neurons and depletion of tissue concentration of norepinephrine, which remains low for several days after discontinuation of the drug. Sensitivity to catecholamines is heightened in effector cells and tissue due to chronic transmitter absence. Guanethidine also directly depresses the myocardium that has been depleted of catecholamines.

Contraindications

— Pheochromocytoma
— Hypersensitivity
— Congestive heart failure not due to hypertension
— Use of monoamine oxidase inhibitors

Warnings

These are essentially the same as for guanadrel (see page 471).

Adverse Reactions

The undesirable effects of guanethidine are quantitative extensions of its useful pharmacological action, related to profound peripheral sympathetic blockage. Annoying side effects have been common, paralleling the popular use of guanethidine in treating severe hypertensive patients not responsive to other drugs. Approximately 15% of hypertensive patients discontinue guanethidine use because of noxious side effects. A diuretic should always be used with guanethidine. This combination minimizes side effects and improves patient compliance. Only 10% of patients discontinue therapy of guanethidine plus a diuretic.

Our review of more than 1,000 patients treated with guanethidine[3] showed that postural hypotension occurred in 37% of the total population of patients treated with guanethidine. The major symptom, dizziness, could not be prevented by altering the times of doses. Orthostatic hypertension is dose-related.[6]

In males, the most frequent side effect, occurring in 52% of male patients, is ejaculatory impairment manifested as retrograde ejaculation with normal achievement of orgasm. Impotence occurred in 31% of male patients. These effects limit the use of guanethidine for male patients.

Severe diarrhea may necessitate discontinuation of medication. Guanethidine has a notable lack of side effects related to the central nervous system. Drug-related allergies, rashes, fever and organ toxicity are essentially unknown.[2]

The frequencies of adverse reactions with guanethidine are given in Table IV.

Drug Interactions

These are the same as with guanadrel (See page 470).

TABLE IV
FREQUENCY OF ADVERSE REACTIONS DUE TO GUANETHIDINE

Frequent (> 5.0%)
    Postural hypotension (dizziness), ejaculatory impairment, impotence, diarrhea, muscle weakness and fatigue, nasal stuffiness, bradycardia, ↑ BUN, ↑ creatinine, weight gain, edema.

Occasional (0.5–5.0%)
    Shortness of breath, mental changes (mainly depression), nocturia, blurred vision, nausea, vomiting, dry mouth, pruritis, congestive heart failure, urinary incontinence.

Rare (< 0.5%)
    Increase in lymphocytes, complete A-V block, scalp hair loss, dermatitis, eyelid ptosis, parotid tenderness, myalgia, muscle tremor, chest paresthesias, angina pectoris, asthma, anemia, leukopenia, thrombocytopenia.

The Nature of Guanethidine Reactions
A. Pharmacological Adverse Reactions of Guanethidine

1. Sexual Dysfunction

The main pharmacologic side effect of guanethidine's adrenergic blockage action is impaired sexual function: retrograde ejaculation, impotence, and diminished libido.

2. Fall in Blood Pressure and Orthostasis

The posture of the patient is a critical determinant of the degree of blood pressure reduction in guanethidine-treated patients.

a. Supine Position

Supine blood pressure is relatively unchanged as compared to erect blood pressure in guanethidine-treated patients. Use of a diuretic with guanethidine does lower supine systolic pressure.

b. Erect Position

Erect blood pressure is normally maintained by the sympathetic nervous system. Guanethidine controls blood pressure by adrenergic blockage. This blockage inhibits reflex sympathetic vasomotor tone and results in a high incidence (37%) of symptoms of orthostatic hypotension. Gordon and Robertson[9] noted that blood pressure is lowest in the morning among guanethidine-treated patients. Exercise augments postural hypotension. Talbot[10] believes that patients with good control of blood pressure at rest should be exercised at the time of maximum drug effect to evaluate exercise hypotension. Exercise induces a further reduction of systolic blood pressure from resting value by 6% and of diastolic pressure by 13%.[11] Louther[12] studied 30 guanethidine-treated patients who were stair-exercised. In all but one patient, there was an additional fall in diastolic pressure of 20-25 mm Hg with exercise, from 90-130 to 70-95 mm Hg.

3. Hemodynamic Effects:

Blood pressure is controlled by cardiac output and peripheral resistance; guanethidine affects both of these factors in lowering blood pressure. After initial guanethidine administration, a fall in cardiac output is evident.[13] With chronic therapy, decreased peripheral resistance is paramount in maintaining reduced blood pressure. The disruption syndrome has been reported in patients upon abrupt halt of guanethidine therapy.[14] This syndrome is characterized by rapidly elevated blood pressure to pre-treatment levels and increased sympathetic activity.

Guanethidine decreases heart rate, stroke volume, and *cardiac output* by depleting the heart's catecholamine stores.

Data from several studies[15-20] indicated that guanethidine decreased *pulse rate* by an average of 11 beats/minute down to 5 to 20 beats/minute. In exercised patients on guanethidine (35 mg/day), Ruedy et al[17] recorded an increase in pulse rate from resting values of only 19 beats/minute, as opposed to a rise of 33 beats/minute in normotensive exercised subjects.

During chronic therapy, fluid collects, which causes manifest edema. Congestive heart failure with increased jugular pressure and peripheral edema developed in four of 80 patients on guanethidine alone. A diuretic must be used with guanethidine.

Adrenergic blockers such as guanethidine decrease plasma renin activity. These drugs should be discontinued at least two weeks before determining plasma renin activity (PRA).

4. Effect of Guanethidine on Renal Function

Guanethidine decreases glomerular filtration rate (GFR) and renal blood flow. Richardson and Magee[21] studied renal function in 27 hypertensive patients on guanethidine. GFR fell in 41% of patients. In the standing position, there was an average decrease in GFR by 25% and of renal blood flow by 17%. In 50% of patients, blood urea nitrogen increased from an average of 26 mg/dl before treatment to 31 mg/dl with guanethidine.

Patients with hypertension due to chronic renal disease, a condition maintained by increased total peripheral resistance, should not receive guanethidine.[22] This drug may worsen their azotemia.

B. Unpredictable Adverse Reactions of Guanethidine

1. Urinary Retention

Moderate doses of guanethidine can cause transient urinary retention in patients with impaired renal function.[23]

2. Complete AV Block

Griffiths[24] believes that guanethidine inhibits catecholamine excitation of the bundle of His, which might lead to a heart block.

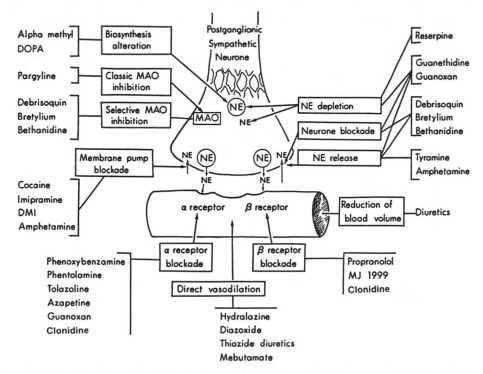

Figure 4: Site of action of peripheral adrenergic blockers (including guanethidine, guanadrel, bethanidine and debrisoquine). These drugs (B) enter the nerve terminal by the NE uptake mechanism. They displace NE from storage vesicles. The NE is then metabolized by MAO. Guanethidine also blocks NE release from the nerve terminal upon stimulation.

BETHANIDINE (Tenathan®, Esbatal)
Introductory year: 1963 (Europe)

INTRODUCTION:

Bethanidine (Figure 5), a guanadine derivative, has been available in Great Britain and many countries for treatment of hypertension for over twenty years,[1,2] but is not available in the U. S. Its adrenergic neuron blocking action and the nature of its side effects are similar to those of guanethidine.

When should the physician consider bethanidine for hypertension?

Bethanidine given with other antihypertensive drugs can be useful in treating moderate to severe hypertension.[3] This drug can improve the response to therapy when added to a treatment regimen that has previously controlled blood pressure poorly. Bethanidine monotherapy is not appropriate for long-term treatment of hypertension,[4] but small doses given with diuretics are often effective and satisfactorily tolerated.

How effective is bethanidine in hypertension?

Bethanidine does lower systolic and diastolic blood pressures in supine and erect positions and can be used for hypertension with other antihypertensive drugs.

In one comparative study,[5] mean arterial pressure fell by at least 10 mm Hg in 70% of the patients on bethanidine and in 84% of the patients on guanethidine. The average drop in pressure by standard auscultatory measurement was about 14/10 mm Hg with bethanidine and 21/17 mm Hg with guanethidine.

Indications for Bethanidine

— Hypertension

Formulation

Tablets .... 10 and 25 mg

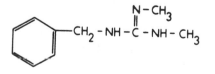

Figure 5: Structure of bethanidine.

Dose in Hypertension

Frequency: two times daily, three times daily for large doses
Initial: ambulatory 20 mg/day (10 mg twice daily)
Range: ambulatory 20–180 mg/day
Usual dose: 25 mg twice daily

● *Ambulatory Patients:*

In ambulatory patients, bethanidine administration should begin with 10 mg doses given twice daily. The dosage may be raised by 10 to 25 mg/day, with at least two or three days between each dose elevation.

● *Hospitalized Patients:*

A bethanidine loading scheme can rapidly lower blood pressure in hospitalized patients. Following an initial dose of 10 mg, the dose can be increased by 10 to 25 mg every four to six hours. Once a single dose is effective, then one-half to two-thirds of this dosage is given two or three times daily to maintain lowered blood pressure. It is important to monitor erect as well as supine blood pressures in these patients and to avoid orthostatic hypotension.

The response to bethanidine is variable. The dosage must be titrated for each patient to achieve a diastolic pressure of 80 to 90 mm Hg with minimal side effects and orthostatic hypotension. The change in diastolic pressure from supine to erect positions reflects the extent of organ perfusion. At a diastolic pressure below 80 mm Hg, inadequate perfusion may amplify pre-existing cerebral, coronary, and renal damage. Patients should be warned of possible postural hypotension.

Diuretics add to bethanidine's antihypertensive effects and help prevent fluid retention. The dosage of the diuretic should be small (e.g., 12.5–25 mg/day of hydrochlorothiazide) to avoid electrolyte imbalance and orthostatic hypotension. It may be necessary to add drugs like propranolol, alpha-methyldopa, or hydralazine. These agents should initially be given at low doses and increased until good blood pressure control is achieved.

Mechanism of Action

The antipressor action of bethanidine is similar to that of guanethidine.[6,7] (see page 478).

Drug Interactions

These are similar to those tested for guanadrel (see page 470).

Contraindications

— Pheochromocytoma
— Hypersensitivity to bethanidine and related compounds, e.g., guanethidine
— Congestive heart failure not due to hypertension
— Use of monoamine oxidase inhibitors

Warnings

These are essentially the same as for guanadrel (see page 471).

Use in Pregnancy

Bethanidine should be used during pregnancy only if there is no better alternative therapy and if the anticipated benefits to the mother outweigh the potential harm to the fetus. In animal studies, bethanidine had no teratogenic effects. However, in rats there is placental drug transfer, diminished placental blood flow, placental necrosis, abortifacient effects, increased stillbirths, and decreased postnatal survival. These effects are possible and should be considered in humans.

Precautions

1. Edema and Congestive Heart Failure:

Bethanidine may decrease cardiac output which leads to sodium and water retention. This could cause resistance or tolerance to bethanidine's antihypertensive action or congestive heart failure. A diuretic should be given with bethanidine to minimize edema formation.

2. In Patients with Congestive Heart Failure:

Bethanidine must be given with great caution since it may interfere with adrenergic compensatory reflexes in these patients.

3. In Patients with Peptic Ulcer:

The relative increase in parasympathetic tone induced by bethanidine can aggravate peptic ulcers and other chronic disorders under autonomic nervous system influence.

4. In Nursing Mothers:

Bethanidine is secreted in mother's milk of rats; it should not be used in nursing mothers.

5. In Pediatric Use:

The safety of bethanidine in children has not been established.

Management of Overdose

Signs and Symptoms:

An overdose of bethanidine is marked by postural hypotension and bradycardia with dizziness and fainting.

Treatment:

Bethanidine should be diminished or discontinued. Patients should remain supine until the drug's effects dissipate. Organ perfusion, especially cerebral, coronary, and renal, should be watched. In extreme responses, vasopressors must be used cautiously since bethanidine augments the cardiovascular response to vasopressors, which leads to arrhythmias. Atrioventricular dissociation has been reported in dogs after bethanidine overdosage.

Absorption, Metabolism, Excretion

Bethanidine is absorbed from the gastrointestinal tract into the circulation. Duration of the drug's action is short. Effects begin within two hours after dosage, peak in four-to-five hours, and are lost after about 12 hours.[7] The drug is excreted by the kidneys. Its half-life is 10–12 hours, much shorter than that of guanethidine.[8]

Adverse Reactions

Side effects are extensions of bethanidine's pharmacological properties.[19] Common complaints, occurring in 20% of patients, are dizziness, nasal stuffiness, lethargy, and sexual dysfunction. These usually diminish with continued therapy and dosage adjustments. In a Veterans Administration comparison of bethanidine and guanethidine, bethanidine caused fewer and less severe complications than guanethidine.[5] There was no diarrhea[1,6] and less dyspnea, depression, and sexual dysfunction with bethanidine than with guanethidine. Bethanidine did cause more lethargy, orthostatic hypotension, and diurnal variation in blood pressure.[5] Dose-related postural hypotension has occurred at doses of only 5 mg/day.[9] Guanethidine and bethanidine have equivalent effects on increased bowel mobility, syncope, and vertigo.

Nature of Bethanidine Reactions

1. Fall in Blood Pressure and Orthostasis:

The extent of blood pressure reduction by bethanidine is posture-dependent. One study reported a larger supine-to-erect pressure drop with bethanidine, by 23/6 mm Hg, than with guanethidine, by 14/2 mm

Hg.[5] Pressure changes throughout the day are controlled less by bethanidine.[10] Inhibition of vascular reflexes by bethanidine[11] lowers systolic and diastolic pressures after exercise.

Orthostatic hypotension, potentiated by blockage of sympathetic vasomotor tone, is greater with bethanidine than with guanethidine.[5]

Abrupt withdrawal of bethanidine can cause severe hypertension characteristic of the disruption syndrome.[12,13] Goldberg has reported pressure of 300/160 mm Hg and ventricular tachycardia, supraventricular tachycardia, and rebound hypertension[14] within 18 hours after stopping bethanidine. This condition can be prevented by gradually removing the drug. Readministration of bethanidine restores lowered blood pressure.

2. Hemodynamic Effects:

Bethanidine lowers blood pressure in a manner similar to guanethidine, chiefly by decreasing peripheral resistance. In a Veterans Administration study,[5] bethanidine increased heart rate by 1.2 beats/min, while guanethidine decreased heart rate by 6 beats/min.

Edema formation caused by bethanidine's action is alleviated with a diuretic.

Although the rapid onset and short duration of bethanidine's effects allow frequent dose adjustment, bethanidine does not smoothly control blood pressure.[15]

DESBRISOQUINE (Declinax®)

Desbrisoquine (Figure 6) is a potent hypotensive agent in the management of moderate to severe hypertension. It is as effective as guanethidine in lowering systolic and diastolic blood pressures[1] and appears to reduce erect pressure more than supine pressure.[2]

Desbrisoquine's short half-life and duration of effect allow it to be given in twice-daily doses.[3] Its mechanism of action is similar to that of

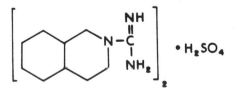

Figure 6: Structure of desbrisoquine.

guanethidine; it interferes with norepinephrine release at postganglionic nerve terminals.

Upon oral ingestion, over 75% of desbrisoquine is absorbed into the plasma circulation.[4,5] It is metabolized by the liver and excreted in the urine. Patient response to desbrisoquine is quite variable; in one study, the drop in erect systolic pressure ranged from 0.3 to 44.4 mm Hg in different subjects each given 40 mg of desbrisoquine/day.[2] In these patients, the degree of response correlated directly with plasma concentration of unchanged drug and inversely with the amount of metabolites, which suggests that the drug's metabolism determines its availability and effectiveness.[2]

The side effects of desbrisoquine are similar but less severe than those of guanethidine.[1,6] The main side effects of desbrisoquine are depression, orthostatic hypotension, and retrograde ejaculation.[7] Guanethidine causes more postural hypotension, nasal stuffiness, weakness, edema, and diarrhea than desbrisoquine.[1] Both drugs diminish libido and impair ejaculation in males.

Desbrisoquine is not available in the United States.

REFERENCES:

Rauwolfia

1. Achor, R. W. O., Hanson, N. O., and Gifford, R. W.: Hypertension treated with rauwolfia serpentina (whole root) and with reserpine. *JAMA*, **159**(9):841, 1955.
2. Quetsch, R. M., Achor, R. W. P., Litin, E. M., and Faucett, R. L.: Depressive reactions in hypertensive patients. *Circulation*, **19**:366, 1959.
3. Wilkins, R. J.: New drug therapies in arterial hypertension. *Ann. Intern. Med.*, **37**:1144, 1952.
4. Veterans Administration Cooperative Study Group on Antihypertensive Agents: Propranolol in the treatment of essential hypertension. *JAMA*, **237**:2303, 1977.
5. Veterans Administration Multi-Clinic Cooperative Study on Antihypertensive Agents: Double-blind controlled study of antihypertensive agents. *Arch. Intern. Med.*, **110**:126, 1962.
6. The effects of treatment on mortality in "mild" hypertension. Results of the Hypertension Detection and Follow-Up program. *N. Engl. J. Med.*, **307**(16):976, 1982.
7. Kuramoto, K., Matsushita, S., et al: Prospective study on the treatment of mild hypertension in the aged. *Jpn. Heart J.*, **22**(1):75, 1981.
8. Goodman, L. S., and Gilman, A.: *The Pharmacological Basis of Therapeutics*, Macmillan, New York, 1975, p. 576.
9. Finnerty, F. A., Gyftopoulos, A., et al: Step 2 regimens in hypertension. An assessment. *JAMA*, **241**(6):579, 1979.

10. Enlund, H., Turakka, H., and Tuomilchto, J.: Combination therapy in hypertension. A population-based study in Eastern Finland. *Eur. J. Clin. Pharmacol.*, **21**(1):1–8, 1981.

11. Opie, L. H.: Hypertension in general practice. Part III. Treatment of hypertensive heart failure and hypertensive emergencies. *S. Afr. Med. J.*, **58**(26):1025–1029, 1980.

12. Veterans Administration Multi-Clinic Cooperative Study on Antihypertensive Agents: A double-blind control study of antihypertensive agents. *Arch. Intern. Med.*, **106**:133, 1960.

13. Tuchman, H., and Crumption, C. W.: A comparison of rauwolfia serpentina compounds, crude root, alseroxylon derivative, and single alkaloid in the treatment of hypertension. *Am. Heart J.*, **49**:742, 1955.

14. Velasco, M., Arbona, J., Guevara, J., and Torres, J.: A randomized double-blind study of furosemide-reserpine in essential hypertension. *Curr. Ther. Res.*, **18**(3):395, 1975.

15. Livesay, W. R., Moyer, J. H., and Miller, S. I.: Treatment of hypertension with rauwolfia serpentina alone and combined with other drugs. *JAMA*, **155**(12):1027, 1954.

16. David, N. A.: Current comment on use of antihypertensives. *Curr. Ther. Res.*, **7**(2):139, 1965.

17. Salmela, P. I., Jounela, A. J., and Karppanen, H.: Double-blind comparison of dihydralazine and prazosin in hypertensive patients on the diuretic-reserpine regimen. *Ann. Clin. Res.*, **13**:433, 1981.

18. Freis, E. D.: Reserpine in hypertension: Present status. *Am. Fam. Physician*, **11**(6):120, 1975.

19. Curry, C. L., and Hosten, A. O.: Current treatment of malignant hypertension. *JAMA*, **232**(13):1367, 1975.

20. Freis, E. D.: Hypertensive crisis. *JAMA*, **208**(2):338, 1969.

21. Iggo, A. and Vogt, M.: Preganglionic sympathetic activity in normal and in reserpine-treated cats. *J. Physiol.* (Lond.), **150**:114, 1960.

22. Chidsey, C. A., Braunwald, W., Morrow, A. G., and Mason, D. T.: Myocardial norepinephrine concentration in man. *N. Engl. J. Med.*, **269**(13):653, 1963.

23. Cohen, S. J., Young, M. W., et al: Effects of reserpine therapy on cardiac output and atrioventricular conduction during rest and controlled heart rates in patients with essential hypertension. *Circulation*, **37**:738, 1968.

24. Viveros, O. H., Argueros, L., et al: Mechanism of secretion from the adrenal medulla — the fate of the storage vesicles following insulin and reserpine administration. *Mol. Pharmacol.*, **5**:69, 1969.

25. Kalsner, S., and Nickerson, M.: Effects of reserpine on the disposition of sympathomimetic amines in vascular tissue. *Br. J. Pharmacol.*, **35**:394, 1969.

26. Carrier, O., and Jurevics, H. A.: The role of calcium in "non-specific" supersensitivity of vascular muscle. *J. Pharmacol. Exp. Ther.*, **184**(1):81, 1973.

27. Leon, A., and Abrams, W. B.: The role of catecholamines in producing arrhythmias. *Am. J. Med. Sci.*, **262**(1):9, 1971.

28. Wilson, B. N., and Wimberley, N. A., Jr.: Production of premature ventricular contractions by rauwolfia. *JAMA*, **159**(14):1363, 1955.

29. Simpson, F. O., and Waal-Manning, H. J.: Hypertension and depression: Interrelated problems in therapy. *J. R. Coll. Physicians Lond.*, **6**(1):14, 1971.

30. Uman, S. J.: Reserpine and Raynaud's phenomenon. *Ann. Intern. Med.*, **77**(6).1005, 1972.

31. Pfeifer, H. J., Greenblatt, D. J., and Koch-Weser, J.: Clinical toxicity of reserpine in

hospitalized patients: A report from the Boston Collaborative Drug Surveillance Program. *Am. J. Med. Sci.*, **271**(3):269, 1976.

32. Hansten, P. D.: *Drug Interactions.* Lea J. Febiger, Philadelphia, 1975, p. 81.
33. Pare, C. M. B.: Psychiatric complications of everyday drugs. *Practitioner*, **210**:120, 1973.
34. Lemieux, G., Davingnon, A., and Genest, J.: Depressive states during rauwolfia therapy for arterial hypertension: A report of 30 cases. *Can. Med. Assoc. J.*, **74**:522, 1956.
35. Smessaert, A. A., and Hicks, R. G.: Problems caused by rauwolfia drugs during anesthesia and surgery. *N. Y. State J. Med.*, July:2399, 1961.
36. Houston, M. C.: Abrupt cessation of treatment in hypertension: Consideration of clinical features, mechanisms, prevention and management of the discontinuation syndrome. *Am. Heart J.*, **102**(3, part 1):415, 1981.
37. Page, I. H., and Dustan, H. P.: Persistence of normal blood pressure after discontinuing treatment in hypertensive patients. *Circulation*, **25**:433, 1962.
38. Ball, J.: Potassium strictures of the upper alimentary tract. *Lancet*, **1**(1957):495, 1976.
39. Learmonth, I., and Weaver, P. C.: Potassium stricture of the upper alimentary tract. *Lancet*, **1**:251, 1976.
40. Martin, J. D.: A critical survey of drugs used in the treatment of hypertensive crises of pregnancy. *Med. J. Aust.*, **2**:252, 1974.
41. Anagnostakis, D., and Matsoniotis, N.: Neonatal cold injury and maternal reserpine administration. *Lancet*, **2**:471, 1974.
42. Forfar, J. O., and Nelson, M. M.: Epidemiology of drugs taken by pregnant women: Drugs that may affect the fetus adversely. *Clin. Pharmacol. Ther.*, **14**(4, Part 2):632, 1973.
43. Desmond, M. M., Rogers, S. F., et al: Management of toxemia of pregnancy with reserpine. *Obstet. Gynecol.*, **10**(2):140, 1957.
44. Gibb, W. R., Malpas, J. S., Turner, P., and White, R. J.: Comparison of bethanidine, alpha-methyldopa, and reserpine in essential hypertension. *Lancet*, **2**:275, 1970.
45. Leighton, P. W.: Problems faced by hypertensive patients. *Med. J. Aust.*, **2**(Suppl):13, 1973.
46. Lambert, M. L., Jr.: Drug and diet interactions. *Am. J. Nurs.*, **75**(3):402, 1975.
47. Loggie, J. M. H., Saito, H., et al: Accidental reserpine poisoning: Clinical and metabolic effects. *Clin. Pharmacol. Ther.*, **8**(5):692, 1967.
48. Loggie, J. M. H.: Hypertension in children and adolescents: Causes and diagnostic studies. *J. Pediatrics*, **74**(3):331, 1969.
49. Rosecrans, J. A.: Effects of route of administration on the chronic toxicity of reserpine. *Psychopharmacologia*, **10**:452, 1967.
50. Elkowitz, E. B.: Hypertension in the elderly: Review of therapy with a hydroflumethiazide-reserpine combination. *J. Am. Geriatr. Soc.*, **27**(11):507, 1979.
51. Aldrich, C. K., and Achor, L.: Psychiatric side effects of drugs, a perspective — commonly encountered reactions. *Drug Ther.*, **3**:31, 1973.
52. McMahon, F. G.: *Management of Essential Hypertension.* Futura Publishing Co., Mount Kisco, N. Y., 1978, pp. 317–354.
53. Blue, J. A.: Rhinitis medicamentosa. *Ann. Allergy*, **26**:425, 1968.
54. Mathov, E., and Misenta, J.: Rhinitis induced by rauwolfia: A cholinergic entity. *Ann. Allery*, **21**(9):481, 1963.
55. Boston Collaborative Drug Surveillance Program: Reserpine and breast cancer. *Lancet*, **2**(7882):669, 1974.
56. Heinonen, O. P., Shapiro, S., et al: Reserpine use in relation to breast cancer. *Lancet*, **2**(7882):675, 1974.

57. Armstrong, B., Stevens, N., and Doll, R.: Retrospective study of the association between use of rauwolfia derivatives and breast cancer in English women. *Lancet,* **2**(7882):672, 1974.

58. Immich, H.: Rauwolfia derivatives and cancer. *Lancet,* **2**(7883):774, 1974.

59. Saxen, E. A.: Rauwolfia derivatives and breast cancer. *Lancet,* **2**(7884):833, 1974.

60. Brown, G. W.: Berkson fallacy and studies on reserpine and breast cancer. *Am. J. Dis. Child.,* **130**:56, 1976.

61. Mann, R. D., Troetel, W. M., and Nadelmann, J.: Rauwolfia derivatives and breast cancer. *Lancet,* **2**(7886):966, 1974.

62. Aromaa, A., Hakama, M., et al: Breast cancer and use of rauwolfia and other antihypertensive agents in hypertensive patients: A nation-wide case-control study in Finland. *Int. J. Cancer,* **18**:727, 1976.

63. Marguardt, H.: Reserpine and chemical carcinogenesis. *Lancet,* **1**(7912):925, 1975.

64. O'Fallos, W. M., and Larbaithe, D. R.: Rauwolfia derivatives and breast cancer. *Lancet,* **2**:292, 1975.

65. Lilienfeld, A. M., Chang, L., et al: Rauwolfia derivatives and breast cancer. *Johns Hopkins Med. J.,* **139**(2):41, 1976.

66. Laksa, E. M., Siegel, C., et al: Matched-pairs study of reserpine use and breast cancer. *Lancet,* **2**:296, 1975.

67. Kewitz, H., Schroter, P. M., et al: Reserpine and breast cancer. *Lancet,* **2**(7998):1296, 1976.

68. Labarthe, D. R., and O'Fallon, W. M.: Reserpine and breast cancer. A community-based longitudinal study of 2,000 hypertensive women. *JAMA,* **243**(22):2304, 1980.

69. Gaffney, T. E.: Antihypertensive effects of reserpine, guanethidine, and methyldopa. *CMD,* **34**(3):492, 1967.

70. Goffney, T. E., Bryant, W., and Brownwall, E.: Effects of reserpine and guanethidine on venous reflexes. *Circ. Res.,* **11**:889, 1962.

71. Moyer, J. H.: Cardiovascular and renal hemodynamic response to reserpine. *Ann. N. Y. Acad. Sci.,* **59**:82, 1954.

72. Chrysant, S. G.: Side effects of antihypertensive drugs. *Am. Fam. Physician,* **9**(1):94, 1974.

73. Camanni, E., Strumia, E., et al: Prolactine secretion during reserpine and syrosingopine treatment. *Eur. J. Clin. Pharmacol.,* **20**:347, 1981.

Guanadrel

1. Chrysant, S. G., and Frohlich, M. D.: Comparison of the antihypertensive effectiveness of guanadrel and guanethidine. *Curr. Ther. Res.,* **19**:379, 1976.

2. Reichgott, M. J.: *Report of a multi-center trial evaluating Hylorel® (guanadrel sulfate) in patients receiving hydrochlorothiazide.* The Hylorel Symposium, Scottsdale, Arizona, Jan. 6–9, 1983.

3. Dunn, M. I., and Dunlap, J. L.: Guanadrel: A new antihypertensive drug. *JAMA,* **245**(16):1639, 1981.

4. Bloomfield, D. K., and Cargiano, J. L.: Guanadrel and guanethidine in hypertension. *Clin. Pharmacol. Ther.,* **11**:200–204, 1970.

5. Sosnow, P. L., and McMahon, F. G.: A two-year comparison of guanadrel sulfate and methyldopa in patients with hypertension. Unpublished data.

6. Hansson, L., Pascual, A., and Julius, S.: Comparison of guanadrel and guanethidine. *Clin. Pharmacol. Ther.,* **14**(2):204, 1973.

7. Nugent, C. A., Palmer, J. D., and Ursprung, J. J.: Guanadrel sulfate compared with methyldopa for mild and moderate hypertension. *Pharmacotherapy,* **2**(6):378, 1982.

8. DeQuattro, V.: *A comparison of Hylorel® (guanadrel sulfate) with Inderal (propranolol) to measure the effects on blood pressure, cardiac function, and peripheral blood flow, at rest and during exercise.* The Hylorel Symposium, Scottsdale, Arizona, Jan. 6–9, 1983.

9. Bloomfield, D. K., and Cargiano, J. L.: Clinical experience with a new antihypertensive agent, guanadrel sulfate. *Curr. Ther. Res.*, 11(12):727, 1969.

10. Mroczek, W. J.: A multi-center, open label comparison of Hylorel® (guanadrel sulfate) vs. Aldomet® (methyldopa) in hypertensive patients. *Clin. Pharmacol. Ther.*, 27(2):272, 1980.

11. Pascual, A. V., and Julius, S.: Short-term effectiveness and hemodynamic actions of guanadrel, a new sympatholytic drug. *Curr. Ther. Res.*, 14(2):333, 1972.

12. Cangiano, J. L., and Bloomfield, D. K.: Hemodynamic effects of a new antihypertensive agent, guanadrel sulfate. *Curr. Ther. Res.*, 11(12):736, 1969.

13. Malinow, S. H.: Comparison of guanadrel and guanethidine efficacy and side effects. *Clin. Ther.*, 5(3):248, 1983.

14. Palmer, J. D.: *Clinical pharmacology and CNS effects of guanadrel sulfate and the major classes of antihypertensive agents.* The Hylorel Symposium, Scottsdale, Arizona, Jan. 6–9, 1983.

Guanethidine

1. Maxwell, R. A., et al: Pharmacology of [2(octahydro-1-azo cinyl)-ethyl]—guanidine sulfate (SU-5864). *J. Pharmacol. Exp. Ther.*, 128:22, 1960.

2. Woosley, R. L., and Nies, A. S.: Medical intelligence, drug therapy: Guanethidine. *N. Engl. J. Med.*, 295(19):1053, 1976.

3. McMahon, F. G.: *Management of Essential Hypertension.* Futura Publishing Co., Inc., Mount Kisco, New York, 1978, pp. 435–436.

4. Mazzaferri, M. L., and Skillman, T. G.: Thyroid storm. *Arch. Intern. Med.*, 124:6, 1969.

5. Rahn, K. H., and Goldberg, L. I.: Comparison of antihypertensive efficacy, intestinal absorption, and excretion of guanethidine in hypertensive patients. *Clin. Pharmacol. Ther.*, 10(6):858, 1969.

6. *Meyler's Side Effects of Drugs*, M. N. G. Dukes (Ed.), Vol. 8, American Elsevier Publishing Co., New York, 1975, pp. 462–465.

7. McMartin, C., et al: The fate of guanethidine in two hypertensive patients. *Clin. Pharmacol. Ther.*, 11(3):423, 1970.

8. Caldwell, J. R.: Drug regimens for long-term therapy of hypertension. *Geriatrics*, 31(1):115, 1976.

9. Gordon, R. D., and Robertson, A. H.: The treatment of severe hypertension with guanethidine. *Med. J. Aust.*, 50(2):134, 1963.

10. Talbot, S., and Gill, G. W.: Excretional hypotension due to post-ganglionic sympathetic blocking drugs. *Postgrad. Med. J.*, 52:487, 1976.

11. Prichard, B. N. C., Johnston, A. W., Hill, I. D., and Rosenheim, M. L.: Bethanidine, guanethidine, and methyldopa in treatment of hypertension: A within-patient comparison. *Br. Med. J.*, 1:135, 1968.

12. Louther, C. P., et al: Guanethidine in the treatment of hypertension. *Br. Med. J.*, 5630:776, 1963.

13. Richardson, D. W., Wyso, E. M., Magee, J. H., et al: Circulatory effects of guanethidine. *Circulation*, 22:184, 1960.

14. Houston, M. C.: Abrupt cessation of treatment in hypertension: Consideration of

clinical features, mechanisms, prevention and management of the discontinuation syndrome. *Am. Heart J.*, **102**(3, part 1):415, 1981.

15. Talbot, S., and Smith, A. J.: Factors predisposing to postural hypotensive symptoms in the treatment of high blood pressure. *Br. Heart J.*, **37**:1059, 1975.
16. Klapper, M. S., and Richard, L.: Guanethidine in hypertension. *South. Med. J.*, **55**:75, 1962.
17. Ruedy, J., et al: A comparative clinical trial of guanoxan and guanethidine in essential hypertension. *Clin. Pharmacol. Ther.*, **8**:38, 1967.
18. Tarpley, E. L.: Controlled trial of guanethidine and methyldopa in moderate hypertension. *Curr. Ther. Res.*, **16**(11):1187, 1974.
19. Glazer, N.: Comparison of guanethidine and methyldopa in essential hypertension: A controlled study. *Curr. Ther. Res.*, **17**:3, 1975.
20. Chrysant, S. G., and Frohlich, M. D.: Comparison of the antihypertensive effectiveness of guanadrel and guanethidine. *Curr. Ther. Res.*, **19**:379, 1976.
21. Richardson, D. W., and Magee, J. H.: Influence of guanethidine on cardiac output and renal function. Symposium on guanethidine. *Ciba*:37, 1960.
22. Swartz, C. D., and Kim, K. E.: Management of hypertension in the patient with chronic renal disease. *Cardiovasc. Clin.*, **9**(1):263, 1978.
23. Bateson, M. C., et al: Guanethidine and retention of urine. *Lancet*, **I**(816):1394, 1973.
24. Griffiths, H. J.: Case of complete AV block produced by guanethidine. *Am. Heart J.*, **75**:371, 1968 (IDIS 5688).

Bethanidine

1. Editorial: Today's drugs. Bethanidine sulfate. *Br. Med. J.*, **2**:865, 1964.
2. Gibb, W. E., Malpos, J. S., et al: Comparison of bethanidine, alpha methyldopa, and reserpine in essential hypertension. *Lancet*, **2**:275, 1970.
3. Johnston, A. W., Prichard, B. N. C., et al: The use of bethanidine in the treatment of hypertension. *Lancet*, **2**:659, 1964.
4. Alexander, W. D.: Guanethidine in hypertension. *Br. Med. J.*, **1**:1341, 1976.
5. Veterans Administration Cooperative Study Group on Antihypertensive Agents: Multiclinic controlled trial of bethanidine and guanethidine in severe hypertension. *Circulation*, **55**(3):579, 1977.
6. Moser, M.: Guanethidine and bethanidine in the management of hypertension. *Am. Heart J.*, **77**(3):423, 1969.
7. Procter, J. D., Evans, E. F., et al: Comparison of bethanidine dosing schedules for rapid control of blood pressure. *Curr. Ther. Res.*, **20**(3):257, 1976.
8. Sandler, G., Leishman, A. W. D., and Humbenstone, P. M.: Guanethidine—resistant hypertension. *Circulation*, **38**:542, 1968.
9. Meyler, L., and A. Herxheimer (Eds.): *Side Effects of Drugs*, Vol. XI, Excerpta Medica, Amsterdam, 1968, p. 208.
10. Gordon, R. D., and Robertson, A. H.: The treatment of severe hypertension with guanethidine. *Med. J. Aust.*, **50**(2):134, 1963.
11. Chalmers, A. G., Hunter, J., et al: A comparison and an investigation of a potential synergistic effect of labetalol and bethanidine in patients with mild hypertension. Macmillan Journals Ltd., *Br. J. Clin. Pharmacol.*, **1**(4):305, 1979.
12. Houston, M. C.: Abrupt cessation of treatment in hypertension: Consideration of clinical features, mechanisms, prevention, and management of the discontinuation syndrome. *Am. Heart J.*, **102**(3): 415, 1981.

13. Goldberg, A. D., Raffery, E. B., and Wilkinson, P.: Blood pressure and heart rate and withdrawal of antihypertensive drugs. *Br. Med. J.*, **1**:1243, 1977.
14. Goldberg, A. D., Wilkinson, P., and Raffery, E. B.: The overshoot phenomenon on withdrawal of clonidine therapy. *Postgrad. Med. J.*, **52**:128, 1976.
15. Rowlands, G., McConachie, N. A., and Currie, W. J. C.: Bethanidine and oxprenolol in hypertension—a study in combination therapy. *Practitioner,* **219**:105, 1977.

Desbrisoquine

1. Adi, F. C., Eze, C. J., et al: Comparison of desbrisoquine and guanethidine in treatment of hypertension. *Br. Med. J.*, **1**:482, 1975.
2. Silas, J. H., Lennard, M. S., et al: Why hypertensive patients vary in their response to oral desbrisoquine. *Br. Med. J.*, **1**:422, 1977.
3. Luria, M. H., and Freis, E. D.: Treatment of hypertension with desbrisoquine sulfate (Declinax). *Curr. Ther. Res.*, **7**:289, 1965.
4. Angelo, M., et al: The metabolism of desbrisoquine in rat and man. *Biochem. Society Transactions,* **4**:704, 1976.
5. Kitchin, A. H., and Turner, R. W. D.: Studies on desbrisoquine sulphate. *Br. Med. J.*, **2**:728, 1966.
6. Heffernan, A. G., and Carty, A. T.: Clinical observations on the use of desbrisoquine sulfate (Declinax) in the treatment of hypertension. *Ir. J. Med. Sci.*, **3**:37, 1970.
7. Messerli, F. H.: Individualization of antihypertensive therapy: An approach based on hemodynamics and age. *J. Clin. Pharmacol.*, **21**:517, 1981.

CHAPTER XIII

POTENT PARENTERAL AGENTS

SODIUM NITROPRUSSIDE (NIPRIDE® OR NITROPRESS®)
DIAZOXIDE (HYPERSTAT®)
TRIMETHAPHAN (ARFONAD®)
LABETALOL (IV) (NORMODYNE®)

I. SODIUM NITROPRUSSIDE (Nipride® or Nitropress®)
Discovery: 1850
Market Introduction: 1974

INTRODUCTION:

Sodium nitroprusside is a powerful direct acting vasodilator which is the most rapidly acting and popular drug for treating hypertensive crises today.

In 1850, sodium nitroprusside (Figure 1) was in use as a chemical color indicator. Then, in 1929, Johnson discovered that intravenous administration of this drug promptly lowered blood pressure.[1] A half-century later, in 1974, the Food and Drug Administration approved it for medical use. Actually, the delay was not due to bureaucratic red tape but rather to a reluctance on the part of any pharmaceutical company to attempt to market a drug which has: (a) the serious intrinsic disadvantages of deteriorating in light; (b) a physician bias about the presence of "toxic cyanide radicals" in the molecule[2-4]; and (c) an apparently limited medical need. Fortunately, the first problem was overcome with the use of amber-colored bottles and aluminum foil,

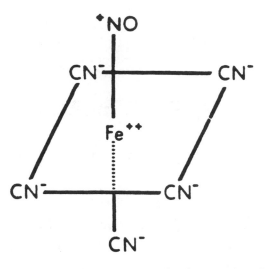

Figure 1: Schematic representation of the iron coordination complex of nitroprusside. Overall complex has a net negative charge and must be associated with cations such as the two sodiums in sodium nitroprusside.[5] Reprinted by permission of *The New England Journal of Medicine* (292:294, 1975).

and the second with physician education about the metabolism and removal of nitroso, thiocynate and cyanide groups (see below). Finally, the third problem seems to have dissipated with the widespread experience and acceptance of this form of treatment of hypertensive emergencies, together with the discovery of new uses for this old drug.

When should the physician consider sodium nitroprusside for hypertension?

● *In virtually all hypertensive crises:*[*6-17]

The infusion of this instantly-acting vasodilator lowers blood pressure to any desired level in very nearly all hypertensive crises, including those due to accelerated and malignant hypertension, pheochromocytoma, monoamine oxidase-induced hypertension, hypertensive encephalopathy,[16] and refractory hypertensive emergencies in pregnancy.[17] Sodium nitroprusside is also used to treat hypertensive crises associated with acute left ventricular failure, aortic dissection, coronary insufficiency and intracranial hemorrhage.[16] During treatment of the above, blood pressure must be monitored precisely and oral antihypertensives should be coadministered as soon as possible, with gradual withdrawal of nitroprusside.

* See Chapter I.

● *In producing controlled hypotension during surgical procedures:*

Sodium nitroprusside is appropriately used to produce controlled hypotension during anesthesia in order to reduce bleeding in surgical procedures.[18-23] The procedures in which it has been used include nephrectomy, cystectomy, prostatectomy, head and neck surgery, middle ear surgery, urological and orthopedic surgery, and pheochromocytoma removal.[16]

● *In cardiac disease:*

Nitroprusside is useful in the treatment of both acute and chronic refractory congestive heart failure. Bed rest, salt restriction, digitalization and diuretics generally restore function and relieve the symptoms in a patient with heart failure. Occasionally, however, chronic heart failure is not benefited by these measures and the patient is hypotensive, dyspneic, weak, oliguric and presents with these manifestations of pump failure. In these cases of low output, sodium nitroprusside can be used to increase cardiac output.[24] Of course, the degree of hypotension may restrict the administration of this intravenous drug but frequently, with careful monitoring in an intensive care unit, cardiac output improves, a diuresis ensues, and the patient responds nicely.[25-27] Nitroprusside has also been suggested for use in treatment of acute myocardial infarction.[28,29] However, this usage has been criticized by some who feel that nitroprusside therapy should only be considered in specific situations after taking into consideration location of infarct, severity of disease and length of time after infarct.

● *In treatment of postoperative hypertension following coronary artery bypass surgery:*

Postoperative hypertension of a sustained duration occurs in 17–73%,[30-33] and Mitchell (1982)[34] estimates that 62% of these patients are treated with nitroprusside.

● *Other uses:*[16,35-38]

Sodium nitroprusside has been used to lower blood pressure during renal angiography and renal biopsy and to treat cardiac tamponade, electroconvulsive shock therapy-induced blood pressure elevations and systemic lactic acidosis.

It is nearly 100% effective in lowering the blood pressure of either hypertensive or normotensive individuals, although its activity is more obvious in the former group.[5,7-11]

The degree of reduction of blood pressure is dose-dependent. However, infusion rates greater than 10 μg/kg/min should not be attempted (see text on Dose, below).

Formulation

Vials .... 50 mg

Dose in Hypertension

The contents of a 50 mg nitroprusside vial should be dissolved in 2 to 3 ml of dextrose in water. No other dilutent should be used. Depending on the desired concentration, all of the prepared stock solution should be diluted in 250 to 1,000 ml of five percent dextrose in water and the infusion container promptly wrapped in aluminum foil or another opaque material to protect it from light. The tubing may be left uncovered to allow for visualization of the drug color. Both the stock solution and the infusion solution should be freshly prepared and any unused portion discarded. The freshly prepared infusion has a very faint brownish tint. If it is highly colored (i.e., blue, green or dark red), it should be discarded. Once prepared, the solution should not be kept or used after 24 hours. The infusion fluid used for the administration of nitroprusside should not be employed as a vehicle for simultaneous administration of any other drug.

In patients who are not receiving other antihypertensive drugs, the average dose of nitroprusside is 3 μg/kg/min (range of 0.5 to 10 μg/kg/min). The initial dosage should be 0.5 μg/kg/min. The dose is then titrated until the desired hypotensive effects are achieved. Usually, at 3 μg/kg/min, blood pressure can be lowered by about 30-40% below the pre-treatment diastolic levels and maintained. In hypertensive patients receiving concomitant antihypertensive medications, smaller doses are required. In order to avoid excessive levels of thiocyanate and to lessen the possibility of a precipitous drop in blood pressure, infusion rates greater than 10μg/kg/min should rarely be used. If, at this rate, an adequate reduction of blood pressure is not obtained within ten minutes, administration of nitroprusside should be stopped. If infusion is to be extended for longer than 24 hours, plasma thiocyanate levels should be monitored, especially if the patient has decreased renal function. Thiocyanate levels of 1.7 mmol/liter (10 mg %) should not be exceeded.

---

1 Vial (50 mg) nitroprusside in 250 ml
    5% dextrose in water .... contains $200 \mu g/ml$

1 Vial (50 mg) nitroprusside in 500 ml
    5% dextrose in water .... contains $100 \mu g/ml$

1 Vial (50 mg) nitroprusside in 1000 ml
    5% dextrose in water .... contains $50 \mu g/ml$

Dose	$\mu g/kg/min$
Average	3
Range	0.5 to 10

The intravenous infusion of nitroprusside should be administered by an infusion pump, micro-drip regulator, or any similar device that will allow precise measurement of the flow rate. Care should be taken to avoid extravasation at the infusion site. The rate of administration should be adjusted to maintain the desired hypotensive effect, as determined by frequent blood pressure determinations. Some tolerance to the drug may develop with extended therapy. During initial treatment it is recommended that systolic pressure not be lowered below 60 mm Hg. In hypertensive emergencies nitroprusside infusion may be continued until the patient can safely be treated with oral antihypertensive medications alone.

In the future, use of closed-loop computer-controlled administration may become the optimal mode of nitroprusside treatment.[16,36,39,40] This method has successfully been used by Hammond and co-workers.[39] However, further studies are needed to determine the reliability of this method.

Mechanism of Action

Sodium nitroprusside is a potent, immediately-acting, intravenous hypotensive agent. Recent evidence[41,42] shows the likely mechanism of action of nitroprusside, as well as other nitrogen oxide-containing vasodilators, is via reaction with cysteine to form nitrosocysteine. Nitrosocysteine, a potent activator of guanylate cyclase, stimulates a cyclic GMP accumulation which, in turn, relaxes vascular smooth muscle and causes the hypotensive effects of nitroprusside.

Both arterial and venous dilatation occur in response to nitroprusside. Thus, there is a decrease in both preload and afterload causing a decreased myocardial oxygen demand. Sodium nitroprusside does not have a direct effect on heart rate. However, a reflex tachycardia follows its hypotensive effects via the baroreceptor mechanism.[43,44] According to Schlant,[45] nitroprusside infusion causes cardiac output to fall or remain the same unless heart failure is present, at which time nitroprusside usually causes an increase in cardiac output.

Nitroprusside, like nitroglycerin, causes vasodilation of coronary vessels. However, research in animals has shown that the actions of nitroprusside and nitroglycerin are different.[46] While nitroglycerin produces its beneficial effects by dilation of the larger conducting coronary arteries, nitroprusside's action appears to be on the smaller resistance vessels. This may imply that nitroprusside will be less effective in treatment of myocardial infarcts because the resistance vessels in the ischemic regions are already maximally dilated. Thus, infusion of nitroprusside may cause blood to be shunted away from the ischemic area as in the coronary steal phenomena. Further studies are needed to prove this theory in humans.

Nitroprusside has been shown to decrease cerebral blood flow in a dose-dependent manner.[47,48] In hypertensive patients, moderate doses of nitroprusside induce renal vasodilation without appreciable increase in renal blood flow or decrease in glomerular filtration. As with other vasodilators, plasma renin activity is increased.

Drug Interactions

1. With *Potent (Loop) Diuretics:*

Nitroprusside's hypotensive activity is increased when given with furosemide or ethacrynic acid.

2. With *Other Antihypertensive Agents:*

An additive effect can be anticipated. Indeed, whenever possible, oral agents should be started simultaneously with the intravenous nitroprusside infusion in order to withdraw the patient eventually from intravenous treatment.

3. With *Ganglionic Blocking Agents:*

The hypotensive effect of nitroprusside is augmented by concomitant administration of trimethaphan.

4. With *Volatile Liquid Anesthetics:*

Halothane and enflurane, for example, will increase the hypotensive effect.

5. With *Clonidine or Methyldopa:*

Abrupt hypotension with myocardial infarction has been reported one or two hours after therapy with nitroprusside and oral clonidine.[49] Three cases have been reported, so this possible interaction should be watched for. A similar report with methyldopa was also reported.[50]

6. With *Tolbutamide:*

Tolbutamide may decrease the effects of nitroprusside.

Contraindications

Nitroprusside should not be used in the treatment of compensatory hypertension, e.g., arteriovenous shunt or coarctation of the aorta.

The use of nitroprusside to produce controlled hypotension during surgery is contraindicated in patients with known inadequate cerebral circulation. Nitroprusside is not intended for use during emergency surgery in moribund patients.

Warnings

If excessive amounts of nitroprusside are used and/or thiosulfate supplies are depleted, cyanide toxicity can occur.

If sodium nitroprusside infusion is to be extended, particularly if renal or hepatic impairment are present, close attention should be given not to exceed the recommended maximum infusion rate of 10 μg/kg/min. If in the course of therapy increased tolerance to the drug develops, it is essential to monitor blood acid-base balance, as metabolic acidosis along with tachyphylaxis are the most reliable signs of cyanide toxicity.

Serum thiocyanate levels should be monitored daily if treatment is to be extended, especially in patients with renal dysfunction. Thiocyanate accumulation and toxicity may manifest itself as tinnitus, blurred vision, delerium.

Use in Pregnancy

Sodium nitroprusside should be given to a pregnant woman only if clearly needed. It is not known whether nitroprusside can cause fetal harm or can affect future reproduction capacity when administered to a pregnant woman. It is also not known whether this drug is excreted in human milk.

Precautions

- Adequate facilities, equipment, and personnel must be available for frequent and precise monitoring of blood pressure. An infusion pump or micro-drip regulator system is highly desirable in order to regulate the rate of infusion.
- Careful monitoring is required when discontinuing infusion, as blood pressure usually begins to rise immediately and returns to pre-treatment levels within one to ten minutes.
- Special care is necessary if there is preexisting liver dysfunction, since cyanide is converted to thiocyanate through the mediation of a hepatic enzyme.
- Special care is needed if there is some impairment of renal function because thiocyanate accumulates.
- Caution should be exercised in using nitroprusside in patients with hypothyroidism since thiocyanate inhibits both the uptake and binding of iodine.
- Geriatric patients may be more sensitive to the hypotensive effects of the drug.
- Patients who are receiving concomitant antihypertensive medications are more sensitive to the hypotensive effects of nitroprusside.
- Since nitroprusside deteriorates in light, care must be taken to prevent the solution from exposure to light. Wrap the infusion bottle in aluminum foil, which is provided in the product carton, or other opaque material. If nitroprusside solution becomes discolored (blue, green or dark red), the solution should be discarded.
- Once dissolved in solution, it should be used or discarded within 24 hours even though protected from light.

Management of Overdosage or Exaggerated Response

The first signs of nitroprusside overdosage are those of profound hypotension. Metabolic acidosis and increasing tolerance to the drug are early indications of overdosage. These may be associated with or followed by dyspnea, headache, vomiting, dizziness, ataxia and loss of consciousness. If these symptoms occur, then nitroprusside should be discontinued. Overdosage may lead to cyanide toxicity if thiosulfate supplies are depleted. Other signs of cyanide poisoning are pink color, widely dilated pupils, distant heart sounds, imperceptible pulse, absent reflexes, shallow breathing, and coma. Oxygen therapy alone will not provide adequate counteractive measures. Nitrites should be administered to induce methemoglobin formation. Combination of methemoglobin with cyanide causes liberation of cytochrome oxidase and the formation of a non-toxic complex, cyanmethemoglobin. Cyanide then gradually dissociates from the complex and, with the administration of thiosulfate, is converted to sodium thiocyanate in the presence of rhodanase.

Use of the following regimen is advocated in cases of massive overdose when signs of cyanide toxicity are present:

- Discontinue nitroprusside infusion.
- Administer amyl nitrite inhalations for 15–30 seconds each minute until sodium nitrite solution is prepared.
- Inject sodium nitrate 3% solution intravenously at a rate not exceeding 5 ml/min, up to a total dose of 10–15 ml.
- Following the above steps, inject sodium thiosulfate intravenously, 12.5 gm in 50 ml of 5% dextrose injection over a ten-minute period.
- Observe patient for several hours for signs of relapse. If signs of overdosage reappear, sodium nitrite and sodium thiosulfate injections are repeated in one-half of the above doses.

Absorption, Metabolism, Excretion

Nitroprusside is very rapid acting. Hypotensive effects appear within seconds after onset of administration and cease immediately following discontinuation. Half-life is reported to be three to four minutes. Sodium nitroprusside is effective only after intravenous administration. When it has been tried orally, it failed to reduce pressure significantly.[7,14] Nitroprusside promptly reacts with sulfhydryl groups in blood and tissues to produce free cyanide ions $(CN)^{51}$ (see Figure 2). These CN groups are then converted to thiocyanate by the enzyme rhodanase which is primarily found in the liver. The rate of conversion of cyanide to thiocyanate is limited by the availability of thiosulfate[51] and in cases of cyanide toxicity, addition of thiosulfate may be therapeutic.

Thiocyanate is excreted unchanged in the urine. This excretion is prolonged in azotemic patients. Thiocyanate, like cyanide, is toxic and

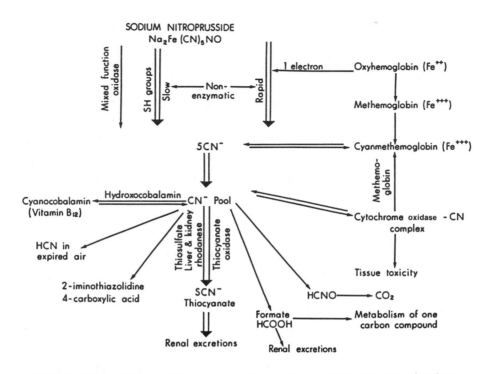

Figure 2: Proposed metabolism and excretion of nitroprusside with sites of actions.

should be monitored in prolonged nitroprusside use. Its toxicity, however, is much less than cyanide.

Adverse Reactions*
A. Pharmacological Side Effects

1. Hypotension or Shock[7,8,12,25]

Accidental acceleration of the intravenous infusion, faulty infusion equipment, or failure to monitor adequately the patient's blood pressure have all been causes of hypotension and shock.

2. Thiocyanate Toxicity[8,12,13,52]

Thiocyanate (SCN-) accumulation after long-term administration can cause hypothyroidism or acute toxic psychosis, particularly if there is renal impairment or hyponatremia. Thiocyanate (SCN-) may cause hypothyroidism by inhibiting iodine uptake and binding. Plasma SCN- levels should be monitored if the drug is needed for several days and levels should be kept < 10 mg/dl. Symptoms of SCN- toxicity include

° See Table I.

fatigue, anorexia, weakness, skin rash and tinnitus. Toxic psychoses with hallucinations may also occur with large doses given for several days. Hemodialysis will promptly remove SCN- groups and relieve these symptoms.

3. Cyanide Poisoning[1-4,12,53-55]

Cyanide poisoning, intuitively feared by medicinal chemists when studying the molecular configuration of sodium nitroprusside decades ago, has indeed occurred, though fortunately rarely. If liver disease exists, CN- levels must be monitored. Also, the physician should be on the alert for signs of cyanide toxicity, including a bitter almond odor on breath, anxiety, headache, dizziness, confusion, stiffness in lower jaw and convulsions. Since hydroxycobalamin (Vitamin B-12a) is an antidote for cyanide, its use may be advisable before and during nitroprusside administration at large doses.[3]

B. Additional Side Effects

The most frequent additional side effects which occur with the infusion of nitroprusside are anorexia, nausea, abdominal cramps, diaphoresis, retching, apprehension, headache, restlessness, dizziness, vomiting, weakness, chills, and palpitations. These symptoms can be reduced or alleviated by slowing the rate of infusion or by discontinuing it altogether. Table I gives the frequency of these and other lesser occurring side effects.

TABLE I
FREQUENCY OF SIDE EFFECTS FROM SODIUM NITROPRUSSIDE*

Frequent ($>$ 5.0%)
Anorexia, nausea, abdominal cramps, diaphoresis, retching, apprehension, headache, restlessness, dizziness, vomiting, weakness, chills, palpitations

Occasional (0.5–5.0%)
Ectopic beats, muscle cramps, hypotension, confusion, warm flushes, chest pain, nasal stuffiness, skin rash, tinnitus, fatigue, irritability

Rare ($<$ 0.5%)
Cyanide toxicity, hypothyroidism, hallucinations, toxic psychosis, blurred vision, intracranial hypertension[56]

---

* Data here were provided principally from the study conducted by I. Tuzel, R. Limjuco, et al.[57]

One case of hypothyroidism following prolonged therapy has been reported. The patient was uremic and received sodium nitroprusside for 21 days. With peritoneal dialysis, the signs of hypothyroidism subsided.

II. DIAZOXIDE (Hyperstat®)
Introductory year: 1973

INTRODUCTION:

Diazoxide is chemically related to the thiazide diuretics (Figure 3), but pharmacologically, it is a smooth muscle relaxant and an antidiuretic with salt-retaining activity.[50,58] It is available in an aqueous solution for intravenous treatment of hypertensive emergencies. This hypotensive activity is associated with a striking increase in both heart rate and cardiac output which may be advantageous for the maintenance of cerebral and renal blood flow. However, the increased cardiac output may place inappropriate stress on the heart of those patients with limited coronary reserve. Thus, proper implementation is essential for the safe use of diazoxide. This means careful monitoring for adverse effects and countering the antidiuresis it induces with the concomitant administration of a potent diuretic agent such as furosemide.

When should the physician consider diazoxide for hypertension?

1. In hypertensive emergencies
2. In severe hypertension with impaired renal function
3. In refractory hypertension

Diazoxide is useful in hypertensive emergencies. However the fact is that in recent years, diazoxide has been replaced in very many emergency rooms by sodium nitroprusside or by the oral administration of such drugs as clonidine (Chapter VI) or beta-blockers (Chapter VII). Nevertheless, diazoxide is useful when the physician must reduce a

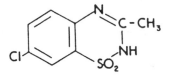

Figure 3: Structural formula of diazoxide.

patient's arterial pressure rapidly. The advantages of diazoxide in this situation are as follows[63]:
— It has a very rapid onset of action.
— It does not require continuous infusion.
— It usually does not cause excessive hypotension.
— Absence of sedative effects enables the physician to evaluate the patient's mental status.
— Drug resistance apparently does not occur, provided that an effective diuretic is given concomitantly.

- *In hypertensive emergencies:*

This is the primary therapeutic indication for diazoxide,[61] and the only use approved by the Food and Drug Administration. Some have considered diazoxide the therapy of choice for hypertensive crises because of its rapid onset of action, its relatively long duration, and its relatively few side effects.[6,64] However, the popularity of diazoxide has decreased due to the ability of nitroprusside to reduce pressure to virtually any desired level in almost 100% of patients. In addition, it is generally safer to give certain oral medications which, though requiring a few hours' time, are quite effective in many emergency room situations. Although most commonly utilized for hypertensive encephalopathy, it is useful in other hypertensive crises (Table II), especially those associated wih collagen vascular disease, renal disease, and toxemia of pregnancy.[65]

In the initial evaluation of the patient with a hypertensive crisis (see Chapter 1, p. 12), the physician must quickly attempt to categorize the crisis before administering diazoxide or any other definitive therapy. As mentioned, diazoxide increases cardiac output while causing generalized vasodilatation, thereby maintaining blood flow to the brain and kidneys[60] as well as the coronary arteries.[63] This rather unique feature can be used to good advantage in specific crisis situations but is deleterious in others, e.g., aortic dissection and intracerebral hemorrhage.

Diazoxide may be used successfully in the management of the acute obstetrical hypertensive emergency. In preeclamptic toxemia and eclampsia, diazoxide promptly controls convulsions.[66,67] It has been suggested that the generalized vasodilation induced by diazoxide benefits maternal renal blood flow and placental perfusion. The most significant side effect has been cessation of labor caused by the relaxant

TABLE II
GUIDELINES FOR THE USE OF DIAZOXIDE IN HYPERTENSIVE CRISES

Diazoxide Indicated	Diazoxide Contraindicated	Diazoxide Not Effective
• Acute hypertensive encephalopathy	• Intracerebral hemorrhage	• Pheochromocytoma
• Toxemia of pregnancy	• Dissecting aortic aneurysm	• Monoamine oxidase inhibitor therapy
• Lupus nephritis or other collagen disease crisis	• Acute myocardial infarction	
	• Aortic coarctation	
	• A-V fistula	
	• Hypertension with acute pulmonary edema	

effect on the smooth muscle of the myometrium, but uterine contractions can be re-established with oxytocin.[58] Hyperglycemia in the mother and infant is only rarely found to be a problem[67,68] (see below "Use in Pregnancy").

• *In severe hypertension associated with impaired renal function:*

This condition requires urgent control—control that is often difficult to achieve with conventional antihypertensive regimens. Total resistance to therapy is not uncommon, and if any degree of control is established, it is often accompanied by disabling postural hypotension.[69] In this situation, a number of investigators[69,70] showed that intravenous diazoxide with oral furosemide is effective. Pohl and Thurston[69] have reported that the elevated blood pressure in these patients can be managed with diazoxide regardless of whether the hypertension constitutes the patient's primary disease or is a complication of renal disease. It is noteworthy that these researchers have also achieved long-term blood pressure control with an oral diazoxide preparation marketed in Europe. Others[71,72] have reported similar successes with oral diazoxide.

In the past, clinicians had been reluctant to lower blood pressure sharply in azotemic hypertensive patients because renal function often rapidly further deteriorated.[73] Evidence, however, has shown that while the blood urea nitrogen (BUN) may initially rise, the lower pressure promotes healing of the vascular lesions, with subsequent improvement in renal function.[64,70,74,75] A study by Mroczek et al[70] suggested that the value of intravenous diazoxide under these circumstances is to lower arterial pressure rapidly in patients who are unresponsive to standard antihypertensive therapy, thus diminishing the danger of developing cerebral complications that are so often fatal. Dosage in uremic patients should be reduced to avoid hypotensive responses.

- *In refractory cases of hypertension:*

When patients occasionally become refractory to triple or quadruple drug therapy, it is usually necessary to admit them to the hospital. In addition to rest and protection from their usual stresses, a 2.0 gm salt diet is frequently needed. Consideration of secondary causes such as renovascular hypertension is also prudent. Outpatient medications may now become effective once again. If not, the administration of diazoxide has been found to be effective in many patients who are otherwise refractory to routine agents,[58,63,70,76] possibly by resetting the baroreceptor response. Others, however, would dispute this claim.[77] Mroczek et al[70] feel that the return to responsiveness is an effect not peculiar to diazoxide, but rather results from maintenance of arterial blood pressure within near-normal ranges. Whatever the explanation, hospitalization and administering diazoxide appear to be good choices for the physician confronted with a refractory hypertensive patient.

How effective is diazoxide in hypertension?

For the emergency reduction of arterial blood pressure, data suggest that intravenous diazoxide is effective in greater than 90% of patients when given in a series of small bolus injections.[78-80] In the past, it was recommended that diazoxide be administered in a 300 mg bolus as a rapid injection. It was believed that this large bolus would cause an overload of the diazoxide plasma binding sites, and thus would be a good means of attaining a high free-drug concentration.[61,62] This high free-drug concentration was hypothesized to cause the sustained hypotensive effects of diazoxide by binding to vascular receptors in a slowly reversible fashion. Today, however, it has been shown by several researchers[81] that plasma diazoxide concentration directly correlates with its hypotensive action whether the injection is fast or slow or given in one large injection or several small miniboli injections. In fact, the use of a large (300 mg) single bolus dose is no longer advocated because it makes no allowance for possible intersubject variability and thus commits the physician and patient to whatever hypotensive effects may ensue, no matter how intense. Several cases of severe hypotension[82] with resultant myocardial ischemia[82,83] and cerebral vascular insufficiency[82,84] have been reported with the use of the 300 mg dose of diazoxide.

Presently, the minibolus application of diazoxide is the most widely preferred because it allows for titration of blood pressure to the desired level. There is also a reduced incidence of side effects.[78-80] Recent studies[78-80] show that the minibolus administration in 1-3 mg/kg doses, repeated at intervals of ten minutes, is effective. While all of the above studies suggest the use of different dosages, it is suggested that the individual dose never be greater than 150 mg (Table III).

Finally, mention should be made of the recent investigations into the efficacy of oral diazoxide. This route has been shown[69,85,86] to have value in the long-term blood pressure control that is necessary in patients with refractory hypertension or toxemia of pregnancy. Oral diazoxide has also been advocated for use in the treatment of primary pulmonary hypertension.[87-89] However, the frequent association of side effects with the oral form has precluded its use as an antihypertensive agent in other instances. Oral diazoxide is available in the U. S., but only for the treatment of hypoglycemia.

There also are many recent studies which suggest that administration of diazoxide by slow-intravenous infusion results in hypotensive effects equal to those achieved with bolus diazoxide. These studies also indicate that there are fewer side effects with slow intravenous infusion than with bolus administration.[90-92] The most commonly used dose for slow infusion diazoxide treatment is 15 mg/min. Ogilvie et al[93] report success with the use of a 7.5 mg/min loading dose. Then, after reduction of blood pressure to a desired level, he suggests use of a maintenance dose equal to 10% of the total loading dose, given every six hours either by bolus injection or continuous infusion. Application of this method may allow for maintenance of lowered blood pressure in a very efficient manner, although further studies are needed before it might be an accepted therapeutic alternative.

TABLE III

SUMMARY OF CLINICAL STUDIES OF THE EFFICACY OF INTRAVENOUS DIAZOXIDE IN THE TREATMENT OF HYPERTENSION

Study (Ref.)	No. of Patients Treated	No. of Patients Unresponsive	Comment	MAP† Pre-Rx (mm Hg)	MAP† Post-Rx (mm Hg)	Decrease in MAP† (mm Hg)
Velasco et al 1976[78]	7	0	Increasing doses given every 10 min (50, 75, 100 mg)	147	111	36
Wilson et al 1980[80]	25(14) (11)	0 0	50 mg every 10 min 75 mg every 10 min	167 159	119 118	48 41
Ram & Kaplan 1979[79]	32(12) (20)	0 0	105 mg followed by 150 mg 150 mg every 5 min	166 163	145* 140*	21 23

† Mean Arterial Pressure
* No minimum post-Rx blood pressure was reported. These are the values following the initial injection.

Formulation

Injectable .... 300 mg/20 ml ampule

Dose in Hypertension

Do not use 300 mg as a single rapid bolus. Severe complications have occurred too frequently. (See Warnings below.)

Bolus: 1 to 3 mg/kg, up to a maximum of 150 mg per injection given as a bolus over a 10 to 30 second interval. May repeat in 10 minutes if needed.

Minibolus: 50 or 75 mg given over 5 to 10 seconds at 10–15 minute intervals until a goal diastolic pressure of 100 mm Hg is obtained. Most patients respond after total doses of 150 to 450 mg, though some require 600 mg or more.[79,80,94] Dosage in uremic patients should be reduced as these individuals have been shown to have an increased hypotensive response to diazoxide.[95]

Frequency: Dosage should be repeated at ten-minute intervals until satisfactory reduction in blood pressure has been obtained.

Mechanism of Action

Diazoxide produces a prompt reduction in blood pressure by acting as a direct vasodilator. The effects of the drug are primarily on the arterial side, as there is little change in venous tone.[96,97] Diazoxide does not have a direct effect on the heart.[98] There is a reflex increase in heart rate and cardiac output which occurs in response to its hypotensive effects. (See Figure 4 for hemodynamic effects of diazoxide.) Importantly, this increase in heart rate and cardiac output allows the cerebral, coronary and renal circulations to be maintained in most cases.[60,63,99,100] The antidiuretic activity of diazoxide results in marked retention of sodium and water,[58,101] and unless this is corrected, tolerance to diazoxide's hypotensive effects rapidly develops.[39] Renin production is usually increased[103,104] with treatment, a response typical of vasodilator drugs.

The exact mechanism by which diazoxide exerts its vasodilatory effects is not known. It has been suggested that because diazoxide attenuates the pressor response to both norepinephrine and angiotensin II, it does not act solely by blocking alpha-adrenergic receptors.[105] There also is evidence that diazoxide's mechanism of action is not strictly beta-adrenergic receptor stimulation, since isoproterenol and

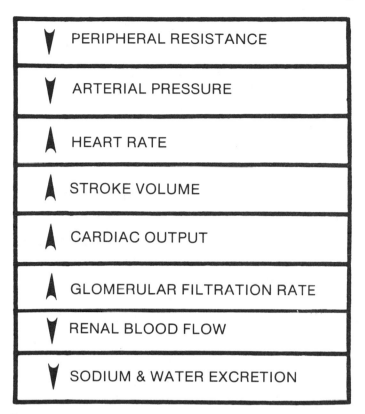

Figure 4: Hemodynamic effects after an effective dose of diazoxide.

propranolol have little effect on its hypotensive effect.[105] Diazoxide's action is involved in some way with calcium ion movement at the receptor site.[99,103,106,108]

Since diazoxide is highly bound to albumin, it has been suggested that rapid bolus injection is the only effective means of obtaining an adequate response. Sellers and Koch-Weser (1969)[107] feel that the use of a rapid bolus injection floods the plasma protein binding sites for diazoxide causing a high concentration of free drug. The free diazoxide can then bind to "slowly reversible" vascular receptors to cause a prolonged hypotensive effect. However, this hypothesis is disputed by other research[105] in which "non-recirculating infusions" of diazoxide produce substantial decreases in vascular resistance which, however, progressively return to control levels following termination of the infusion. In addition, Crout and co-workers[81] showed that a given dose of diazoxide was associated with the same hypotensive effects regardless of whether the intravenous administration was rapid or slow.

Drug Interactions

1. Plus *Propranolol*

Propranolol potentiates the hypotensive effects of diazoxide. Concomitant use of propranolol and diazoxide has been recommended for use in patients with angina pectoris or acute myocardial infarctions because propranolol prevents the increase in cardiac output caused by diazoxide and only causes a slight further reduction in blood pressure.[109,110]

2. Plus *Thiazides or Other Potent Diuretics*

The use of diazoxide with these agents may potentiate its hyperglycemic, hyperuricemic, and antihypertensive effects.[111]

3. Plus *Other Vasodilators or Catecholamine-depleting Agents*

Drugs which potentiate the hypotensive action or diminish the reflex cardiac stimulation of diazoxide may lead to severe hypotension.[112] Thus, drugs such as hydralazine, aminophylline, reserpine and methyldopa should not be ordinarily given concurrently with diazoxide.[113,114]

4. Plus *Diphenylhydantoin*

When giving phenytoin to a patient on diazoxide therapy, it has been observed that therapeutic serum levels of phenytoin may not be achieved despite administration of adequate doses of the drug.[115]

5. Plus *Coumarin Anticoagulants*

Since diazoxide is highly bound to serum albumin, it may displace other substances or drugs which are also bound to albumin[102] (e.g., bilirubin or coumarin and its derivatives), thus enhancing their pharmacologic activity. Therefore, reduction in anticoagulant dosage may be required; however, no cases of excessive bleeding after diazoxide therapy have been reported.[63]

6. Plus *Chlorpromazine*

Chlorpromazine enhances the hyperglycemic action of diazoxide.[116]

Contraindications

— Diazoxide should not be used in the treatment of compensatory hypertension, such as is associated with aortic coarctation, arteriovenous shunts, or aortic dissection.[100]

— Its use is contraindicated in patients with intracerebral hemorrhage[58] or acute pulmonary edema.[101]

— The drug should not be used in patients hypersensitive to diazoxide, other thiazides,[102] or to other sulfonamide-derived drugs, unless the potential benefits outweigh the risks.

— Diazoxide should be avoided in patients with postoperative bleeding.[58,117]

Warnings

- Serious hypotension, myocardial infarction, angina pectoris, arrhythmias, electrocardiographic abnormalities, strokes, coma and seizures have all been reported after patients received a rapid 300 mg bolus. Usually cardiovascular or cerebrovascular disease preexists.[80]

- Diazoxide causes marked sodium and water retention, which can cause serious problems in patients predisposed to circulatory overload. To avoid volume expansion and congestive heart failure, and to discourage the development of drug resistance, a potent diuretic such as furosemide should be administered concomitantly.[62,63] With this combination, however, the physician should expect potentiation of diazoxide's hypotensive, hyperglycemic and hyperuricemic effects.

- Postural hypotension may occur if plasma and extracellular volumes have been markedly reduced previously by vigorous diuretic therapy[63,102]; therefore, it is recommended that patients avoid the erect position for eight to ten hours after combined therapy. Ordinarily, postural hypotension does not occur with diazoxide treatment because the sympathetic nervous system is intact.

- Severe hypotension, although rare, has been reported with the use of diazoxide. It will usually respond to administration of adrenergic agents such as levarterenol bitartrate[63] or norepinephrine.

- The risk of myocardial ischemia with the use of diazoxide is especially hazardous in patients with limited coronary reserve. Thus, hypertensive patients with known coronary arterial disease or even subclinical coronary insufficiency should be managed with extreme caution.[52,80,118] The reflex tachycardia induced by diazoxide may blunt its blood pressure lowering effect and be responsible in some instances for angina pectoris after therapy.[119] The ischemia in these patients is believed to be due to an increased myocardial demand and a decrease in coronary blood flow that results from the hypotensive effects of diazoxide.[83] Similarly, diazoxide can precipitate cerebral ischemia[120] in patients with impaired cerebral circulation. Consequently, all patients receiving diazoxide should remain recumbent and should be monitored closely for the first 15–30 minutes following injections.

- Diazoxide causes hyperglycemia in most patients[72,85] and commonly produces hyperuricemia as well.[85] Both of these effects are generally mild and do not interfere with the usual therapeutic administration of diazoxide for a few days. The hyperglycemic rarely needs to be treated,[58] but glucose levels should be monitored, especially in patients who have compromised renal functions, diabetes mellitus or another disorder of carbohydrate metabolism.[58,121] Failure to recognize and treat hyperglycemia in such patients has led to diabetic ketoacidosis[122] and nonketoacidotic hyperosmolar syndrome[123] in a few cases. Hyperglycemia during diazoxide therapy responds to the usual management, including insulin when necessary.[58] Diabetic patients may require an adjustment in dosages of hypoglycemic drugs during diazoxide therapy.[63]

- Because the diazoxide solution is so alkaline (pH = 11.6), extravasation can cause severe local pain and cellulitis, although no sloughing has been reported. To prevent this complication, the injection should be made into an established intravenous line.

- Diazoxide is a powerful relaxant of uterine smooth muscle and, as such, may arrest labor when used in the hypertensive crises of pregnancy.[58,106,124,125] Uterine contractions can be reestablished with oxytocin.

- Diazoxide can displace coumarin anticoagulants from serum albumin.[102] Therefore, reduction of anticoagulant dosage may be necessary during diazoxide therapy, particularly if the patient is hypoalbuminemic. However, there have been no clinical reports of excessive bleeding in patients receiving these drugs concomitantly.[63]

Use in Pregnancy

The safety of diazoxide has not yet been fully established,[58,103,126] nevertheless, several authors suggest that it be used in the treatment of the hypertension associated with severe preeclampsia and eclampsia.[123,127-129]

There are several side effects associated with its use in pregnancy. It is not known whether or not diazoxide passes into breast milk, although it has been shown that diazoxide crosses the placenta where it can cause fetal or neonatal hyperglycemia and hyperbilirubinemia.[58,]

[103,130] Diazoxide use is also associated with neonatal hypotension and shock.[128] Uterine hypotonia and cessation of labor occur very commonly following diazoxide administration due to its relaxant action on uterine smooth muscle.[124,125] This side effect can, however, be counteracted by the administration of oxytocin.

Notwithstanding the above side effects, diazoxide can be used to treat extreme hypertension in pregnancy. It is cautioned, however, that treatment with diazoxide should only be attempted when electronic fetal monitoring is available.

Finally, it is advised that the former 300 mg bolus injection used in the past is excessive.[124,128,131] Use either the minibolus or infusion methods described above.

Management of Overdosage or Exaggerated Response

Overdosage with diazoxide may cause undesirable hypotension. Usually this can be controlled with a sympathomimetic agent such as norepinephrine. Failure of the blood pressure to rise in response to such an agent suggests that the hypotension may have been caused by something other than diazoxide. Excessive hyperglycemia from diazoxide therapy will respond to conventional therapy of hyperglycemia. Finally, diazoxide can be removed by peritoneal dialysis or hemodialysis, but dialysis is relatively slow due to the extensive binding of diazoxide to plasma albumin.

Absorption, Metabolism, Excretion

Following a bolus infusion, blood pressure usually falls in response to diazoxide within one minute and reaches a nadir within five minutes. The half-life of diazoxide is relatively long due to its being highly protein bound. According to Ogilvie et al,[93] diazoxide levels following a bolus injection decline biphasically with the early-distribution phase having a half-time of 0.09 hours and the late-elimination phase having a half-time of 47.6 hours. The apparent volume of distribution of diazoxide at steady state is approximately 20% of body weight,[132] and plasma clearance has been reported in the 5 to 7 ml per minute range.[93,132]

Diazoxide is metabolized in the liver to hydroxy-methyl and carboxy-methyl derivatives which do not have any known cardiovascular activity.[133] These derivatives, as well as the parent compound, have been shown to be eliminated in the urine[134] with unchanged drug accounting for approximately one-third of plasma clearance. Uremic patients are likely to have an increased response to diazoxide and thus the dosage should be reduced in these patients.[95,135] It is not known whether or not diazoxide induces the metabolism of other drugs,[133] although it appears to decrease the serum level of phenytoin in man.[115]

Adverse Reactions

There are three usual side effects of diazoxide: fluid retention, hyperglycemia, and tachycardia.[6] When fluid retention occurs, it can usually be overcome by concomitant use of a potent diuretic.[6,103] The hyperglycemia which is mild and transitory usually presents no problems.[136] However, it does occasionally require treatment, and in such cases (usually diabetic patients), the elevated blood glucose can generally be managed with either insulin or oral hypoglycemic agents.[6,63,100] A few cases of severe disturbances in carbohydrate metabolism resulting from diazoxide therapy have been reported, i.e., hyperglycemic hyperosmolar coma[123] and diabetic ketoacidosis.[122] These cases, however, only occurred in patients who were predisposed to carbohydrate intolerance. Diazoxide also commonly causes mild hyperuricemia, but this generally does not require treatment.[100,102]

Diazoxide regularly induces tachycardia, which can precipitate angina pectoris, especially in predisposed individuals. Excessive hypotension is an infrequent effect of diazoxide,[6,137] rarely severe enough to require treatment with a sympathomimetic agent such as norepinephrine.[103] Nonetheless, the potent hypotensive effect may diminish coronary and cerebral blood flow; thus, some risk of myocardial ischemia and cerebral ischemia is associated with its use,[83,103,118] particularly in patients with pre-existing vascular disease. Ordinarily such ischemic effects are transient, but angina pectoris, atrial and ventricular arrhythmias, and EKG changes can develop.[82,102,103] More serious but fortunately less frequent are the reports of serious cerebral and myocardial sequelae of diazoxide therapy.[82,118] Myocardial infarction has been reported in isolated cases, occurring not only in patients with previous histories of angina pectoris, but also in patients having either no evidence of coronary artery disease or a subclinical form of it.[82,83,103]

Other potentially serious adverse reactions that may occur with diazoxide include unconsciousness, convulsions, paralysis, retention of nitrogenous wastes after repeated injections, and hypersensitivity reactions (including rash, leukopenia, and fever).[63,103] Fortunately these effects are uncommon.

Although orthostatic hypotension has been reported in patients receiving diazoxide alone,[60] it is much more commonly associated with the combined therapy of diazoxide plus a potent diuretic. Many believe that the orthostatic hypotension observed in this situation is caused more by the volume depleting effects of the diuretic than by diazoxide.[63,101]

Diazoxide, when used in eclampsia, commonly interrupts labor (in up to 50% of patients[138]); however, uterine contractions can be reestablished with oxytocin.[58,63,66] Numerous other side effects from the use of diazoxide have been reported in the literature including the following: gastrointestinal disturbances (i.e., nausea, vomiting, anorexia, and abdominal pain); vasodilative phenomena such as flushing, generalized or localized sensations of warmth, headache, and sweating; dizziness and weakness of short duration; supraventricular tachycardia and palpitations; non-anginal chest discomfort; and pain or cellulitis (without sloughing) from extravasation at the injection site. Less commonly reported are: alteration in taste, abnormal odors and auditory phenomena; hyperpnea; dyspnea and choking sensations; apprehension, malaise, blurred vision, and blindness; parotid swelling, salivation, lacrimation, and xerostomia; tinnitus; bradycardia; muscle cramps and back pain; ileus, diarrhea, constipation, and rectal burning; pruritus, increased nocturia; drowsiness, and euphoria.[58,63,66,77,102,103,136,139-141] However, for brief treatment periods, very few patients[82,119,123] have required discontinuation of diazoxide because of noxious side effects.

The Nature of Diazoxide Reactions
A. Predictable Pharmacological Reactions

1. Effects of Diazoxide on the Cardiovascular System

Diazoxide induces tachycardia and increases cardiac output[142] as a reflex response to the rapid fall in arterial pressure.[97] Following mini-bolus diazoxide, increases in heart rate from 6–31% have been reported.[79,143]

The potent vasodilatative and hypotensive effects of diazoxide may explain many of its adverse effects such as angina pectoris, EKG changes, severe hypotension, headaches, palpitations, convulsions, dizziness, dyspnea and so forth. Ischemic symptoms are not common after diazoxide injection, probably because excessive hypotension is rare and cardiac output is increased.[58] Even though cerebral and myocardial circulations are thought to be maintained after diazoxide,[60,63] a sudden significant fall in blood pressure may cause excessive reductions in blood flows in patients with cerebral vascular and coronary artery disease because their circulations are critically dependent on blood pressure.[59,84,143] Kanada et al[83] have demonstrated that the electrocardiographic changes sometimes seen with diazoxide have greater statistical correlation with the hypotensive effects of the drug than with the tachycardia it induces. Nevertheless, deleterious changes were observed in some patients who did not show a steep fall in blood pressure. Thus, it seems that the ischemic episodes following diazoxide treatment are due to a combination of the increased cardiac work and the hypotensive effects of diazoxide.

2. Effects of Diazoxide on Sodium Excretion

Marked sodium and water retention are associated with the repeated use of diazoxide and result in the development of tolerance to the drug's hypotensive effects unless prevented by prior concomitant administration of a potent diuretic.[102] Diazoxide enhances reabsorption of sodium in the proximal tubules and decreases delivery of salt and water to the distal portions of the nephron.[99]

3. Effects of Diazoxide on Serum Uric Acid

Diazoxide has been shown to induce mild hyperuricemia by inhibition of the tubular excretion of uric acid.[85,144]

4. Effect of Diazoxide on Blood Glucose

Diazoxide causes mild, usually transitory, hyperglycemia primarily by acting directly on the pancreatic beta cells to decrease insulin secretion.[145,146] It also increases catecholamine release which is believed to reinforce its direct effects on insulin secretion[62,146] and at the same time to induce lipolysis leading to increased serum fatty acid levels. The elevation in serum catecholamines causes a further increase in blood glucose by enhancing glycogen degradation and decreasing glycogen synthesis. Conditions such as diabetes mellitus, liver disease, or uremia, and concomitant use of drugs like diuretics or gluconeogenic steroids, etc., will enhance the hyperglycemic effects of diazoxide.

5. Effects of Diazoxide on the Uterus

Diazoxide has a direct and immediate relaxant effect on the smooth muscle of the myometrium,[58] just as it does on the smooth muscle of the peripheral vessels where the effect is thought to be due to an interaction with calcium ions at the receptor sites.[99,103,106] The rapid relaxation produced by diazoxide is similar to that induced by magnesium salts, which probably also act by a calcium interaction.[147] Consequently, diazoxide causes cessation of myometrial contractility. Uterine contractions can, however, be reestablished with oxytocin.[58,63,66]

6. Other Pharmacological Effects of Diazoxide

Gastrointestinal disturbances such as nausea and vomiting are relatively common. They are probably manifestations of diazoxide's relaxant effect on the smooth muscle of the stomach wall.[148] More serious gastrointestinal complaints such as abdominal pain and anorexia may occur[63] but are more often associated with oral diazoxide.

Occurring very infrequently and reported only with the use of oral diazoxide are various hematological reactions. Diazoxide is similar in structure to dapsone, a well-recognized oxidant drug that will produce a compensated hemolytic state in normal individuals, probably owing to stress on aging erythrocytes.[149] Consequently, hemolysis with diazoxide therapy can occur and has indeed been reported.[149] In addition, there have been isolated cases of neutropenia and thrombocytopenia,[150,151] probably as hypersensitivity phenomena.[63]

B. Unpredictable Adverse Reactions to Diazoxide

Many other infrequently-mentioned side effects may occur following administration of intravenous diazoxide. These include sensory phenomena such as alteration in taste, abnormal odors, and auditory sensations; gastrointestinal disturbances like diarrhea, constipation, rectal burning, and ileus; skeletomuscular complaints such as muscle cramps and back pain; respiratory distress of various types; and others (Table IV).

Another group of adverse effects should be mentioned. These occur predominantly after the use of oral diazoxide and have not been reported in association with intravenous use of the drug for brief periods.[63] Included is hypertrichosis lanuginosa, a common adverse effect that occurs after the long-term use of oral diazoxide for the management of juvenile hypoglycemic states.[63,152] Alopecia and hypertrichosis have been observed in the offspring of women who were given diazoxide orally during the last 19–60 days of pregnancy for treatment of preeclampsia.[63,153] Extrapyramidal symptoms have also been reported following the use of oral diazoxide.[58,154]

TABLE IV
FREQUENCY OF ADVERSE REACTIONS DUE TO DIAZOXIDE

Frequent ($>$ 5.0%)
- Hyperglycemia, hyperuricemia, sodium and water retention, tachycardia, interruption of labor, hypertrichosis, alopecia

Occasional (0.1–5.0%)

GI: Nausea, vomiting, constipation

CV: Angina pectoris, electrocardiographic changes, atrial or ventricular arrhythmias, palpitations, non-anginal chest discomfort, headache, dizziness, weakness, diaphoresis, transient hemiparesis, hypotension, orthostatic hypotension

CNS: Extrapyramidal symptoms (with oral diazoxide), tinnitus

DERM: Flushing, warmth, sweating

METABOLIC: ↑BUN and creatinine

MISC: Pain and cellulitis from extravasation at injection site, lacrimation, blurred vision, back pain, xerostomia

Rare ($<$ 0.1%)
- Anorexia, abdominal pain, diarrhea, rectal burning, ileus, salivation
- Myocardial infarction, bradycardia, convulsions, paralysis, unconsciousness, dyspnea, hyperpnea, choking sensation
- Sensory phenomena, drowsiness, euphoria
- Hyperosmolar coma, ketoacidosis
- Hemolysis, platelets, and white blood cells (with oral diazoxide)
- Increased nocturia, muscle cramps, malaise, parotid swelling, salivation, hypersensitivity reactions, rash, pruritis

Use of Diazoxide as an Oral Hyperglycemic

Diazoxide (Proglycem® Capsules or Suspension [Schering]) may be used to control hyperglycemia. It appears to exert direct alpha-adrenergic-like actions on the pancreatic islet B cell. It also stimulates the release of endogenous catecholamines. For this use diazoxide is available in 50 and 100 mg capsules and in an oral suspension (5 mg/ml). The usual daily dose for adults and children is 3–8 mg/kg, divided into two or three equal portions; for neonates and infants, the usual daily dose is 8–15 mg/kg.

III. TRIMETHAPHAN CAMSYLATE

Indications for Trimethaphan

- Hypertensive crisis, particularly when associated with:

— dissecting aortic aneurysm,
— encephalopathy,
— subarachnoid hemorrhage,
— acute pulmonary edema associated with pulmonary and systemic hypertension.

How Effective is Trimethaphan?

It is effective in all forms of hypertension. It will reduce anyone's blood pressure to any level desired, depending upon the rate of infusion and the concentration used. It is optimally effective when the patient's head is elevated. Orthostatic hypotension is to be expected.

Pharmacological Effects

It is a ganglionic-blocking agent, blocking both adrenergic and cholinergic ganglia. Trimethaphan also has direct vasodilating action which enhances its hypotensive effects. Its principal effects are as follows:

- arteriolar dilatation, increased peripheral blood flow, reduced blood pressure (particularly in erect position);
- venous dilatation, decreased venous return, decreased cardiac output;
- tachycardia and palpitations;
- mydriasis and cycloplegia, amblyopia;
- reduced gut motility, constipation;
- urinary retention;
- xerostomia;
- anhidrosis;
- histamine-release.

Dosage and Administration

Trimethaphan is available in 10 ml vials at a concentration of 50 mg/ml. When 1 ampule (10 ml) is added to 500 ml of 5% dextrose in water, the concentration becomes 0.1% (1 mg/ml). The rate of infusion is determined by the patient's response, but initially it is recommended that 2 to 4 mg/min (45-60 drops/min) be given. Systolic pressure should not be allowed to fall below 60 mm Hg systolic for hypotensive surgery. The fall in pressure is largely dependent upon posture, so 4 to

6 inch blocks should always be placed under the head of the bed prior to infusing trimethaphan.

Side effects include those expected by the nature of the ganglionic blockade: mydriasis, cycloplegia, orthostatic hypotension, adynamic ileus, constipation, urinary retention, xerostomia, nausea, vomiting, anorexia.

Continued infusion is essential for its antihypertensive effect, so one should always try to initiate oral agents when starting this agent parenterally. It is best given via an infusion pump or a micro-drip apparatus. After 48 hours, patients may become refractory. Blood pressure must be monitored constantly. Tachyphylaxis develops frequently, chiefly after two days of infusions, and the dose may need to be increased proportionately.

Formulation
Injectable .... 10 ml ampules (50 mg/ml)

Drug Interactions
1. Plus *Antihypertensive Agents*

Trimethaphan should be used with care in patients who have been receiving antihypertensive drugs, since an additive hypotensive effect may occur.

2. Plus *Diuretics*

Diuretic agents may enhance markedly the responses evoked by ganglionic-blocking agents.

3. Plus *Anesthetic Agents*

Trimethaphan should be used with caution with anesthetic agents, especially spinal anesthetics which themselves may produce hypotension.

Concomitant therapy with other drugs can modify materially the dose of trimethaphan necessary to achieve the desired response.

Contraindications
Trimethaphan is contraindicated in those conditions where hypotension may subject the patient to undue risk, e.g.:

— uncorrected anemia,

— hypovolemia,

— shock (both incipient and frank),

— asphyxia,

— uncorrected respiratory insufficiency,

— inadequate availability of fluids and inability to replace blood for technical reasons.

Warnings

Trimethaphan is a powerful hypotensive drug and should always be diluted before use.

● *In Patients Undergoing Surgery:*

It is recommended that the use of trimethaphan to produce hypotension in surgical or medical indications be limited to physicians with proper training in this technique. Adequate facilities, equipment and personnel should be available for vigilant monitoring of the circulation since trimethaphan is an extremely potent hypotensive agent. Adequate oxygenation must be assured throughout the treatment period, especially in regard to coronary and cerebral circulation. For surgical use, administration of trimethaphan should be stopped prior to wound closure in order to permit blood pressure to return to normal. A systolic pressure of 100 mm Hg will usually be attained within 10 minutes after stopping trimethaphan.

● *In Patients with these Concurrent Illnesses:*

Trimethaphan should be used with extreme caution in patients with arteriosclerosis, cardiac disease, hepatic or renal disease, degenerative disease of the central nervous system, Addison's disease, diabetes, and patients who are under treatment with steroids.

Use in Pregnancy

Induced hypotension may have harmful consequences upon the fetus.

Precautions

Trimethaphan should be used with care in patients who have been receiving antihypertensive drugs, since an additive hypotensive effect may occur. It should be used with caution in the following situations: (1) with anesthetic agents, especially spinal anesthetics which themselves may produce hypotension; (2) in the elderly or debilitated; (3) in children; and (4) in allergic individuals because trimethaphan liberates histamine. Concomitant therapy with other drugs can modify materially the dose of trimethaphan necessary to achieve the desired response.

Diuretic agents may enhance markedly the response evoked by ganglionic-blocking drugs. *Note: Pupillary dilation does not necessarily indicate anoxia or the depth of anesthesia, since trimethaphan appears to have a specific effect on the pupil.*

Some animal studies indicate that aggressive dosage administrations may result in respiratory arrest. Rare cases of respiratory arrest in humans have been reported although a casual relationship has not been established. It is recommended that the patient's respiratory status be monitored closely, particularly if large doses of trimethaphan are used.

Management of Overdosage or Exaggerated Response

Vasopressor agents may be used to correct undesirable low pressures during surgery or to effect a more rapid return to normotensive levels. Phenylephrine HC1 or mephentermine sulfate should be tried initially and norepinephrine should be reserved for refractory cases.

LABETALOL (Normodyne®)

Labetalol (see Chapter VII) is a new alpha-plus-beta-blocking agent available for both oral and intravenous administration. The latter preparation is being used more and more for the emergency treatment of hypertensive crisis.

Initially, infuse 20 mg over 2–4 minutes followed 20 minutes later by a 40 mg bolus, and subsequently by 80 mg boluses at 20-minute intervals until blood pressure is controlled. Oral labetalol regimens then provide satisfactory maintenance therapy (see Chapter VII).

Because labetalol has both alpha-blocking and beta-blocking activity, it does not cause significant increases in cardiac output. Some authorities prefer giving infusions of 20 mg/hour, then doubled doses each hour until results are satisfactory. Generally, these practices have produced neither significant side effects nor postural hypotension. It is best to give furosemide concurrently for its own diuretic action as well as the enhancement of the overall antihypertensive effect of labetalol. Because it has beta-blocking action, labetalol should not be used in patients with congestive heart failure, AV block greater than first degree or asthmatics.

REFERENCES:

1. Johnson, C. C.: The actions and toxicity of sodium nitroprusside. *Arch. Int. Pharmacodyn. Ther.*, **35**:480, 1929.
2. Medical News Report about F. M. Smith (University of Ottawa, Toronto, Canada) et al: Dosage of hypertensive agents may be too high. *JAMA*, **235**(15):1547, 1977.
3. Posner, M. A., et al: Nitroprusside-induced cyanide poisoning. *Anesthesiology*, **44**(4):330, 1976.
4. Davies, D. W., Kadar, D., et al: A sudden death associated with sodium nitroprusside in anesthesia. *Can. Anesth. Soc. J.*, **22**(5):547, 1975.
5. Palmer, R. F., and Lasseter, K. C.: Sodium nitroprusside. In Medical Intelligence, Drug Therapy. *N. Engl. J. Med.*, **292**(6):294, 1975.
6. Dranov, J., Skyler, J. S., Gunnells, J. C., and Durham, N. C.: Malignant hypertension. *Arch. Intern. Med.*, **133**:794, 1974.
7. Gifford, R. W.: Hypertensive emergencies and their treatment. *Med. Clin. N. Am.*, **45**:44, 1961.
8. Ahearn, D. J., and Grim, C. E.: Treatment of malignant hypertension with sodium nitroprusside. *Arch. Intern. Med.*, **133**:187, 1974.
9. Finnerty, I. A.: Hypertensive crises. *JAMA*, **229**:1479, 1974.
10. Koch-Weser, J.: Hypertensive emergencies. *N. Engl. J. Med.*, **290**:211, 1974.
11. Grenfell, R. G.: Treatment of hypertensive crises. *Chest*, **2**:212, 1971.
12. Cecace, L., and Thomas, T.: Treatment of hypertensive emergencies with sodium nitroprusside. *Drug Intl. Clin. Pharm.*, **4**:187, 1970.
13. Mani, M. K.: Nitroprusside revisited. *Br. Med. J.*, **3**:407, 1971.
14. Goodman, L. S., and Gilman, A.: *The Pharmacological Basis of Therapeutics*, 4th edition, Macmillan, New York, 1970, p. 487.
15. Vesey, C. J., et al: Some metabolic effects of sodium nitroprusside in man. *Br. Med. J.*, **2**:140, 1974.
16. Hammond, J. J.: Sodium nitroprusside today: A review of its clinical applications and a discussion of problems associated with its use. *Tex. Med.*, **74**:65–70, 1978.
17. Stempel, J. E., O'Grady, J. P., Morton, M. J., and Johnson, K. A.: Use of nitroprusside in complications of gestational hypertension. *Obstet. Gynecol.*, **60**(4):533–538, 1982.
18. Styles, M., et al: Some hemodynamic effects of sodium nitroprusside. *Anesthesia*, **38**:178, 1973.
19. Jones, F. O. M., and Cole, P.: Sodium nitroprusside as a hypotensive agent. *Br. J. Anesth.*, **40**:804, 1968.
20. Mueller, H., et al: Metabolic changes in ischemic myocardium by nitroprusside. *Am. J. Cardiol.*, **33**:158, 1974.
21. Wildsmith, J. A., et al: Hemodynamic effects of sodium nitroprusside during nitrous oxide/halothane anesthesia. *Br. J. Anesth.*, **45**:71, 1973.
22. Siegel, R., Moraca, P. P., and Green, J. R.: Sodium nitroprusside in surgical treatment of cerebral aneurysms and arteriovenous malformations. *Br. J. Anesth.*, **43**:790, 1971.
23. Taylor, T. H., Styles, M., and Lamming, A. J.: Sodium nitroprusside as a hypotensive agent in general anesthesia. *Br. J. Anesth.*, **42**:859, 1970.
24. Franciosa, J. A., and Silverstein, S. R.: Hemodynamic effects of nitroprusside and furosemide in left ventricular failure. *Clin. Pharmacol. Ther.*, **32**(1):62–69, 1982.

25. Cohn, J., and Franciosa, J.: Vasodilator therapy of cardiac failure. *N. Engl. J. Med.*, **297**(5):254, 1977.

26. Miller, R. R., et al: Clinical use of nitroprusside in refractory heart failure: Ventricular unloading by systemic arterial and venodilation. *Clin. Res.*, **22**:148A, 1974.

27. Rowe, G. G., and Henderson, R. H.: Systemic and coronary hemodynamic effects of sodium nitroprusside. *Am. Heart J.*, **87**:83, 1974.

28. Durrer, J. D., Lie, K. I., and van Capelle, F. J.: Treatment of acute myocardial infarction with sodium nitroprusside during 24 hours, followed by isosorbide dinitrate. *Acta Med. Scand.* (Suppl), **651**:163, 1980.

29. Durrer, J. D., Lie, K. I., van Capelle, F. J. L., and Durrer, D.: Effect of sodium nitroprusside on mortality in acute myocardial infarction. *N. Engl. J. Med.*, **306**(19):1121–1128, 1982.

30. Estafanous, F. G., Tarazi, R. C., Viljoen, J. F., and Tawil, M. Y.: Systemic hypertension following myocardial revascularization. *Am. Heart J.*, **85**(6):732–738, 1973.

31. Hoar, P. F., Hickey, R. F., and Ullzot, D. J.: Systemic hypertension following myocardial revascularization. *J. Thorac Cardiovasc. Surg.*, **71**:859–864, 1976.

32. Reves, J. G., Lell, W. A., McCracken, L. E., Kravetz, R. A., and Prough, D. S.: Comparison of morphine and ketamine anesthetic technics for coronary surgery: A randomized study. *South. Med. J.*, **71**(1):33–46, 1978.

33. Wallach, R., Karp, R. B., Reves, J. G., et al: Mechanism of hypertension after saphenous vein bypass surgery. (Abstract) *Circulation*, **3**:141, 1977.

34. Mitchell, R. R.: The need for closed-loop therapy. *Crit. Care Med.*, **10**(12):831–834, 1982.

35. Ciraulo, D., Lind, L., Salzman, C., Pilon, R., and Elkins, R.: Sodium nitroprusside treatment of ECT-induced blood pressure elevations. *Am. J. Psychiatry*, **135**(9):1105–1106, 1978.

36. Elberg, A. J., Gorman, H. M., Baker, R., and Strauss, J.: Use of sodium nitroprusside during kidney biopsy in a 9-year-old boy. *Clin. Nephrol.*, **14**(2):104–105, 1980.

37. Fowler, N. O., Gabel, M., and Holmes, J. C.: Hemodynamic effects of nitroprusside and hydralazine in experimental cardiac tamponade. *Circulation*, **57**(3):563–567, 1978.

38. Fowler, N. O.: Volume expansion and nitroprusside compared with pneucardiocentesis in acute cardiac tamponade. *N. Engl. J. Med.*, **308**(5):283, 1983.

39. Hammond, J. J., Kirkendall, W. M., and Calfee, R. V.: Hypertensive crisis managed by computer controlled infusion of sodium nitroprusside: A model for the closed loop administration of short acting vasoactive agents. *Comput. Biomed. Res.*, **12**:97–108, 1979.

40. Sheppard, L. C.: Computer control of the infusion of vasoactive drugs. *Ann. Biomed. Engr.*, **8**:431, 1980.

41. Ignarro, L. J., Lippton, H., et al: Mechanism of vascular smooth muscle relaxation by organic nitrates, nitrites, nitroprusside and nitric oxide: Evidence for the involvement of S-Nitrosothiols as active intermediates. *J. Pharmacol. Exp. Ther.*, **218**(3):739–749, 1981.

42. Gruetter, C. A., Gruetter, D. Y., Lyon, J. E., Kadowitz, P. J., and Ignarro, L. J.: Relationship between cyclic guanosine 3':5'-monophosphate formation and relaxation of coronary arterial smooth muscle by glyceryl trinitrate, nitroprusside, nitrite and nitric oxide: Effects of methylene blue and methemoglobin. *J. Pharmacol. Exp. Ther.*, **219**(1):181–186, 1981.

43. Chen, R. Y. Z., Fan, F., Schnessler, G. B., and Chien, S.: Baroreflex control of heart

rate in humans during nitroprusside-induced hypotension. *Am. J. Physiology*, **243**:R19–R24, 1982.

44. Chiba, S., Kozu, T. M., and Watanabe, H.: Analysis of cardiac actions of nitroprusside in intact dogs and in isolated atria. *Jpn. Heart J.*, **23**(4):613–621, 1982.

45. Schlant, R. C., Tsagaris, T. S., and Robertson, R. J.: Studies on the acute cardiovascular effects of intravenous sodium nitroprusside. *Am. J. Cardiol.*, **9**:51–59, 1962.

46. Macho, P., and Vatner, S. F.: Effects of nitroglycerin and nitroprusside on large and small coronary vessels in conscious dogs. *Circulation*, **64**(6):1101–1107, 1981.

47. Henribesen, L., Paulson, O. B., and Lauritzen, M.: The effects of sodium nitroprusside on cerebral blood flow and cerebral venous blood gases. *Eur. J. Clin. Invest.*, **12**:383–387, 1982.

48. Henrikson, L., and Paulson, O. B.: The effects of sodium nitroprusside on cerebral blood flow and cerebral venous blood gases. *Eur. J. Clin. Invest.*, **12**:389–393, 1982.

49. Cohen, I. M., Mottet, M. M., et al: Danger in nitroprusside therapy. *Ann. Intern. Med.*, **85**(2):205, 1976.

50. Berdoff, R. L., et al: Hazards in antihypertensive therapy. *Ann. Intern. Med.*, **86**(1):111, 1977.

51. Ivankovich, A. D., Miletich, D. J., and Tinker, J. H.: Sodium nitroprusside: Metabolism and general considerations. *Int. Anesthesiol. Clin.*, **16**(2):1–29, Summer 1978.

52. Chrysant, S. G., and Frohlich, E. D.: Side effects of antihypertensive drugs. *Am. Fam. Physician*, **9**(1):99, 1974.

53. Page, T. H., et al: Cardiovascular action of nitroprusside in animals and hypertensive patients. *Circulation*, **11**:188, 1955.

54. Lazarus, A., Barlow, P., and Norman, G.: Fatal doses of poisoning with sodium nitroprusside. *Br. Med. J.*, **2**:407, 1941.

55. Kim, Y. H., Foo, M., and Terry, R. D.: Cyanide encephalapathy following therapy with sodium nitroprusside. *Arch. Pathol. Lab. Med.*, **106**:392–393, 1982.

56. Cottrell, J. E., Potel, K., et al: Intracranial pressure changes induced by sodium nitroprusside in patients with intracranial mass lesions. *J. Neurosurg.*, **48**:329, 1978.

57. Tuzel, I., Limjuco, R., et al: Sodium nitroprusside in hypertensive emergencies. *Curr. Ther. Res.*, **17**(1):95, 1975.

58. Koch-Weser, J.: Drug therapy: Diazoxide. *N. Engl. J. Med.*, **294**(23):1271, 1976.

59. Nayler, W. G., McInnes, I., Swann, J. B., et al: Some effects of the hypotensive drug diazoxide on the cardiovascular system. *Am. Heart J.*, **75**:223, 1968.

60. Hamby, W. M., Jankowski, G. J., Pouget, J. M., et al: Intravenous use of diazoxide in treatment of severe hypertension. *Circulation*, **37**:169, 1968.

61. Mroczek, W. G., Leibel, B. A., Davidov, M., and Finnerty, F. A.: The importance of rapid intravenous administration of diazoxide in accelerated hypertension. *N. Engl. J. Med.*, **285**(11):603, 1971.

62. Koch-Weser, J.: Vasodilator drugs in the treatment of hypertension. *Arch. Intern. Med.*, **133**:1017, 1974.

63. Drug Commentary, Dept. of Drugs: Evaluation of diazoxide (Hyperstat IV). *JAMA*, **224**(10):1422, 1973.

64. Curry, C. L., and Hosten, A. O.: Current treatment of malignant hypertension. *JAMA*, **232**(13):1367, 1975.

65. Page, L. B., and Sidd, J. J.: Primary hypertension. *N. Engl. J. Med.*, **287**(21):1077, 1972.

66. Pennington, J. C., and Picker, R. H.: Diazoxide in the treatment of the acute hypertensive emergency in obstetrics. *Med. J. Aust.*, **2**:1051, 1972.

67. Michael, C. A.: The control of hypertension in labour. *Aust. N. Z. J. Obstet. Gynaec.*, **12:**48–54, 1972.
68. Milsap, R. L., and Auld, P. A. M.: Neonatal hyperglycemia following maternal diazoxide administration. *JAMA*, **243**(2):144–145, 1980.
69. Pohl, J. E. F., and Thurston, H.: Use of diazoxide in hypertension with renal failure. *Br. Med. J.*, **4:**142, 1971.
70. Mroczek, W. J., Davidov, M., Gavrilovich, L., and Finnerty, F.: The value of aggressive therapy in the hypertensive patient with azotemia. *Circulation*, **40:**893, 1969.
71. Hutcheon, D. E., and Barthalmus, K. S.: Antihypertensive action of diazoxide: A new benzothiadiazine with antidiuretic properties. *Br. Med. J.*, **2:**159, 1962.
72. Okun, R., Russell, R. P., and Wilson, W. R.: Use of diazoxide with trichlormethiazide for hypertension. *Arch. Intern. Med.*, **112:**882, 1963.
73. Langford, H. G., and Bonar, J. R.: Treatment of the uremic hypertensive patient. In G. W. Pickering, W. I. Cranston, and M. A. Pears (Eds.): *Treatment of Hypertension,* (No. 434, American Lectures in Living Chemistry), Charles C. Thomas, Springfield, Illinois, 1961, p. 68.
74. Pickering, G.: Reversibility of malignant hypertension: Follow-up of three cases. *Lancet*, **1:**413, 1971.
75. Woods, J. W., Blythe, W. B., and Huffines, W. D.: Malignant hypertension and renal insufficiency. *N. Engl. J. Med.*, **291:**10, 1974.
76. Finnerty, F. A., Jr., Kakaviatos, N., Tuckman, J., et al: Clinical evaluation of diazoxide: A new treatment for acute hypertension. *Circulation*, **28:**203, 1963.
77. Beamer, V. L., and McDonald, R. I. I., Jr.: Failure of repeated diazoxide injections to modify the course of severe hypertension. *Am. Heart J.*, **79**(6):742, 1970.
78. Velasco, M., Gallardo, E., et al: A new technique for safe and effective control of hypertension with intravenous diazoxide. *Curr. Ther. Res.*, **19**(2):185, 1976.
79. Ram, C. V. S., and Kaplan, N. M.: Individual titration of diazoxide dosage in the treatment of severe hypertension. *Am. J. Cardiol.*, **43:**627, 1979.
80. Wilson, D. J.: Lewis, R. C., and Vidt, D. G.: Control of severe hypertension with pulse diazoxide. *Cardiovasc. Clin.*, **12**(2):79–91, 1982.
81. Crout, J. R., Andreasen, F. V. V., Parks, R. I., and Heimbach, D. M.: Intravenous diazoxide in hypertension. *Clin. Res.*, **18:**337, 1970.
82. Kumar, G. K., Dastoor, F. C., Rabayo, J. R., and Razzaque, M. A.: Side effects of diazoxide. *JAMA*, **235**(3):275, 1976.
83. Kanada, S. A., Kanada, D. J., Hutchinson, R. A., and Wu, D.: Angina-like syndrome with diazoxide therapy for hypertensive crisis. *Ann. Intern. Med.*, **84**(6):696, 1976.
84. Ledingham, J. G. G., and Rajagoplan, B.: Cerebral complications in the treatment of accelerated hypertension. *Q. J. Med.*, **48**(189):25–41, 1979.
85. Lockwood, C. H., Nicholls, D. M., Troop, V. L., et al: Diazoxide therapy in hypertension. *Am. J. Med. Sci.*, **246:**312, 1963.
86. Fang, P., MacDonald, I., Laver, M., Hua, A., and Kincaid-Smith, P.: Oral diazoxide in uncontrolled malignant hypertension. *Med. J. Aust.*, **2:**621, 1974.
87. Honey, M., Cotler, L., Davies, N., and Denison, D.: Clinical and haemodynamic effects of diazoxide in primary pulmonary hypertension. *Thorax*, **35:**269–276, 1980.
88. Klinke, W. P., and Bilbert, J. A. L.: Diazoxide in primary pulmonary hypertension. *N. Engl. J. Med.*, **302**(2):91–92, 1980.
89. Hall, D. R., and Petch, M. C.: Remission of primary pulmonary hypertension during treatment with diazoxide. *Br. Med. J.*, **282:**1118, 1981.
90. Garett, N. G., and Kaplan, N. M.: Efficacy of slow infusion of diazoxide in the

treatment of severe hypertension without organ hypoperfusion. *Am. Heart J.*, **103**(3):390–394, 1982.

91. Huysmans, F. T. M., Thien, T., and Koene, R. A.: Acute treatment of hypertension with slow infusion of diazoxide. *Arch. Intern. Med.*, **143**:882–884, 1983.

92. Johnson, B. F., and Kapur, M.: The influence of rate of injection upon the effects of diazoxide. *Am. J. Med. Sci.*, **263**(6):481–488, 1972.

93. Ogilvie, R. I., Nadeau, J. H., and Sitar, D. S.: Diazoxide concentration response relation in hypertension. *Hypertension*, **4**(1):167–173, 1982.

94. Jellet, L. B., Dye, M. S., Michelakis, A. M., and Oates, J. A.: Individual titration of intravenous diazoxide therapy in patients with severe hypertension (abstr). *Clin. Exp. Pharmacol. Physiol.*, **2**:423, 1975.

95. Pearson, R. M., and Breckenridge, A. M.: Renal function, protein binding and pharmacological response to diazoxide. *Br. J. Clin. Pharmacol.*, **3**:169–175, 1976.

96. Bahlman, J., Brod, J., and Cachovan, M.: Effect of diazoxide on capacitance vessels. *Eur. J. Clin. Pharmacol.*, **13**:321–323, 1978.

97. Thirwell, M. P., and Zsoter, T. T.: The effect of diazoxide on the veins. *Am. Heart J.*, **83**(4):512–517, 1972.

98. Koch-Weser, J.: Myocardial inactivity of therapeutic concentrations of hydralazine and diazoxide. *Experientia*, **30**(2):170–171, 1974.

99. Moser, M.: Diazoxide—an effective vasodilator in accelerated hypertension. *Am. Heart J.*, **87**(6):791, 1974.

100. Vidt, D. G.: Diazoxide for hypertensive crisis. *Am. Fam. Physician*, **11**(5):128, 1975.

101. Finnerty, F. A.: Hypertensive encephalopathy. *Am. J. Med.*, **52**:672, 1972.

102. Koch-Weser, J.: The vasodilator antihypertensives. *Drug Ther.*, **5**:74, 1975.

103. Nussar, D. A., and Wang, R. I. H.: Review of recently introduced drugs. *Drug Ther.*, **4**(6):69, 1974.

104. Baer, L., Goodwin, F. J., and Laragh, J. D.: Diazoxide-induced renin release in man: Dissociation from plasma and extracellular fluid volume changes. *J. Clin. Endocrinol. Metab.*, **29**:1107, 1969.

105. Powell, J. W., Green, R. M., Whiting, R. B., and Sanders, C. A.: Action of diazoxide on skeletal muscle vascular resistance. *Clin. Res.*, **28**:167–178, 1971.

106. Landesman, R., Coutinho, E. M., Wilson, K. H., and Lopes, A. C. V.: The relaxant effect of diazoxide on nongravid human myometrium in vivo. *Am. J. Obst. Gynecol.*, **102**(8):1080, 1968.

107. Sellers, E. M., and Koch-Weser, J.: Protein binding and vascular activity of diazoxide. *N. Engl. J. Med.*, **281**:1141, 1969.

108. Wohl, A. J., Hausler, L. M., and Franklin, E. R.: Studies on the mechanism of antihypertensive action of diazoxide: In vitro vascular pharmacodynamics. *J. Pharmacol. Exp. Ther.*, **158**(3):531–539, 1967.

109. Huysmans, F. T. M., Thien, T. A., and Koene, R. A. P.: Combined intravenous administration of diazoxide and beta-blocking agent in acute treatment of severe hypertension or hypertensive crisis. *Am. Heart J.*, **103**(3):395–400, 1982.

110. Mroczek, W. J., Lee, W. R., Davidov, M. E., and Finnerty, F. A.: Vasodilator administration in the presence of beta-adrenergic blockade. *Circulation*, **53**(6):985–988, 1976.

111. Nanster, P. D.: *Drug Interactions*. Lea and Febiger, Philadelphia, 1975, p 72.

112. Hemrich, W. L., Cronin, R., Miller, P. D., and Anderson, R. J.: Hypertensive sequelae of diazoxide and hydralazine. *JAMA*, **237**(3):264, 1977.

113. Davey, M., Moodley, J., and Soutler, P.: Adverse effects of a combination of diazoxide and hydralazine therapy. *S. Afr. Med. J.*, **59**:496–497, 1981.
114. Henrich, W. L., Cronin, R., Miller, P. D., and Anderson, R. J.: Hypotensive sequelae of diazoxide and hydralazine therapy. *JAMA*, **237**(3):264–265, 1977.
115. Roe, T. F., Podosin, R. L., and Blaskovics, M. E.: Drug interaction: Diazoxide and diphenylhydantoin. *J. Pediatr.*, **87**:480, 1975.
116. Aynsley-Green, A., and Illig, R.: Enhancement by chlorpromazine of hyperglycemic action of diazoxide. *Lancet*, **2**(7936):658–659, 1975.
117. Paulissian, R.: Diazoxide. *Int. Anesthesiol. Clin.*, **16**(2):201–237, (Summer) 1978.
118. Mroczek, W. J., and Lee, W. R.: Diazoxide therapy: Use and risks (Comment). *Ann. Intern. Med.*, **85**(4):529, 1976.
119. Rosove, M. H.: Diazoxide and myocardial ischemia (Comment). *Ann. Intern. Med.*, **85**(3):395, 1976.
120. *Medical Letter:* Diazoxide (Hyperstat). **15**:13 (Issue 377), 1973.
121. Danforth, E., Jr.: Hyperglycemia after diazoxide. (Letter to the Editor) *N. Engl. J. Med.*, **285**(26):1487, 1971.
122. Updike, S. J., and Harrington, A. R.: Acute diabetic ketoacidosis—a complication of intravenous diazoxide treatment for refractory hypertension. *N. Engl. J. Med.*, **280**(14):768, 1969.
123. Charles, M. A., and Danforth, E., Jr.: Nonketoacidotic hyperglycemia and coma during intravenous diazoxide therapy in uremia. *Diabetes*, **20**:501, 1971.
124. MacLean, A. B., Doig, J. R., Chatfield, W. R., and Aickin, D. R.: Small dose diazoxide administration in pregnancy. *Aust. N. Z. J. Obstet. Gynaec.*, **21**:7–10, 1981.
125. Newman, J., Weiss, B., Rabello, Y., Cabal, L., and Freeman, R. K.: Diazoxide for the acute control of severe hypertension complicating pregnancy: A pilot study. *Obstet. Gynecol.*, **53**(3)Suppl:50–55, 1979.
126. Editorial: Use of diazoxide for hypertensive disorders of pregnancy. *Am. J. Obstet. Gynecol.*, **129**(2):234–236, 1977.
127. Morris, J. A., Arce, J. J., et al: The management of severe preeclampsia and eclampsia with intravenous diazoxide. *Obstet. Gynecol.*, **49**(6):675–680, 1977.
128. Redmann, C. W. G.: Treatment of hypertension in pregnancy. *Kidney Int.*, **18**:267–278, 1980.
129. Pohl, J. E. F., Thurston, H., Davis, D., and Morgan, M. Y.: Successful use of oral diazoxide in the treatment of severe toxemia of pregnancy. *Br. Med. J.*, **2**:586, 1972.
130. Boulos, B. M., Davis, L. E., Almond, C. H., et al: Placental transfer of diazoxide and its hazardous effect on the newborn. *J. Clin. Pharmacol.*, **11**:206, 1971.
131. Barr, P. A., and Gallery, E. D. M.: Effect of diazoxide on the antepartum cardiotocograph in severe pregnancy-associated hypertension. *Aust. N. Z. J. Obstet. Gynaec.*, **21**:11–15, 1981.
132. Gilman, A. G., Goodman, L. S., and Gilman, A.: *The Pharmacological Basis of Therapeutics,* Macmillan, 6th Ed., 1980, p. 802.
133. Dayton, P. G., Pruitt, A. W., Faraj, B. A., and Israili, Z. H.: Metabolism and disposition of diazoxide. (A mini-review) *Drug Metab. Dispos.*, **3**(3):226, 1975.
134. Pruitt, A. W., Faraj, B. A., and Dayton, P. G.: Metabolism of diazoxide in man and experimental animals. *J. Pharmacol. Exp. Ther.*, **188**:248, 1974.
135. O'Malley, K., Velasco, M., Pruitt, A., et al: Decreased plasma protein binding of diazoxide in uremia. *Clin. Pharmacol. Ther.*, **18**:53, 1975.

136. Miller, W. E., Gifford, R. W., Humphrey, D. C., and Vidt, D. G.: Management of severe hypertension with intravenous injections of diazoxide. *Am. J. Cardiol.*, **24**:870, 1969.

137. Tansey, W. A., Williams, E. G., Kanderman, R. H., et al: Diazoxide. *JAMA*, **225**:749, 1973.

138. Finnerty, F. A., Jr.: Hypertensive emergencies. *Am. J. Cardiol.*, **17**:652, 1966.

139. Saker, B. M., Mathew, T. H., Eremin, J., and Kincaid-Smith, P.: Diazoxide in the treatment of acute hypertensive emergency. *Med. J. Aust.*, **1**:592–593, 1968.

140. Food and Drug Administration, Medical Officer's Summary of NDA 16-996 (Sponsor: Schering Corp.) 1–6, 1972.

141. Cove, D. H., Seddon, M., Fletcher, R. F., and Dukes, D. C.: Blindness after treatment for malignant hypertension. *Br. Med. J.*, **2**:245, 1979.

142. Finnerty, F. A., Jr., Davidov, M., and Kakaviatos, N.: Hypertensive vascular disease: The long-term effect of rapid repeated reductions of arterial pressure with diazoxide. *Am. J. Cardiol.*, **19**:377, 1967.

143. Goldberg, H. J., Cadario, R. A., Banka, R. S., and Reivich, M.: Patterns of cerebral dysautoregulation in severe hypertension to blood pressure reduction with diazoxide. *Acta Neurol. Scand.* (Suppl), **56**(64):64–65, 1977.

144. Johnson, B. F.: Diazoxide and renal function in man. *Clin. Pharmacol. Ther.*, **12**:815, 1971.

145. Robb, G. H.: A fatal reaction to diazoxide. *Postgrad. Med. J.*, **45**:43, 1969.

146. Today's Drugs: Diazoxide. *Br. Med. J.*, **4**:417, 1972.

147. Coutinho, E. M.: The effect of magnesium on the staircase phenomenon of the rat uterus. *Acta Physiol. Lat. Am.*, **16**:318, 1966.

148. Finnerty, F. A., Jr.: Hypertension in pregnancy. *Clin. Obstet. Gynecol.*, **18**(3):145, 1975.

149. Best, R. A., and Clink, H. M.: Haemolysis associated with diazoxide, used for the control of hypertension. *Postgrad Med. J.*, **51**:402, 1975.

150. Combs, J. J., Grunt, J. A., and Brandt, I. K.: Hematological reactions to diazoxide. *Pediatrics*, **40**:90, 1967.

151. Wales, J. K., and Wolff, F.: Hematological side effects of diazoxide. *Lancet*, **1**:53, 1967.

152. Ehrlich, R. M.: Hypoglycemia in infancy and childhood. *Arch. Dis. Child.*, **46**:716, 1971.

153. Milner, R. D. G., and Chouksey, S. K.: Effects of fetal exposure to diazoxide in man. *Arch. Dis. Child.*, **47**:537, 1972.

154. Neary, D., Thurston, H., and Pohl, J. E. F.: Development of extra-pyramidal symptoms in hypertensive patients treated with diazoxide. *Br. Med. J.*, **3**:474, 1973.

CHAPTER XIV

NEW DRUGS

INTRODUCTION

> Perhaps within the next few decades, the genetic factors
> which predispose so many of us to develop essential
> hypertension will be identified on a biochemical
> level, and with appropriate genetic-splicing,
> the disease will be preventable.

Because hypertension is mankind's most common serious illness, new pharmacological agents continue to appear. Perhaps within the next few decades, the genetic factors which predispose so many of us to develop essential hypertension will be identified on a biochemical level, and with appropriate genetic-splicing, the disease will be preventable. Until then, we must continue to use the present agents we have and the new ones that are being developed. Indeed they are saving lives and reducing morbidity, specifically because they are effective. We can now successfully lower blood pressure in virtually everyone. However, there are always side effects associated with drug therapy. Although patients must be willing to accept some side effects for the benefits received, the search continues, and we must continue to find agents with better benefit:risk ratios. Often, what initially appears to be a "me-too" drug may, with clinical experience, develop into a drug of choice for various subpopulations of hypertensive patients. We have attempted to provide a brief description of same of these newer agents, as listed in Table I.

TABLE I
NEW ANTIHYPERTENSIVE DRUGS

Alpha-adrenergic agonists
  Catapres-TTS®
  Guanfacine
  Urapidil
  Tiamenidine
Alpha-adrenergic blockers
  Indoramin (Baratol®)
  Tiodazosin
Beta-adrenergic blockers
  Betaxolol
  Sotalol (Beta-Cardone®, Sotacor®)
  Oxprenolol (Trasicor®)
  Pronethalol
  Alprenolol
  Bevantolol HCl

Calcium channel blockers
  Nitrendipine
  Nicardipine
Diuretics
  Indacrinone (MK-196)
  Piretanide (Arlix®)
  Muzolimine (Edrul®)
Serotonin Antagonist
  Ketanserin
Vasodilators
  Guancydine
  Pinacidil

ALPHA-ADRENERGIC AGONISTS

CATAPRES TRANSDERMAL THERAPEUTIC SYSTEM®

Good patient compliance is one of the most difficult problems in the management of hypertension. In an effort to ease this problem, Catapres-TTS®, a new delivery system based on the most advanced physical-chemical and biopharmaceutic technology, has been developed. This consists of minute microcrystals of clonidine embedded in a Band-Aid-like four-layer patch adhering well to the skin. From this patch, clonidine is released in fixed amounts and absorbed through the skin at a rate yielding constant plasma levels. When a single patch is applied once a week to a hairless area of the upper chest or arms, blood levels equivalent to those provided by an oral dose of 0.1 mg/day are obtained. Therapeutic plasma clonidine levels are reached 48–72 hours after application. After the seventh day, plasma levels gradually fall over a period of 24–48 hours, avoiding any possible side effects of an abrupt cessation of treatment.

Catapres-TTS® patches will be available in three sizes: 3.5, 7.0, and 10.5 cm², which contain sufficient clonidine to deliver 0.1, 0.2, and 0.3 mg/day, respectively, for one week. The patches are designed not to separate from the skin with bathing or perspiring. The patient is relieved of the worry over whether he has remembered to take his pill in the morning or at night. Patches are removed and new ones applied to a different area of the skin at seven-day intervals.

Weber et al[1] have reported results of a five-center study in which 85 patients with diastolic pressures of 90–105 mg Hg were treated with one to three 3.5 cm² (0.1 mg/day) TTS patches. During a three-month stable-dose treatment period the patients removed and reapplied their own patches at weekly intervals and were examined monthly at their respective clinics. Seventy-six patients completed this course. Mean blood pressures declined from 147/97 to 137/87 mm Hg. Two-thirds of the patients (54) had excellent responses, reaching diastolic pressures below 90 mm Hg. These results were obtained with a single TTS disc in 17 patients, while 27 patients required two discs and 10 needed three. Males responded somewhat better than females to the lowest dose, as did white compared with black patients, and also older as compared with younger patients. The antihypertensive effect of clonidine persisted for the full three months. Cholesterol, triglyceride and HDL-cholesterol levels were not significantly changed. Mild drowsiness occurred in 16% and dry mouth in 31% of the patients, which means that the incidence of these side effects was approximately half that which has been reported with oral clonidine. They also were milder than the reactions to oral clonidine. During chronic therapy many patients experienced episodes of mild pruritis or localized erythema, associated with week-long skin occlusion. These reactions generally resolved within 24 hours of removal of the system, and placement of a new system on a different area of skin. Five of 85 patients (6%) had significant skin reactions secondary to allergic contact sensitization which required discontinuation of therapy. After removal of the last patch, the blood level of clonidine declined over a period of three to four days. No hypertension or rebound symptoms were noted.

That this new method of clonidine administration was found to be convenient and well accepted by nearly all the patients in this study and comparable in efficacy to the conventional oral treatment has been confirmed by other studies published in this country and abroad.[2-4]

GUANFACINE

Guanfacine is an effective new antihypertensive agent which has a mechanism of action similar to clonidine. A guanidine derivative, guanfacine lowers blood pressure by stimulating central alpha-2-adrenergic receptors. Its hypotensive effect is associated with a fall in peripheral vascular resistance, heart rate, and cardiac output.[1] Guanfacine is usually administered with a diuretic.

Clinical studies in man have shown guanfacine to be effective at doses ranging from 0.5 to 6 mg daily, with the initial dose being 1 mg/day given at bedtime. In a two-year follow-up study with 11 patients, Titschen showed guanfacine to be effective and well tolerated, reducing blood pressure 28/20 mm Hg.[2] Zamboulis and Reid found a significant decline in blood pressure (42/24 mm Hg) and heart rate (12 bpm) with single doses of 2–4 mg daily.[3] Jerie and Tasence demonstrated guanfacine's long duration of action with low dose monotherapy, a mean of 2.2 mg daily, resulting in 75% normotension among 36 patients.[4] In a multi-investigator study coordinated by Hutcherson, 1.0 mg of guanfacine administered once daily with a diuretic reduced the mean blood pressure in 60 patients by 13/13 mm Hg.[5] In comparative studies with clonidine and methyldopa, guanfacine has been reported as equal in efficacy and well tolerated.[6-9] The most common side effects are dry mouth, somnolence, dizziness and asthenia.[1,4,6,10,11] Other adverse reactions reported are constipation, orthostatic symptoms, sexual dysfunction, insomnia, and sweating. Few adverse reactions appear with doses of 2 mg or less.

Nami et al[12] compared clonidine 0.15 mg three times daily with guanfacine 0.5 mg once daily in an open label study with ten patients in each group. They found equal antihypertensive effects but more side effects with clonidine (likely related to the large doses employed). Urinary norepinephrine levels returned to baseline within two days of abrupt clonidine cessation, compared with a more gradual return in 4–5 days after guanfacine. Headache, palpitations and sweating were more frequent after discontinuation of clonidine, but unfortunately, the study was not blinded.

Guanfacine appears to be a safe and effective addition to the class of centrally-acting alpha-agonist drugs. Further experience will be needed to discuss any unique advantages over other members of this group.

URAPIDIL

Urapidil is a new antihypertensive agent discovered and developed in Germany. It has both alpha-2 agonist activity in the central nervous system and peripherally (like clonidine), but also postganglionic alpha-1 antagonist action. It reduces peripheral vascular resistance and reduces blood pressure with 30 mg doses orally without appreciable change in heart rate. As with other alpha-blocking agents, postural hypotension and dizziness may occur. Doses used in Europe ranged from 30 to 120 mg/day given in divided daily doses. Efficacy data from abroad show an 88.2% "moderate to good" response. Side effects include dizziness (3.7%), nausea (1.4%), fatigue (1.4%), headache (1.1%), dyspepsia (0.7%), orthostasis (0.5%), and drowsiness (0.5%).

TIAMENIDINE

Tiamenidine is a central alpha-2 agonist with antihypertensive activity like clonidine. It is rapidly and well absorbed with peak plasma levels occurring between 0.5 and 2.2 hours, and a plasma half-life of 4 hours. It is excreted essentially unchanged in the urine. The dose range is 0.25 to 1.5 mg twice daily. Rebound hypertension, after abrupt cessation of therapy, appears to be more frequent than with other agents. Dry mouth and drowsiness also appear to be significant side effects.

ALPHA-ADRENERGIC BLOCKERS

INDORAMIN (Baratol®)

INTRODUCTION

Indoramin is a new antihypertensive agent with a peripheral vasodilator effect due to a selective post-synaptic alpha-1 adrenoceptor antagonistic function. Indoramin has been advocated for the treatment of mild and moderate essential hypertension. The use of classical alpha-adrenoceptor blockers such as phentolamine and phenoxybenzamine has been advocated for the treatment of hypertension.[1] However, due to the severity of its associated side effects, the most important of which are postural hypotension[2,3] and reflex tachycardia, alpha-blockade has not gained widespread acceptance. Indoramin is an alpha-blocker that counteracts and prevents these reflex responses.[4-14]

Significant decreases in blood pressure with indoramin administration have been reported in all species studied.[15-17] Long-term studies of indoramin in hypertensive patients have demonstrated clinically important falls in blood pressure without any increase in heart rate.[18-24] Clinical trials by Gould et al[25] demonstrated that after six weeks of treatment of hypertensive patients with twice daily indoramin administration, significant reductions in blood pressure were obtained throughout 24-hour periods of intra-arterial ambulatory blood pressure monitoring. Reductions were also seen in the early morning phase of rising blood pressure just prior to awakening.

Indications for Indoramin

Indoramin is indicated for the control of mild and moderate essential hypertension. There are no contraindications for the use of indoramin as sole therapy, although it is too early to define the true place of indoramin in the management of hypertension. To date, indoramin has been useful as a Step-2 drug.[15] Indoramin may be indicated for use, in combination with a diuretic, in patients in whom beta-receptor blocking drugs are contraindicated because of increased airway resistance, heart failure, or concurrent vasospastic conditions. In other patients who have not responded satisfactorily to a beta-blocker plus a diuretic, indoramin may play a valuable role as a third-line treatment. In the management of severe hypertension, indoramin is indicated as an alternative to other alpha-blockers or labetalol[26] in therapeutic regimens including combined alpha- and beta-blockade.[27] Indoramin is also indicated in patients with mild hypertension in whom other antihypertensives are contraindicated because of asthma or interactions with tricyclic antidepressant drugs.[28] Therapy for hypertension requires that the conditions of each patient be carefully monitored and examined. A reassessment of treatment may be necessary as those conditions will undoubtedly fluctuate.

Formulation

Tablets .... 25 mg

Dose in Hypertension

Frequency: usually twice daily in the first 48 hours, increasing by 25 mg increments at not less than two-week intervals to a maximum of 75–100 mg/day. *

Initial: 25 mg twice daily

Range: 25–100 mg/day

Usual dose: 25–50 mg twice daily

Mechanism of Action

As already mentioned, alpha-blockade is believed to play a major role in controlling essential hypertension. The bis-indoles have been shown to exert an alpha-blocking action.[29] Indoramin is synthesized[4] when a benzamido group is substituted for one indolyl-ethyl group of the bis-indole. Thus indoramin exerts not only its alpha-blocking action with a bis-indole backbone, but also a myocardial-stabilizing action with the incorporation of a benzamido moiety.

Blood pressure response after indoramin administration is in contrast to the effects of conventional alpha-adrenoceptor blockade. As mentioned, postural hypotension and reflex tachycardia are serious drawbacks when administering phentolamine and phenoxybenzamine. The incidence of postural hypotension with indoramin is minimal.[30] This is attributed to the selective alpha-1-adrenoceptor blockade leaving the alpha-2-adrenoceptors open to stimulation.

The increase in heart rate and the relative ineffectiveness in lowering blood pressure when using the classical alpha-blockers are attributed to their unselectivity at the pre- and post-synaptic sites. These unselective alpha-blockers interfere with the negative feedback control of noradrenaline release leaving the post-synaptic beta-receptors in the heart and the alpha-receptors in the blood vessels open to greater sympathetic stimulation. By preserving the alpha-2 mediated pre-synaptic feedback loop, indoramin prevents excessive noradrenaline release into the synaptic cleft thereby inhibiting the excess sympathetic activity. In this manner, indoramin resembles another antihypertensive—prazosin.[31]

Indoramin appears to exert an apparently greater activity in resistance than in capacitance vessels.[32] This helps explain the absence of a reflex tachycardia, yet alternative explanations have been proposed.

* This regimen has been shown to provide satisfactory 24-hour control of blood pressure.[25]

The resemblance of indoramin to procainamide,[33] a potent myocardial membrane stabilizing agent, may explain the local anesthetic properties[34-36] on the conducting system of the heart. Evidence exists to show that there is a significant decrease in the rate of depolarization with indoramin in canine myocardial strips.[35] This *in vivo* evidence of a direct effect on the heart supports the results in isolated tissues.[37]

Drug Interactions

There have been relatively few reports to date with indoramin in combination with other drugs in the treatment of hypertension. One study[38] indicated that indoramin in combination with a thiazide diuretic reduced diastolic blood pressure an average of 20 mm Hg in 76% of 199 patients treated. In combination with the thiazide diuretic, the dose of indoramin was lowered from 125 mg/day to 75 mg/day. The decreased dose of indoramin when used with a diuretic should presumably decrease the occurrence of unwanted side effects.[23,25,27,39,40]

The effects of indomethacin on the reduced efficacy of diuretics and beta-blocking drugs[41] have yet to be examined with indoramin. Gaddie et al[42] have reported that intravenous indoramin administration to asthmatic hypertensive patients, in combination with aerosol salbutamol, increased FEV_1 (forced expiratory one-second volume) and FVC (forced vital capacity), the indoramin-salbutamol values being greater than salbutamol alone.

In a long-term clinical study of indoramin administered alone and in combination with a thiazide diuretic, the addition of propranolol to the regimen was efficacious in producing the desired antihypertensive effects in those patients failing to respond to an indoramin-diuretic combination therapy.[43] The results of this study are summarized in Table II.

The hypotensive effects of adrenergic blocking agents can be antagonized by drugs that inhibit monamine uptake at the synaptic site. It appears that these drugs do not interfere with the action of indoramin.[25]

Contraindications

Renal failure is a contraindication to the use of indoramin.[23] Blood urea estimates and urine analysis should be performed frequently when indoramin is administered to hypertensive patients. Caution is also urged before presenting indoramin to patients with a history of depressive illness.[44]

TABLE II
PATIENTS COMPLETING 12 MONTHS OF TREATMENT
ON INDORAMIN, DIURETIC AND PROPRANOLOL (N = 29)

Treatment	Mean Supine Blood Pressure (+/−s.d.) (mm Hg)	
	Systolic	Diastolic
Pre-treatment	186.9+/−8.1	118.8+/−5.5
Indoramin alone for 6 weeks	173.9+/−16.3	110.5+/−9.5†
Indoramin and a diuretic at week 10	172.6+/−18.2**	107.1+/−9.8††
Indoramin, diuretic and propranolol at 12 months	142.8+/−15***	85.5+/−13.2†††

  * P < 0.002 compared with pre-treatment value.
  ** NS compared with indoramin alone.
  *** P < 0.00001 compared with indoramin and diuretic.
  † P < 0.001 compared with pre-treatment value.
  †† P < 0.02 compared with indoramin alone.
  ††† P < 0.00001 compared with indoramin and diuretic.

Use in Pregnancy

The effects of indoramin are unknown in the management of hypertension in pregnant women. It may be that indoramin crosses the placental barrier and appears in cord blood. Although no effects of indoramin during pregnancy have been reported, the possibility of fetal injury cannot be excluded.

Management of Overdosage

To date, only one fatal case of self-poisoning with indoramin has been reported.[40] Toxicology reports at admission confirmed an indoramin plasma level to be 50–200 times greater than therapeutic values (plasma indoramin concentration after an oral dose of 100 mg is 0.03–0.12 mg/L). Complicating the deep sedative effects of the high indoramin concentrations was the fact that the patient had consumed a large volume of alcohol (plasma ethanol concentration was 225 mg/dl). The patient had a previous history of moduretic and ethanol overdose and self-mutilation of her wrist. Along with the deep sedation, the main clinical features were respiratory depression, hypotension and convulsions. The depressed state of the central nervous system was resistant to treatment and proved fatal.

Although untried, intravenous administration of alpha-adrenoceptor agonists may prove beneficial in counteracting the effect of high plasma concentrations of indoramin self-poisoning. Prompt treatment of indoramin overdose should include a gastric lavage, diazepam for convulsions and circulatory support to control the induced hypotensive state.[44] Exaggerated responses to indoramin may be alleviated by a reduction in dosage which may lead to disappearance of the side effects without any appreciable reduction in blood pressure control.

Absorption, Metabolism, Excretion

Indoramin is a lipid soluble drug which is readily absorbed from the gastrointestinal tract after oral administration and is almost completely metabolized.[45] It is likewise readily absorbed from parenteral sites of injection. Peak plasma levels of both indoramin and its metabolites occur one to two hours after dosage, with the maximal lowering of blood pressure occurring at this time.[45] These studies also show that less than four percent of an oral dose of $[^{14}C]$-labeled indoramin is recovered unchanged in the feces as is less than two percent of the radioactivity detected in the urine.

Kinetic studies in intravenous indoramin administration indicate a high apparent volume of distribution and a mean clearance of 1.43 L/min,[45] which is of the same order as liver blood flow. These studies confirm that there exists a high first-pass hepatic metabolism for indoramin, similar to that described for propranolol.[46]

The indoramin–metabolite concentration in the plasma exceeds that of the parent drug by tenfold and is the most significant consequence of the hepatic first-pass effect for indoramin. (The range of plasma–indoramin concentration following a 60 mg oral dose is 13–45 ng/ml one hour after administration, while that of the plasma-metabolites is 200–300 ng/ml.) However, no distinction can be made between the pharmacological activity of indoramin and its metabolites because of the near parallel relationship exhibited by the two following oral dosage.

Several investigators report that there are no drug-related effects on biochemical or hematologic values when using indoramin to treat hypertension.[18,20-23] There are also no reported urinalysis abnormalities in patients taking indoramin.[22]

Precautions and Adverse Reactions

Marked orthostatic hypotension and syncope have been reported to occur at the onset of treatment with prazosin,[47-50] a drug rather similar to indoramin in that it is also a selective alpha-1 adrenoceptor blocking agent. These adverse "first dose phenomenon" effects appear not to occur with indoramin.[40] In long-term clinical trials, tolerance to indoramin does not develop.[19-25] Johnson reports that continuous indoramin administration for 12 months was not significantly different from only three months of indoramin treatment, indicating that the antihypertensive effect did not diminish during long-term therapy.[39]

There have been many mild adverse effects reported with the use of indoramin, the most frequent of these being sedation, lethargy and drowsiness, dizziness and failure of ejaculation.[19,25,39,43] Table III summarizes the major side effects reported with indoramin administration. Small reductions in the indoramin dosage may lead to a disappearance of these side effects (especially sedation when it appears to be dose-related) without reducing blood pressure control. Other less frequently occurring side effects include headache, depression, weight gain, fluid retention, and palpitations.

No other significant side effects, including electrocardiographic changes or biochemical side effects,[19] have appeared with prolonged indoramin use. Abrupt withdrawal of some antihypertensives may have been associated with a rebound hypertension (acute withdrawal syndrome). This has not been the case with indoramin where abrupt discontinuance has not been associated with this syndrome.[19,23,24]

TIODAZOSIN

Tiodazosin is a peripherally-acting new antihypertensive resembling prazosin with its alpha-2 blocking action. It must not be confused with trimazosin. It decreases peripheral vascular resistance without affecting cardiac output or heart rate. It reduces blood pressure at doses of 6 to 60 mg/day given in three divided doses. First dose syncope, as with prazosin, does not appear to be a problem. Orthostasis and dizziness occasionally occur. Vardon et al[1] found only seven of ten patients responding and they felt the 30% failure rate, together with the profound orthostatic hypotension in one patient, make the drug offer "little advantage" over existing drugs.

TABLE III
SIDE EFFECTS OF INDORAMIN

Study (Ref.)*	No. of Patients	Mean Dosage (mm Hg)	Impotence and/or Failure of Ejaculation	Sedation	Lethargy/ Drowsiness	Dizziness	Depression	Dry Mouth	Increased Appetite
Gould[25]	27	120	4/9	—	12	—	—	—	—
Coleman[21]	11	20**	—	—	***	—	—	—	—
Rosendorf[22]	19	158	—	—	6	2	1	1	—
Yajnik[19]	48	93	—	***	***	—	***	—	—
Shah[24]	41	72	3/31	4	—	2	1	—	—
Zacharias[51]	21	80	—	—	11	—	—	***	15
DeOliveria[43]	108	100–200	37/86	29	57	—	—	—	—
Stokes[27]	6	76	—	3	—	—	—	—	—
Fitzgerald[18]	122	95	***	17	—	5	9	—	—
Totals	403		44/126	53/277	75/175	9/182	11/182	1/19	15/108
Percentage			35	19	43	5	6	5	14

* See reference section for complete information on sources.
** Dose given intravenously.
*** Reported as "present."

BETA-ADRENERGIC BLOCKERS

BETAXOLOL

Betaxolol is a new beta-1 or cardioselective adrenergic blocking agent manufactured by Lorex Pharmaceuticals in the U. S. An excellent monograph has recently been published by Morselli et al[1] delineating the animal and clinical activity including pharmacodynamic and pharmacokinetic effects of this drug. It has virtually complete oral absorption, very little first-pass effect, high oral bioavailability, a half-life of 16–22 hours, protein binding of about 50%, and essentially no active metabolites. Published reports clearly indicate that 10 or 20 mg given once daily is effective in the reduction of mild-moderate hypertension. Although the side effects of betaxolol appear thus far to be mild and similar to other beta-1 blocking agents, further clinical experience is necessary to adequately define its safety and its proper position in the long-term management of hypertensive patients.

SOTALOL

Sotalol is another beta-adrenergic-blocking agent which, like timolol, has no local anesthetic action (membrane-stabilizing activity) and lacks sympathomimetic activity.[1,2] The relative potency of sotalol as a beta-blocker in comparison to propranolol is one-tenth. Its half-life is 12 hours, so it may provide the convenience of once-daily administration.[3] Sotalol was compared with placebo in 30 patients with angina pectoris.[4] In 24 (80%), sotalol decreased the number of angina attacks by more than 50% as well as improving exercise tolerance and the electrocardiogram. Three of 30 had dyspnea, but all symptoms were mild. The dose used was 320 mg/day given in two equal doses.

OXPRENOLOL (Trasicor®)

Oxprenolol is a non-selective beta-blocking agent that also possesses intrinsic sympathomimetic (ISA) or partial agonist activity. Although it blocks both beta-1 and -2 adrenergic receptors, it also has a significant stimulant effect on the myocardium. It is widely used in Europe but is not yet available in the U. S. Friedman[1] recently reviewed the U. S. experience with oxprenolol in hypertension. Compared with placebo, 48 patients had their pressures reduced by 9/9 mm Hg vs. placebo which lowered pressure 1/4 mm Hg (p < 0.001). The average dose used was 426 mg/day given in a twice daily dosage schedule. Forty percent of patients attained satisfactory control. In a comparison with propranolol (both groups also received hydrochlorothiazide), oxprenolol reduced final pressure by 23/20 mm Hg (in 57 patients) compared with propranolol, which combination reduced pressure 25/20 mm Hg (in 71 patients). Doses were 60–480 mg/day (given three times daily) for both drugs. When oxprenolol vs. hydrochlorothiazide was studied, the former reduced pressure 14/11 mm Hg compared with 20/13 mm Hg in the diuretic-treated group. Among black hypertensives, oxprenolol (as with all beta-blockers) reduced pressure much less than did the diuretics: 6/7 vs. 20/13 mm Hg.

The side effects of oxprenolol are similar to those of propranolol and other beta-blocking agents. However, bradycardia is somewhat less (the pulse decreased 13/min in one study vs. 19/min on propranolol). Lethargy, dizziness, paresthesia and wheezing also appeared to occur less frequently with oxprenolol in the Friedman review.

Controversy exists about the clinical significance of ISA. Perhaps some of the side effects, like bradycardia, are fewer but the overriding purpose of administering beta-blocking drugs is to dampen sympathet·ᵉ drive of the heart.

Other recent reviews of oxprenolol are contained in *The American Journal of Cardiology*.[2]

Use in Pregnancy

Fidler et al[3] studied 100 pregnant women with diastolic pressures above 94 mm Hg, randomly treated with either methyldopa or oxprenolol. Patients entered before 32 weeks gestation required larger doses of drugs for pressure control. Hydralazine was added after 640 mg/day oxprenolol or 3 gm methyldopa failed to reduce the pressure below 95 mm Hg. Twenty of 22 patients receiving methyldopa before 32 weeks of pregnancy achieved good blood pressure reductions, whereas only 15 of 24 on oxprenolol did so before hydralazine or very large drug doses were necessary. The eventual outcome for all patients was similar with both drugs: birth weight, placental weights, head circumference, and Apgar scores were similar and no stillbirths occurred.

PRONETHALOL AND ALPRENOLOL

Pronethalol and alprenolol are two new non-selective beta-adrenergic blocking agents which are similar inasmuch as they all have been shown to possess intrinsic sympathomimetic activity as well as potent membrane-stabilizing activity. Preliminary clinical trials have shown these agents to be effective in the therapy of essential hypertension.

Alprenolol (Betaptin®, Aplin®)—which is prototypical of this group—has a relative potency of 1.0 when compared to propranolol, and has also been shown to be effective in angina pectoris, cardiac arrhythmias and neurocirculatory asthenia. In a double-blind crossover study comparing alprenolol and propranolol in equipotent beta-blocking doses (150 mg three-times daily and 60 mg three-times daily, respectively), alprenolol and propranolol had almost identical blood-pressure-reducing effects. Propranolol, however, did reduce the heart rate significantly more than alprenolol.[1] Another study by Tibblin and Ablad[2] showed that 400 mg alprenolol daily produced statistically significant reductions of about 20 mm Hg systolic and 10 mm Hg diastolic in the supine as well as standing and sitting positions. Berglund and Hansson,[3] in a within-patient comparison of alprenolol and propranolol, found propranolol more effective in causing a significantly greater reduction of arterial pressure both in the supine and erect positions. In another study in which the antihypertensive efficacy of alprenolol (400 mg daily) was compared to chlorthalidone (50 mg daily), the latter was found to reduce blood pressure more than alprenolol.[4] Although the exact mechanism by which beta blockers exert their antihypertensive effect is not specifically known and may indeed vary from one blocker to another, it has been shown that alprenolol does reduce plasma renin activity but does not affect renal plasma flow or glomerular filtration rate.[5,6]

Side effects associated with alprenolol include headache, dizziness, weakness, angina, bradycardia, urticaria, breathlessness, rhinitis, and dyspnea—most of which were also seen with placebo.

BEVANTOLOL HCl

Bevantolol hydrochloride is a cardioselective beta-blocker. In animals, bevantolol selectively blocks the positive chronotropic and inotropic action of isoproterenol and is essentially devoid of intrinsic sympathomimetic activity, producing about the same degree of modest negative inotropic activity as does propranolol.[1] Its beta-selectivity is demonstrated by a dose-related blockade of myocardial beta-receptors coupled with poor blockade of bronchial and tracheal beta-receptors against agonist effects.[1]

In clinical studies, oral bevantolol is rapidly absorbed, with peak dose-related plasma levels around one hour. Preliminary results of a multicenter controlled double-blind study in mild to moderate hypertensive patients (diastolic blood pressure 100–115 mm Hg) have revealed that about 70% of patients given dialy oral doses of 100 to 400 mg of bevantolol hydrochloride (Cl-775), once daily or in two divided doses, have reduction and maintenance of diastolic blood pressure below 95 mm Hg compared with about 20% of the placebo-treated patients. The combination of bevantolol HCl with hydrochlorothiazide (200/25 mg) is currently being studied in 240 patients with mild to moderate (World Health Organization Stage-1 and -2) hypertension, with the aim that once-daily doses of the combination may improve compliance and provide optimal blood pressure control.

Preliminary experience in 218 patients has demonstrated the additive blood pressure lowering effects of the combination from 25/15 mm Hg 25 mg bid to 18/10 mm Hg without clinically significant adverse effects. The incidence of possibly drug-related adverse effects was 15% on bevantolol alone and 10% on combination therapy. Side effects associated with combination therapy included headaches, fatigue, dizziness, myalgias, and in males, possible impotence.

There are a number of other beta-adrenergic-blocking agents in various stages of development.[2] Many will never be marketed. While each may have some particular advantage associated with its use, each will have to be tested and compared with propranolol, the clinical prototype, to determine its advantages as an antihypertensive in terms of efficacy and associated side effects.

CALCIUM CHANNEL BLOCKERS

NITRENDIPINE

Nitrendipine (Bay e 5009) is a potent new calcium channel blocker. We carried out a double-blind comparison of the safety and antihypertensive efficacy of nitrendipine, combined with low doses of hydrochlorothiazide, in 20 patients with mild to moderate essential hypertension. Our results were as follows: mean reductions in supine blood pressure on 5 mg/day were 0/2 mm Hg, on 10 mg/day—4/5 mm Hg, on 20 mg/day—5/5 mm Hg and on 20 mg twice daily 8/7 mm Hg.

Patients receiving a combination of nitrendipine and hydrochlorothiazide 25 to 50 mg/day showed a mean reduction of 18/12 mm Hg. Side effects during the study were as follows: 6/20 patients complained of headaches, 1 patient developed pretibial, pitting edema, one developed a mild skin rash with pruritis and another patient developed a transient ischemic attack, probably unrelated to therapy. In patients with severe hypertension (i.e., supine diastolic blood pressure > 115 mm Hg), 10 mg/day of nitrendipine reduced blood pressure by 7/7 mm Hg, 20 mg produced a reduction in blood pressure of a 17/8 mm Hg, 40 mg reduced the pressure by 22/12 mm Hg and with a 30 mg twice-daily dose of nitrendipine, pressure fell by 26/14 mm Hg.

NICARDIPINE

Nicardipine is a new calcium slow-channel blocking agent, structurally related to nifedipine. It is a potent vasodilator of both the coronary and peripheral arteries. Like nifedipine and unlike verapamil, nicardipine administration does not inhibit the reflex tachycardia; therefore, a mild increase in heart rate is often noted. Jain et al,[1] Jones et al,[2] Taylor[3] and Bowles[4] have all reported on its usefulness in treating hypertension or angina pectoris. Our experience giving 20, 30, and 40 mg doses three times daily,[1] with increasing doses given after three-to-five days of placebo treatment to 10 patients hospitalized for 14 days, indicated a good dose response. Mean diastolic pressures were reduced by 6, 10 and 11 mm Hg ($p < 0.05$) and no significant effect was noted on heart rate. All doses were well tolerated. In the Jones study,[2] 14 patients received doses of 20 or 40 mg twice daily with direct brachial artery monitoring of blood pressure. Blood pressure decreased from 184/110 mm Hg to 167/102 mm Hg. Dynamic exercise produced significantly reduced hypertension on drug compared with placebo, and the tachycardia from exercise was unchanged by drug. Four of 14 patients withdrew, two with palpitations, headache and edema, one with lethargy and anxiety and one with muscle cramps. Other side effects noted were generally mild.

DIURETICS

INDACRINONE (MK-196)

A large percentage of hypertensive patients have hyperuricemia and many more have this condition following diuretic treatment. Although few patients actually develop gout, hyperuricemia is usually listed as a minor risk factor for the development of cardiovascular disease. Tricrynafen lowered uric acid by as much as 40%, whereas crinone in the racemic mixture employed is virtually isouricemic.

Indacrinone is a new diuretic with natriuretic and uricosuric activity developed by Merck Sharp and Dohme Research Laboratories. In man it is more potent and has a more gradual onset and longer duration of action than furosemide. As a loop-acting diuretic, it is useful in congestive heart failure and in other edematous states. However, because of the unique pharmacologic properties of its two enantiomers, the (−) enantiomer of the racemic compound is significantly more potent as a *natriuretic* agent than the (+), and the (+) enantiomer possesses more *uricosuric* action. Clinical studies by Jain et al[1] confirmed that by altering the ratio of (+) to (−) from its naturally occurring racemate, it was possible to produce a drug which would enhance the uricosuric action while maintaining the potent antihypertensive action.

This was a double-blind placebo-controlled study of 37 patients. A control diastolic pressure of 90–104 mm Hg was criterion for inclusion into the study. Diastolic blood pressures were reduced by 25/10 mm Hg after treatment with a $(-)$ 10/$(+)$ 80 ratio of indacrinone. The serum uric acid changes after 12 weeks were virtually identical to the placebo group.

When amiloride, the potassium sparing drug, is combined with indacrinone, the resulting drug combination is essentially isouricemic and isokalemic.

When amiloride, the potassium sparing drug, is combined with indacrinone, the resulting drug combination is essentially isouricemic and isokalemic. This combination is now under clinical investigation. Irvin et al[2] reported the clinical results of a metabolic study utilizing 2.5 and 5.0 mg doses of amiloride, hydrochlorothiazide and placebo, confirming the benefit of this potassium sparing agent given with a balanced ratio of indacrinone enantiomers.

Numerous clinical studies have been conducted and are ongoing with a final balanced ratio of enantiomers of indacrinone of $(-)$10/$(+)$90. Doses of 50 mg (5:45) or 100 mg (10:90) (a 10:90 ratio) once daily appear to be both effective in hypertension while maintaining relative isouricemia. This new drug promises to be an important addition to our therapeutic armamentarium.

PIRETANIDE (Arlix®)

Piretanide is a new diuretic-antihypertensive pharmacologically similar to furosemide. As such, it causes urinary excretion of sodium, potassium and calcium, with a rapid onset of diuresis at doses of 6 to 24 mg. The initial dose is 6 mg once daily. Piretanide is 96% albumin bound. It is well absorbed, reaching peak levels at 1-2 hours. As with other diuretics, the principal side effects are biochemical. Hypokalemia, hyperglycemia, hyperuricemia and occasionally hypochloremic-hypokalemic alkalosis may occur.

We studied piretanide in 32 patients with mild hypertension in a double-blind study using placebo and three doses of drug. We found 6 mg given twice daily reduced blood pressure comparable to standard diuretics. Side effects were minimal, and mild biochemical changes occurred, such as an increase in serum uric acid and glucose with a reduction of serum potassium.

MUZOLIMINE (Edrul®)

Muzolimine is a new diuretic-antihypertensive with much similarity to furosemide, but with a prolonged duration of action. Its diuretic effect peaks in 60–180 minutes and persists for 6 to 12 hours. A 30 mg dose of muzolimine is equivalent to 40 mg of furosemide. In the treatment of hypertension, doses of 15–60 mg/day are recommended. The usual dose is 20 mg/day, and decrements in the range of 20–30 systolic and 10–12 mm Hg diastolic are produced. Side effects have been mild in clinical studies thus far and include dizziness, headache, nausea, diarrhea, rash and fatigue. The biochemical changes have been characteristic of diuretics: hypokalemia, hyponatremia, hyperuricemia and also elevation of serum creatinine.

SEROTONIN ANTAGONIST

KETANSERIN

Ketanserin is the first selective serotonin antagonist which blocks serotonin at the $5\text{-}HT_2$ receptor without any effect on the $5\text{-}HT_1$ receptor. Chemical analogues like methylsergide, LSD and cyproheptadine have both $5\text{-}HT_1$ and $5\text{-}HT_2$ in vitro binding profiles as well as some serotonergic agonist activity. The $5\text{-}HT_2$ receptor is found in small muscles of arteries, bronchi and on platelets. Serotonin is released by the chromoffin cells of the gut and is normally rapidly removed by the hepatic and pulmonary beds. However, susceptibility to serotonin is felt to increase with aging and atherosclerosis, so its constrictor effects on both vascular and bronchial smooth muscles are felt to be factors in hypertension and diminished pulmonary function. Serotonin also amplifies some of the vasoconstricting and platelet-aggregatory effects of catecholamines, angiotensin II and prostaglandins.

Ketanserin, given either parenterally or orally, clearly lowers blood pressure. Its hypotensive effect is greater on the diastolic pressure than on the systolic, although both are reduced. Reflex sympathetic tachycardia does not occur as with most other vasodilators. There is little or no increase in heart rate or cardiac output. Postural hypotension has not occurred. It raises plasma renin activity, aldosterone levels and catecholamines. Although renal vascular resistance is reduced, no effect on either glomerular filtration rate or renal blood flow has been noted. The drug is 63% albumin bound. Peak blood levels occur in one hour after oral administration and it is 50% bioavailable.

The effective oral dose is 20 to 40 mg (tablets) given twice or three times daily with meals. Since an initial "hangover" effect may occur, particularly during the first week or two of treatment, small initial doses are recommended. The principal side effects consist of dizziness, fatigue, lightheadedness, headaches, polyuria and drowsiness. Venous blood turns cherry-red after the intravenous or oral administration. A significant rise in venous pO_2 explains this color change.

Besides its potential use in hypertension, ketanserin shows promise in many peripheral vascular disorders, such as Raynaud's disease, intermittent claudication, etc. Plethysmographic studies indicate increased blood flow to the extremities. Intravenous ketanserin has been used successfully to relieve acute asthmatic attacks, to treat acute thrombophlebitis and pulmonary emboli. Obviously this new drug has multiple potential uses, but further controlled clinical studies are required before its actual benefit-to-risk status can be determined.

VASODILATORS

GUANCYDINE

Guancydine is a new vasodilator reported to have significant antihypertensive action, blocking the vasoconstrictor effects of angiotensin-II and decreasing those of norepinephrine.[1,2] Freis and Hammer[3,4] report a hydralazine-like effect on the systemic circulation which suggests a peripheral site of action. However, guancydine differs from hydralazine in that it dilates both capacitance and resistance vessels, causing a reduction in right atrial pressure rather than an elevation as seen with hydralazine.

Clinical studies have shown guancydine to be an effective antihypertensive agent[3,5-8] in doses ranging from 500 to 1,000 mg daily. Compared with hydralazine, guancydine produces a greater reduction in diastolic pressure.[4] Fluid retention is especially prominent unless given with diuretics.[4,8] Because sympathetic reflexes are not blocked, both heart rate and cardiac output increase through baroreceptor reflexes. The tachycardia may be blunted by giving concurrent beta-blockers.[4,9] Headaches appear to be less severe and less frequent after guancydine than after hydralazine. Other adverse effects include epigastric burning, disorientation, hallucinations, feelings of being intoxicated, nausea, vomiting, congestive heart failure, paresthesias, depression, constipation, and urinary retention.[3,4,6,8]

PINACIDIL

(racemic N" -cyano-N'-4-pyridyl-N-1,2,-trimethylpropyl-guanidine monohydrate)

Pinacidil is a new potent direct vasodilator synthesized in 1978 by Dr. A. J. Peterson[1] together with Drs. C. Kaehgaard-Nielsen[2] and E. Arrigani-Mantelli.[3] It belongs to the N-alkyl-N"-cyano-N'-pyridylguanidine series of drugs. It acts predominantly on the arterial smooth muscle vasculature and has minimal orthostatic effects on blood pressure.

Pinacidil causes a dose-dependent reduction in blood pressure and has little effect on the supine heart rate. A moderate increment of heart rate is noted in erect posture, although there is no significant difference in erect and supine blood pressures. The potency is 6.9 times that of hydralazine (molar ratio) or 4.2 times on the basis of mass. The n-oxide metabolite of the drug has about one-third the hypotensive effect of pinacidil. In an acidic stomach, a hydrochloride is formed that is soluble and rapidly absorbed. Maximum serum concentrations are observed at an average of 0.9 hours. The drug is eliminated mainly through the kidneys as an n-oxide metabolite. Due to the rapid absorption, shorter duration of action, higher incidence of dizziness and syncope and marked inter-individual variability in absorption, a retarded dissolution capsule has been developed and is undergoing clinical trials at various centers.

The effective oral dose appears to be between 12.5 mg to 50 mg given twice daily. Headaches, dizziness, asthenia, edema, anemia, hirsutism and, rarely, syncope have been reported.

Although no teratogenic effects were seen in animal testing, the safety of pinacidil in pregnancy has not been established. Pinacidil is not recommended during pregnancy unless the potential benefit outweighs potential risk to mother and fetus.

Pinacidil has several advantages over hydralazine. It is more potent, has a longer duration of action, a lower incidence of tachycardia and causes no rise in antinuclear antibody titers. Animal studies have indicated no lowering of renal or coronary blood flow in high doses, as does with hydralazine. Long-term clinical studies in all forms of hypertension are ongoing at various centers, including ours, todetermine the safety and efficacy of this promising drug.

REFERENCES:

Catapres TTS

1. Weber, M. A., Drayer, T. I. M., McMahon, F. G., et al: Transdermal administration of clonidine for the treatment of high blood pressure. *Arch. Intern. Med.*, (in press).
2. Popli, S., and Stroke, G.: Transdermal clonidine for hypertensive patients. *Clin. Ther.*, **5**:624–628, 1983.
3. Mroczek, W. J., Ulrych, M., and Yoder, S.: Weekly transdermal clonidine administration in hypertensive patients. *Clin. Pharmacol. Ther.*, **31**(2):252, 1982.
4. Fleuckiger, A.: Transdermale therapeutische system. *Pharama-Kritik*, **4**:49–52, 1982.

Guanfacine

1. Dollery, C. T., and Davies, D. S.: Centrally acting drugs in antihypertensive therapy. *Br. J. Clin. Pharmacol.* **10**:5–12, 1980.
2. Titschen, G.: Experience with guanfacine in a two-year follow-up study. *Br. J. Clin. Pharmacol.*, **10**(Suppl 1):83s–84s, 1980.
3. Zamboulis, C., and Reid, J. F.: Effects of single and multiple doses of guanfacine in essential hypertension. *Clin. Pharmacol. Ther.*, **28**:715–721, 1980.
4. Jerie, P., and Lasance, A.: Guanfacine in the treatment of hypertension: Two years' experience with low dose monotherapy. *Int. J. Clin. Pharmacol.*, **19**:279–287, 1981.
5. Hutcherson, S. T.: A multi-investigator, double-blind, randomized and parallel clinical study of guanfacine versus placebo for treatment of essential hypertension (not published).
6. Roeckel, A., and Heidland, A.: Comparative studies of guanfacine and methyldopa. *Br. J. Clin. Pharmacol.*, **10**:55–59, 1980.
7. Rengo, F., Ricciardelli, B., et al: Long-term comparative study of guanfacine and alpha-methyldopa in essential hypertension. *Arch. Int. Pharmacodyn.*, **244**:281–291, 1980.
8. Bune, A. J., Chalmers, J. P., et al: Double-blind trial comparing guanfacine and methyldopa in patients with essential hypertension. *Eur. J. Clin. Pharmacol.*, **19**:307–315, 1981.
9. Lauro, R., Reda, G., et al: Hypotensive effect of guanfacine in essential hypertension: A comparison with clonidine. *Br. J. Clin. Pharmacol.*, **10**:81–82, 1980.

10. Dugler, J., Seus, R., et al: Difference in psychic performance with guanfacine and clonidine in normotensive subjects. *Br. J. Clin. Pharmacol.*, **10**:71–82, 1980.
11. Distler, A., Kirch, W., and Luth, B.: Antihypertensive effect of guanfacine: A double-blind crossover trial compared with clonidine. *Br. J. Clin. Pharmacol.*, **10**:49–53, 1980.
12. Nami, R., Bianchini, C., Fiorella, G., Chiorichetti, S., and Gennari, C.: Comparison of effects of guanfacine and clonidine. *J. Cardiovasc. Pharm.*, **5**(4):546–551, 1983.

Indoramin

1. Majid, P. A., Meeran, M. K., Benaim, M. E., Sharma, B., and Taylor, S. H.: Alpha- and beta-adrenergic receptor blockade in the treatment of hypertension. *Br. Heart J.*, **36**:588–596, 1974.
2. Mayer, J. H., and Caployitz, C.: The clinical results of oral and parenteral administration of 2-(N^{1}p-Tolyl-N-m-hydroxyphenylaminoethy) imidazoline hydrochloride (Regitine) in the treatment of hypertension and an evaluation of the cerebral hemodynamic effects. *Am. Heart J.*, **45**:602–610, 1953.
3. Beilen, L., and Juel-Jensen, B. E.: Alpha and beta-adrenergic blockade in hypertension. *Lancet*, **i**:979–982, 1972.
4. Archibald, J. L., Alps, B. J., Cavalla, J. F., and Jackson, J. L.: Synthesis and hypotensive activity of benzamidopiperidylethylindoles. *J. Med. Chem.*, **14**:1054–1059, 1971.
5. Carballo, R., Conde, L., Lapelle, M. M., and Suarez, J.: The treatment of arterial hypertension with a new alpha-blocker, indoramin. *Curr. Med. Res. Opin.*, **2**:437–443, 1974.
6. Kramer, R., Rosendorff, C., and Bloom, D.: Clinical evaluation of indoramin as the sole agent for the treatment of hypertension. *S. Afr. Med. J.*, **48**:1569, 1974.
7. Faerchtein, L., Rouque, A. F., Kastansky, I., Campos, J. C., and Puppin, S.: A placebo-controlled trial of the alpha-blocker, indoramin, in the treatment of arterial hypertension. *Curr. Med. Res. Opin.*, **3**:675–684, 1975.
8. Lewis, P., George, C. F., and Dollery, C. T.: Evaluation of indoramin, a new antihypertensive agent. *Eur. J. Clin. Pharmacol.*, **6**:211–216, 1973.
9. Klahr, L., Salazar, A., Almeida, D., and Brandy, S.: The effects of indoramin in essential arterial hypertension: A placebo controlled trial. *Curr. Med. Res. Opin.*, **3**:685–692, 1976.
10. Ramirez, J.: Indoramin in the treatment of hypertension: A placebo-controlled trial. *Curr. Med. Res. Opin.*, **4**:177–184, 1976.
11. Faerchtein, I., Roque, A. F., Kastansky, I., Campos, J. C., and Puppin, S.: A placebo controlled trial of the alpha-blocker, indoramin, in the treatment of arterial hypertension. In M. Velasco (Ed.): Excerpta Medica, Amsterdam, Oxford, 1977, pp. 1957–1966.
12. Ramirez, J., Kalahr, L., and Faerchtein, I.: Clinical studies with an alpha-blocker in the treatment of arterial hypertension. Multi-center, double-blind study of indoramin versus placebo. In M. Velasco (Ed.): Excerpta Medica, Amsterdam, Oxford, 1977, pp. 120–128.
13. Carballo, R.: Clinical studies of an alpha-blocker: A double-blind comparison with alpha-methyldopa. In M. Velasco (Ed.): Excerpta Medica, Amsterdam, Oxford, 1977, pp. 129–138.
14. Rosendorff, C.: Clinical studies with an alpha-blocker in arterial hypertension. In M. Velasco (Ed.): Excerpta Medica, Amsterdam, Oxford, 1977, pp. 129–138.

15. Archibald, J. L., and Turner, P.: Indoramin in the treatment of hypertension. A mini-review and update. *S. Afr. Med. J.*, **63**:307–309, 1983.

16. Alps, B. J., Borrons, E. T., Johnson, E. S., Staniforth, M. W., and Wilson, A. B.: A comparison of the cardiovascular actions of indoramin, propranolol, lignocaine and guinidine. *Cardiovasc. Res.*, **6**:226–234, 1972.

17. Baum, T., Shropshire, A. T., and Eckfeld, D. K.: Studies relating to the antihypertensive and antidysrhythmic action of indoramin. *Arch. Int. Pharmacodyn. Ther.*, **204**:390–406, 1973.

18. Fitzgerald, M. V.: A long-term open evaluation of indoramin in hypertension. *Br. J. Clin. Pharmacol.*, **12**(Suppl 1): 117s–124s, 1981.

19. Yajnik, V. H., and Patel, S. C.: Long-term efficacy of indoramin in hypertension. *Br. J. Clin. Pharmacol.*, **12**(Suppl 1): 125S–130S, 1981.

20. Coltart, J.: Clinical pharmacological studies of indoramin in man. *Br. J. Clin. Pharmacol.*, **12**(Suppl 1):49S–60S, 1981.

21. Coleman, A. J.: Evidence for increase in peripheral blood flow by indoramin in man. *Br. J. Clin. Pharmacol.*, **12**(Suppl 1):89S–93S, 1981.

22. Rosendorff, C.: Indoramin in hypertension: Clinical studies. *Br. J. Clin. Pharmacol.*, **12**(Suppl 1):89S–93S, 1981.

23. Yajnik, V. H., Chaubey, B. S., Thiruvengadam, K. V., and Bhatia, M. L.: A comparison of indoramin and methyldopa in patients pretreated with a thiazide diuretic. *Br. J. Clin. Pharmacol.*, **12**(Suppl 1):101S–104S, 1981.

24. Shah, K. D.: Open assessment of the long-term efficacy and tolerance of indoramin in hypertension. *Br. J. Clin. Pharmacol.*, **12**(Suppl 1):101S–104S, 1981.

25. Gould, B. A., Mann, S., Davies, A., Altman, D. G., and Rafter, E. B.: Indoramin: 24 hour profile of intra-arterial ambulatory blood pressure, a double-blind placebo-controlled crossover study. *Br. J. Clin. Pharmacol.*, **12**(Suppl 1):67S–73S, 1981.

26. Morgan, T., Gillies, A., Morgan, G., and Adam, W.: The effect of labetalol in the treatment of severe drug-resistant hypertension. *Med. J. Aust.*, **1**:393–396, 1978.

27. Stokes, G. S., Frost, G. W., Grahm, R. M., and MacCarthy, E. P.: Indoramin and prazosin as adjuncts to beta adrenoceptor blockade in hypertension. *Clin. Pharmacol. Ther.*, **25**:783–789, 1979.

28. White, C. de B., Royds, R. B., and Turner, P.: Some clinical pharmacological studies with indoramin, with observations on its therapeutic usefulness. *Postgrad. Med. J.*, **50**:729–733, 1974.

29. Archibald, J. L., Baum, T., and Childress, S. J.: 1,4-Bis(2-indol-3-ylethyl) piperidines. *J. Med. Chem.*, **13**:138–140, 1970.

30. Lewis, P. J., George, C. F., and Dollery, C. T.: Clinical evaluation of indoramin, a new antihypertensive agent. *Eur. J. Clin. Pharmacol.*, **6**:211–216, 1973.

31. Davey, M. J.: Relevant features of the pharmacology of prazosin. *J. Cardiovasc. Pharmacol.*, **2**:S287–S298, 1980.

32. Collis, M. G., and Alps, B. J.: The evaluation of the alpha-adrenoceptor blocking action of indoramin, phentolamine and thymoxamine on the rat and guinea-pig isolated mesenteric vasculature and aortic spiral preparations. *J. Pharm. Pharmacol.*, **25**:621–628, 1973.

33. Archibald, J. L.: Medicinal chemistry and animal pharmacology of indoramin. *Br. J. Clin. Pharmacol.*, **12**(Suppl 1):45S–47S, 1981.

34. Alps, B. J., Johnson, E. S., and Wilson, A. B.: Cardiovascular actions of Wy. 21901, a new hypotensive and anti-arrhythmic agent. *Br. J. Pharmacol.*, **40**:151–152, 1970.

35. Coltart, D. J., Meldrum, S. J., and Royds, R. B.: Myocardial effects of indoramin, a new hypotensive agent. *Br. J. Pharmacol.*, **42**:664, 1971.
36. Alps, B. J., Hills, M., Fidler, K., Johnson, E. S., and Wilson, A. B.: The reversal of experimental arrhythmias by indoramin. *J. Pharm. Pharmacol.*, **23**:678–686, 1971.
37. Algate, D. R., Rashid, S., and Watertall, J. F.: Cardioregulatory properties of indoramin in the rat. *J. Pharm. Pharmacol.*, **33**:236–239, 1981.
38. Bednavek, M. R., and Schoeman, H. S.: Indoramin as an antihypertensive agent in the treatment of essential hypertension. A multicentre trial. *S. Afr. Med. J.*, **63**:398–400, 1983.
39. Johnson, E. S.: Indoramin in essential hypertension: A survey of the patient records from long-term clinical trials. *Br. J. Clin. Pharmacol.*, **12**(Suppl 1):131S–137S, 1981.
40. Nicholls, D. P., Harron, D. W. G., and Shanks, R. G.: Acute and chronic cardiovascular effects of indoramin and prazosin in normal man. *Br. J. Clin. Pharmacol.*, **12**:61S–66S, 1981.
41. Watkins, J., Abbott, E. C., Hensby, C. N., Welster, J., and Dollery, C. T.: Attenuation of hypotensive effect of propranolol and thiazide diuretics by indomethacin. *Br. Med. J.*, **281**:702–705, 1980.
42. Gaddie, J., Skinner, C., and Palmer, K. N.: Intravenous indoramin and aerosol salbutamol in bronchial asthma. *Br. J. Clin. Pharmacol.*, **12**:85S–87S, 1981.
43. DeOliveria, J. M., and Ortega-Recio, J. C.: Three years of experience with indoramin. *Br. J. Clin. Pharmacol.*, **12**:111S–114S, 1981.
44. Hunter, R.: Death due to overdose of indoramin. *Br. Med. J. [Clin. Res.]*, **285**(6347):1011, 1982.
45. Draffan, G. H., Lewis, P. J., Firmin, J. L., Jordan, T. W., and Dollery, C. T.: Pharmacokinetics of indoramin in man. *Br. J. Clin. Pharmacol.*, **3**:489–495, 1976.
46. Shand, D. O., Nuckolls, E. M., and Oates, J. A.: Plasma propranolol levels in adults. *Clin. Pharmacol. Ther.*, **11**:112–120, 1970.
47. Rubin, P. C., and Blaschke, T. F.: Studies on the clinical pharmacology of prazosin. I: Cardiovascular, catecholamine and endocrine changes following a single dose. *Br. J. Clin. Pharmacol.*, **10**:23–32, 1980.
48. Verbesselt, R., Mullie, A., Tjandramage, T. B., DeSchepper, P. J., and Dessain, P.: The effect of food intake on the plasma kinetics and toleration of prazosin. *Acta Ther.*, **2**:27–39, 1976.
49. Grahm, R. M., Thornell, I. R., et al: Prazosin: The first-dose phenomenon. *Br. Med. J.*, **2**:1293–1294, 1976.
50. Rosendorff, C.: Prazosin: Side-effects are dose dependent. *Br. Med. J.*, **2**:508, 1976.

Tiodazosin

1. Vardon, S., Smulyon, H., Mookherjee, S., and Eich, R.: Effects of tiodazosin, a new antihypertensive, hemodynamic and clinical variable. *Clin. Pharmacol. Ther.*, **34**(3):290–295, 1983.

Betaxolol

1. Morselli, P. L., Kilborn, J. R., Cavero, I., Harrison, D. C., and Langer, S. Z. (Eds.): *Betaxolol and Other Beta-1-Adrenoceptor Antagonists*, Vol. 1, Raven Press, New York, N. Y., 1983.

Sotalol

1. Lish, P. M., Weikel, J. M., et al: Pharmacological and toxicological properties of two new beta-adrenergic-blocking antagonists. *J. Pharmacol. Exp. Ther.*, **149**:161, 1965.
2. Svedyr, N., Malmberg, R., et al: The hemodynamic effects of sotalol and propranolol in man. *Eur. J. Pharmacol.*, **8**:79, 1979.
3. Shaw, H. L.: Once-daily treatment of hypertension. *Br. Med. J.*, **2**:46, 1976.
4. Slome, R.: Sotalol in angina pectoris. *S. Afr. Med. J.*, **50**:469, 1976.

Oxprenolol

1. Friedman, B., Gray, J. M., Gross, S., and Levit, S. A.: United States experience with oxprenolol in hypertension. *Am. J. Cardiol.*, **52**:43D–48D, 1983.
2. Symposium on the Role of Oxprenolol (Transicor®) in Systemic Hypertension. In A. V. Chobanian, H. M. Perry, Jr., H. G. Langford, S. H. Taylor, (Eds.) *Am. J. Cardiol.*, **52**(9):1D–65D, 1983.
3. Fidler, J., Smith, V., Fayers, P., and De-Swift, M.: Randomized controlled comparative study of methyldopa and oxprenolol in treatment of hypertension in pregnancy. *Br. Med. J.*, **286**:1927–1930, 1983.

Pronethalol-Alprenolol

1. Bengtsson, C.: Comparison between alprenolol and propranolol as antihypertensive agents. *Acta Med. Scand.*, **192**:41, 1972.
2. Tibblin, G., and Ablad, B.: Antihypertensive therapy with alprenolol a beta-adrenergic receptor antagonist. *Acta Med. Scand.*, **193**:547, 1973.
3. Berglund, G., and Hansson, L.: A within-patient comparison of alprenolol and propranolol in hypertension. *Acta Med. Scand.*, **191**:433, 1972.
4. Bengtsson, C.: Comparison between alprenolol and chlorthalidone as antihypertensive agents. *Acta Med. Scand.*, **191**:433, 1972.
5. Castenfors, J., Johnsson, H., et al: Effects of alprenolol on blood pressure and plasma renin activity in hypertensive patients. *Acta Med. Scand.*, **193**:189, 1973.
6. Pederson, E. B.: Glomerular filtration rate and renal plasma flow in patients with essential hypertension before and after treatment with alprenolol. *Acta Med. Scand.*, **198**(5):365, 1975.

Bevantolol HCl

1. Summary for Investigators, bevantolol Hcl (CI-775). Parke Davis/Warner Lambert, data on file.
2. Hansson, L., and Werko, L.: Beta-adrenergic blockade in hypertension. *Am. Heart J.*, **93**(3):394, 1977.

Nicardipine HCl

1. Jain, A. K., Glick, A., et al: Nicardipine hydrochloride, a new calcium channel blocking agent in the treatment of essential hypertension. (Unpublished data.)
2. Jones, R. I., Hornung, R. S., Sonecha, T., and Raftery, E. B.: The effect of a new calcium channel blocker nicardipine on 24-hour ambulatory blood pressure and the pressor response to isometric and dynamic exercise. *J. Hypertension*, **1**:85–89, 1983.

3. Taylor, S. H., Silke, B., Ahuja, R. C., and Okoli, R.: Influence of nicardipine on the blood pressure at rest and on the pressor responses to cold, isometric exertion, and dynamic exercise in hypertensive patients. *J. Cardiovasc. Pharm.*, 4:803–807, 1982.
4. Bowles, M. J., Subramanian, V. B., Khurmi, N. S., Davies, A. B., and Raftery, E. B.: Efficacy of a new calcium blocking agent nicardipine in chronic stable angina.*Br. J. Clin. Pharmacol.*, 13:590, 1982.

Indacrinone

1. Jain, A. K., Michael, R., Ryan, J. R., and McMahon, F. G.: Antihypertensive and biochemical effects of variable rations of indacrinone enantiomers in hypertensive patients. (In press.)
2. Irvin, J., McMahon, F. G., et al: Effects of amiloride on the natriuretic and kaliuretic activity of the (-)10/(+)90 ratio of indacrinone enantiomers. *Clin. Pharmacol. Ther.*, 33(2):265, 1983.

Guancydine

1. Freis, E. D., and Hammer, J.: Guancydine, a new type of antihypertensive agent. *Med. Ann. DC*, 38:69, 1969.
2. Cummings, J. R., Welter, A. N., et al: Angiotension-blocking actions of guancydine. *J. Pharmacol Exp. Ther.*, 170:334, 1969.
3. Cummings, J. R., Welter, A. N., Grace, J. L., Jr., et al: Cardiovascular actions of guancydine in normotensive and hypertensive animals. *J. Pharmacol. Exp. Ther.*, 161:88–97, 1968.
4. Hammer, J., Ulrych, M., et al: Hemodynamic and therapeutic effects of guancydine in hypertension. *Clin. Pharmacol. Ther.*, 12(1):78, 1971.
5. Stenbert, J., Sannerstedt, R., et al: Hemodynamic studies on the antihypertensive effect of guancydine. *Eur. J. Clin. Pharmacol.*, 3:63, 1971.
6. Clark, D. W., and Goldberg, T. I.: Guancydine: A new antihypertensive agent, use with quinethazone and guanethidine or propranolol. *Ann. Intern. Med.*, 76:579, 1972.
7. Russo, C., and Mendlowitz, M.: The effects of guancydine on blood pressure, vascular reactivity, and norepinephrine uptake in essential hypertension. *Clin. Pharmacol. Ther.*, 13(6):875, 1972.
8. Villarreal, H., Arcila, H., et al: Effects of guancydine on systemic and renal hemodynamics in arterial hypertension. *Clin. Pharmacol. Ther.*, 12(5):838, 1971.
9. Gilmore, E., Weil, J., et al: Treatment of essential hypertension with a new vasodilator in combination with beta-adrenergic blockade. *N. Engl. J. Med.*, 282:521, 1970.

Pinacidil

1. Petersen, H. J., et al: Synthesis and hypotensive activity of N-alkyl-N"-cyano-'-pyridylguanidines. *J. Med. Chem.*, 21:773–781, 1978.
2. Nielson, C. K., and Arrigoni-Martelli, E.: Effect of a new vasodilator, pinacidil (P1134), on potassium, noradrenaline and serotonin induced contractions in rabbit vascular tissues. *Acta Pharmacol. et Toxicol.*, 49:427–431, 1981.
3. Arrigoni-Martelli, E., et al: N"-cyano-N-4-pyridyl-N'-1,2,2-trimethylpropylguanidine, monohydrate (P1134): A new potent vasodilator. *Experientia*, 36:445–447, 1980.

INDEX

A

Acidosis, and amiloride, 190
Acute myocardial infarction, and hypertensive crisis, 27
Acute toxicity syndrome, and hydralazine, 373
Acute withdrawal reaction, and beta-adrenergic blocking drugs, 308
Adolescents
  and clonidine, 225–226
  and thiazides, 92
Adrenergic blocking agents, and sexual dysfunction, 20–21 *see also* Sexual dysfunction
Afferent input mechanism, effect of beta-adrenergic blocking drugs, 291
Age, and renin production, 24
Alcohol, 64–66
  and beta-adrenergic blocking agents, 295
  and drug interaction, 32
  and guanadrel, 470
Aldactone® *See* Spironolactone
Aldomet® *See* Methyldopa
Aldoril® *See* Hydrochlorothiazide
Aldosteronism
  and renin production, 24
  and spironolactone, 201
Allergy
  and furosemide, 136–137
  and thiazides, 90, 112
Alpha-adrenergic agonists, 536–539
Alpha-adrenergic blocking agents, 339–356, 539–546, 558–560
Alpha-beta blocking drugs, 277–338
  and mild hypertension, 15–16
Alpha-methyldopa, and nifedipine, 409
Alpha$_2$ agonists, 215–276
Alprenolol, 549, 561
Amenorrhea, and spironolactone, 207–208
American Heart Association, 1
Amiloride, 185–192, 208–209
  absorption, 191–192
  acidosis, 190
  contraindications, 189
  distribution, 191–192
  dosage, 188
  drug interactions, 188–189
  excretion, 191–192
  formulation, 188
  indications, 188
  and liver or kidney dysfunction, 31
  metabolism, 191–192
  overdose management, 190–191
  precautions, 190
  and pregnancy, 189–190
  sensitivity, 189
  structure, 185
  use, 186
Amphetamines, and methyldopa, 244
Analgesics
  and beta-adrenergic blocking drugs, 324
  and guanabenz, 259
Anemia, and hydralazine, 376

Anesthesia
  and beta-adrenergic blocking drugs, 294, 298, 324
  and methyldopa, 244
  and sodium nitroprusside, 500
  and trimethaphan, 524
Angina pectoris
  and beta-adrenergic blocking drugs, 296–297, 325
  and labetolol, 325
  and minoxidil, 380
Angiotensin II blocking agents, 425–456
Anhydron® *See* Cyclothiazide
Antidepressants, and beta-adrenergic blocking drugs, 324
Antidiabetic drugs, and furosemide, 122–123
Antihypertensive agents
  and amiloride, 189
  and hydralazine, 366
  and methyldopa, 242–244
  and minoxidil, 380
  and reserpine, 460
  and sodium nitroprusside, 500
  and spironolactone, 203
  and triamterene, 195
  and trimethaphan, 524
Anti-inflammatory agents
  and beta-adrenergic blocking drugs, 324
  and furosemide, 124
  and thiazides, 89
Anxiolytics, and guanabenz, 259
Apresoline® *See* Hydralazine
Aquatag® *See* Benzthiazide
Arfonad® *See* Trimethaphan
Arlix® *See* Piretanide
Arterioles, effect of beta-adrenergic blocking drugs, 288
Asthma
  and beta-adrenergic blocking drugs, 297
  and guanadrel, 471
Atenolol, 312
  and alcohol, 295
  dosage, 285
  formulations, 285
  and left ventricular hypertrophy, 10
  and liver or kidney dysfunction, 31
  molecular structure, 278
  pharmacokinetics, 292
  pharmacologic properties, 323
  side effects, 299
Atrial fibrillation, and verapamil, 411
Atrial flutter, and verapamil, 411
Atrioventricular block
  and guanethidine, 482
  and verapamil, 411–412
Atropine, and beta-adrenergic blocking drugs, 294
Australian Therapeutic Trial, 7–8, 11–12
Azotemia, and thiazides, 106

B

Baratol® *See* Indoramin
Barbiturates, and methyldopa, 244

Baroreceptor mechanism, effect of beta-adrenergic blocking drugs, 290
Bartter's syndrome, and renin production, 24
Bendroflumethiazide, 77, 342, 345
Benzthiazide, 77
Beta-adrenergic blocking agents, 277–338, 546–550, 560–561
  absorption, 291–293, 325–326
  acute withdrawal reaction, 308
  advantages, 305
  adverse reactions, 298–308
  afferent input mechanism, 291
  and alcohol, 295
  beta-receptor blockage, 286–288
  comparative pharmacology, 293
  contraindications, 310, 311, 324
  disadvantages, 305
  dosages, 285
  drug interactions, 293–296, 324
  effect on arterioles, 288
  effect on the heart, 288
  effect on the kidneys, 288–289
  effect on the lungs, 289
  excretion, 291–293, 325–326
  formulations, 285
  indications for use, 279
  metabolism, 291–293, 325–326
  overdose management, 310–312
  pharmacokinetics, 292
  pharmacologic properties, 323
  physiologic effects, 288
  and postpartum, 325
  precautions, 309–310
  and pregnancy, 308–309, 325
  use, 277–286
  warnings, 296–298, 324–325
Beta-blocking agents
  and captopril, 435
  and clonidine, 232
  versus diuretics, 82
  and left ventricular hypertrophy, 11
  and mild hypertension, 16, 18
  and second drug therapy, 18–19
  and Stepped-Care therapy, 15
  and verapamil, 409
Betaxolol, 547, 560
  availability, 285
  dosage, 285
  and liver or kidney dysfunction, 31
  pharmacokinetics, 292
Bethanidine, 483–487, 493–494
  absorption, 486
  adverse reactions, 486–487
  contraindications, 485
  dosage, 484
  drug interactions, 484
  excretion, 486
  formulation, 483
  indications, 483
  mechanism of action, 484
  metabolism, 486
  molecular structure, 483
  overdose management, 486
  and Stepped-Care therapy, 15
  use in pregnancy, 485
  warnings, 485
Bevantolol hydrochloride, 550, 561
Biofeedback, 61–63
Black patients
  and captopril, 427

Black patients (continued)
  and hydrochlorothiazides, 93
  and thiazides, 91–92, 93
Bladder, obstruction, and furosemide, 138
Blindness
  and malignant hypertension, 25
  and thiazides, 112
Blocadren® *See* Timolol
Blood dyscrasia, and methyldopa, 247
Blood glucose
  and beta-adrenergic blocking drugs, 304
  and diazoxide, 520
  and thiazides, 106
Blood pressure, 32
  and captopril 431, 432
  and enalapril, 444
  and guanadrel, 474
  and guanethidine, 480, 486–487
  and minoxidil, 380–381
Blood urea nitrogen (BUN), and triamterene, 199–200
Bone marrow, and triamterene, 200
British Medical Research Council (MRC), 111
Bronchial asthma, and thiazides, 90
Bronchospastic disease
  and beta-adrenergic blocking drugs, 325
  and labetalol, 325
Bumetamide, and furosemide, 124
BUN *See* Blood urea nitrogen

C

Calan®*See* Verapamil
Calcium, 63–64
  and furosemide, 135
  and thiazides, 107–108
Calcium channel blocking agents, 393–424, 551–552, 561
  absorption, 414–416
  adverse reactions, 416–418
  and beta-adrenergic blocking drugs, 295
  cardiovascular effects, 394
  contraindications, 410
  dosage, 405
  drug interactions, 407–410
  excretion, 414–416
  formulations, 405
  and hypertensive crisis, 28
  indications, 403–405
  and malignant hypertension, 28
  mechanism of action, 405–407
  metabolism, 414–416
  and mild hypertension, 15–16
  monotherapy, 396–398
  overdose management, 414
  precautions, 413
  and pregnancy, 412–413
  and refractory hypertension, 30
  as second drug therapy, 18
  and sexual dysfunction, 21
  side effects, 417–418

Calcium channel blocking agents (continued)
  structure, 395
  warnings, 410–412
Capoten® *See* Captopril
Captopril, 425–439, 448–453
  absorption, 438–439
  adverse reactions, 439, 440
  contraindications, 436
  dosage, 433
  drug interactions, 435–436
  excretion, 438–439
  formulations, 433
  interference with laboratory tests, 436
  and left ventricular hypertrophy, 10
  and liver or kidney dysfunction, 31
  mechanism of action, 434–435
  metabolism 438–439
  and mild hypertension, 15–16
  molecular structure, 425
  and multi-drug therapy, 430
  precautions, 438
  and refractory hypertension, 30
  results of treatment, 428
  as second drug therapy, 18–19
  and sexual dysfunction, 21
  side effects, 439
  and Stepped-Care therapy, 15
  use in pregnancy, 437–438
  warnings, 436–437
Cardiac arrhythmia, diuretic-induced, 177–179
Cardiac conduction, and diltiazem, 412
Cardiac failure
  and beta-adrenergic blocking drugs, 296, 324
  and digitalis with labetalol, 324
  and labetalol, 324
Cardiac function, and beta-adrenergic blocking drugs, 300–302
Cardiac mechanism, effect of beta-adrenergic blocking drugs, 288–289
Cardiovascular disease (CVD), 8, 9
  and hydralazine, 375
  risk, 12–14
Cardiovascular effects, and thiazides, 109–110
Cardiovascular mechanism, effect of beta-adrenergic blocking drugs, 289
Cardiovascular system, and diazoxide, 519
Cardizem® *See* Diltiazem
Cardivar® *See* Trimazosin
Catapres® *See* Clonidine
Catapres-TTS®, 536–537, 557
Catecholamines
  and diazoxide, 513–514
  and renin production, 24
  and thiazides, 89
Cation-exchange resins, and thiazides, 89
  effect of beta-adrenergic blocking drugs, 290, 303–304
  and furosemide, 137–138
Cephalosporins, and furosemide, 122
Cerebral insufficiency, and guanadrel, 471
Chloral hydrate, and furosemide, 124

Chlorothiazide, 77
Chlorpromazine, and diazoxide, 514
Chlorthalidone, 77, 85
  antihypertensive effect, 79
  and clonidine, 222
  dosage, 86
  efficacy in black patients, 93
  and left ventricular hypertrophy, 10
  as second drug therapy, 18
Cholesterol, 32
  and mild hypertension, 12–13
Cholestyramine, and thiazides, 89
Chronic obstructive pulmonary disease (COPD), and beta-adrenergic blocking drugs, 297
Cigarettes *See* Smoking
Cimetidine, and beta-adrenergic blocking drugs, 294–295, 324
Cirrhosis, and renin production, 24
Clofibrate, and furosemide, 124
Clonidine, 215–234, 261–267
  absorption, 218
  and adolescents, 225–226
  adverse reactions, 234
  and azotemic hypertension, 29
  and beta-adrenergic blocking drugs, 293–294
  cardiac variables, 220
  contraindications in hypertensive crises, 27
  distribution 218
  dosage, 219–225
  drug interactions, 231–232
  and emergency room treatment, 26, 28
  excretion, 218
  and hypertensive urgencies, 228–230
  and left ventricular hypertrophy, 10, 11
  and liver or kidney dysfunction, 31
  mechanism of action, 216–217
  metabolism, 218
  and mild hypertension, 15–16, 18
  and post-treatment syndrome, 232–233
  precautions, 231
  and refractory hypertension, 30
  renal variables, 220
  and reserpine, 460
  as second drug therapy, 18
  and sodium nitroprusside, 501
  and Stepped-Care therapy, 15
  structure, 216
  use in special subgroups, 225–228
CNS depressant drugs
  and guanabenz, 259
  and clonidine, 232
  and reserpine, 461
Coffee, 66
Colestipol, and thiazides, 89
Collagen disease, and malignant hypertension, 24–25
Coma, and thiazides, 110
Combination therapy, effects of thiazides, 84
Combipres® *See* Chlorthalidone
Community Hypertension Evaluation Clinic Program, 2
Congestive heart failure
  and bethanidine, 485
  and captopril, 427
  and diltiazem, 412
  and guanadrel, 472

Congestive heart failure (continued)
 and minoxidil, 380
 and renin production, 24
Converting enzyme inhibitors, 425–456
 and left ventricular hypertrophy, 11
 and mild hypertension, 16
 and renin production, 24
 and sexual dysfunction, 21
Coombs' test, and methyldopa, 245–246,
 250–251
COPD *See* Chronic obstructive pulmonary
 disease
Corgard *See* Nadolol
Coronary artery disease
 and beta-adrenergic blocking drugs, 296–297
 and guanadrel, 471
Coronary insufficiency, and hypertensive crisis, 27
Corticosteroids
 and furosemide, 123
 and renin production, 24
 and thiazides, 89
Coumarin, and diazoxide, 514
Cyanide poisoning, and sodium nitroprusside,
 504–505
Cyclothiazide, 77

D

Death
 and beta-adrenergic blocking drugs, 306
 and thiazides, 110
Declinax® *See* Desbrisoquine
Dehydration, and amiloride, 190
Desbrisoquine, 487–488, 494
 molecular structure, 487
 side effects, 88
Deserpidine, formulations, 459
Diabetes mellitus
 and amiloride, 190
 and beta-adrenergic blocking drugs, 297
 and clonidine, 228
 and mild hypertension, 16
Dialysis, and azotemic hypertension, 29
Diazoxide, 506–522
 absorption, 517
 and acute glomerulonephritis, 27
 and acute hypertensive encephalopathy, 27
 adverse reactions, 517–522
 clinical studies, 511
 contraindications, 27, 514
 dosage, 510, 512
 excretion, 517
 formulations, 510
 and hypertensive crisis, 28–29, 507–508
 and liver or kidney dysfunction, 31
 and lupus nephritis, 27
 and malignant hypertension, 25
 mechanism of action, 512–514
 metabolism, 517
 overdose management, 516–517
 pharmacological effects, 520–521
 and postoperative hypertension, 27
 structure, 506
 and thiazides, 89
 use in pregnancy, 516
 warnings, 514–516

Dibenzyline® *See* Phenoxybenzamine HCL
Dietary fat, 58–61
Digitalis
 and beta-adrenergic blocking drugs, 294,
 324
 and furosemide, 123
 and guanagenz, 259
 and nifedipine, 408
 and reserpine, 461
 and thiazides, 88
 and verapamil, 409
Diltiazem
 absorption, 415–416
 adverse reactions, 416–418
 cardiovascular effects, 394
 contraindications, 410
 dosage, 405
 excretion, 415–416
 formulations, 405
 indications, 405
 and liver or kidney dysfunction, 31
 metabolism, 415–416
 monotherapy, 400
 precautions, 413
 and pregnancy, 413
 and Stepped-Care therapy, 15
 structure, 395
 warnings, 412
Diphenylhydantoin, and diazoxide, 514
Disopyramide, and verapamil, 410
Dissecting aortic aneurysm, and hypertensive
 crisis, 27
Diucardin® *See* Hydroflumethiazide
Diulo® *See* Metolazone
Diuresis, and furosemide, 135
Diuretics, 75–155, 552–554, 562
 and amiloride, 189   –
 and beta-adrenergic blocking drugs, 293,
 324
 and captopril, 435
 and cardiac arrhythmias, 177–179
 and diazoxide, 513
 and furosemide, 122
 and guanabenz, 259
 and guanadrel, 470
 and indoramin, 542, 543
 and methyldopa, 242–244
 and nifedipine, 408
 potassium-retaining, 183–213
 and renin production, 24
 and reserpine, 460
 and sodium nitroprusside, 500
 and spironolactone, 203
 and triamterene, 194–195
 and trimethaphan, 524
 and verapamil, 410
Diuril® *See* Chlorothiazide
Drug interactions *See* Alcohol; specific drug
 names
Drugs, new, 535–563 *see also* specific drug
 names
Dyrenium® *See* Triamterene

E

Edema
 and bethanidine, 485
 and furosemide, 138

Edema (continued)
  and guanadrel, 472
  and hypertensive crisis, 27
  and nifedipine, 413
Edrul® *See* Muzolimine
Electrolytes, and furosemide, 136
Enalapril, 439–445, 454
  and blood pressure, 444
  case studies, 443
  dosage, 445
  and left ventricular hypertrophy, 10
  and liver or kidney dysfunction, 31
  and mild hypertension, 15–16
  and refractory hypertension, 30
  results of treatment, 443
  structure, 441
Encephalopathy, and hypertensive crisis, 27
Enflurane, and sodium nitroprusside, 500
Ephedrine, and methyldopa, 244
Epinephrine, and hydralazine, 367
Esbatal® *See* Bethanidine
Esidrix® *See* Hydrochlorothiazide
Estrogen, and renin production, 24
Ethanol, and alcohol, 295
Exercise, 24, 51
Exna® *See* Benzthiazide

F

Fenfluramine, and thiazides, 89
Flurbiprofen, and furosemide, 124
Food *See* Nutrition
Framingham Studies, 6
Furosemide, 115–138, 149–155
  absorption, 129
  and acute glomerulonephritis, 27
  and acute pulmonary edema, 27
  adverse reactions, 129–138
  and allergic reaction, 136–137
  and azotemic hypertension, 29
  contraindications, 125
  and dissecting aortic aneurysm, 27
  drug interactions, 122–124
  efficacy, 119
  formulations, 121
  and liver or kidney dysfunction, 31
  and lupus nephritis, 27
  mechanism of action, 121–122
  metabolism excretion, 129
  oral dosage, 121
  precautions, 127–128
  use in pregnancy, 126–127
  and refractory hypertension, 30
  structure, 117
  and thiazides, 120
  warnings, 125–126

G

Gallamine, and thiazides, 88
Ganglionic blocking agents, and sodium nitro-
    prusside, 500
Gastric disturbances, and furosemide, 138
Gastrointestinal catecholamines, and
    guanadrel, 475
Gastrointestinal system, and spironolactone,
    207

Geriatrics
  and amiloride, 190
  and beta-adrenergic blocking drugs, 295–296
  and clonidine, 225
  and thiazides, 92–94
Glomerulonephritis, and hypertensive crisis,
    27
Guanabenz, 255–261, 275–276
  absorption, 260–261
  adverse reactions, 261
  contraindications, 259
  distribution, 260–261
  dosage, 258
  drug interactions, 259
  excretion, 260–261
  formulations, 258
  indications for use, 258
  and liver or kidney dysfunction, 31
  mechanism of action, 258–259
  metabolism, 260–261
  molecular structure, 255
  overdose management, 260
  precautions, 260
  and pregnancy, 259–260
  and refractory hypertension, 30
  and Stepped-Care therapy, 15
Guanadrel, 465–475, 491–492
  absorption, 472–473
  adverse reactions, 473–475
  and alcohol, 470
  blood pressure response, 467, 468
  contraindications, 470–471
  dosage, 469
  drug interactions, 470
  excretion, 472–473
  formulations, 469
  and liver or kidney dysfunction, 31
  mechanism of action, 469–470
  metabolism, 472–473
  overdose management, 472
  precautions, 472
  and Stepped-Care therapy, 15
  structure, 466
  use in pregnancy, 471
  warnings, 471
Guancydine, 555–556, 562
Guanethidine, 476–482, 492–493
  absorption, 477–478
  adverse reactions, 479–482
  contraindications, 27, 479
  dosage, 477, 478
  drug interactions, 479
  excretion, 477–478
  and fixed-combination therapy, 20
  formulation, 477
  indications, 477
  and liver or kidney dysfunction, 31
  mechanism of action, 478–479
  metabolism, 477–478
  and minoxidil, 380
  and refractory hypertension, 30
  and reserpine, 460
  and sexual dysfunction, 20–21
  and Stepped-Care therapy, 15
  structure, 476
  warnings, 479
Guanfacine, 538, 557
Gynecomastia, and spironolactone, 207

H

Haloperidol, and methyldopa, 245
Halothane
    and beta-adrenergic blocking drugs, 324
    and sodium nitroprusside, 500
HANES Survey, 1, 2
Harmonyl® *See* Deserpidine
HDFP *See* Hypertension Detection and Follow-up Program
Heart
    effect of beta-adrenergic blocking drugs, 288
    failure, and verapamil, 411
    rate, and hydralazine, 366
Hematologic reactions
    and beta-adrenergic blocking drugs, 306
    and furosemide, 137
    and thiazides, 111
Hemodynamic effects
    and blood pressure, 481
    and guanadrel, 475
    and guanethidine, 487
Hemolytic anemia, and methyldopa, 250–251, 252
Hemorrhage, and hypertensive crisis, 27
Heparin, and reserpine, 461
Hepatic disease
    and methyldopa, 253–254
    and thiazides, 90
Hepatic function, and verapamil, 413
Hepatic injury
    and diltiazem, 412
    and thiazides, 111
Homeostasis, 160–161
Hormones, and beta-adrenergic blocking drugs, 324
Hydralazine, 357–377, 382–390
    absorption, 369–370
    and acute glomerulonephritis, 27
    and acute toxicity syndrome, 373
    adverse reactions, 370–377
    and azotemic hypertension, 29
    contraindications, 27, 367
    distribution, 369–370
    dosage, 364–365
    drug interactions, 366–367
    effect on heart rate, 366
    efficacy, 359, 360, 362, 363, 366
    excretion, 369–370
    and fixed combination therapy, 20
    formulations, 364
    and liver or kidney dysfunction, 31
    and lupus nephritis, 27
    mechanism of action, 365–366
    metabolism, 369–370
    overdose management, 368–369
    precautions, 368
    predisposition to toxicity, 374
    and pregnancy, 368
    and refractory hypertension, 29–30
    and reserpine, 460
    and sexual dysfunction, 21
    side effects, 347, 371–373
    and Stepped-Care therapy, 15
    structure, 358
    warnings, 367–368
Hydrex® *See* Benzthiazide

Hydrochlorothiazide, 77, 85
    antihypertensive effect, 78
    efficacy in black patients, 93
    and guanadrel, 468
Hydrochlorothiazine, and left ventricular hypertrophy, 10
Hydrodiuril® *See* Hydrochlorothiazide
Hydroflumethiazide, 77
Hydromox® *See* Quinethazone
Hygroton® *See* Chlorthalidone
Hylorel® *See* Guanadrel
Hyperglycemia
    and furosemide, 135
    and triamterene, 199
Hyperkalemia
    and amiloride, 189
    and triamterene, 199
Hyperpyrexia, and methyldopa, 254
Hyperstat® *See* Diazoxide
Hypertension
    azotemic, 29
        and captopril, 426
    borderline, and clonidine, 226–227
    and captopril, 426
    definition, 1–3
    drug selection, 18–19
    emergency, 24–29
    fixed-combination therapy, 19–20
    initial medical evaluation, 12–13
    left ventricular hypertrophy, 8–11
    and liver or renal insufficiency, 30–32
    malignant, 24–29
        and renin production, 24
    mild
        and clonidine, 230
        and guanabenz, 257
        initial therapy, 17
        and methyldopa, 236
    moderate
        and clonidine, 230
        and methyldopa, 237
    mortality, 4
    natural course of the disease, 11–12
    non-drug treatment, 13–14, 37–73
    postoperative, 27
    and PRA determination, 23–24
    and prazosin, 345
    preoperative patients, and guanadrel, 471
    refractory, 29–30
        and diazoxide, 509–510
    renovascular, and captopril, 426
    risks, 3–8
    and role of renin, 22–23
    severe, 3
        and captopril, 430
        and clonidine, 228–230
        and diazoxide, 508
        and methyldopa, 237
    and sexual dysfunction, 20–21
    Stepped-Care technique, 14–18
    therapeutic goal, 21–22
    withdrawal, and thiazides, 111
Hypertension Detection and Follow-up Program (HDFP), 7
Hypertensive crises, 27
Hypertrophy, left ventricular, 8–11, 12–14
Hyperuricemia, 104–106
    and furosemide, 134
    and thiazides, 104–106

Hyperuricemia (continued)
and triamterene, 199
Hypnotics, and beta-adrenergic blocking drugs, 324
Hypochloremia, and furosemide, 134
Hypoglycemia, and beta-adrenergic blocking drugs, 294, 297, 324
Hypokalemia, 101
and furosemide, 134
and renin production, 24
and spironolactone, 201-202
versus potassium deficiency, 161-163
Hypomagnesemia, and thiazides, 108
Hyponatremia
and furosemide, 122-134
and thiazides, 107
Hypotension
and diltiazem, 412
and guanadrel, 471
and nifedipine, 413
and prazosin, 345
and sodium nitroprusside, 503-504
and verapamil, 411

I

Ibuprofen, and furosemide, 124
Imipramine, and methyldopa, 244
Impotency *See* Sexual dysfunction
Indacrinone, 552-553, 562
Indapamide, 114-115, 148-149
efficacy, 116
Inderal® LA *See* Propranolol
Inderal® *See* Propranolol
Indomethacin
and beta-adrenergic blocking drugs, 294
and captopril, 436
and furosemide, 124
and indoramin, 542
and thiazides, 89
Indoramin, 539-546, 558-560
absorption, 544
adverse reactions, 544-545
contraindications, 542
dosage, 541
drug interactions, 542
excretion, 544
formulation, 540
indications, 540
mechanism of action, 541-542
metabolism, 544
overdose management, 543-544
precautions, 544-545
side effects, 546
use in pregnancy, 543
Insulin
and beta-adrenergic blocking drugs, 294
and thiazides, 88
Ischemic heart disease
and beta-adrenergic blocking drugs, 325
and labetalol, 325
Ismelin® *See* Guanethidine
Isoptin® *See* Verapamil

J

Joint National Committee on Detection, Evaluation and Treatment of High Blood Pressure, 219-221

K

Ketanserin, 554-555
Kidneys, effect of beta-adrenergic blocking drugs, 288-289

L

Labetalol, 526
absorption, 325-326
and acute hypertensive encephalopathy, 27
adverse reactions, 326-327
and alcohol, 295
contraindications, 27, 324
dosage, 320
drug interactions, 324
excretion, 325-326
hemodynamic effects, 321, 322
indications for use, 316-320
and liver or kidney dysfunction, 31
mechanism of action, 320-324
metabolism, 325-326
molecular structure, 317
overdosage, 326
pharmacologic properties, 323
precautions, 326
and pregnancy, 325
and refractory hypertension, 30
Laboratory tests
and captopril, 436
and hydralazine, 374
Late toxicity syndrome, and hydralazine, 373
L-DOPA
and methyldopa, 244
and reserpine, 461
Leukopenia, and methyldopa, 252
Levodopa, and clonidine, 232
Libido *See* Sexual dysfunction
Licorice, and renin production, 24
Lipids
and beta-adrenergic blocking drugs, 307-308
and furosemide, 135-136
and thiazides, 108-109
Lithium
and amiloride, 189
and furosemide, 123-124
and methyldopa, 244
and thiazides, 88, 90
Liver
disorders, and methyldopa, 246-247
enzymes, and verapamil, 411
Loniten® *See* Minoxidil
Lopressor® *See* Metoprolol
Lozol® *See* Indapamide
Lungs, effect of beta-adrenergic blocking drugs, 289
Lupus nephritis, and hypertensive crisis, 27

M

Magnesium, and furosemide, 135
MAO inhibitors
and hydralazine, 367
and reserpine, 460-461
Medical Directors of Insurance Companies' Report, 1975, 2
Meditation, 61-63
Menstruation, and spirololactone, 207-208

Mesenteric infarction, and furosemide, 138
Metahydrin® *See* Trichlormethiazide
Metaraminol, and reserpine, 461
Methyldopa, 234–255, 267–275
    absorption, 248–249
    and acute glomerulonephritis, 27
    adverse reactions, 249–254
    and azotemic hypertension, 29
    contraindications, 27, 245
    and dissecting aortic aneurysm, 27
    dosage, 239–240
    drug interactions, 242–245
    effect on mild hypertension, 236
    effect on moderate hypertension, 237
    effect on severe hypertension, 237
    excretion, 248–249
    and fixed-combination therapy, 19–20
    formulations, 239
    indications for use, 235–239
    interference with laboratory tests, 245
    and left ventricular hypertrophy, 10, 11
    and liver or kidney dysfunction, 31
    and lupus nephritis, 27
    mechanism of action, 240
    metabolism, 248–249
    and postoperative hypertension, 27
    precautions, 247–248
    and pregnancy, 247
    and refractory hypertension, 30
    and reserpine, 460
    as second drug therapy, 19
    side effects, 250
    and sodium nitroprusside, 501
    and Stepped-Care therapy, 15
    structure, 235
    warnings, 245–247
Metolazone, 77, 85, 112–114, 115
    dosage, 86
    and furosemide, 123
Metoprolol, 312–313
    and alcohol, 295
    dosage, 285
    formulations, 285
    and liver or kidney dysfunction, 31
    metabolism, 291
    molecular structure, 278
    pharmacokinetics, 292
    pharmacologic properties, 323
    side effects, 299
Midamor® *See* Amiloride
Minipress® *See* Prazosin
Minoxidil, 377–383, 390–391
    absorption, 381
    adverse reactions, 381–382
    contraindications, 380
    dosage, 378
    drug interactions, 380
    efficacy, 379
    excretion, 381
    formulations, 378
    mechanism of action, 379–380
    metabolism, 381
    and pregnancy, 381
    and refractory hypertension, 30
    side effects, 382
    and Stepped-Care therapy, 15
    structure, 377
    warnings, 380–381
Moderil® *See* Rescinnamine

Monoamine oxidase inhibitors
    and guanadrel, 470
    and methyldopa, 244
MRC *See* British Medical Research Council
Multicenter Diuretic Cooperative Study
    Group, 187
Musculoskeletal disturbances, and furosemide,
    138
Muzolimine, 554

N

Nadolol, 313
    and alcohol, 295
    dosage, 285
    formulations, 285
    and liver or kidney dysfunction, 31
    pharmacokinetics, 292
    pharmacologic properties, 323
    side effects, 299
    structure, 278
Naqua® *See* Trichlormethiazide
Naturetin® *See* Bendroflumethiazide
Nephrectomy, and azotemic hypertension, 29
Nephrosclerosis, 21–22
Nephrosis, and renin production, 24
Neurologic effects, and thiazides, 112
Nicardipine, 551–552, 562
Nifedipine
    absorption, 414–415
    adverse reactions, 416–418
    and beta-adrenergic blocking drugs, 295
    cardiovascular effects, 394
    contraindications, 410
    dosage, 405
    drug interactions, 407–409
    efficacy, 402
    excretion, 414–415
    formulations, 405
    indications, 403
    and liver or kidney dysfunction, 31
    metabolism, 414–415
    and mild hypertension, 15–16
    monotherapy, 397
    precautions, 413
    and pregnancy, 412
    and sexual dysfunction, 21
    side effects, 417–418
    and Stepped-Care therapy, 15
    structure, 395
    warnings, 410–411
Nipride® *See* Sodium nitroprusside
Nitrates
    and nifedipine, 408
    and verapamil, 410
Nitrendipine, 551
Nitropress® *See* Sodium nitroprusside
Nitroprusside *See* Sodium nitroprusside
Non-occlusive mesenteric infarction, and thi-
    azides, 112
Norepinephrine
    and guanadrel, 470, 475
    and reserpine, 461
    and spironolactone, 203
Normodyne® *See* Labetalol
Nursing mothers
    and bethanidine, 485
    and guanadrel, 472

Nutrition
  and alcohol, 64–66
  and beta-adrenergic blocking drugs, 295
  calcium, 63–64
  coffee, 66
  dietary fat, 58–61
  potassium 54–58
  and potassium supplements, 157–182
  role of diet in potassium regulation, 164–168
  sodium restriction, 38–45
  vegetarian diet, 58–61

O

Oral anticoagulants, and thiazides, 88–89
Oretic® *See* Hydrochlorothiazide
Orthostasis
  and guanadrel, 474–475
  and guanethidine, 486–487
Ototoxicity, and furosemide, 136
Ouabain, and reserpine, 461
Oxprenolol, 547–549, 561

P

Pancreatitis, and thiazides, 111
Pancytopenia, and hydralazine, 376
Papilledema, and malignant hypertension, 25
Parenchymal disease, and renin production, 24
Parenteral agents, 495–533
Pediatrics
  and amiloride, 189
  and bethanidine, 485
  and captopril, 427
  and thiazides, 92
Peptic ulcer
  and bethanidine, 485
  and guanadrel, 472
Pericardial effusion, and minoxidil, 380–381
Peripheral adrenergic blocking agents, 457–494
Peripheral vascular system, and beta-adrenergic
    blocking drugs, 302–303
Phenobarbital, and methyldopa, 244
Phenothiazines
  and guanadrel, 470
  and methyldopa, 244
Phenoxybenzamine HCL, 352–353
  and pheochromocytoma, 27
Phentolaminine HCL, 352–353
  and pheochromocytoma, 27
Pheochromocytoma
  and beta-adrenergic blocking drugs, 325
  and guanadrel, 471
  and hypertensive crisis, 27
  and labetalol, 325
  and renin production, 24
Physical activity, and blood pressure, 51–54
  see also Exercise
Pinacidil, 556–557, 562
Pindolol, 313
  dosage, 285
  formulations, 285
  and liver or kidney dysfunction, 31
  metabolism, 291
  molecular structure, 278
  pharmacokinetics, 292
  pharmacologic properties, 323
  side effects, 299

Piretanide, 553–554
Polythiazide, 77
Post-treatment syndrome, and methyldopa, 253
Potassium, 54–58
  and amiloride, 188
  and captopril, 436
  risk factors, 163–164
  role of and diet regulation, 164–168
  and thiazides, 88
  total body (TBK), 99–110
Potassium-retaining diuretics, 183–213
  guidelines for use, 184
Potassium supplements, 157–182
  and amiloride, 189
  dosage, 168–169
  indications, 168
  side effects, 169–177
  and spironolactone, 203
  toxicity, 169–177
  and triamterene, 195
Prazosin, 339–350, 354–356
  absorption, 341–345
  dosage, 340
  drug interactions, 345
  effectiveness, 342–345
  efficacy, 343, 344
  excretion, 341–345
  formulations, 340
  and liver or kidney dysfunction, 31
  and mean arterial pressure, 345
  mechanism of action, 340–341
  metabolism, 341–345
  and mild hypertension, 15–16
  molecular structure, 340
  overdose management, 346–347
  and pregnancy, 346
  receptor classification, 348–350
  and refractory hypertension, 30
  and reserpine, 460
  side effects, 347–348
  and Stepped-Care therapy, 15
  warnings, 345–346
Pregnancy
  and amiloride, 189–190
  and beta-adrenergic blocking drugs, 308–309,
    325
  and bethanidine, 485
  and calcium channel blocking agents, 412–413
  and captopril, 437–438
  and diazoxide, 516
  and diltiazem, 413
  and furosemide, 126–127
  and guanabenz, 259–260
  and guanadrel, 471
  and hydralazine, 368
  and indoramin, 543
  and labetalol, 325
  and methyldopa, 247
  and minoxidil, 381
  and nifedipine, 412
  and oxprenolol, 548
  and prazosin, 346
  and renin production, 24
  and reserpine, 462
  and sodium nitroprusside, 501
  and spironolactone, 204
  and thiazides, 90–91
  and triamterene, 196
  and trimethaphan, 525

Pregnancy (continued)
and verapamil, 412–413
Pre-synaptic receptor mechanism, effect of beta-adrenergic blocking drugs, 290–291
Procardia® *See* Nifedipine
Proglycem® *See* Diazoxide
Pronethalol, 536, 549, 561
Propranolol, 314
adverse reactions, 302
and alcohol, 295
contraindications in hypertensive crises, 27
and diazoxide, 513
dosage, 285
and fixed-combination therapy, 19–20
formulations, 285
versus hydrochlorothiazide use, 281
and indoramin, 543
and liver or kidney dysfunction, 31
metabolism, 291
pharmacokinetics, 292
pharmacologic properties, 323
and pheochromocytoma, 27
and prazosin, 345
side effects, 299
structure, 278
Prostaglandins, and beta-adrenergic blocking drugs, 294
Pulmonary edema, and thiazides, 111
Pyridoxine, and hydralazine, 367

Q

Quinethazone, 77
Quinidine
and reserpine, 461
and verapamil, 410

R

Raudixin® *See* Rauwolfia
Rauwolfia, 457–465, 488–491 *see also* Reserpine
contraindications in hypertensive crises, 27
formulations, 459
and liver or kidney dysfunction, 31
reactions, 464–465
and Stepped-Care therapy, 15
Rauwolfia serpentina, 457
Regitine® *See* Phentolamine
Relaxation, 61–63 *see also* Meditation
Renal colic, and thiazides, 110
Renal disease
and hydralazine, 375
and methyldopa, 238, 254–255
and thiazides, 90
Renal failure
and captopril, 431, 432
and clonidine, 227–228
and guanadrel, 472
Renal function
and amiloride, 189
and guanadrel, 475
and guanethidine, 481–482
and verapamil, 413
Renal reactions, and beta-adrenergic blocking drugs, 306–307
Renese® *See* Polythiazide
Renin-angiotensin-aldosterone system, 22, 23
Renin

Renin (continued)
factors that alter production, 24
and hypertension, 22–23
mechanism, effect of beta-adrenergic blocking drugs, 289–290
Renovascular disease, and renin production, 24
Rescinnamine, formulations, 459
Reserpine
absorption, 463–464
adverse reactions, 464
and beta-adrenergic blocking drugs, 293–294
contraindications, 461–462
and dissecting aortic aneurysm, 27
distribution, 463–464
dosage, 459–460
drug interactions, 460–461
excretion, 463–464
formulations, 459
and guanadrel, 470
indications, 459
mechanism of action, 460
metabolism, 463–464
molecular structure, 458
overdose management, 463
and postoperative hypertension, 27
precautions, 462–463
and pregnancy, 462
warnings, 462
Reserpine methyldopa, and acute pulmonary edema, 27
Retinopathy, 21–22

S

Salicylates, and furosemide, 122
Salt, and renin production, 24
Saluron® *See* Hydroflumethiazide
Sandril® *See* Reserpine
Saralasin, 445–448, 455–456
test, 447–448
Sarenin® *See* Saralasin
Second Joint National Committee on Detection, Evaluation, and Treatment of High Blood Pressure, 80–81
Serotonin antagonist, 554–555
Serpasil® *See* Reserpine
Serum potassium, and spironolactone, 206–207
Sexual dysfunction, 20–21
from antihypertensive agents, 20–21
and captopril, 21
and guanadrel, 474
and guanethedine, 20–21, 480
and hydralazine, 21
and nifedipine, 21
and spironolactone, 207
SHEP *See* Systolic Hypertension in the Elderly Program
Shock, and sodium nitroprusside, 503–504
Skeletal muscle relaxants, and furosemide, 123
Skin, and spironolactone, 207
Smoking, 32, 66–67
and beta-adrenergic blocking drugs, 295
and mild hypertension, 12–14, 16
Sodium nitroprusside, 495–505
absorption, 503
and acute glomerulonephritis, 27
and acute hypertensive encephalopathy, 27
and acute myocardial infarction, 27

Sodium nitroprusside (continued)
 and acute pulmonary edema, 27
 adverse reactions, 503–505
 and captopril, 436
 contraindications, 501
 and coronary insufficiency, 27
 and diazoxide, 519–520
 and dissecting aortic aneurysm, 27
 dosage, 498–499
 drug interactions, 500–501
 excretion, 503
 formulations, 498
 and hypertensive crisis, 28
 and intracerebral hemorrhage, 27
 and liver or kidney dysfunction, 31
 and lupus nephritis, 27
 and malignant hypertension, 25, 28
 mechanism of action, 499–500
 metabolism, 503
 overdose management, 502–503
 and pheochromocytoma, 27
 and postoperative hypertension, 27
 precautions, 501–502
 schematic representation, 496
 side effects, 505
 and subarachnoid hemorrhage, 27
 use, 495–497
 use in pregnancy, 501
 warnings, 501
Sodium, restriction, 38–45
Sotalol, 547, 560–561
 and alcohol, 295
Spastic craniofacial syndrome, and thiazides,
  111–112
Spironolactone, 200–208, 210–213
 absorption, 205
 adverse reactions, 205–208
 and aldosteronism, 201
 contraindications, 203–204
 distribution, 205
 dosage, 202
 drug interactions, 203
 excretion, 205
 formulations, 202
 indications for use, 202
 and liver or kidney dysfunction, 31
 mechanism of action, 202–203
 metabolism, 205
 molecular structure, 200
 overdose management, 205
 precautions, 204–205
 and pregnancy, 204
 side effects, 206
 use, 200–202
 warnings, 204
Stepped-Care technique, 14–18, 92
Succinylcholine, and thiazides, 88
Sudden death, 18, 136 *see also* Death
Sulindac, and thiazides, 89
Surgery
 and beta-adrenergic blocking drugs, 298
 and trimethaphan, 525–526
Sympatholytics, contraindications in hypertensive crises, 27
Sympathomimetics
 and guanadrel, 470
 and methyldopa, 244
Syncope, and prazosin, 345–346

Systemic lupus erythematosus
 and hydralazine, 367, 376
 and malignant hypertension, 25
 and methyldopa, 253
 and thiazides, 90
Systolic Hypertension in the Elderly Program
  (SHEP), 80

T

Tachycardia, and minoxidil, 380
Tamponade, and minoxidil, 380–381
Task Force on Blood Pressure Control in Children, 92
TBK *See* Potassium, total body
Tenathan® *See* Bethanidine
Tenormin®. *See* Atenolol
Thalidone® *See* Chlorthalidone
Thiazides, 77, 138–148
 absorption, 95–96
 and adolescents, 92
 adverse reactions, 96–112, 113, 114
 allergic reaction, 90, 112
 and captopril, 435
 contraindications, 89
 and diazoxide, 513
 distribution, 95–96
 dosage, 85–86
 drug interactions, 88–89
 efficacy, 362, 363, 364
  in black patients, 91–92, 93
 and excretion, 95–96
 and fixed-combination therapy, 19–20
 formulations, 85
 and guanadrel, 470
 indications, 85
 and indoramin, 542
 and liver or kidney dysfunction, 31
 mechanism of action, 86–88
 and metabolism, 95–96
 for mild hypertension, 14–15, 16, 17
 overdose management, 95
 precautions, 94–95
 and second drug therapy, 18–19
 side effects, 97–99
 and Stepped-Care technique, 15
 and total body potassium (TBK), 99–110
 use in pregnancy, 90–91
 warnings, 90
Thiocyanate, and sodium nitroprusside, 504
Thrombocytopenia, and methyldopa, 252
Thyrotoxicosis, and beta-adrenergic blocking
  drugs, 298
Tiamenidine, 539
Timolol, 314–316
 and alcohol, 295
 dosage, 285
 formulations, 285
 and liver or kidney dysfunction, 31
 metabolism, 291
 and mild hypertension, 18
 pharmacokinetics, 292
 pharmacologic properties, 323
 side effects, 299
 structure, 278
Tiodazosin, 545, 560
Tobacco *See* Smoking
Tobocurarine, and furosemide, 123

Tolbutamide, and sodium nitroprusside, 501
Toxicity
    and hydralazine, 375, 376–377
    and sodium nitroprusside, 504
Trandate® *See* Labetalol
Tranquilizers, and beta-adrenergic blocking
        drugs, 324
Trasicor® *See* Oxprenolol
Trauma, and renin production, 24
Triamterene, 192–200, 209–210
    absorption, 197–198
    adverse reactions, 197, 198–200
    contraindications, 195
    dosage, 194
    drug interactions, 194–195
    excretion, 197–198
    formulations, 194
    indications for use, 193
    and liver or kidney dysfunction, 31
    mechanism of action, 194
    metabolism, 197–198
    molecular structure, 192
    precautions, 196–197
    and pregnancy, 196
    warnings, 195–196
Trichlormethiazide, 77
Tricyclic and antidepressants
    and clonidine, 231–232
    and drug interaction, 32
    and guanadrel, 470
    and methyldopa, 244
    and reserpine, 461
Trimazosin, 350–352, 356
    dosage, 351
    formulations, 351
    and liver or kidney dysfunction, 31
    and mild hypertension, 15–16
    molecular structure, 352
    and refractory hypertension, 30
Trimethaphan, 522–525
    and acute hypertensive encephalopathy, 27
    and acute pulmonary edema, 27
    administration, 523
    contraindications, 27, 524
    and dissecting aortic aneurysm, 27
    dosage, 523
    drug interactions, 524
    effectiveness, 522
    formulations, 524
    indications, 522
    and intracerebral hemorrhage, 27
    overdose management, 526
    pharmacological effects, 522–523
    precautions, 525–526
    and subarachnoid hemorrhage, 27
    use in pregnancy, 525
    warnings, 525
Tubocurarine, and thiazides, 88

U

U. S. Health Survey, 1
U. S. Public Health Service Hospital Trial, 8,
    12

Urapidil, 539
Uric acid, and diazoxide, 520
Urine, retention, and guanethidine, 482
Uterus, and diazoxide, 520

V

Vasodilator agents, 555–556
    and beta-adrenergic blocking drugs, 295
    and diazoxide, 513–514
    direct, 357–391
    oral, 357–391
    and renin production, 24
    and sexual dysfunction, 21
Vasoril® *See* Enalapril
Verapamil
    absorption, 415
    adverse reactions, 416–418
    and beta-adrenergic blocking drugs, 303
    cardiovascular effects, 394
    contraindications, 410
    dosage, 405
    drug interactions, 409–410
    excretion, 415
    formulations, 405
    indications, 403
    and liver or kidney dysfunction, 31
    metabolism, 415
    and mild hypertension, 15–16
    monotherapy, 399
    precautions, 413
    and pregnancy, 412–413
    side effects, 418
    and Stepped-Care therapy, 15
    structure, 395
    warnings, 411
Veteran's Administration Cooperative Study
        Group on Antihypertensive Agents, 81, 91–92,
        361–362
Veterans Administration Multiclinic Study
        Group, 18–19, 426
Visken® *See* Pindolol

W

Warfarin
    and furosemide, 124
    and thiazides, 88–89
Weight
    and guanadrel, 472
    reduction, 45–51
WHO *See* World Health Organization
Wolff-Parkinson-White syndrome, and beta-
        adrenergic blocking drugs, 298
World Health Organization (WHO), 1
Wytensin® *See* Guanabenz

Z

Zaroxolyn® *See* Metolazone
Zinc, and thiazides, 108